Handbook of Clinical Endocrinology

a LANGE medical book

2nd Edition

Handbook of Clinical Endocrinology

PAUL A. FITZGERALD, MD
Associate Clinical Professor
Department of Medicine and Metabolic Research Unit
University of California School of Medicine, San Francisco

APPLETON & LANGE
Norwalk, Connecticut/San Mateo, California

92 93 94 95 96 / 10 9 8 7 6 5 4 3 2 1

Prentice Hall International (UK) Limited, *London*
Prentice Hall of Australia Pty. Limited, *Sydney*
Prentice Hall Canada, Inc., *Toronto*
Prentice Hall Hispanoamericana, S.A., *Mexico*
Prentice Hall of India Private Limited, *New Delhi*
Prentice Hall of Japan, Inc., *Tokyo*
Simon & Schuster Asia Pte. Ltd., *Singapore*
Editora Prentice Hall do Brasil Ltda., *Rio de Janeiro*
Prentice Hall, *Englewood Cliffs, New Jersey*

ISBN: 0-8385-3615-8
ISSN: 1057–5669

Developmental Editor: Carol Vartanian
Sponsoring Editor: Nancy Evans

To our patients and families

Contents

Preface

Handbook of Clinical Endocrinology is an unusually practical text-book covering most topics in **endocrinology and metabolism** of interest to clinicians. Both **pediatric and adult** endocrine disorders are discussed in a decidedly **problem-oriented** manner.

This text concentrates a tremendous amount of useful information in one place. The authors are outstanding clinicians who describe what really works in practice and offer many **clinical pearls.**

Relevant anatomy and physiology are clearly reviewed in each chapter. **Clinical problems are then presented with endocrine conditions discussed as diagnostic possibilities.** For example, the evaluation of short stature includes discussions of Turner's syndrome and growth hormone deficiency; the evaluation of hyperthyroidism includes discussions of Graves' disease and subacute thyroiditis; the evaluation of hypertension is followed by discussions of pheochromocytoma and Conn's syndrome; and the evaluation of hypoglycemia includes a discussion of insulinoma.

Handbook of Clinical Endocrinology **covers other common problems** that are only sometimes caused by endocrine disorders, such as premenstrual syndrome, dysmenorrhea, erectile dysfunction, infertility, and nephrolithiasis. **Comprehensive tables** present differential diagnoses for common electrolyte and mineral abnormalities (eg, hyponatremia, hypo- or hyperkalemia, hypo- or hypercalcemia). **Treatment sections present detailed information** (eg, doses of medications, tablet sizes, side effects) that facilitates prescribing.

This handbook also provides reference features **useful for treating children,** such as normal height and weight curves, growth velocity curves, and height prediction tables. **Recommended diets** are included for patient use (eg, low fat diet for hyperlipidemia, low iodine diet for 131-I treatment of thyroid cancer).

In short, we have tried to give this book a convenient, practical quality not usually found in other endocrine texts featuring the molecular biology of relatively rare disorders.

AUDIENCE

Handbook of Clinical Endocrinology will be **helpful to any health professional caring for patients.** Medical students and house officers will find the text readable, useful, and portable. Its handy size allows it to be discretely carried to hospitalized patients and to rounds by fellows, endocrinologists and others. This book will allow internists, family physicians, pediatricians, nurse practitioners, and subspecialists to remain up-to-date in practical endocrinology and metabolism.

OUTSTANDING FEATURES

- Concise, portable, and affordable
- Practical and problem-oriented
- Acronyms listed in each chapter
- Extensive quick-reference tables
- Illustrative scans, figures and photographs
- Current references following each chapter
- Large appendix containing testing protocols, specimen collection procedures, normal laboratory values expressed in conventional and SI units with conversion factor
- Detailed Table of Contents highlights disorders discussed in each chapter

ACKNOWLEDGMENTS

I am grateful to the authors for their excellent contributions and to our colleagues at the campuses of the University of California and Harvard University for their helpful comments.

Paul A. Fitzgerald, MD
San Francisco, California
October, 1991

Authors

Thomas P. Bersot, MD, PhD
Associate Clinical Professor, Department of Medicine; Gladstone Foundation Laboratories; Cardiovascular Research Institute; Chief Lipid Clinic, San Francisco General Hospital; University of California School of Medicine, San Francisco.

Paul M. Copeland, MD
Assistant Clinical Professor of Medicine, Harvard Medical School; Clinical Associate in Medicine, Massachusetts General Hospital, Boston.

Michael W. Draper, MD, PhD
Assistant Professor of Medicine, Indiana University School of Medicine; Director, Internal Medicine; Lilly Research Laboratories, Indianapolis.

Paul A. Fitzgerald, MD
Associate Clinical Professor, Department of Medicine and Metabolic Research Unit, University of California School of Medicine, San Francisco.

Philip H. Frost, MD
Professor of Medicine, Cardiovascular Research Institute, University of California School of Medicine, San Francisco.

Mara Lorenzi, MD
Associate Professor of Ophthalmology, Harvard Medical School; Clinical Associate in Medicine, Massachusetts General Hospital; Senior Scientist, Eye Research Institute.

Robert D. Nachtigall, MD
Associate Clinical Professor of Obstetrics and Gynecology, University of California School of Medicine, San Francisco.

Henry F. Safrit, MD
Clinical Professor of Medicine, University of California School of Medicine, San Francisco.

Ira D. Sharlip, MD
Assistant Clinical Professor of Urology, University of California School of Medicine, San Francisco.

Dolores Shoback, MD
Assistant Professor of Medicine, University of California School of Medicine, San Francisco.

Dennis M. Styne, MD
Professor and Chair, Department of Pediatrics, University of California School of Medicine, Davis.

Pituitary Disorders | 1

Paul A. Fitzgerald, MD

ANATOMY OF THE PITUITARY

The pituitary (**hypophysis**) has profound effects upon the body and other endocrine glands. The gland is small—its entire mass averages only about 600 mg but may double during pregnancy, primary hypothyroidism, primary hypogonadism, or Addison's disease—and consists of 2 adjacent but distinct parts.

The **anterior pituitary** (**adenohypophysis**) normally accounts for about 75% of the gland's mass and is mainly composed of glandular cells. It is embryologically derived from Rathke's pouch, an upward invagination of the oropharynx, and is connected to the hypothalamus only by a plexus of portal veins (pars tuberalis) surrounding the neural stalk.

The **posterior pituitary** (**neurohypophysis**) normally accounts for about 25% of the gland's mass and is mainly composed of nerve cells. It is embryologically derived from a downward protrusion of the floor of the third ventricle and remains connected to the hypothalamus by a neural stalk (infundibulum).

The pituitary and surrounding structures are visualized by computerized tomography (CT) in Figs 1–1 and 1–2 and by magnetic resonance imaging (MRI) in Figs 1–3 and 1–6.

The **sella turcica** (Turkish saddle) holds the pituitary and comprises anteriorly, the tuberculum sellae and the 2 anterior clinoids; posteriorly, the dorsum sellae and the 2 posterior clinoids; and inferiorly, the floor of the sella, which is one wall of the sphenoid sinus. The shape of the normal sella and its pituitary usually conform to each other and may be round or irregularly oval. The dimensions of the normal sella ordinarily do not exceed 19 mm (in width), 17 mm (anteroposteriorly), or 14 mm (vertically).

The **cavernous sinuses** border the pituitary laterally; these are extradural venous plexuses that drain blood from anterior structures into the inferior and superior petrosal sinuses and hence into the internal jugular veins. Within each cavernous sinus is a tortuous

1

SOME ACRONYMS USED IN THIS CHAPTER

ACTH	Adrenocorticotropic hormone
ADH	Antidiuretic hormone
AVP	Arginine vasopressin
CBG	Cortisol–binding globulin
CRH	Corticotropin–releasing hormone
CT	Computerized tomography
CVP	Central venous pressure
DDAVP	1–Desamino–8–D–arginine vasopressin (desmopressin)
DHEA	Dehydroepiandrosterone
DHEAS	DHEA sulfate
DI	Diabetes insipidus
FSH	Follicle–stimulating hormone
GH	Growth hormone
GHRH	Growth hormone–releasing hormone
GnRH	Gonadotropin–releasing hormone
hCG	Human chorionic gonadotropin
hMG	Human menopausal gonadotropin
hPL	Human placental lactogen
IGF-I	Insulinlike growth factor I, somatomedin C
ITT	Insulin tolerance test
LH	Luteinizing hormone
MRI	Magnetic resonance imaging
OT	Oxytocin
PET	Positron emission tomography
PIF	Prolactin–inhibiting factor
POMC	Pro–opiomelanocortin
PRL	Prolactin
RIA	Radioimmunoassay
SHBG	Sex hormone–binding globulin
SIADH	Syndrome of inappropriate antidiuretic hormone
ST	Somatostatin
T_3	Triiodothyronine
T_4	Thyroxine
TRH	Thyrotropin–releasing hormone
TSH	Thyroid–stimulating hormone
VLDL	Very low density lipoprotein

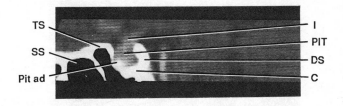

Figure 1–1. CT scan of the parasellar region. Saggital view. A 22-year-old woman with amenorrhea, galactorrhea, and hyperprolactinemia. An 8-mm calcified necrotic tumor was removed surgically. I = infundibulum (pituitary stalk thickened in this case); PIT = normal pituitary; DS = dorsum sellae; C = clivus; Pit ad = pituitary adenoma; SS = Sphenoid sinus; TS = tuberculum selae. (Courtesy of David Norman, MD.)

section of the carotid artery that carries blood to the circle of Willis; the carotid arteries have a plexus of sympathetic nerves that supply the pupils (to dilate) and lacrimal glands (to inhibit tearing). Also lying along the cavernous sinuses are cranial nerves: III (oculomotor, levator palpebrae), IV (trochlear), and VI (abducens), as well as the first division of V (trigeminus). The 2 cavernous sinuses are often connect-

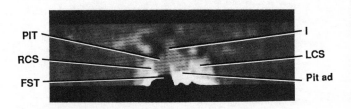

Figure 1–2. CT scan of the parasellar region. Coronal view. Same patient as in Fig. 1–1. I = infundibulum (pituitary stalk; unusually thick); LCS = left cavernous sinus; Pit ad = pituitary adenoma; FST = floor of sella turcica; RCS = right cavernous sinus; PIT = normal pituitary. (Courtesy of David Norman, MD.)

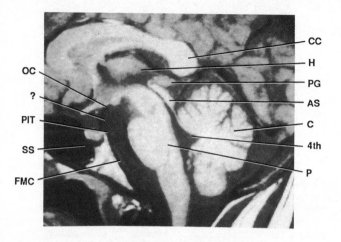

Figure 1–3. MRI of the parasellar region. Sagittal view (T1 = weighted). A 19-year-old male with hypopituitarism and diabetes insipidus following a motorcycle accident. CC = corpus callosum; H = hypothalamus surrounding 3rd ventricle; PG = pineal gland; AS = aqueduct of silvius; C = cerebellum; 4th = fourth ventricle; P = pons; FMC = fatty marrow in clivus; SS = sphenoid sinus; PIT = pituitary (the missing posterior pituitary "bright spot" is characteristic of diabetes insipidus); ? = area where infundibulum (pituitary stalk) is usually visualized (it was severed by head trauma); OC = optic chiasm. (Courtesy of T. Hans Newton, MD.)

ed by an intercavernous venous sinus that runs through the sella, around the pituitary.

The **diaphragma sellae** usually encloses the pituitary superiorly; this membrane is a reflection of the dura and is continuous with the capsule encasing the pituitary like a bag, while allowing the pituitary stalk (infundibulum) to pass through. Defects in the diaphragma sellae are found in as many as 54% of normal individuals and allow cerebrospinal fluid to enter the sella, compress the pituitary, and sometimes expand the sella, creating variable degrees of an empty sella. Just anterior to the pituitary stalk is the optic chiasm, the crossing fibers of which account for temporal vision.

The **arterial blood supply** to the posterior pituitary comes directly from the inferior hypophyseal artery, a branch of the intracavernous internal carotid artery. The anterior pituitary receives no direct arterial blood. Instead, the internal carotid sends the superior hypophyseal artery to join with arteries from the circle of Willis to form a portal

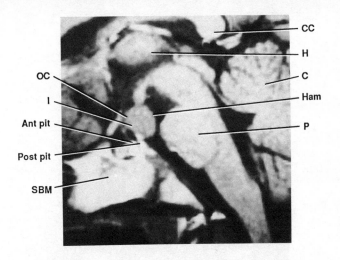

Figure 1–4. MRI of the parasellar region. Sagittal view (T1-weighted). Child with precocious puberty due to a tumor (hamartoma) of the tuber cinereum. CC = corpus callosum; H = hypothalamus surrounding 3rd ventricle; Ham = hamartoma of tuber cinereum; C = cerebellum; P = pons; SBM = spheroid bone marrow; Post pit = posterior pituitary "bright spot"; Ant pit = anterior pituitary; I = infundibulum (pituitary stalk); OC = optic chiasm. (Courtesy of William Dillon, MD.)

plexus of veins in the hypothalamus that runs down the pituitary stalk to the anterior pituitary. Blood flows down this venous plexus at a high rate, carrying hormones and releasing or inhibiting factors from the hypothalamus and systemic circulation that serve to "feed back" and modulate the anterior pituitary's own hormone secretions.

The **venous drainage** from the anterior pituitary connects with the posterior pituitary's capillary bed and veins and then follows 2 major routes: (1) some veins drain directly into the nearby cavernous sinuses; (2) other veins form a portal plexus along the posterior aspect of the pituitary stalk and carry blood back up to the hypothalamus.

NEURORADIOLOGY OF THE PITUITARY

The pituitary is best visualized radiologically with either magnetic resonance imaging (MRI) or computerized tomography (CT). MRI is generally preferred.

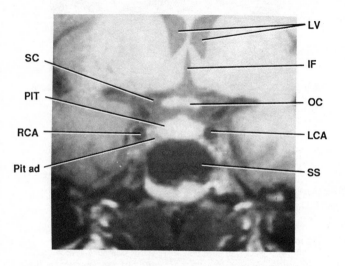

Figure 1–5. MRI of the parasellar region. Coronal view (T1-weighted). Woman with Cushing's disease due to a 3-mm pituitary microadenoma. LV = lateral ventricles; IF = interhemispheric fissure; OC = optic chiasm; LCA = left carotid artery (in cavernous sinus); SS = spheroid sinus; Pit ad = pituitary adenoma; RCA = right carotid artery (in cavernous sinus); PIT = pituitary gland; SC = suprasellar cistern. (Courtesy of William Dillion, MD.)

COMPUTERIZED TOMOGRAPHY

CT scan data recorded from multiple adjacent axial cuts may be reformatted to provide multiple coronal and sagittal images of the area. Such CT images of a normal young individual are shown in Figs 1–1 to 1–3. A CT scan of the pituitary may also be performed with direct coronal cuts for which the patient must hyperextend the neck in the scanner.

In CT images, bone appears dense (white) and other tissues appear less dense (dark) in a manner similar to conventional x-ray films. The CT scan should be done with intravenous contrast, as such contrast-enhanced CT scans allow better visualization of vessels and improve contrast (density differences) between tumors and adjacent tissue.

The normal pituitary generally appears homogeneous in density. Alterations in density may provide clues to diagnosis.

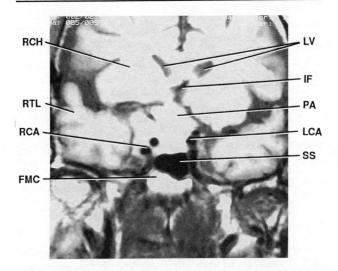

Figure 1–6. MRI of the parasellar region. Coronal view (T1 = weighted). Man with hypogonadism, headache, and visual field defects due to an invasive class IV pituitary prolactinoma. LV = lateral ventricles; IF = interhemispheric fissure; PA = pituitary (macro) adenoma; LCA = left carotid artery; SS = sphenoid sinus; FMC = fatty marrow in clivus; RCA = right cerebral artery (tortuous portion) encased in tumor; RTL = right temporal lobe; RCH = right cerebral hemisphere.

Hypodense lesions measuring 3–10 mm in diameter within the substance of the pituitary on contrast-enhanced CT scan occur in as many as 20% of normal individuals. About half of these lesions are pars intermedia cysts, while the others are areas of focal hyperplasia or adenomas which are usually asymptomatic but which come to clinical attention if they are hypersecretory. Hypodense lesions measuring more than 6 mm in diameter are most likely adenomas. Lesions 6 mm or less are a diagnostic problem, but the occurrence of such a lesion with endocrinologic evidence of hypersecretion is reasonable additional evidence that a discrete adenoma is present. Such small adenomas cause convexity of the pituitary's upper surface, although a microadenoma may be present even in an empty sella. Other causes for hypodense lesions within the pituitary include arachnoid or pars intermedia cysts, anterior recesses of the third ventricle extending into the sella, and many of the mass lesions noted in Table 1–4 (p 38). The empty sella is discussed below.

Radiologic artifacts may also produce intrasellar low-density areas that may sometimes be mistaken for pituitary adenomas. Such artifacts may be caused by substandard equipment, poor technique, or patient movement. Axial cuts that pass through both petrous bones may cause an artifact (high-spatial-frequency artifact) in the sellar fossa that is of low density. Coronal cuts that pass through dental hardware will also be distorted.

Isodense lesions on contrast-enhanced CT scan are occasionally tumors. An adenoma is suspected if there is lateral deviation of the pituitary stalk, if the gland height is more than 7 mm, or if the upper border of an adult's pituitary is convex (young patients normally have plump glands). However, primary hypothyroidism, primary hypogonadism, Addison's disease, and pregnancy also produce pituitary enlargement that may enlarge the sella and even appear to erode the sella floor. Therefore, these conditions must always be considered in the differential diagnosis of a homogenous-appearing mass on CT scan in patients having no sign of acromegaly, Cushing's disease, or a prolactinoma.

Hyperdense lesions on contrast-enhanced CT scan can be either large tumors, vascular tumors, or aneurysms. An aneurysm is more likely if the pituitary tumor is nonfunctioning and the detected mass enhances homogeneously and intensely and extends beyond the sella. Aneurysms and pituitary tumors are not mutually exclusive and may coexist. When there is any question of whether a contrast-enhancing lesion is an aneurysm, arteriography or MRI will make the distinction.

Calcifications within the sella may be due to pituitary adenomas and have the appearance of an intrasellar stone. Calcifications are usually due to craniopharyngiomas, meningiomas, or aneurysms. They can usually be distinguished, since meningiomas may form a rather solid calcification, whereas craniopharyngiomas are often speckled, and aneurysm calcification often conforms to the vascular pattern. Intrasellar calcifications have also been reported with hamartomas and chordomas. Hypothalamic calcifications also occur in hypoparathyroidism.

CT scans may be windowed or photographed to reveal soft tissue lesions or osseous abnormalities (**bone visualization**). Soft tissue images may give a false appearance of erosion of the sellar floor. Bone windows give a more accurate assessment of surrounding bone and should be ordered to aid the surgeon's approach if transsphenoidal surgery is planned.

MAGNETIC RESONANCE IMAGING

Magnetic resonance imaging works by using strong magnetic fields and radiofrequency energy to detect the density and behavior of protons within tissues. Unlike CT scanning, where tissue contrast is dependent on a single tissue property (electron density), magnetic resonance image contrast is dependent on 3 tissue properties (proton density and T1 and T2 relaxation times). T1-weighted MRIs are shown in Figs 1–3 to 1–6.

Images may be acquired to emphasize either T1 or T2 proton relaxation characteristics. The approximate order of signal intensity from tissues on heavily **T1-weighted images** is as follows: *No signal*—bone and rapidly flowing blood. *Low signal*—cerebrospinal fluid, acute hemorrhage, and most pathologic lesions (tumors, ischemia, infection, demyelination). *Intermediate signal*—gray matter. *High signal*—fat, subacute hemorrhage, white matter, and tissue-secreting antidiuretic hormone (ADH).

The approximate order of signal intensity from tissues on heavily **T2-weighted images** is as follows: *No signal*—bone and rapidly flowing blood. *Low signal*—fat. *Intermediate signal*—brain. *High signal*—cerebrospinal fluid, acute hemorrhage, and most pathologic lesions.

MRI is useful in identifying tumor as well as vascular abnormalities such as aneurysms and arteriovenous malformations. However, about 15% of normal individuals have some "abnormal" reading.

MRI that is T1-weighted usually portrays pituitary microadenomas as small masses with lower signal intensity than the surrounding pituitary tissue. Pituitary macroadenomas are easily seen with MRI. Their impingement upon surrounding structures is better seen with MRI than with CT. Areas of necrosis and hemorrhage within such macroadenomas may also be distinguished. Gadolinium-enhanced MRI is helpful for distinguishing tumors from edema and detecting microadenomas if noncontrast studies are not definitive. The adenoma does not take up contrast.

MRI has the advantage of not exposing the patient to x-rays or intravenous contrast agents that can cause adverse reactions. It produces no side effects but ordinarily cannot be performed on patients with cardiac pacemakers or some intracranial metal aneurysm clips that could undergo torque when exposed to the intense magnetic field. No adverse effects have been noted in pregnant patients.

POSITRON EMISSION TOMOGRAPHY

Positron emission tomography (PET) using fluorine-18-2-fluoro-deoxyglucose (FDG) can be employed to detect pituitary microadenomas, albeit with less resolution than MRI or CT. Certain microadenomas of Cushing's disease have been detected by PET that were not visible on MRI. False-positive studies appear to be less frequent.

THE EMPTY SELLA

Larger hypodense areas not within the substance of the gland may be due to cerebrospinal fluid. Some cerebrospinal fluid is found within the sella in at least 50% of individuals. This condition is commonly called a partially empty sella (arachnoidocele) and is due to an opening in the diaphragma sellae that allows a herniation of arachnoid and cerebrospinal fluid downward into the sella, compressing the normal pituitary. Most empty sellas are only partial, but as many as 5% of individuals have an enlarged sella that is virtually filled with cerebrospinal fluid, the normally functioning pituitary being flattened to a barely visible 2-mm thickness along the sella floor. The empty sella is usually a normal variant, but it is more frequently seen in obese women and in such conditions as prior pituitary surgery, radiation, infarction, and idiopathic nontumorous hypopituitarism.

An empty sella per se does not appear to cause local symptoms or pituitary functional impairment. Reports that patients with an empty sella have headaches, neurologic abnormalities, diabetes mellitus, or hypertension may represent an aberration secondary to referral patterns.

In an empty sella, the pituitary usually retains a midline stalk that is visible by CT scan on direct coronal views or coronal re-formations. An empty sella can usually be distinguished from a cystic pituitary adenoma, which ordinarily displaces or obscures the stalk. MRI can usually make the distinction based on differences in signal intensity (see above). A CT scan following the introduction of water-soluble iodinated contrast material (metrizamide) into the subarachnoid space is usually diagnostic. Contrast enters an empty sella or surrounds a low-density mass. A metrizamide study cannot always distinguish between a low-density mass and a cerebrospinal fluid recess or cyst that fails to communicate with the subarachnoid space.

CLINICAL CORRELATIONS

Many lesions other than pituitary tumors can produce pituitary masses (Table 1–4). The grading and staging of pituitary tumors are described in Table 1–6. Although the definitive diagnosis must usually be endocrinologic or histologic, the diagnosis can often be inferred from the radiologic appearance, association with other abnormalities, or clinical presentation. The symptoms of excess hormone secretion are discussed later in this chapter. Sarcoidosis is usually systemic and has a proclivity to involve the pituitary stalk with a contrast-enhancing mass. An optic glioma is usually associated with visual field loss and may be traced by CT scan to the optic nerve. Chordomas and cholesteatomas usually cause gross bony erosions. Lesions of Langerhans' cell granulomatosis generally produce diabetes insipidus and destruction of other areas of the skull. Autoimmune hypophysitis usually occurs in pregnant women nearing term or immediately post partum. The bones of the skull should be considered in assessing pituitary conditions: acromegaly causes enlarged bones and frontal sinuses, whereas Cushing's syndrome causes osteopenia.

Many secretory microadenomas may not be visible on CT or MR scan (**negative scan**). An empty sella may also harbor such small tumors. Such invisible microadenomas occur in about 44% of patients with Cushing's disease. Negative neuroradiologic studies also occur in about 15–20% of patients with symptomatic prolactinomas and in about 5–10% of acromegalics.

NORMAL PHYSIOLOGY OF THE PITUITARY

The pituitary gland secretes polypeptide hormones that circulate unbound and act on receptors located on the surface of target cells. The activation of the receptor involves changing the molecular shape of an N protein in the adjacent cell membrane. The activated N protein in turn activates cell membrane adenyl cyclase, which in turn catalyzes intracellular ATP to form cAMP. The cAMP causes phosphorylation of intracellular structural and enzymatic proteins, thereby changing their activity to produce the final effect.

ANTERIOR PITUITARY

The anterior pituitary synthesizes and secretes many polypeptide hormones, of which 6 are of major clinical importance (Table 1–1). GH and PRL act directly on target tissues and are simple peptides of similar structure. Four hormones (ACTH, TSH, LH, FSH) act by stimulating other endocrine glands. ACTH is a simple polypeptide hormone. The latter 3 hormones (TSH, LH, FSH) are glycopeptides having 2 subunits that are synthesized separately and then linked. The β-subunits of each are different and confer affinity to different target cells' receptors. The α-subunits are identical in each and stimulate the target endocrine cell.

Table 1–1. Pituitary hormones.

	Structure	Serum Half-life (approximate)
Anterior pituitary		
Growth hormone (GH)*	Polypeptide 191 amino acids	35 minutes
Prolactin (PRL)	Polypeptide 198 amino acids	35 minutes
Adrenocorticotropic hormone (ACTH)	Polypeptide 39 amino acids	10 minutes
Thyroid-stimulating hormone (TSH)	Glycopeptide α-subunit, 89 amino acids β-subunit, 112 amino acids	50 minutes
Luteinizing hormone (LH)†	Glycopeptide α-subunit, 89 amino acids β-subunit, 115 amino acids	50 minutes
Follicle-stimulating hormone (FSH)	Glycopeptide α-subunit, 89 amino acids β-subunit, 115 amino acids	50 minutes
Posterior pituitary		
Arginine vasopressin (AVP)‡	Ringed polypeptide 9 amino acids	4 minutes
Oxytocin (OT)	Ringed polypeptide 9 amino acids	4 minutes

* GH closely resembles human placental lactogen (hPL).
† LH closely resembles human chorionic gonadotropin (hCG).
‡ AVP is synonymous with antidiuretic hormone (ADH).

Growth Hormone (GH)

A. Secretion: GH secretion is stimulated mainly by growth hormone releasing hormone (GHRH), a polypeptide secreted by the hypothalamus. GH release is inhibited by somatostatin (ST), a 14-amino acid peptide secreted by the hypothalamus that inhibits most other hormones as well. ST is also found in other tissues such as the intestinal mucosa and pancreatic islets.

GH levels are increased by many physiologic factors. Normal serum levels have a diurnal pattern: sleep induces a rise in GH, which peaks about 1.5 hours after the onset of sleep and then declines over 2 hours. Increases in the serum level of amino acids cause an increase in GH about 2.5 hours after meals containing protein and during intravenous infusions of amino acids such as arginine. Exercise and stress also stimulate GH secretion; such stresses may by psychological or physical (eg, trauma, hypoglycemia).

Drugs that increase GH levels include estrogens, dopamine agonists (eg, clonidine), and β-adrenergic blockers (eg, propranolol). Other conditions producing elevated serum levels of GH include protein starvation, anorexia nervosa, and chronic renal failure. These stimuli of GH do not lead to actual increased growth, however. Pituitary adenomas can produce excessive GH and lead to gigantism and acromegaly.

Factors inhibiting GH release include GH itself, acute hyperglycemia, progesterone, glucocorticoids, dopamine blockers (eg, phenothiazines), α-adrenergic blockers (eg, phentolamine), β-adrenergic agonists (eg, isoproterenol, amphetamines), and serotonin antagonists (eg, methysergide). GH response to stress (eg, hypoglycemia) is inhibited by obesity.

B. Effects: GH produces growth via the stimulation of insulinlike growth factor (IGF-I; somatomedin C) by the liver and possibly other tissues. GH acts directly on adipose tissue to break down triacylglycerols to fatty acids, a fuel source. It thus spares the catabolism of muscle and encourages its growth.

Prolactin (PRL)

A. Secretion: The pituitary would spontaneously secrete PRL in large amounts, but it is normally inhibited by dopamine (prolactin-inhibiting factor, PIF) from the hypothalamus. Although PRL secretion can be stimulated by thyrotropin-releasing hormone (TRH) from the hypothalamus, this effect is not physiologically significant unless the patient has primary hypothyroidism. During pregnancy, high estrogen levels stimulate PRL secretion. Other causes of hyperprolactinemia are listed in Table 1–7.

B. Effects: High levels of PRL stimulate the secretory apparatus of the breast in preparation for lactation, doing so in concert with other hormones—hPL, cortisol, insulin, progesterone, and estrogen. The high estrogen level of pregnancy promotes breast development but inhibits actual lactation. Estrogen levels fall precipitously postpartum and no longer antagonize the effect of PRL on the alveolar cells of the breast to synthesize milk, which thereby ''comes in.''

Postpartum, baseline serum PRL levels fall to less than 20 ng/mL within 3 weeks but rise as high as 400 ng/mL during suckling, although this response diminishes as nursing continues. The frequent spikes in PRL levels serve to maintain the breasts' secretory capacity; concurrent oxytocin secretion produces actual ejection. Even in normal nonpuerperal women, nipple stimulation for just 5 minutes causes increases in serum PRL of up to 170 ng/mL. Such women who allow infants to suckle frequently may even develop lactation. If postpartum nursing is rather constant (ie, no bottles or pacifiers), ovulation is inhibited. Intensive breast feeding is thus a potent but imperfect contraceptive.

In men, PRL has no known function and is not increased by nipple stimulation.

Prolactin levels are high in newborns, having been stimulated by high estrogen levels in utero, which accounts for the occasional transient lactation found in newborns known commonly as "witches' milk."

Adrenocorticotropic Hormone (ACTH)

A. Secretion: A large precursor molecule, pro-opiomelanocortin (POMC), is broken and sections of it are found in the serum (Fig 1–7). The major sections consist of ACTH, an N-terminal fragment, and β-lipotropin, a fragment of which (β-endorphin) is an endogenous opiate. ACTH secretion is stimulated by corticotropin-releasing hormone (CRH), a hypothalamic polypeptide of 41 amino acids. CRH stimulates ACTH secretion from the pituitary by increasing the set point, ie, the level of cortisol necessary to inhibit ACTH secretion. ACTH is secreted in periodic bursts and is particularly stimulated by stresses of many kinds. ACTH secretion is inhibited by cortisol and synthetic glucocorticoids which "feed back" on both the pituitary and hypothalamus.

B. Effects: ACTH exerts most of its activity through its stimulation of cortisol production by the adrenals. ACTH also stimulates adrenal production of androgens. Chronically high ACTH levels may increase skin pigmentation; however, this effect is insignificant at normal plasma ACTH levels.

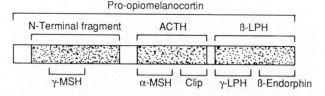

Figure 1–7. Pro-opiomelanocortin and its sections. ACTH = adrenocorticotropic hormone; β-LPH = β-lipotropin; γ-MSH = γ-melanocyte–stimulating hormone; α-MSH = α-melanocyte–stimulating hormone (fetus only); CLIP = corticotropinlike intermediate lobe peptide (fetus only); γ-LPH = γ-lipotropin.

Thyroid-Stimulating Hormone (TSH)

A. Secretion: TSH secretion is rather constant and is stimulated by thyrotropin-releasing hormone (TRH), a small hypothalamic peptide of 3 amino acids. T_4 and T_3 suppress TSH secretion by direct negative feedback on the pituitary thyrotrope cells as well as on the hypothalamic TRH cells.

B. Effects: TSH stimulates the thyroid to (1) take up iodine, (2) link iodine to tyrosine to form T_4 and T_3, and (3) secrete the T_4 and T_3.

GONADOTROPINS

The gonadotropins, FSH and LH, are glycopeptide hormones that are usually secreted from the same pituitary gonadotrope cells. These cells are able to segregate or combine these hormones in cytoplasmic granules, the secretion of which is modulated by complex factors. Both FSH and LH are stimulated by a 10-amino-acid hypothalamic gonadotropin-releasing hormone (GnRH), but only when the latter is secreted in a pulsatile manner. The different effects of these hormones are discussed separately below. Further discussions are found later in this book regarding their effects in children, women, and men.

Luteinizing Hormone (LH)

A. Secretion and Effects in Children: LH levels are generally suppressed in the fetus and newborn, being inhibited by the high serum estradiol levels of pregnancy. LH secretion then increases during the first 2 years of life and reaches pubertal levels. In boys, this causes the testes to produce pubertal levels of testosterone at age 3–6 months. This brief exposure to testosterone produces no ill effects. From about age 3–10 years, LH and FSH are both suppressed by unknown factors, even in hypogonadal children, delaying the onset of adolescence until the usual time.

B. Secretion and Effects in Women: During the follicular phase of the menstrual cycle, LH secretion gradually increases, being stimulated by rising levels of estradiol secreted by the ovary that has some inherent cyclicity. Once a critical level of serum estradiol occurs, LH surges and, along with a smaller surge in FSH, causes ovulation. LH then maintains the ovarian corpus luteum's secretion of progesterone, which prepares the endometrium for implantation. As LH levels fall during the luteal phase of the menstrual cycle, the corpus luteum becomes atretic unless rescued by hCG secretion that causes a corpus luteum of pregnancy.

C. Secretion and Effects in Men: LH secretion remains relatively constant in men. It stimulates the Leydig cells in the testis to produce the testosterone necessary for both masculinization and sperm production. The testosterone in turn inhibits excessive LH secretion from the pituitary.

Follicle-Stimulating Hormone (FSH)

A. Secretion and Effects in Children: FSH levels are generally inhibited in the fetus and newborn by the high serum estradiol levels of pregnancy. FSH secretion then increases during the first 2 years of life, temporarily reaching pubertal levels. In girls, this causes the ovaries to produce pubertal levels of estradiol at age 6–12 months. This brief exposure to estradiol produces no ill effects except for occasional premature telarche in infant girls. From about age 3–10 years, FSH and LH are both suppressed by unknown factors, even in hypogonadal children, delaying the onset of adolescence until the usual time.

B. Secretion and Effects in Women: During the menstrual cycle, FSH secretion gradually increases. FSH causes development of the ovarian follicle and stimulates estradiol and progesterone levels that occur later in the menstrual cycle and is suppressed during pregnancy. Menopause and ovarian disorders causing estradiol deficiency stimulate compensatory hypersecretion of FSH.

C. Secretion and Effects in Men: FSH secretion remains relatively constant in men. It stimulates the Sertoli cells in the testes to produce local sex hormone–binding globulin (SHBG). This allows the high concentrations of testosterone in the testis that are required for sperm production. The Sertoli cells produce a hormone called **inhibin**, which inhibits excessive FSH secretion from the pituitary.

POSTERIOR PITUITARY

The posterior pituitary secretes arginine vasopressin and oxytocin, which are synthesized in the hypothalamus by different neurons and are each transported down axons to nerve endings in the posterior pituitary and stalk.

Arginine Vasopressin (AVP)

A. Secretion: AVP is produced along with its binding protein, neurophysin II, in nerve cell bodies located in the hypothalamus. The AVP–neurophysin II secretory material is transported from the supraoptic and paraventricular nuclei lining the third ventricle down axons to nerve terminals in the posterior pituitary and stalk. AVP and its inactive neurophysin are then secreted in response to nerve impulses caused by hypotension or extracellular hyperosmolality.

The major stimulant for AVP secretion (and later, thirst) is an increase in extracellular osmolality, mainly caused by an increase in serum sodium. In normal individuals, the sodium level stimulating AVP release is slightly lower than that causing thirst. AVP levels and thirst drive usually remain low, since obligate water loss is largely balanced by water derived from oxidative metabolism and from drinking for social reasons or to aid food ingestion.

Serum sodium and plasma osmolality are kept remarkably constant in a given individual and rarely vary more than 2%. However, during pregnancy, serum sodium drops about 4 mEq/L and plasma osmolality drops about 10 mOsm/kg, and at high altitude, the plasma osmolality rises about 10 mOsm/kg. There are differences in the osmolar set points among individuals such that the normal serum sodium is between 136 and 145 mEq/L and the normal plasma osmolality is between 280 and 300 mOsm/kg water.

Plasma osmolality determinations can often be misleading. A high plasma osmolality does not necessarily indicate dehydration, since osmolality may be increased by other solutes that, unlike sodium, permeate central nervous system cells rather freely. Plasma osmolality can be measured by freezing-point depression on heparinized plasma (not EDTA) but also may be calculated by the following formula:

$$\text{Plasma osmolality (mOsm/kg water)} =$$
$$2[Na^+(mEq/L) + K^+(mEq/L)] + [Glucose (mg/dL)/18] +$$
$$[BUN (mg/dL)/2.8] + [ETOH (mg/dL)/4.6]$$

As is apparent from the above formula, a high plasma osmolality measurement should not be interpreted as showing dehydration if obtained in a patient with hyperglycemia, azotemia, or alcohol intoxication.

B. Effects: AVP acts mainly upon the renal collecting duct epithelium, which is otherwise impermeable to water. The kidneys might excrete as many as 20 L of dilute urine daily were it not for the action of AVP. AVP causes an increase in the epithelium's permeability, allowing water to diffuse from the dilute urine into the hypertonic interstitial fluid of the renal medulla. The urine flowing out of the collecting duct thereby becomes more concentrated and decreases in volume. Some individuals having no detectable AVP concentrate their urine by unknown means.

Oxytocin (OT)

A. Secretion: OT is produced along with its binding protein, neurophysin I, in nerve cell bodies located in the hypothalamus. The OT–neurophysin I secretory material is transported down axons to nerve terminals in the posterior pituitary and stalk. OT and its inactive neurophysin are secreted in response to distention of the lower uterus, cervix, and vagina during parturition. It also is secreted during suckling and at ejaculation.

B. Effects: OT causes the uterus to contract more strongly and is one factor that facilitates delivery. Suckling stimulates OT secretion, which helps lactation by causing milk ejection from the nipple.

HYPOPITUITARISM

Hypopituitarism refers to deficiency of one or more pituitary hormones. Symptoms depend on the specific deficiencies and their severity, the duration of the deficiency, and the cause. Cases due to a secretory pituitary adenoma or hypothalamic injury may demonstrate a combined deficiency/excess syndrome. Certain hormone deficiencies may be partial and produce symptoms that are overshadowed by more severe deficiencies or nonendocrine symptoms associated with the underlying cause (Table 1–2).

Therefore, when one pituitary hormone deficiency is diagnosed, other deficiencies may be present and must be searched for vigilantly, and the underlying cause must be determined. *This requires CT or MRI of the pituitary.* MRI may show a destructive lesion or attenuation or absence of the pituitary stalk; the visual posterior pituitary "bright spot" may be absent or present superiorly (ectopic neurohypophysis). Patients with a normal pituitary scan should be screened for **hemochromatosis** with serum measurements of ferritin and transferrin saturation. Hemochromatosis may be confirmed by CT, MRI, or biopsy of the liver.

In β-thalassemia major, hypogonadotropic hypogonadism due to transfusion-caused iron overload can be prevented in 90% by beginning deferoxamine administration before puberty.

Patients with diseases known to cause hypopituitarism (Table 1–4) require ongoing evaluation in order to diagnose endocrine deficiencies early in their course. Patients with a slowly destructive process in the pituitary may lose pituitary hormones in a serial manner and in any combination, but most often beginning with GH, followed by LH/FSH, and then TSH, and finally ACTH. Patients with generalized anterior pituitary insufficiency are said to have **panhypopituitarism**. Children with panhypopituitarism generally present with signs of growth hormone deficiency. Neonates may have hypoglycemia and prolonged jaundice. Children are pudgy, appear doll-like, and have growth failure.

Table 1–2. Manifestations of pituitary and hypothalamic disease.

Endocrine deficiencies
  GH (micropenis, hypoglycemia, short stature, obesity)
  PRL (inability to lactate)
  ACTH (hypoadrenalism)
  TSH (hypothyroidism)
  FSH, LH (hypogonadism or delayed adolescence)
  AVP (diabetes insipidus)
  OT (inability to lactate)

Endocrine excesses
  Pituitary tumor secretion
    ACTH (Cushing's disease or Nelson's syndrome)
    GH (gigantism or acromegaly)
    PRL (amenorrhea, galactorrhea, impotence)
    TSH (hyperthyroidism—rare)
  Hyperprolactinemia (hyperplastic) (amenorrhea and galactorrhea)
  hCG from a germinoma in the hypothalamus or pineal region—
    pseudoprecocious puberty in boys
  Excess AVP or CNS natriuretic factor (hyponatremia)

Hypothalamic neurologic damage
  Hypodipsia (recurrent hypernatremia)
  Memory impairment (especially short-term)
  Sleep disorders (somnolence, coma)
  Eating disorders (morbid obesity, anorexia)
  Temperature disorders (hypothermia, poikilothermia, hyperthermia)
  Epilepsy
  Autonomic nervous system (cardiac dysrhythmias, pulmonary edema)
  Psychiatric disorders (rage attacks, hallucinations)

Familial syndromes
  See Table 1–4.

Mass effect
  Headache
  Visual field abnormalities
  Cranial nerve damage (II, III, IV, VI)
  Hydrocephalus
  Perinaud's syndrome
  Cerebrospinal fluid leak
  Nasal airway obstruction

Laboratory abnormalities
  Hyperuricemia
  Abnormalities of endocrine deficiency or excess

Adults with panhypopituitarism generally present with symptoms of fatigue and generalized lassitude as well as amenorrhea (women) and decreased libido. Adults with long-standing panhypopituitarism lose body and sexual hair and develop characteristic facial features consisting of fine wrinkles, mild myxedema, somewhat pallid-colored fawny-textured skin, and an apathetic countenance. Men have diminished beard growth. Patients may have clinical diabetes insipidus if there has been hypothalamic damage or a high stalk section.

Because the presentation of hypopituitarism can be quite varied, the diagnosis and treatment of each hormonal deficiency are described separately below.

ANTERIOR PITUITARY DEFICIENCIES

Prolactin Deficiency

Women with PRL deficiency have normal breast enlargement during pregnancy due to the effects of high levels of estradiol, progesterone, and human placental lactogen (hPL). These women cannot lactate post partum. PRL deficiency is never isolated and is found along with other pituitary hormone deficiencies in hypopituitarism caused by pituitary destruction. Ironically, hypopituitarism caused by damage to the stalk or hypothalamus produces an increase in PRL owing to diminished prolactin-inhibiting factor (dopamine). PRL deficiency causes no known symptoms in men. It is impractical to evaluate or treat any patient for PRL deficiency.

Growth Hormone Deficiency

The diagnosis and treatment of GH deficiency in children are discussed in Chapter 3.

GH deficiency is common in adults, occurring in up to one-third of the elderly. No destructive pituitary or hypothalamic lesions are visible, although conditions listed in Table 1–4 must be considered. GH deficiency may contribute to "aging." Elderly patients with low IGF-I (< 350 U/L) treated with GH, 0.03 mg/kg (0.06 U/kg) 3 times weekly intramuscularly for 6 months, have increased lean body mass, decreased adiposity, increased skin thickness, and improved cognitive function and vitality. Complications are unusual and dose-related and include carpal tunnel syndrome, hypertension, peripheral edema, and arthralgias. Older patients with GH deficiency whose epiphyses have fused cannot have further longitudinal growth. Owing to cost considerations, it is impractical to evaluate or treat most adults for GH deficiency unless they have hypoglycemia, which may respond to GH therapy.

Adrenocorticotropic Hormone Deficiency

A. Symptoms and Signs: ACTH deficiency causes secondary hypoadrenalism with resultant deficiencies of cortisol and adrenal androgens. Some patients have no symptoms, but most exhibit anorexia, nausea, vomiting, abdominal pain, weight loss, fatigue, weakness, and malaise. Some patients present with hypotension, anemia, sexual hair loss, delirium, or hyponatremia. Patients may develop hypoglycemia, especially if they have concurrent GH deficiency. Infants with panhypopituitarism are especially prone to hypoglycemia and neuroglycopenic seizures. Hypotension and hyponatremia are usually less common or severe than in primary adrenal insufficiency, since the renin-angiotensin mechanism for aldosterone secretion remains intact in ACTH deficiency. Rarely, patients may exhibit the **stiff-man syndrome**, with progressive muscle stiffness and pain and an EMG showing continuous muscle activity at rest. Muscle spasms improve dramatically with hydrocortisone replacement.

ACTH deficiency causes decreased adrenal androgen secretion. Serum DHEA and DHEAS are low, possibly adding to a tendency to asthenia. Children of both sexes with ACTH deficiency usually also have concurrent FSH/LH deficiency; the resultant hypogonadism results in combined total deficit in androgens of adrenal as well as gonadal origin. This produces diminished axillary and pubic hair growth in both sexes, as well as decreased beard in men and decreased phallic growth in boys. Boys develop adequate (but often subnormal) sexual hair growth once adequate testosterone replacement therapy is begun. Girls given the usual estrogen/progestin replacement may menstruate normally and have adequate breast development but persist in a total lack of body sexual hair unless given small doses of androgens. Some of these children have an aversion to becoming adults (**Peter Pan syndrome**).

Secondary adrenal insufficiency that develops during adulthood produces similar symptoms of androgen deficiency if gonadal function is also impaired. In that case, men and women gradually lose their body sexual hair.

ACTH deficiency usually occurs with other pituitary deficiencies but may be isolated as part of lymphocytic hypophysitis or polyglandular autoimmune failure or may be idiopathic.

B. Diagnosis: The quickest and safest way to diagnose ACTH deficiency is with the brief cosyntropin (ACTH$_{1-24}$) stimulation test. Glucocorticoids, if being taken, are switched to hydrocortisone, the last dose of which is taken more than 12 hours before the test. (See Appendix for protocol.) In addition, baseline morning DHEAS is subnormal (for age) in over 90% of affected patients.

The cosyntropin stimulation test is a perfectly acceptable (albeit indirect) way to assess ACTH reserve and an individual's response to stress, since ACTH stimulation from the pituitary is required to keep the adrenal cortex primed for episodic surges in ACTH. The adrenal cortex becomes physiologically atrophic within 4 weeks after ACTH deficiency begins; therefore, cosyntropin testing should be held off that long after a known pituitary insult (eg, surgery); in the meantime, physiologic doses of hydrocortisone are prophylactically given (eg, 20 mg at 8 AM and 10 mg at 5 PM) and do not significantly suppress endogenous ACTH and cortisol production over 4–6 weeks.

If the cosyntropin stimulation test is distinctly abnormal, adrenal insufficiency is documented. If it occurs in the setting of obvious pituitary pathology (eg, pituitary surgery or radiation), a plasma ACTH level is not required to distinguish primary adrenal insufficiency (Addison's disease). In primary adrenal insufficiency, ACTH is elevated, whereas in secondary adrenal insufficiency the ACTH level is normal or low.

The insulin tolerance test (ITT) and the overnight metyrapone stimulation test (see Appendix) may also be used to diagnose ACTH/cortisol deficiency. The ITT is more sensitive than the cosyntropin test for uncovering milder deficiencies that are rarely of clinical importance. ITT produces unpleasant symptoms that make it less desirable for outpatients. The metyrapone test is not superior to the cosyntropin test, and results may be delayed. Furthermore, coexistent hypothyroidism may cause a low basal cortisol and an abnormal ITT and 24-hour metyrapone test (which are corrected by thyroid hormone replacement) while the cosyntropin test remains normal.

C. Treatment: Secondary adrenal insufficiency is usually permanent if caused by a destructive process and transient if caused by glucocorticoid feedback inhibition. Patients need to wear an identification bracelet or neck-chain stating "Adrenal insufficiency. Takes hydrocortisone." In the event of serious trauma, the recommended dosage of hydrocortisone is 100 mg (hemisuccinate or phosphate) given intramuscularly. Perioperative hydrocortisone replacement is frequently excessive but it may be given as follows for an uncomplicated but *major* surgical procedure. The adult regimen is as follows:

Day of surgery: 100 mg intramuscularly on call to the operating room, then 50 mg intramuscularly or intravenously every 6 hours beginning in the recovery room or intraoperatively if the procedure takes more than 6 hours.

First day postoperatively: 40 mg every 6 hours, intramuscularly, intravenously, or orally.

Second day postoperatively: 30 mg every 6 hours, intramuscularly, intravenously, or orally.

Third day postoperatively: 20 mg every 6 hours, intramuscularly, intravenously, or orally.

Fourth day postoperatively: 10 mg every 6 hours, intramuscularly, intravenously, or orally.

Subsequently: If the patient is eating food well, give 20 mg orally at 8 AM and 10 mg at 5 PM or usual replacement dose. If the patient is taking nothing by mouth, give 10 mg intravenously every 8 hours.

For illnesses not requiring hospitalization, a patient with chronic secondary adrenal insufficiency is advised to triple the usual replacement dose of hydrocortisone and see a physician within 3 days, or immediately if the illness is especially severe or nausea occurs. Any patient who hikes or travels to remote areas is prescribed parenteral hydrocortisone (100-mg vial, syringe, and needle) for emergency use. Hydrocortisone is the replacement glucocorticoid of choice. Prednisone (about 5 mg daily) is an alternative. Hydrocortisone dosage is easier to adjust than dexamethasone whose long duration of action predisposes the patient to a cumulative overdosage of glucocorticoid, resulting in iatrogenic Cushing's syndrome.

The optimal dose of hydrocortisone varies among individuals and must be adjusted carefully according to the patient's clinical response. Many patients may become cushingoid on chronic daily doses of only 30 mg of hydrocortisone. Such patients may do better on only 15–20 mg of hydrocortisone daily (10 mg at 8 AM; 5 mg at 5 PM). Children must be maintained on low doses of hydrocortisone (2.5–5 mg twice daily) to avoid growth inhibition. Patients who become fatigued in the afternoon may require a midday dose of hydrocortisone. Patients doing intermittent heavy labor or exercise may avoid exhaustion by taking an additional 5–10 mg prophylactically 1 hour before the activity. Patients who always arise from sleep very tired are advised to keep their medication on the bedside and take their prescribed dose upon first awakening. Only rarely do patients require chronic replacement hydrocortisone of more than 30 mg/d; such patients include those with intestinal malabsorption.

Thyroid-Stimulating Hormone Deficiency

A. Symptoms and Signs: Symptoms and signs of TSH deficiency in adults are generally similar to those of primary hypothyroidism. Children frequently have no signs aside from delayed growth. The potential for severe hypothyroidism or myxedema coma is not as great, since the thyroid produces some T_4 and T_3 spontaneously. Adults may have fatigue, mental slowing, apathy, cold intolerance, dry skin, constipation, and bradycardia. Over time, patients may gain weight (especially if GH deficiency is also present) unless concomitant secondary adrenal insufficiency has produced anorexia. Patients may also develop a myxedematous facial appearance characteristic of panhypopituitarism. If TSH deficiency occurs acutely, hypothyroidism develops gradually over the ensuing 6 weeks; symptoms do not develop acutely due to the long half-life of the T_4 already in circulation. Therefore, after an event such as pituitary surgery, postoperative evaluation for hypothyroidism (and hypoadrenalism) is usually delayed 4–6 weeks (sooner if symptomatic).

B. Diagnosis: Evaluation for secondary hypothyroidism involves obtaining a serum T_4 and resin T_3 uptake (RT_3U) to calculate a free thyroxine index. Alternatively, free T_4 may be measured directly by radioimmunoassay (RIA) if a reliable assay is available.

Since TSH is low in secondary hypothyroidism, patients lack goiter (which is a frequent finding in primary hypothyroidism) unless some intrinsic thyroid pathology is incidentally present as well. Unfortunately, conventional RIA using polyclonal antibodies for TSH has not proved of value in making the diagnosis of secondary hypothyroidism. More sensitive RIA using monoclonal antibodies for TSH may be more helpful. The TSH response to TRH is discussed in the Appendix.

The lack of having TSH as a marker for secondary hypothyroidism poses no problem for patients with obvious hypopituitarism and a definitely low free thyroxine index. However, patients with mild secondary hypothyroidism may have vague symptoms and low-normal serum T_4 levels. Following correction of any other deficiencies, these patients may remain simply fatigued. The serum level of T_4 may also be in the low-normal range, but lower than a T_4 obtained previously.

C. Differential Diagnosis: Factors that may depress serum T_4 without affecting clinical status are listed in Table 5–1. During very severe illness, the serum free T_4 may be depressed without any rise in TSH; physiologic secondary hypogonadism may also be present. It is important to distinguish whether such patients truly have secondary hypothyroidism that may be worsening their clinical condition or have hypothyroxinemia of nonthyroidal disease; patients receiving phenytoin (Dilantin) may also have depressed T_4 levels due to accelerated metabolism of T_4 to T_3. Thyroxine replacement is not given to these patients unless they have (1) hypothyroidism diagnosed prior to the illness, (2) unmistakable clinical signs of hypothyroidism, (3) secondary hypoadrenalism or diabetes insipidus, or (4) an illness affecting the central nervous system that is also a common cause of hypopituitarism.

D. Treatment: Since TSH is a complex glycopeptide, it is digested if given orally, has a short half-life, and cannot be economically produced. Therefore, L-thyroxine is given as replacement therapy. The dose of L-thyroxine requires clinical judgment, especially since TSH levels will not be elevated if the dose is inadequate. As in primary hypothyroidism, the starting dose should be low if the hypothyroidism has been long-standing and the patient is over 50 years of age or has a known coronary insufficiency. In that clinical situation, the usual starting dose of L-thyroxine is 0.025–0.05 mg/d and is increased by 0.025–0.05 mg monthly until the patient is clinically euthyroid. In acute pituitary insufficiency and in young adult patients without coronary disease, begin treatment with L-thyroxine, 0.1–0.15 mg/d. Some adult patients ultimately require 0.175 or 0.2 mg daily and rarely more. If a patient has a low-normal T_4 level but has symptoms or signs of hypothyroidism in a clinical setting predisposing to secondary hypothyroidism, an empiric trial of L-thyroxine therapy (eg, 0.1–0.15 mg/d) for 2 months is indicated. If the patient shows no symptomatic improvement, the L-thyroxine is simply discontinued.

The recommended preparations of L-thyroxine are Synthroid and Levothroid. Some generic L-thyroxine preparations vary in potency as does desiccated thyroid. T_3 or synthetic combinations of T_4 and T_3 produce wider daily fluctuations of T_3 levels and are not recommended.

If thyroxine replacement is to be given to such a patient or if the diagnosis of secondary hypothyroidism is uncertain, a cosyntropin stimulation test is performed. While the results are pending, hydrocortisone may be given. If the condition is acute, however (less than 4 weeks' duration), not enough time may have elapsed for the adrenals to become unresponsive to ACTH. In that case, physiologic glucocorticoid replacement may be given for 1 month and the cosyntropin stimulation test then repeated. The presence of hypoadrenalism helps confirm the diagnosis of hypopituitary hypothyroidism; in that case, both medications are continued. If the patient recovers and the diagnosis of secondary hypothyroidism made during the illness was at all tenuous, then thyroxine replacement may be withdrawn later under close observation.

Luteinizing Hormone and Follicle-Stimulating Hormone Deficiency

A. Symptoms and Signs: Symptoms and signs of secondary hypogonadism are essentially the same as those of primary hypogonadism in men or women. Symptoms include decreased libido and infertility. Axillary and pubic hair decreases gradually in both men and women owing to decreased testicular and ovarian androgens. Total lack of sexual hair does not occur unless hypoadrenalism is concurrently present. Both male and female patients with chronic untreated hypogonadism may develop osteoporosis and prematurely wrinkled skin. Some lassitude may occur.

Women have amenorrhea and other symptoms of hypoestrogenism such as vasomotor instability (sweats and hot flashes), decreased vaginal lubrication with resultant dyspareunia, and a decrease in clitoral erectile function and orgasmic potential. Emotional depression and instability are common.

Men may note diminished beard growth, impotence, and a hematocrit below male normals (which is higher than that of female normals owing to the erythropoietic effect of androgens). Severe diaphoresis may also occur in hypogonadal men.

Isolated gonadotropin deficiency usually presents as absence of puberty. Such patients have a deficiency in hypothalamic GnRH, which classically results in deficiency of both FSH and LH; since GH and the other pituitary hormones are not affected, such patients develop eunuchoid proportions if left untreated; the epiphyses fail to fuse at the appropriate times and the longitudinal growth of long bones continues, producing span:height and pubis-floor:pubis-head ratios of more than 1. This same eunuchoid stature is also seen in cases of primary hypogonadism, except for patients with Klinefelter's syndrome, who tend to have relatively short arms and a span:height ratio of less than 1 despite isolated primary hypogonadism. Thus, this difference in span:height ratio may be of some value in distinguishing hypothalamic hypogonadism from the common Klinefelter's syndrome if serum measurements of FSH and LH have not been obtained. Isolated GnRH deficiency may also present in adulthood after a normal puberty.

Cases of isolated LH deficiency have been reported in men whose intact FSH allows adequate spermatogenesis despite low serum LH and testosterone levels that produce a eunuchoid appearance (**fertile eunuch syndrome**). Likewise, men may sometimes become fertile during testosterone treatment for hypogonadotropic hypogonadism. Therefore, fertility cannot be accurately predicted without a semen analysis.

In women, isolated LH deficiency might cause amenorrhea or irregular menses and infertility in an otherwise normally feminized woman. Cases of isolated FSH deficiency have rarely been reported but might present as decreased spermatogenesis and infertility in otherwise normally masculine men. It would cause women to have hypogonadism.

B. Diagnosis: Secondary hypogonadism is confirmed by a normal or low serum FSH level in the presence of a low estradiol level in women or a low testosterone level in men. Serum LH is usually low. The GnRH test has not proved helpful owing to commonly misleading results. Coexistent hypothyroidism and hypocortisolism must be ruled out.

C. Differential Diagnosis: In addition to the usual causes of hypopituitarism noted in Table 1–4, isolated FSH and LH deficiency may be caused by systemic disease, obesity or weight loss, alcoholism, and hyperprolactinemia (either physiologic or due to pituitary adenomas). In women, lesser degrees of FSH or LH deficiency may nonetheless cause amenorrhea or infertility and may be caused by physical or emotional stress or vigorous exercise. FSH and LH are normally suppressed by high levels of estrogens and progestins found in women who are pregnant or taking oral contraceptives.

D. Treatment: Treatment consists of replacing the gonadal hormone; gonadotropes are replaced only for induction of fertility. Vasomotor hot flashes can be controlled by estrogen or testosterone replacement. Other therapies for hot flashes include clonidine, cyproterone acetate, and a mixture of ergotamine, belladonna, and phenobarbital.

1. Women–In women, estrogen replacement therapy may consist of an oral estrogen preparation taken once daily on days 1–25 of each calendar month. Usual preparations include conjugated estrogens (0.625 or 1.25 mg) or ethinyl estradiol (0.02 or 0.05 mg). Some women with hypopituitarism develop hot flashes and moodiness during days when not receiving estrogen. This may be treated with low estrogen doses (eg, 0.3 mg) on days 26–30. In chronic hypopituitarism, begin with the lower dose to prevent breast discomfort. To produce normal menses, an oral progestational agent should be added once daily on days 16–25 of the month. The usual dosage consists of medroxyprogesterone acetate, 5 or 10 mg. No increased risk of breast or endometrial carcinoma is associated with cycled estrogen/progestin replacement. Libido may remain depressed in women with hypopituitarism owing to the absence of adrenal androgens from coexistent ACTH-adrenal insufficiency and can be restored by giving low doses of androgen (eg, testosterone cypionate, 25 mg intramuscularly every 1–2 months, or fluoxymesterone, 2–5 mg orally once or twice weekly), being careful to keep the dose low enough to avoid hirsutism and acne.

In women with infertility due to hypothalamic hypopituitarism (ie, with a structurally intact pituitary), ovulation may be induced with clomiphene citrate, 50 mg/d orally for 5 days monthly for 2 courses; if no ovulation occurs, increase the dose to 100 mg. The use of gonadotropins to induce ovulation in patients with functional or organic hypopituitarism should be undertaken only by those experienced in their use because of the danger of multiple births (20%), painful ovarian enlargment (20%), and hyperstimulation syndrome (1.3%). The protocol is described more fully in Chapter 9.

2. Men–In men, the preferred testosterone replacement therapy is testosterone enanthate or testosterone cypionate, 300 mg intramuscularly every 2–4 weeks. In chronic hypopituitarism, begin with a 100-mg dose to reduce priapism, acne, gynecomastia, and disruptive mood changes. The oral androgen preparation fluoxymesterone (Halotestin, 5–10 mg/d orally) is less effective than the parenteral preparation and may rarely produce peliosis hepatis.

Men with isolated GnRH deficiency but an intact pituitary may have fertility induced by GnRH delivered subcutaneously by a programmed infusion pump. The GnRH is given every 2 hours in pulse doses ranging from 25 to 600 ng/kg; the larger doses are required for patients with smaller initial testicular volume. Optimal dosing is determined by monthly monitoring of LH, testosterone, testis growth, and ultimately seminal fluid. Most patients require a minimum of 2 years' treatment to achieve maximum testis growth and spermatogenesis. Spermatogenesis occurs in more than two-thirds of noncryptorchid patients after 18–139 weeks of therapy. Patients with an initial testis volume > 6 mL tend to have faster onset of spermatogenesis. Most patients reach sperm counts that are subnormal but adequate for fertility. In one series, preconception counts ranged from 1 to 68 million/mL with 75% occurring at < 15 million/mL.

Men with prepubertal onset of hypogonadotropic hypogonadism may have fertility induced by first stopping testosterone therapy and giving hCG (20,000 IU/10-mL ampule) 2000 IU intramuscularly 3 times weekly. A serum testosterone is obtained after 2 months, and hMG (Pergonal) 75 IU intramuscularly 3 times weekly is added to the regimen. After another 4 months, the hMG dose is increased to 150 IU 3 times weekly. If the serum testosterone level is not well within the normal range, the hCG dosage is increased to 5000 IU intramuscularly 3 times weekly. Such a regimen has induced fertility in 6 of 8 men without prior cryptorchidism, but in only 1 of 7 men with prior cryptorchidism.

Men with postpubertal onset of hypogonadotropic hypogonadism may have fertility induced by first stopping testosterone therapy and giving hCG, 2000 IU intramuscularly 3 times weekly. A serum testosterone is obtained after 2 months. If the serum testosterone level is not well within the normal range, the hCG dose is increased to 5000 IU intramuscularly 3 times weekly. hCG therapy alone has restored fertility in all 6 men in one series. hMG is usually unnecessary.

The success of therapy in such men is monitored by periodic sperm counts. The hCG and hMG doses may be individualized according to the patient's response. The protocol is discussed further in Chapter 8.

POSTERIOR PITUITARY DEFICIENCIES

Polyuria & Central Diabetes Insipidus
(Arginine Vasopressin Deficiency)

Central diabetes insipidus (DI) is caused by deficient secretion of arginine vasopressin (AVP, antidiuretic hormone) at an individual's usual plasma osmolality. The plasma osmolality threshold required for

AVP release rises *above* that stimulating thirst. Thirst-induced polydipsia keeps the plasma osmolality below that required for AVP release; polyuria results.

Polyuria may be arbitrarily defined in the adult as the excretion of urine of more than 2000 mL/24 h. The severity of polyuria may be classified as mild (urine output 2,000–4000 mL/24 h), moderate (urine output 4000–6000 mL/24 h), or severe (urine output > 6000 mL/24 h). Polyuria in infants and young children is more difficult to define and quantitate, especially in children with enuresis. Urine volume in infants may be measured via a urine collection bag or approximated by weighing diapers before and after use, separating contaminants.

It is usually possible to distinguish the cause of polyuria (Table 1–3) by thoughtfully considering these possibilities and by screening the patient's plasma for K^+, Ca^+, Na^+, and blood urea nitrogen and urine for glucose and timed volume. Still, distinguishing the cause for polyuria may sometimes be difficult. The measurement of serum AVP is usually not necessary and is often misleading.

T1-weighted MRI of the pituitary in a patient with DI generally shows an absent or diminished posterior pituitary "bright spot."

Table 1–3. Differential diagnosis of polyuria.

Central diabetes insipidus

Vasopressin-induced
(especially in last trimester of pregnancy and puerperium, often with preeclampsia or hepatic dysfunction)

Excessive fluid intake
  Intravenous
  Psychogenic polydipsia
  Central nervous system sarcoidosis

  Thioridazine (Mellaril)
  Lithium

Nephrogenic diabetes insipidus
  Renal disease
  Chronic myeloma
  Sjögren's syndrome
  Sickle cell anemia
  Protein malnutrition
  Hereditary (usually males)
  Hypercalcemia
  Hypokalemia

  Diuretics (acutely)
  Lithium
  Demeclocycline
  Glucocorticoid excess
  Aminoglutethimide
  Methicillin
  Foscarnet

Resolution of edema

Osmotic diuresis
  Glycosuria
  Intravenous solutes (mannitol, glycerol, contrast)

A. Diagnosis of Central DI in Alert Patients Drinking Fluids:
Patients who are alert with normal thirst and access to fluids have polyuria and polydipsia. Some patients with chronic DI adapt amazingly well to their polydipsia and polyuria. Other patients complain bitterly of their incessant thirst. Nocturnal thirst and polyuria produces insomnia in adults or enuresis in children and mentally deficient patients. Many patients develop a craving for ice water.

Serious ill effects from chronic untreated DI include occasional hydroureters and hydronephrosis. Dehydration may occur in patients who lose their thirst sensation, have increased fluid losses due to diarrhea or sweating, or are unable to consume adequate fluids because of unavailability, nausea, or coma. DI is exacerbated by glucocorticoid administration or other conditions causing nephrogenic DI.

Patients should be asked if they are deliberately drinking large quantities of fluids for some specific reason (eg, dry mouth due to medications or other conditions). Then an accurate 24-hour urine collection should be performed during ad libitum fluid intake; urine should be measured for total volume, glucose, and creatinine to ensure an accurate collection. Patients must be questioned about and screened for any other cause of polyuria.

1. Conditions implicating central DI–Most conditions with mass lesions of the hypothalamus or pituitary can cause DI; however, pituitary adenomas rarely cause significant DI unless they are quite massive. Many of the conditions without mass lesions cause DI as well as anterior pituitary insufficiency. Head trauma, surgical injury, newborn conditions, infection, vascular insults, and hereditary deficiency of AVP all may cause DI. However, local radiation therapy and hemochromatosis do not themselves cause DI. It is more difficult to document idiopathic DI, since it does not occur in circumstances that implicate the diagnosis.

Neonatal DI may be spontaneous but is usually seen with intracranial defects, such as septo-optical dysplasia (de Morsier's syndrome: nystagmus, hypoplastic optic nerves), holoprosencephalopathy, meningitis, listerial sepsis, trauma, tumors, or brain death.

Central DI that is first noted about the second year of life may be familial and inherited as an autosomal dominant trait. It is caused by postnatal degeneration of neurosecretory neurons. Polyuria frequently remits after age 40. Some family members without DI may have "imitative" polydipsia. Patients often have partial DI and usually do not consider their polyuria a disease. In one kindred, only 3% of affected family members had been treated. In the absence of a family history of DI, however, other destructive lesions of the hypothalamus and pituitary must be considered. Langerhans cell granulomatosis (histiocytosis X) frequently presents with DI. In children and young adults, germinomas and craniopharyngiomas are especially common causes of DI. In older patients, DI is more likely due to metastatic carcinoma, accidental or surgical trauma, autoimmune hypophysitis, meningitis, sarcoidosis or vascular insult, or it may be idiopathic. A variety of different types of hypothalamic brain tumors may also be responsible for DI.

DI is also seen in Wolfram syndrome, an autosomal recessive disorder with *d*iabetes *i*nsipidus, *d*iabetes *m*ellitus, *o*ptic *a*trophy, *d*eafness (DIDMOAD), neurogenic bladder, and cerebellar ataxia.

In addition, certain patients may have combined lesions (eg, patients taking lithium may have both psychogenic polydipsia and nephrogenic DI). Distinguishing these 3 conditions is often difficult.

2. Plasma and urine osmolality testing–Baseline plasma osmolality (pOsm) and urine osmolality (uOsm) during ad libitum fluid intake may help determine the cause of polyuria. Patients with DI frequently have a pOsm > 290 mOsm/kg (serum Na > 143 mEq/L) and a uOsm < 290 mOsm/kg. In such cases, psychogenic polydipsia is unlikely. If the pOsm is > 300 mOsm/kg with a uOsm < 100 mOsm/kg, the diagnosis of central DI is most likely. Central DI can usually be distinguished from nephrogenic DI by considering the clinical setting, patient's sex (hereditary nephrogenic DI is usually X-linked and rare in females), or response to vasopressin or chlorpropamide. A plasma vasopressin measurement may be helpful (see below).

Polyuric patients having a normal pOsm and serum Na may have either compensated DI or psychogenic polydipsia. These conditions are more difficult to distinguish for reasons described below. In addition, some cases of psychogenic polydipsia may actually represent a pathologic decrease in the thirst osmostat with a normal vasopressin osmostat; polyuria in this case may also respond to DDAVP treatment.

3. MRI scan–T1-weighted MRI of the pituitary shows absence of the usual pituitary "bright spot" in patients with central DI owing to diminished neurosecretory granules. MRI is thus useful in the diagnosis of DI and also helps establish the cause.

4. Vasopressin challenge test–The best pragmatic test for suspected central DI therefore appears to be an inpatient test challenge with vasopressin during ad libitum fluid intake under close supervision for several days. Any diuretics, smoking, or other confounding medications should be stopped and the patient's serum electrolytes and volume status normalized. DDAVP, 0.05 mL, is then given intranasally once daily in the evening while urine volumes and serum electrolytes and/or plasma osmolality and body weights are measured daily. The dose of DDAVP may be increased by 0.05 mL daily to a maximum of 0.2 mL twice daily or until (1) urine volumes are reduced to normal while serum electrolytes remain normal (central DI); (2) urine volumes decline but serum sodium and osmolality become subnormal (psychogenic polydipsia or central nervous system natriuresis and occasional patients with true central DI who have become habitual water drinkers); or (3) urine volumes do not decline to normal and serum electrolytes remain normal (nephrogenic DI). Patients with true central DI will usually confirm the diagnosis by their gratitude.

No single testing protocol for DI is completely accurate, so other testing procedures may be utilized when the cause of a polyuric state remains unclear.

5. Water deprivation test–The water deprivation test (Miller-Moses test) has been the standard test used to diagnose DI by distinguishing it from other polyuric states (see Appendix for protocol). Unfortunately, there is a misdiagnosis rate of about 30% when this test is used alone.

Factors that confound the water deprivation test are (1) Individuals with any type of polyuria develop renal medullary washout within days, from which substantial recovery also requires several days. Therefore, during the test, the urine often gradually becomes more concentrated over many hours, prolonging the test to the consternation of the treating physician and patient alike. Patients with moderate to severe DI may become seriously dehydrated prior to substantial recovery from medullary washout. (2) Most patients with central DI actually have a reset osmostat for release of vasopressin. They release enough vasopressin to concentrate their urine reasonably well but only at higher than normal levels of osmolality, at which time thirst has already been stimulated. When they are water-deprived, however, their urine often becomes concentrated to as high as 800 mOsm/kg and does not respond dramatically to exogenous vasopressin even though their polyuric state is corrected by vasopressin treatment. (3) Patients with nephrogenic DI may have a small further increase in urine concentration after vasopressin administration, especially in high doses. Variations such as laboratory accuracy and normal small fluctuations of urine osmolality during fluid deprivation may make the urine appear to become more concentrated in the hour after vasopressin administration. (4) Patients with psychogenic polydipsia may go to great lengths to drink water surreptitiously, making their test results uninterpretable.

The water-deprivation test is therefore reserved for patients with polyuria in whom the diagnosis is not clear. In infants and children, an overnight water-deprivation test is usually not done because of the danger of serious dehydration. Instead, a modified water-deprivation test may be employed during the daytime under close observation for periods of 3 hours (Richman test) or 7 hours (Frasier test).

Polyuric patients having a high pOsm or serum sodium in the baseline or water-deprived state are considered dehydrated. A plasma vasopressin level less than 4 pg/mL at such times is additional but not definitive evidence for central DI.

6. Chlorpropamide test—Central DI may be distinguished from nephrogenic DI by administration of chlorpropamide, 250 mg daily for 2 weeks. Patients with central DI, even of severe degree, may concentrate and decrease urine volume in response to chlorpropamide, whereas patients with nephrogenic DI or psychogenic polydipsia will not. However, a lack of response to chlorpropamide does not exclude the diagnosis of central DI.

B. Diagnosis of Central DI in Patients Taking Nothing by Mouth: Polyuria may first present while a patient is unconscious or unable to take fluids by mouth. Patients who are obtunded or who lack normal thirst or access to fluids develop dehydration and hypernatremia despite usual intravenous fluids. Additional intravenous fluids, given to correct the volume depletion of hypernatremia, produce polyuria. It is critical to make a quick and accurate diagnosis in such patients to avoid serious dehydration. The setting may be one in which central DI is expected, such as following head trauma or cardiopulmonary resuscitation. Such patients with central DI have a serum sodium greater than 150 mEq/L and plasma osmolality greater than 290 mOsm/kg at the time of diagnosis; hypovolemia and hypotension may be present. At the time of discovery of hypernatremia, or during the attempt to correct it with intravenous 5% dextrose or 0.45 N saline, an inappropriately high urine excretion rate will be noted, as will an inappropriately low urine sodium or osmolality (ie, < 285 mOsm/kg) unless hypernatremia has reached the threshold that has finally triggered adequate AVP secretion.

In such a situation, other causes of polyuria (Table 1–3) must be considered and excluded. An empiric trial of parenteral DDAVP or aqueous vasopressin may then be given.

C. Treatment of Central DI: For a patient with DI who is hypernatremic and not drinking, treatment consists of the administration of sufficient and appropriate intravenous fluids, usually consisting of 0.45 N NaCl. To calculate the approximate water deficit in a hypernatremic adult:

$$\text{Water deficit (L)} = [\text{wt (kg)} \times 0.6] - [\text{wt (kg)} \times 83/\text{serum Na}]$$

Fluid should be replaced quickly to reverse shock and then more gradually to reverse persistent hypernatremia. Never infuse 5% dextrose intravenously at more than 150 mL/h, since higher rates may produce hyperglycemia and a solute diuresis. Follow serum electrolytes, blood pressure, and body weights carefully. Parenteral DDAVP (4 μg/mL), 1–2 μg, may be given as an empiric trial intravenously or intramuscularly every 8–24 hours. Alternatively, vasopressin is given as aqueous vasopressin (Pitressin, 10–20 U/ampule), 5–10 U subcutaneously every 4–8 hours. The criterion for administration of

DDAVP for DI initially is hypernatremia itself; once under treatment, the criteria are hypernatremia or a urine volume greater than 200 mL/h (adults) or 100 mL (children) without glycosuria. Once antidiuresis is established, the intravenous rate may be reduced when the serum sodium becomes normal. The above regimen is adjusted according to individual response.

Chronically, all patients with DI should be offered treatment, even those who appear to be coping well with their degree of polyuria and polydipsia. Some patients with mild or even moderate DI will elect to treat themselves only periodically. For patients with impaired thirst as well as DI, rigid adherence to the established regimen must be stressed to prevent serious dehydration and hypernatremia. Serum electrolytes should be measured in any patient with DI who feels ill and periodically even in patients who appear to have their DI well-controlled.

Hyponatremia may occur during treatment of DI. Although cumulative overdosage with DDAVP is the usual cause, other causes must be considered (Table 1–10) and treated.

The following treatments are available:

1. DDAVP–DDAVP (1-desamino-8-D-arginine vasopressin; desmopressin). The elimination of the NH_2 group from the 1–amino acid prolongs this compound's duration of action to 12–24 hours. Substitution of the D-isomer for the natural L-isomer of arginine at the eighth amino acid eliminates vasopressor activity and produces a synthetic hormone with almost entirely antidiuretic activity. DDAVP may be administered either intranasally or parenterally. It is the treatment of choice for central DI. It is also used for DI during pregnancy (where the DI appears to be due to high vasopressinase activity, which destroys native vasopressin but not DDAVP). Intractable enuresis may also respnd to DDAVP at bedtime. Because of its expense and occasional adverse reactions, other forms of treatment are also discussed below.

(a) Nasal DDAVP–DDAVP for nasal insufflation comes in a 2.5-mL vial containing 100 µg DDAVP/mL. The vials have a malleable plastic teat from which the preparation is carefully squeezed into an accompanying small plastic curved tube called a rhinyle. The calibrated rhinyle is filled to the desired dose. The calibrated end is then inserted 3 cm into the nose and the patient blows on the other end, delivering the DDAVP onto the mucous membrane. DDAVP is also available as a unit dose nasal spray delivering 0.1 mL per spray. The starting dose is usually 0.05 mL every evening, although infants may require less; in that case, an insulin or tuberculin syringe may be used to get a more exact dosage into the rhinyle.

The dosage may be adjusted according to the clinical response. Up to 0.2 mL may be required for adequate antidiuresis. About 25% of patients require only an evening dose, but the rest require a dose twice daily. The dosage should be the minimum required to produce an adequate effect; in that way overdosage with hyponatremia is avoided, since patients usually remain mildly polyuric. A few patients may become episodically hyponatremic on a twice daily DDAVP regimen; such patients may be protected against this event by reducing the DDAVP dose and omitting a daytime dose about once weekly in order to allow diuresis and thirst to occur.

(b) Parenteral DDAVP–This product is distributed as 1-mL and 10-mL vials containing 4 μg/mL. The 1-mL vials are used for DI, and the required dosage varies from 1 to 4 μg every 12–24 hours. The duration of action is about the same as that of the nasal preparation. The preparation may be safely given by direct intravenous bolus or subcutaneously. Nephrogenic DI may be treated with DDAVP, 8–16 μg parenterally, but such large doses are expensive and frequently cause gastrointestinal side effects. DDAVP, 6 μg parenterally, is synergistic with indomethacin, 50 mg orally twice daily, for treatment of lithium-induced nephrogenic DI.

2. Lysine vasopressin–Substitution of lysine for arginine at the 8-position of human arginine vasopressin produces lysine vasopressin. This form of vasopressin is naturally produced in pigs. It is marketed as Diapid, which comes as a liquid nasal spray. The dosage must be individualized and varies from 1 to 4 sprays in each nostril. The duration of action is only 6–8 hours, even when administered at maximum dosage. Some patients with mild DI may do well with Diapid alone and find the preparation more convenient to administer than DDAVP if they only administer it before bedtime, trips, or social events. However, for constant antidiuresis it must be taken about 4 times daily. Its potency is much less than DDAVP, and it is expensive. Some patients take both DDAVP and Diapid, using the shorter-acting Diapid on occasion when DDAVP's effect wanes prematurely. Most patients can be managed on DDAVP alone, and the use of Diapid has decreased since DDAVP's release.

3. Aqueous vasopressin–This preparation of AVP is generally available as Pitressin. It comes in 10-U and 20-U ampules, It is so short-acting (4–8 hours) that it is used only in acute situations to help establish the diagnosis or after pituitary surgery when the duration of the DI is uncertain. Aqueous Pitressin has been largely supplanted by parenteral DDAVP. Starting dose is 0.05–0.1 U/kg administered subcutaneously. Higher doses should be administered cautiously, since it does have vasoconstricting action and may rarely cause angina in predisposed patients.

4. Chlorpropamide–This medication is generally available as Diabinese and comes as 100-mg and 250-mg scored tablets. Its overwhelming use has been for diabetes mellitus. Its effectiveness in central DI appears due to direct renal action, since it is often effective even in patients with severe central DI having no detectable plasma levels of AVP.

The starting dose in adults is 250 mg orally once daily. It may require several days for full effectiveness. The dose should be kept to the minimum effective dose. The main advantage is its low cost and once daily administration. Many patients with central DI will not have an adequate response to chlorpropamide, but the only way to determine if it will work is to try it. *The main disadvantage is its hypoglycemic effect.* Patients taking chlorpropamide must be repeatedly reminded of the drug's hypoglycemic effect. A serum glucose should be obtained at each ofice visit to screen for early, unperceived hypoglycemia. Patients should wear a medical identification tag listing any other endocrine deficiencies or major medical problems along with "Takes chlorpropamide; may become hypoglycemic; administer sugar."

Some patients taking chlorpropamide may have systemic allergies, gastrointestinal intolerance, or a disulfiram like reaction when they drink alcoholic beverages.

Side effects make chlorpropamide a less desirable treatment than DDAVP. However, it is the drug of choice for patients with central DI who also have an impaired thirst center as part of a destructive hypothalamic process. Such patients develop recurrent hypernatremia despite free access to water. Chlorpropamide often restores appropriate thirst perception in such individuals.

Chlorpropamide is not effective for nephrogenic DI, and a definite response to it effectively rules out that condition. Some patients with hypothalamic obesity may develop diabetes mellitus in addition to DI; chlorpropamide is especially useful for such patients.

5. Diuretics–By causing a mild sodium deficiency and decreased intravascular volume, diuretics produce decreased free water clearance. After the initial diuresis, diuretics lead to an improvement in polyuria in patients with either central or nephrogenic DI. The improvement may be as much as 50% reduction in baseline urine excretion. In some patients with mild DI, this effect may be all that is required to make their condition tolerable. Most patients with moderate to severe DI still have excessive polyuria and need other treatment. Nevertheless, some patients may want to combine a diuretic with chlorpropamide to produce an additive, more satisfactory effect or more commonly to add a diuretic to vasopressin therapy to reduce the dose of the more costly drugs.

The choice of diuretics to promote improvement in DI has traditionally been of the thiazide type, usually hydrochlorothiazide, although others may be effective. The starting dose is 50 mg of hydrochlorothiazide once daily, but this may be reduced or increased as indicated by the clinical response after about 1 week. The patient must restrict dietary sodium to about 2 g/d for antidiuresis to occur. Thiazides promote renal potassium loss, and the resultant hypokalemia may interfere with renal concentrating capacity, an undesirable effect. Therefore, when thiazides are given for DI, a potassium supplement is ordinarily given prophylactically from the start unless contraindicated.

Oxytocin Deficiency

Oxytocin deficiency is rarely diagnosed. It may present as inadequate milk ejection during breast feeding. In such cases, empiric treatment may be given with oxytocin nasal spray (Syntocinon, 40 μ/mL), 1 spray 2–3 minutes before nursing.

DISORDERS CAUSING HYPOPITUITARISM

Hypopituitarism can be caused by many conditions. The causes differ especially according to the age at which the deficiency presents. The major causes are listed in Table 1–4.

PITUITARY LESIONS

Pituitary tumors may be classified both according to the amount of sellar destruction (grade) and extrasellar extension (stage) according to modified Hardy criteria (Table 1–5).

Pituitary Adenomas

These lesions are the most common cause of pituitary insufficiency and pituitary masses in adults. They account for about 12% of intracranial tumors presenting clinically and are usually histologically benign. They produce anterior pituitary deficiencies but rarely cause diabetes insipidus.

A. Histologic Types: The most common pituitary adenoma in adults is the prolactin cell adenoma (29%), followed by the nonsecreting (null cell or oncocytic) adenoma (25%), growth hormone cell adenoma (16%), ACTH cell adenoma (14%), plurihormonal adenoma (12%), gonadotrope cell adenoma (3%), and thyrotrope cell adenoma (1%). Of the plurihormonal adenomas, most secrete PRL and GH, but other rare combinations include GH and TSH; PRL and TSH; PRL and ACTH; and PRL, ACTH, and TSH. Of the nonsecreting adenomas, a few actually secrete an inactive α-subunit. No pituitary tumors secrete AVP or OT.

Table 1–4. Causes of hypopituitarism.

Conditions with mass lesions

Pituitary adenomas*
  Secretory (prolactinoma, acromegaly, Cushing's disease; rarely TSH, LH, FSH)
  Nonsecretory

Brain tumors

Craniopharyngioma* (common)	Hamartoma	Angioma
Hemangioma (especially < 2 yrs)	Medulloblastoma	Lipoma
Glioma (especially optic < 12 yrs)	Ganglioneuroma	Sarcoma
Infundibuloma (especially < 12 yrs)	Pinealoma	Neuroblastoma
Ependymoma (especially < 12 yrs)	Meningioma	Glioblastoma
Germinoma* (especially < 25 yrs)	Colloid cyst	Cholesteatoma
Dermoid (especially < 25 yrs)	Lymphoma	Chordoma
Rathke's pouch cyst (especially < 25 yrs)	Plasma cytoma	

Metastatic carcinoma
  Leukemia (especially < 12 yrs)
  Gastrointestinal tract, breast, lung, other
Abscess (bacterial or fungal)
Parasitic (eg, cysticercosis)
Sarcoidosis and idiopathic granuloma
Wegener's granulomatosis
Tuberculoma
Autoimmune hypophysitis (especially peripartum women), polyglandular failure
Sheehan's syndrome (postpartum pituitary necrosis)
Pituitary apoplexy (hemorrhagic infarction)
Aneurysm or arteriovenous malformation
Multifocal Langerhans' cell (eosinophilic) granulomatosis (previously called histiocytosis X): deficiencies other than diabetes insipidus are uncommon. Triad of skull lesion, diabetes insipidus (42%), and exophthalmos in some cases (Hand-Schüller-Christian syndrome). Lesions often not visible.

Conditions without mass lesions

Trauma to head
Surgical or radiation injury to pituitary/hypothalamus*
Physiologic inhibition:
  Glucocorticoids suppress ACTH, GH, and LH
  Thyroxine suppresses TSH
  Estrogen and testosterone suppress LH
  Stress (chronic illness, weight loss, etc) may suppress FSH and LH
  Severe illness may suppress TSH, FSH, and LH
  GnRH analogue suppresses LH and FSH
  Aging often results in GH deficiency

(continued)

Table 1–4. (*Continued*)

Conditions in newborns:
  Intraventricular hemorrhage
  Kernicterus
  Hydrocephalus
  Basal encephalocele
  Midline defects: cleft lip; single central incisor
Septo-optic dysplasia with variable anterior (especially GH) and posterior
  pituitary deficiency (de Morsier's syndrome)
Meningitis/encephalitis
Hemochromatosis—primary or secondary (eg, thalassemia)
Vascular
  Subarachnoid hemorrhage
  Stroke (thrombotic, embolic, or anoxic)
Selective congenital deficiencies (may be familial)
  GH—hypoglycemia, slow growth, micropenis in boys
  TSH—hypothyroidism
  FSH, LH—hypogonadism
  AVP—diabetes insipidus after age 2
  Wolfram syndrome (diabetes insipidus, diabetes mellitus, optic atrophy,
    deafness, neurogenic bladder, ataxia)
Familial syndromes with pituitary deficiency:
  FSH, LH (hypogonadotropic hypogonadism)
    Kallman's (anosmia)
    Noonan's (short stature, ptosis, webbed neck, pulmonary stenosis)
    Prader-Willi (obesity, mental retardation, hypotonia)
    Laurence-Moon-Bardet-Biedl (obesity, mental retardation, polydactyly,
      renal anomalies, retinitis pigmentosa)
    Biemond's (obesity, diabetes mellitus, polydactyly, iritis colobomata)
  Panhypopituitarism (variable degrees)
    Myotonic dystrophy (muscular dystrophy, mental retardation, premature
      balding, diabetes mellitus). Men usually have primary testicular
      failure.
    Fanconi's syndrome (short stature, radius malformations, bone marrow
      hypoplasia, skin pigmentation, diabetes mellitus)
Idiopathic (sometimes associated with empty sella)

*See text.

B. Endocrine Manifestations: The tumors secreting active hormones may present with a purely hormonal excess syndrome or a combined excess/deficiency syndrome. Hypopituitarism is most commonly caused by nonsecreting tumors and prolactinomas (in men), since they remain endocrinologically silent until they produce symptoms due to local destruction. Women with prolactinomas who are postmenopausal may have no endocrine symptoms unless estrogen replacement therapy is given, at which time they may develop galactorrhea; men may have only decreased libido or impotence. Secreting adenomas can produce hypopituitarism owing to destruction or excess

Table 1–5. Grading and staging of pituitary tumors.

Degree of sella destruction (grade)

Grade I: Tumor < 10 mm. The sella may be normal or focally expanded.

Grade II: Tumor ≥ 10 mm. The sella is enlarged.

Grade III: Tumor has focally perforated the dura and bone of the sella's anterior wall or floor, and there is limited extension into the sphenoid sinus.

Grade IV: Tumor has diffusely destroyed the sella and extended into the sphenoid sinus.

Grade V: Tumor has distant metastases via the blood or cerebrospinal fluid.

Degree of extrasellar extension (stage)

Stage 0: Tumor is confined within the sella.

Stage A: Tumor extends into the suprasellar cistern but has not deformed the third ventricle.

Stage B: Tumor has obliterated the anterior recesses of the third ventricle.

Stage C: Tumor has elevated the floor of the third ventricle.

Stage D: Tumor has intracranial extension.

D_1—anterior fossa.

D_2—middle fossa.

D_3—posterior fossa.

Stage E: Tumor has perforated the lateral dural envelope of the sella and extends into one or both cavernous sinuses.

hormone secretion; eg, Cushing's disease and prolactinomas may cause hypogonadism. Any patient presenting with a pituitary mass must be screened endocrinologically (Table 1–6) even though a hormone excess or deficiency syndrome may not yet be clinically apparent.

C. Nonendocrine Manifestations: Of patients with clinically significant pituitary adenomas, about 9% have visual field defects and 1% ocular motility problems. Pituitary tumors that are large and invasive enough to destroy the normal pituitary often have suprasellar extension and may compress the optic chiasm; a small number (5%) invade laterally into the cavernous sinus and may cause other cranial nerve palsies (especially III). They may even grow into the sphenoid and maxillary sinuses and rarely can present with nasal airway obstruction.

Endocrine changes may be overlooked and the presenting complaint may be one of impaired vision or of headaches. Of patients with significant **visual field defects**, about 30% are unaware of the defect. Only 30% of patients with visual field defects complain of headaches. Of patients with nonsecreting tumors, about 60% have visual field

Table 1–6. Screening tests for patients with
pituitary/hypothalamic/pineal lesions.

General tests
   24-hour urine for volume and creatinine. Serum sodium, blood urea
      nitrogen, calcium, glucose, liver enzymes, complete blood count
   T_4, T_3RU
   Cosyntropin stimulation test
   Testosterone (men)
   Estradiol (nonmenstruating women aged 14–50)
   Growth curve (children and adolescents)
   Visual fields

Lesions involving pituitary—additional tests
   TSH, PRL, LH, FSH, ACTH (α-subunit if available)
   hCG (women)
   Growth hormone suppression test
   Dexamethasone suppression test (1 mg overnight)

Lesions involving hypothalamus/pineal—additional tests
   hCG
   Alpha-fetoprotein

defects, whereas about 7% of patients with prolactinomas or acromegaly have such defects; visual field defects are uncommon in patients with Cushing's disease.

Any mass lesion may cause a visual field defect. Growth of a mass lesion must be distinguished from optic nerve necrosis due to radiation therapy, which also may produce visual field defects. This can occur acutely even up to 6 years following irradiation.

D. Asymptomatic Adenomas: Pituitary mass lesions may be discovered accidentally during a diagnostic x-ray performed for a different reason. All such patients need thorough endocrinologic evaluation, follow-up, and treatment, if indicated. A patient with a truly incidental asymptomatic pituitary microadenoma should ordinarily receive a full workup, careful follow-up, and a scan in 4–6 months. No immediate treatment is mandated, since such small lesions are common, with an incidence of 8–27% in different unselected autopsy series. Pituitary macroadenomas (>10 mm) are more likey to grow and should be treated and followed carefully.

E. Pituitary Apoplexy: Most pituitary adenomas are rather slow growing. Spontaneous necrosis is common in larger adenomas and causes areas of liquefaction and cysts. Clinical manifestations may thus fluctuate in some patients. Spontaneous hemorrhage within an adenoma is also common and often subclinical. A major hemorrhage (apoplexy), however, can cause abrupt onset of headache or visual field defects as well as hypopituitarism. The treatment of a major pituitary apoplectic event usually entails glucocorticoid administration and prompt transsphenoidal surgical decompression. Pituitary function improves in most patients after decompression.

Craniopharyngiomas

Craniopharyngiomas are found in the pituitary (5%), hypothalamus (25%), or both areas (70%). They are the most common mass causing hypopituitarism between the ages of 2 and 25 and account for 4% of all intracranial neoplasms. They tend to have different presenting symptoms in different age groups.

A. Clinical Features:

1. Infants–Infants with craniopharyngioma usually present with altered behavior owing to hydrocephalus and/or blindness due to chiasmal compression. Young patients with craniopharyngioma may present with symptoms of hydrocephalus owing to obstruction of the foramen of Monro or third ventricle: patients may present with vomiting and lethargy (42%) or with symptoms caused by optic nerve compression such as blurred vision and visual field defects (35%).

2. Children and adolescents–Approximately 20% present with complaints attributable to hormonal deficiency, although in retrospect at the time of diagnosis over 80% of these children and adolescents are found to have some pituitary hormone deficiency. More than 50% of the younger children prior to expected adolescence are found to have slowed growth usually attributable to GH and/or thyroid hormone deficiency. About 50% of young patients are found to have delayed (ie, boys over age 14, girls over age 13), slowed, or arrested sexual maturation. Occasionally children may have precocious puberty. About 15% of patients have diabetes insipidus at the time of diagnosis although DI is more likely to be a presenting complaint. Fewer than 10% of patients are hypothyroid or hypoadrenal at the time of diagnosis.

3. Adults–In adults, craniopharyngiomas may present at any age, and patients usually have visual field complaints, headache, symptoms of hypogonadism and/or diabetes insipidus, sometimes accompanied by thirst impairment and consequent hypernatremia.

About 3% of relatively asymptomatic craniopharyngiomas are discovered incidentally when routine skull films are obtained for other reasons. Craniopharyngiomas have calcified elements in about 66% of patients ≤ 20 yrs and in about 33% of adult patients. They can be detected by CT or MRI at the time of presenting symptoms in more than 90% of patients. They may be distinguished from other tumors in the region by their usual appearance as a mass with cystic elements, often with calcifications, invading both the pituitary and hypothalamus. Calcifications are not visible with MRI.

B. Treatment: The diagnosis of craniopharyngioma should be confirmed by surgical biopsy, at which time major cysts can be decompressed. Radical surgery usually is not successful in completely excising craniopharyngiomas and produces significant neurologic deficit. For this reason, a transsphenoidal surgical procedure with biopsy and conservative decompression is usually preferable to craniotomy if the tumor is accessible by the former approach. Adequate decompression will usually cause partial or total improvement in any optic nerve compression, and the improvement in any preoperative visual deficits is usually apparent immediately postoperatively. If the patient has hydrocephalus that is not relieved by conservative decompressive surgery, a ventriculoperitoneal shunt may then be placed. Decompressive surgery does not ordinarily improve any preexisting endocrine deficiencies and might worsen them.

Radiation therapy is given about 4 weeks postoperatively to most patients with a craniopharyngioma except young children, and it prevents recurrence in all but about 20% of patients. Radiation therapy is not benign, so small craniopharyngiomas should be completely resected if possible.

HYPOTHALAMIC LESIONS

Injury to the hypothalamic region of the brain by any of the factors listed in Table 1–4 can cause endocrine deficiencies from destruction of the nuclei secreting releasing factors (GnRH, TRH, CRH, GHRH) for the anterior pituitary as well as the nuclei producing AVP and OT, which are transported to the posterior pituitary for release. Hypothalamic lesions may also cause hormone excess syndromes: pseudoprecocious puberty can be produced in male children by hCG-secreting germinomas, and hyperprolactinemia can be produced by diminished hypothalamic dopamine secretion. Extension of the disease process into the pituitary itself also causes direct destruction. Craniopharyngiomas typically have both pituitary and hypothalamic components. Distinguishing pituitary functional impairments from actual destruction is not currently of clinical importance. Hypothalamic injury produces a combination of endocrine deficiencies and other neurologic manifestations that together constitute a hypothalamic syndrome. Nonendocrine neurologic disorders are listed in Table 1–2. The exact combination of manifestations differs in each individual depending on the areas of the hypothalamus most severely affected.

PINEAL AREA TUMORS

The pineal gland is a small gland averaging about 140 mg found above the midbrain at its junction with the aqueduct of Silvius; its name is derived from its shape, which is like that of a pine cone. It has no known functional significance in humans although it secretes many different substances. Tumors in this region are uncommon, representing only about 0.5% of all brain tumors in the USA and about 4% in Japan. The pineal gland is of endocrinologic interest because germinal tumors are common in this region and may secrete hCG, which stimulates pseudoprecocious puberty in male children and serves as a tumor marker. Other types of tumors include pineal parenchymal tumors such as pinealoma, 19% (pinealoblastoma, chemodectoma, ganglioglioma, or mixed); or glial tumors, 27% (astrocytoma, ependymoma, mixed, etc). Other neoplasms of this region include meningiomas, hemangiopericytomas, cysts, and cavernous hemangiomas.

Pineal tumors ordinarily do not present with endocrine symptoms unless they invade the hypothalamus or are hCG-secreting germinomas. Instead, they usually cause hydrocephalus owing to blockage of the aqueduct of Sylvius. Patients may have a variety of central nervous system and visual disturbances. About 50% of patients with pineal tumors have Parinaud's syndrome (paralysis of upward gaze, lack of ocular convergence, and absent pupillary light reflex.)

Germ Cell Tumors

Germ cell tumors ordinarily present in childhood or adolescence. Central nervous system tumors are histologically identical with those that arise in the testis or mediastinum. They may be histologically classified as germinomas or teratomas. Many secrete hCG, whose LH-like activity stimulates testicular testosterone production in boys (FSH is required for ovarian estradiol production). The majority of these tumors arise in the pineal area. Germinomas are found so commonly in the pineal area that those located in the hypothalamus or pituitary are sometimes referred to confusingly as ectopic pinealomas. They are locally invasive, especially in the hypothalamic area, but may also spread to other areas of the brain and spinal cord. Extracranial metastasis to liver and skin has been reported as well as metastasis to the peritoneum through ventriculoperitoneal shunts placed for the treatment of hydrocephalus.

Germinomas are sensitive to radiation therapy. The diagnosis is usually confirmed by biopsy; however, germinomas are so common in the pineal region (especially in Japan) that pineal tumors of childhood and adolescence are often radiated without histologic diagnosis. Tumor shrinkage can be observed after as little as 2000 rads and generally confirms the diagnosis in the absence of hCG or alpha-fetoprotein, which would suggest the presence of a trophoblastic tumor. Alternatively, some neurosurgeons recommend a microsurgical exploration for pineal tumors using a supracerebellar, infratentorial approach. Tumors that appear to be germinomas on histologic evaluation are treated with biopsy or subtotal removal and subsequent radiation therapy, whereas radiation-resistant pineal tumors are totally resected if possible.

HYPERPROLACTINEMIA

CLINICAL FEATURES

Prolactin-secreting pituitary adenomas are the most common type of pituitary tumors and are found eight times more frequently in women than in men. Although they may occur at any age, they are commonly detected between the ages of 20 and 40.

As with any pituitary tumor, prolactin-secreting pituitary adenomas may present with headaches or neurologic deficits, especially visual field abnormalities or third cranial nerve palsies. Grade IV tumors may produce nasal airway obstruction.

Women

In women, the presenting symptoms are most often irregular menses or amenorrhea and/or galactorrhea, and many experience emotional lability or weight gain. Women with amenorrhea and hypoestrogenism also have bone demineralization. Of women with nongestational secondary amenorrhea, about 30% have hyperprolactinemia, while of women with nonpuerperal secondary amenorrhea plus galactorrhea, about 70% have hyperprolactinemia. These symptoms of amenorrhea and galactorrhea used to be known as the Chiari-Frommel syndrome if they persisted post partum, or the Forbes-Albright syndrome if they were unrelated to pregnancy. Not infrequently, these symptoms of prolactin excess occur after discontinuation of estrogen-containing oral contraceptives, in which case, the estrogen is thought to have stimulated the growth of a prolactinoma while inhibiting galactorrhea, as in pregnancy.

Men

In men, prolactinomas generally present with features of local invasion although patients usually also have some degree of decreased libido, hypogonadism, gynecomastia, or erectile dysfunction. Of men presenting with erectile dysfunction, fewer than 5% have hyperprolactinemia, but they often have other physical causative factors.

DIAGNOSIS

A serum PRL level is determined in women between ages 15 and 40 with infrequent menses or amenorrhea, in all nulliparous women with galactorrhea, and in multiparous women in whom significant lactation persists for more than 6 months following cessation of breast feeding.

If a patient has symptoms only of prolactin excess but no local neurologic symptoms (such as headache or visual field impairment), any drugs known to cause hyperprolactinemia should be discontinued if possible prior to the PRL determination, to be sure that any detected hyperprolactinemia is not drug-induced.

Many nontumorous conditions and drugs cause hyperprolactinemia (Table 1–7). However, if the serum PRL level is higher than 200 ng/mL, the diagnosis of a prolactin-secreting tumor is most likely.

Table 1–7. Causes of hyperprolactinemia.

Physiologic
  Pregnancy
  Suckling
  Nipple stimulation
  Sexual intercourse (women)
  Neonatal
  Exercise (acute)
  Sleep

Physical stress
  Surgery
  Myocardial infarction
  Hypoglycemia
  Seizures

Thoracic and pleural lesions
  Thoracotomy
  Mastectomy
  Burns
  Herpes zoster
  Mesothelioma

Spinal cord lesions

Hypothyroidism

Renal failure

Pituitary adenoma
  Prolactinoma
  Acromegaly
  Cushing's disease

Drug-induced
  Estrogens
  Progestins
  Phenothiazines
  Butyrophenones
  Metoclopramide
  Reserpine
  Methyldopa
  Opiates
  Methadone
  Cimetidine
  Beer
  Hydroxyzine
  Amphetamines
  Verapamil
  Sulpiride
  Domperidone
  Tricyclic antidepressants
  Nicotine

Hypothalamic damage
  Tumor, sarcoid, tuberculosis
  Radiation
  Infarction
  Surgery
  Pituitary stalk section

Cirrhosis
  Idiopathic

In any event, *all patients with hyperprolactinemia must have screening tests for hypothyroidism and all women should have a screening test for pregnancy before any neuroradiologic examinations or treatments are performed.* The thyroid function tests should include a TSH assay as a sensitive screening test for primary hypothyroidism and as a safeguard against mistaken interpretation of low serum thyroxine levels as hypopituitarism in cases of primary hypothyroidism with pituitary enlargement due to TSH-cell hyperplasia.

A CT scan or MRI of the pituitary is performed in all patients with possible local neurologic symtoms, with PRL $\geq$ 200 ng/mL, and with lower elevations in PRL after exclusion of other causes of hyperprolactinemia. Patients taking phenothiazines or butyrophenones so often develop symptoms of hyperprolactinemia that, unless neurologic signs are present, no serum PRL or scan is indicated. Treatment of galactorrhea in these patients may begin directly with bromocriptine.

TREATMENT

Prolactin-secreting pituitary tumors may be treated effectively with bromocriptine or transsphenoidal pituitary surgery, or both. Bromocriptine has the advantage of negligible serious morbidity but the disadvantages of side effects, expense, and chronic treatment. Surgery has the advantage of offering a drug-free remission but the disadvantages of expense and surgical morbidity.

PRL-Cell Hyperplasia

If hyperprolactinemia is obviously caused by pituitary-cell hyperplasia (eg, postpartum or drug-induced hyperprolactinemia), treatment with bromocriptine is indicated at a dose sufficient to alleviate clinical symptoms (eg, in women for relief of mastalgia, amenorrhea, or infertility; in men for relief of gynecomastia, hypogonadism, or impotence). CT or MRI is not indicated unless the patient has local symptoms.

Idiopathic Hyperprolactinemia

Patients with symptomatic spontaneous hyperprolactinemia frequently (about 20%) do not have a discrete prolactinoma visible on CT scan or MRI and are classified as *idiopathic* cases. Most such patients have a small microadenoma, but since there is less certainty in distinguishing an adenoma from hyperplasia, such patients are ordinarily just followed or treated with bromocriptine for relief of symptoms or infertility. With no treatment, most patients remain stable or even improve; PRL levels normalize in about 20% of women. Patients may also be treated with ergoloid mesylates (Hydergine; 1-mg tablets), 2 mg three times a day, if PRL is < 100 ng/mL. Occasional mild nausea or hypotension occurs, but the drug may be better tolerated than bromocriptine. Progression of an unseen microadenoma is unusual (less than 5%) and does not occur without concomitant rising PRL levels. Transsphenoidal exploration is reserved strictly for patients with unremitting symptoms who cannot tolerate medical treatment.

Visible Prolactin-Secreting Microadenomas

Patients with definite microadenomas are given an informed choice of initial treatments:

A. Medical Treatment: Many patients choose to have a trial of bromocriptine or congeners, which is continued if well tolerated (see p 60). Bromocriptine may safely be given to induce fertility in such women. It is discontinued once conception occurs. Significant adenoma growth occurs in less than 5%. Most patients may also safely breast-feed. Patients should be followed carefully. Ergoloid mesylates may be tried for patients who are intolerant to bromocriptine.

B. Surgery: Some of these patients find that their symptoms have improved but cannot tolerate the drug; bromocriptine is then discontinued and a repeat PRL is obtained about 2 months later. If symptoms and hyperprolactinemia recur, a repeat CT scan is obtained followed by transsphenoidal surgery (see p 61). Most of these patients experience a long-term remission, especially if their postoperative PRL level is below 10 ng/mL. These patients also require long-term observation; if symptoms and hyperprolactinemia recur, bromocriptine therapy is given.

Prolactin-Secreting Macroadenomas

Patients with PRL-secreting macroadenomas (> 1 cm in diameter) are treated primarily with bromocriptine, surgery, or both. Radiation therapy is used only as adjunctive therapy for patients in whom the primary treatment is inadequate.

A. Medical Treatment: To be a candidate for bromocriptine therapy (see p 60) without surgery, a patient with a macroadenoma should have serum PRL measurements consistently above 150 ng/mL, an important criterion, since some nonsecreting macroadenomas cause milder hyperprolactinemia through stalk or hypothalamic dysfunction. Similarly, other conditions may cause milder hyperprolactinemia (Table 1–7). Pregnant patients can have higher serum PRL levels (see Appendix).

For patients with macroadenomas, bromocriptine treatment is aggressive. The starting dose is 1.25 mg/d, but the dose is increased if tolerated over 10 days to 7.5 mg/d, administered as 2.5 mg, 3 times daily. If the serum PRL level has not returned to normal over the next several weeks, the dose is increased stepwise until either normal PRL levels are achieved, or a maximum bromocriptine dosage of 20 mg/d is reached, or the patient experiences intolerable side effects.

Using bromocriptine alone, normal PRL levels can be achieved in 67% of patients. PRL levels fall to 11% or less of basal values in 85–90%.

A reduction in PRL levels always precedes any tumor shrinkage. A detectable decrease in tumor size occurs within 6 weeks in 70% of patients. In the remaining 30%, shrinkage may not be noted until up to 6 months. The reduction in tumor size can be dramatic: in one series, 46% of tumors shrank more than 50%; 18% of tumors shrank about 50%; 36% shrank 10–25%. Recurrent growth of the tumor usually occurs if bromocriptine is stopped. Therefore, bromocriptine is continued indefinitely, although a carefully supervised trial off the drug may be considered after about 5 years.

Visual field impairments improve in 90% but may not return to normal. Some patients with destruction of the sellar floor develop cerebrospinal fluid rhinorrhea as the tumor shrinks.

Once a good response has been achieved, progression of a prolactinoma occurs in only 2% of patients as long as bromocriptine is continued. Apparent enlargement in such circumstances may represent a second neoplasm. However, testosterone or estrogen therapy may cause growth of prolactinomas whose secretion is incompletely suppressed by bromocriptine.

Patients who cannot tolerate bromocriptine are candidates for surgery and postoperative radiation therapy (see p 61–67) if necessary.

B. Surgery: Patients with severe or rapidly progressive visual field or other neurologic deficits should be treated with urgent transsphenoidal surgery (see p 61–65). Craniotomy is ordinarily not performed, since the transsphenoidal approach offers better and safer decompression. Bromocriptine is used as adjunctive therapy preoperatively. It is continued in patients postoperatively in whom a complete surgical resection is not obtained and when the diagnosis of PRL-secreting tumor has been established by either a preoperative PRL higher than 150 ng/mL or by positive immunoperoxidase staining of the tumor tissue for PRL.

Certain huge PRL-secreting tumors (eg, grade IV, stage C–E) are so invasive at the time of diagnosis that craniotomy or transsphenoidal surgery carries little benefit and incurs a high risk of hemorrhage and other complications owing to the distortion of usual surgical landmarks. Such patients are best treated directly with bromocriptine; decompressive transsphenoidal surgery may be attempted if there is symptomatic progression of the tumor or inadequate neurologic improvement despite bromocriptine.

C. Radiation Therapy: Patients with aggressive prolactinomas may receive conventional radiation therapy (see p 65) if bromocriptine or congeners are ineffective or not tolerated and if surgery is contra-indicated or ineffective.

GIGANTISM & ACROMEGALY

CLINICAL FEATURES

Excessive exposure to growth hormone (GH) produces gigantism in youths prior to epiphyseal fusion and acromegaly in adults. About 99% of cases are caused by a primary pituitary tumor, and only rarely have cases been discovered of ectopic production of GH or growth hormone releasing hormone (GHRH). Excessive exogenous GH administration could also produce the syndrome.

GH-secreting pituitary tumors ordinarily grow slowly. Symptoms of GH excess are listed in Table 1–8; they usually begin in the third or fourth decade and progress insidiously. The mean age at diagnosis is 42 years. Men and women are affected with equal frequency. Many patients consider the coarsening of their facial features to be due to normal aging and may not come to medical attention for many years until growth of the tumor finally produces headache, visual field changes, or hypopituitarism. The disease may be first suspected by a dentist who notes malocclusion due to prognathism and increasing separation of the teeth. Other manifestations may provide the first clue, eg, carpal tunnel syndrome, diabetes mellitus, headache, skin tags (acrochordons), or spinal stenosis.

It is important to treat gigantism or acromegaly early in its course, since bony disfigurement is not reversible and patients have increased morbidity and mortality from cardiovascular disease, especially when diabetes or hypertension is present. Acromegalic patients have increased mortality from respiratory disease and cancer (especially gastrocolic).

DIAGNOSIS

In normal persons, fasting serum GH levels are usually less than 5 ng/mL. GH is more than 10 ng/mL in 90% of patients with acromegaly. However, since GH is secreted episodically in normal individuals, a single elevated serum level is not optimal supporting evidence for gigantism or acromegaly. RIAs for GH done during pregnancy may give falsely elevated results owing to cross-reactivity with human placental lactogen (hPL).

Table 1–8. Manifestations of acromegaly.*

Facial changes
  Coarsening of features
  Prognathism
  Increased spacing between teeth
	Local effects of pituitary tumor
	  Headaches
	  Hypopituitarism
	  Visual field impairment
	  Spinal fluid rhinorrhea

Acral changes
  Increased ring sizes
  Hands are large, soft, doughy, moist
  Increased shoe size (especially width)
  Tufting of distal phalanges on x-ray
  Thick heel pads
	Changes in libido
	  Decreased
	  Increased
	
	Fatigue
	
	Hypertension

Skin changes
  Increased sweating
  Molluscum fibrosum
  Sebaceous cysts
  Hypertrichosis
	Deep gravelly voice
	
	Bone changes
	  Enlarged
	  Osteoporosis due to hypogonadism
	  Polyostotic fibrous dysplasia (if McCune-Albright syndrome)
	  Arthropathy

Visceromegaly
  Goiter
  Cardiomegaly
  Macroorchidism
  Hepatomegaly	

Neuropathies
  Carpal tunnel syndrome
  Peripheral neuropathy
  Spinal cord or nerve root compression from bony overgrowth
	Laboratory
	  Hyperglycemia (diabetes mellitus)
	  Hyperphosphatemia
	
	Concomitant PRL excess
	  Galactorrhea
	  Amenorrhea

*Most patients have only a few of these manifestations.

Glucose Suppression Test

The diagnosis of gigantism or acromegaly is best confirmed by the glucose suppression test: 100 g of glucose syrup is administered orally to a patient after an overnight fast, and a single measurement of serum GH level is obtained 60 minutes later; the diagnosis is confirmed by finding a GH level higher than 2 ng/mL in males or 5 ng/mL in females. In the presence of typical clinical manifestations of acromegaly, an abnormal glucose suppression test is sufficient laboratory evidence of a GH-secreting tumor that a scan of the pituitary should be performed. The CT scan or MRI will document the presence of a pituitary adenoma in more than 90% of patients with acromegaly or gigantism.

In certain patients, the diagnosis of gigantism or acromegaly is less clear. In young patients with apparent gigantism it is especially

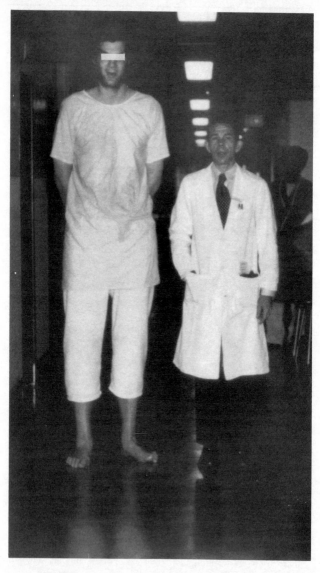

Figure 1–8. Patient with gigantism due to a pituitary adenoma stands next to his neurosurgeon. (Courtesy of C. Wilson, MD.)

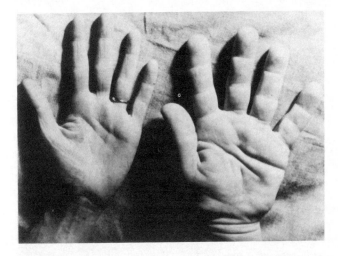

Figure 1–9. Hand of a patient with acromegaly compared with a normal hand. Both bony and soft tissue changes are present. The hand is enlarged, doughy, and diaphoretic. Median nerve compression at the wrist has produced carpal tunnel syndrome and thenar atrophy. Ring size has increased (patient is unable to wear her wedding ring).

important to consider the differential diagnosis and evaluation of tall stature as outlined in Table 3–5. In adults with possible but not florid acromegaly, other causes of elevated GH levels must be considered, eg, chronic renal or hepatic failure, malnourishment, any acute illness, exercise, a protein-rich meal just prior to the test, estrogen or β-blocker treatment, acute agitated states, and diabetes mellitus. Patients with diabetes mellitus frequently have an abnormal glucose suppression test of GH, but seldom have any clinical manifestations suggestive of acromegaly. Some patients have many features of acromegaly but normal GH, somatomedin-C levels and pituitary CT scans, and these patients are considered to have cerebral gigantism and usually require no treatment. Certain very unusual patients with GH-secreting pituitary tumors have normal baseline or glucose-suppressed GH levels.

Serum IGF-I

Serum insulinlike growth factor (IGF-I; somatomedin C) is an indirect measure of GH secretion. Reliable assays are available from

Nichols Institute and Endocrine Science. The blood specimen may be drawn at any time. Most acromegalics have an elevated serum level of IGF-I. Levels of IGF-I are also increased during pregnancy.

TRH & GnRH Tests

After TRH is administered as a 500-μg intravenous bolus, or GnRH as a 100-μg intravenous bolus, GH increases in most patients with acromegaly. However, since TRH causes GH release in 28% of normal individuals also, it is not especially helpful.

Heel Pad Measurement

The heel pad thickness in most acromegalic patients is more than 22 mm and usually exceeds 30 mm. It may be measured with lateral radiographs.

TREATMENT

Transsphenoidal Pituitary Surgery

The preferred treatment for gigantism and acromegaly is the transsphenoidal selective resection of the pituitary tumor by a skilled surgeon who can leave the normal pituitary intact. Perioperatively, these patients are managed like others having pituitary surgery (see p 61). Transsphenoidal surgery is successful in about 90% of patients with adenomas smaller than 2 cm in diameter and GH levels below 50 ng/mL preoperatively. Symptoms of diaphoresis and carpal tunnel syndrome usually remit by the next day. Soft tissue overgrowth regresses quickly, and the regression continues at a slower rate for several months. Glucose intolerance usually improves but may persist in milder form postoperatively. Hypertension, present in about 30%, resolves in only a minority of cases. About 30% of patients gain weight after surgery. Surgical treatment is considered successful if symptoms remit and the baseline or random GH level falls to less than 10 ng/mL. Some patients with good clinical remissions still have an abnormal GH suppression test and still retain paradoxical GH increase after intravenous TRH.

Patients are followed clinically for persistence or recurrence of symptoms. Random GH levels are also checked routinely to detect any rising levels characteristic of a recurring tumor. The patient is assessed clinically and by GH measurement at 2 months, then every 6 months for about 3 years, and yearly thereafter if feeling well otherwise. Repeat visual fields are determined postoperatively and then yearly. Repeat CT scan or MRI is ordinarily performed at about 2 months, 1 year, and 3 years postoperatively and at any time when clinical conditions imply recurrence of the tumor.

Most patients with acromegaly who have surgical resections of large but noninvasive tumors have a good clinical remission and GH less than 10 ng/mL. Postoperative radiation therapy is reserved for patients who do not have clinical remission and have invasive tumors or progressive tumor growth.

Radiation Therapy

Conventional radiation therapy is inferior to selective pituitary surgery as the primary treatment for gigantism and acromegaly. Not only is hypopituitarism often produced, but also radiation therapy takes many months or years for maximum clinical effect. A remission (fasting GH ≤ 10 ng/mL) occurs in 38% of patients after 2 years, 73% after 5 years, and 81% after 10 years, usually at the cost of pituitary hormone deficiencies. Thus, conventional radiation is used only as an adjunct to transsphenoidal surgery that has failed to control the acromegaly. (see p 65)

Heavy particle radiation therapy to the pituitary has been used to treat acromegaly. Remissions occur more quickly than with conventional radiation therapy, but pituitary hormone deficiencies of some degree ultimately occur in about 50% of patients. Complete clinical remission occurs in about 70% after 2 years and 80% after 5 years. This form of treatment is available currently at the MIT-Harvard cyclotron in Boston. It cannot be used for tumors with suprasellar extension owing to the danger of chiasm irradiation.

Medical Treatment

Bromocriptine (see p 60) may be used to treat acromegaly when given in doses of 10-20 mg/d. It requires lifetime treatment and has generally proved inferior to surgery in terms of rate and degree of remission; only about 50% of acromegalic patients have an adequate response to bromocriptine alone. For this reason, it is used as adjunctive therapy. In patients with large adenomas with large suprasellar extension, bromocriptine may be given for 2 months in an effort to shrink the tumors, making them more amenable to complete surgical resection.

Following radiation therapy, bromocriptine is used to treat patients with persistent symptoms, since remission following radiation is uncertain and may require months or years. Patients taking bromocriptine who have had their acromegaly treated with pituitary radiation may have the bromocriptine discontinued about once yearly for 1 month or until symptoms recur, at which time a GH level is determined.

Patients for whom dopamine agonist therapy is contemplated may have an acute test with bromocriptine (2.5 mg) or lisuride (0.3 mg) (not available in the USA) given orally to a fasting patient. Serum GH is measured before and 3, 4, and 5 hours after drug administration. Responders are patients who have a reduction in GH of 50% or more; such patients are much more likely to respond symptomatically to chronic therapy, although only 10% have significant tumor shrinkage.

Somatostatin Analogs

Acromegaly may also be treated with somatostatin analog (octreotide; Sandostatin), from 50 mg twice a day (usual dose) to 250 mg four times a day subcutaneously, which appears to be more frequently effective than bromocriptine; combined use is even more effective. Continuous subcutaneous infusion of somatostatin analog (600 mg/d tapered to 100 mg/d, if possible) appears to be even more effective, and tumor shrinkage has been noted. In one series, 13 of 15 patients responded. It is most effective in patients with serum GH levels below 30 mg/mL. Inconvenience and expense limit use. Side effects include diarrhea, flatulence, and cholelithiasis.

Malignancy Screening

Acromegalic patients require annual physical examination, chest radiography, mammography (females), and at least sigmoidoscopy. Patients at high risk for colon polyps and cancer (over age 50, more than 3 skin tags, disease duration over 10 years, previous polyps) should have a full colonoscopy every 3–5 years.

CUSHING'S DISEASE

Cushing's disease refers to pituitary ACTH secretion causing manifestations of adrenal hypercortisolism and hyperandrogenism. It should be distinguished from the broader term **Cushing's syndrome**, which refers to the manifestations of glucocorticoid excess from any cause.

In adults, spontaneous hypercortisolism may be due to Cushing's disease (68%), ectopic ACTH-producing tumor (15%), adrenal tumor or bilateral macro- or micronodular adrenal hyperplasia with undetectable ACTH (< 1%).

In children, spontaneous hypercortisolism may be due to Cushing's disease (50–70%), ectopic ACTH (2%), adrenal neoplasm (30–50%), or bilateral micronodular hyperplasia without ACTH (1%).

In Cushing's disease, the excessive ACTH is secreted by pituitary adenoma in about 90% of cases and by a hyperplastic pituitary in about 10%. (See pp 249–265 for the evaluation and treatment of hypercortisolism.)

Treatment for Inappropriate Secretion of TSH

A. Neoplastic Inappropriate Secretion of TSH (NIST): Some patients have pituitary tumors that secrete TSH. This frequently produces hyperthyroidism without ocular signs of Graves' disease. Treatment consists of transsphenoidal resection followed by radiation therapy when appropriate. Treatment with bromocriptine or somatostatin analog may be tried. Serum α-subunit levels may be high.

B. Nonneoplastic Inappropriate Secretion of TSH (NNIST): Some patients have an enlarged pituitary owing to hyperplasia of TSH cells despite normal or high serum levels of thyroxine. This condition has variable causes, may be familial, or may be due to prolonged untreated primary hypothyroidism, especially in youth. Goiter may be present. TSH levels may be high or normal (with high T_4). Symptomatic patients are treated with radioactive iodine, antithyroid drugs, or thyroid surgery.

HYPONATREMIA & SIADH

SIADH (syndrome of inappropriate antidiuretic hormone) is manifested by a serum sodium (Na) of less than 136 mEq/L. It is not of clinical significance unless serum Na drops below 130 mEq/L. Symptoms of lethargy and weakness may begin to occur with serum Na concentrations of 120–125 mEq/L. Below a serum Na of 120 mEq/L, there is a danger of seizures and coma due to cerebral edema. Acute hyponatremia is much more dangerous than chronic hyponatremia in which the gradual loss of intracellular KCl by the brain reduces the amount of cellular swelling owing to extracellular hypoosmolality; chronically, serum Na levels as low as 110 mEq/L may be tolerated.

DIAGNOSIS

A serum vasopressin level is not helpful in diagnosing SIADH. In fact, some patients fulfilling the criteria for SIADH have undetectable plasma vasopressin levels.

SIADH is an overdiagnosed condition. It must be distinguished from other causes of hyponatremia (Table 1–9). Hyponatremia must be corrected for hyperglycemia: a given sodium may be corrected for hyperglycemia in a hypovolemic patient by adding 2 mEq/L per 100 mg/dL rise in glucose; in a euvolemic patient, add 1.6 mEq/L per 100 mg/dL rise in glucose; in a hypervolemic patient, add 1.2 mEq/L per 100 mg/dL rise.

Table 1–9. Differential diagnosis of hyponatremia.*

Artifactual: hyperglycemia, hypertriglyceridemia

Syndrome of inappropriate ADH release or action (SIADH)
   Central nervous system lesions; reset osmostat
   Pulmonary lesions
   Other: acute intermittent porphyria, positive pressure breathing
   Ectopic ADH production: especially small-cell carcinoma of the lung
   Drug-induced SIADH (direct renal effect in some)

Chlorpropamide	Vincristine
Amitriptyline	Vinblastine
Clofibrate	Cyclophosphamide
Carbamazepine	Vasopressin
Phenothiazines	Oxytocin
Barbiturates	Melphalan
Morphine	Ifosfamide
Thiothizene	Trimethoprim-sulfamethoxazole (intravenous)

Hyponatremia with hypervolemia
   Decreased water excretion; natriuresis from atriopeptin
      Congestive heart failure
      Cirrhosis
      Renal failure
   Excessive water intake
      Restriction of dietary salt without water restriction
      Compulsive water drinking
      Intravenous water

Hyponatremia due to sodium depletion
   Renal losses
      Diuretics
      Addison's disease; congenital adrenal hyperplasia; selective
         hypoaldosteronism
      Renal diseases: tubulo-interstitial disease, renal tubular acidosis
      Central nervous system–induced natriuresis (associated with central
         nervous system injury, especially subarachnoid hemorrhage and
         also pituitary surgery)
      Nonsteroidal anti-inflammatory agents, ACE inhibitor

Gastrointestinal losses	Third-space losses
Vomiting	Burns
Diarrhea	Pancreatitis
Fistulas	Crush injuries
	Major surgery

Hypothyroidism

Severe illness

*Two or more conditions may coexist.

Hyponatremia with normal serum osmolality may also be caused by elevations of triacylglycerol-containing VLDL or chylomicrons. The serum appears turbid, and the osmolality is normal. Triacylglycerol elevation of 1000 mg/dL spuriously lowers Na slightly.

For the diagnosis of SIADH to be reasonably secure, the following criteria should be considered: (1) serum sodium < 136 mEq/L, (2) normal or increased weight, (3) absence of significant thirst, (4) lack of edema or edema-causing conditions, (5) correct for serum glucose, (6) correct for serum triacylglycerols, (7) lack of elevated blood urea nitrogen or uric acid, (8) euthyroid state, (9) lack of adrenal insufficiency, (10) lack of renal disease, (11) no history of diuretics, angiotensin-converting enzyme (ACE) inhibitors, fluphenazine (Prozac), or nonsteroidal anti-inflammatory (NSAI) agents, (12) no history of excessive water intake, (13) urine Na > 20 mEq/L. Two or more conditions causing hyponatremia may coexist, thus clouding the diagnosis.

TREATMENT OF HYPONATREMIA CAUSED BY SIADH

Fluid Restriction

Restrict fluids to below 800 mL/d or less if severe hyponatremia is present without hypovolemia or thirst. Keep fluid intake to no more than urine output acutely. Chronically, if patient is not eating, restrict fluid to less than the sum of urine output plus insensible fluid losses (400 mL/m^2/24 h).

Intravenous 3% NaCl Plus Furosemide

For symptoms in patients with serum Na below 120 mEq/L, 3% NaCl (513 mEq/L), 100–200 mL, is administered as an intravenous bolus if the patient has no signs of edema or congestive heart failure; furosemide (to 1 mg/kg) is given intravenously, and fluid is restricted. Intravenous 3% saline with KCl is given at about 20–40 mL/h until serum Na = 125 mEq/L. Avoid excessive correction of Na, which may cause central pontine gliosis.

Drug Treatment

Chronic treatment of hyponatremia due to SIADH is best done with fluid restriction alone. The underlying cause must be corrected if possible. Children and some adult patients may be unable to adhere to the fluid restriction. They may be given a trial of furosemide with sodium and potassium supplementation if needed. Patients in whom this form of treatment is inadequate may be given a drug causing nephrogenic diabetes insipidus. Demeclocycline (Declomycin; 300-mg tablets) is the best drug to use and is given in doses of 1–2 g/d orally. The renal concentrating defect is reversible, but the drug is nephrotoxic and the serum blood urea nitrogen and creatinine must be determined frequently. Lithium carbonate has a similar effect but is less commonly used owing to its toxicity at effective doses.

TREATMENT OF HYPONATREMIA DUE TO CENTRAL NERVOUS SYSTEM–INDUCED NATRIURESIS

Patients who become hyponatremic following a brain lesion or pituitary surgery should not be assumed to always have SIADH. If signs of intravascular volume depletion are present (eg, weight loss, increased thirst, orthostatic hypotension) and other factors noted in Table 1–9 are absent, the diagnosis of an ill-defined syndrome known as cerebral salt wasting (central nervous system–induced natriuresis) must be considered. Treatment consists of fluid and salt replacement. This may be done with intravenous 3% or 0.9 N NaCl for serious hyponatremia; alternatively, salt tablets (1 g NaCl/tablet = 17 mEq Na$^+$), 1–2 tablets 4 times daily, may be given along with fluids orally. Diuretics are discontinued. The salt tablets are gradually tapered as serum sodium levels permit. Hyponatremia also responds to fludrocortisone, 0.1–0.4 mg/d.

TREATMENT OF PITUITARY LESIONS

BROMOCRIPTINE THERAPY

Bromocriptine is an ergot derivative with dopamine agonist (prolactin inhibition) action. It is marketed as Parlodel in the USA (2.5-mg scored tablets and 5-mg capsules). It is extremely effective in reducing prolactin levels of any cause and in shrinking most, but not all, prolactin-secreting pituitary adenomas. It is somewhat effective in treating acromegaly.

Side effects occur in about 50% of patients taking bromocriptine. Nausea, vomiting, fatigue, and orthostatic hypotension are most frequently seen. These side effects can be minimized if the medication is begun in small doses and increased to the minimum effective dose. Give half of a 2.5-mg tablet at dinner. Caution the patient to arise very slowly the next morning, since transient nausea and retching are exacerbated by orthostatic hypotension caused by bounding out of bed. Psychiatric side effects including mania, hallucinations, paranoia, delusions, depression, and anxiety are not dose-related and may persist for weeks after discontinuing the drug. Erythromelalgia also occurs rarely. Gastrointestinal side effects have been relieved by intravaginal administration of bromocriptine in a few women.

Once it is clear that the patient tolerates the 1.25-mg dosage of bromocriptine, it is increased to one 2.5-mg tablet at dinner. The dosage should be increased in stepwise fashion. PRL levels generally fall maximally within a week. Tumor shrinkage generally occurs within 1 month but may require as long as 6 months. Suppression may persist for 6 weeks once bromocriptine is stopped. About 20% of patients with prolactin tumors have persistent improvement after long-term treatment (years). For daily dosages greater than 5 mg/d, administration should be divided into twice daily doses (after dinner and breakfast). In patients with physiologic hyperprolactinemia or a micro-adenoma, the end point for dosage is that which alleviates symptoms; the PRL level may still remain somewhat elevated but is usually found to be suppressed below the pretreatment level. For women desiring maximum fertility, the PRL should be suppressed into the low-normal range (ie, less than 10 ng/mL). Ordinarily, doses of between 2.5 and 10 mg of bromocriptine are adequate; most patients require between 5 and 10 mg/d. Women taking bromocriptine for suppression of postpartum lactation should have their blood pressure monitored, since significant hypertension may rarely result.

For patients with PRL macroadenomas, bromocriptine should be increased until PRL levels are suppressed into the low-normal range or the patient has reached the maximum tolerated dose. Transsphenoidal pituitary surgery and/or radiation may be recommended if the tumor is invasive or the patient has an adverse reaction to bromocriptine.

A minority of PRL-secreting tumors are relatively resistant to bromocriptine. Dosage must then be increased with careful attention to PRL levels in order to ascertain whether the increased dosage is effective. Only very rarely are doses of more than 20 mg/d required. Above that dose, side effects such as ergotism and reversible pulmonary infiltrates become more common.

Bromocriptine may also be useful for treating FSH, LH, TSH, or α-subunit–secreting tumors in addition to prolactinomas and acromegaly.

Other dopamine agonists are becoming available that, like bromocriptine, are ergot derivatives. Pergolide, lisuride, and cabergoline (not yet available in the USA) appear to be more potent than bromocriptine on a dosage basis. Cabergoline at doses of 0.3 and 0.6 mg orally twice weekly appears to have fewer side effects in preliminary studies. Ergoloid mesylates are sometimes useful.

TRANSSPHENOIDAL PITUITARY SURGERY

When surgery is indicated for a pituitary tumor, the transsphenoidal approach is the procedure of choice for virtually all these tumors except for the rare patient whose tissue is largely aberrant with eccentric suprasellar extension that requires craniotomy.

Preoperative Evaluation & Management

Some suggested screening tests are presented in Table 1–5. The patient should be screened preoperatively for any hypothyroidism which, if present, should at least partially be corrected. Undetected secondary hypothyroidism is usually relatively mild, with only slightly higher morbidity due to anesthesia. If immediate surgery is indicated, it may be done relatively safely in such patients before euthyroidism is restored by giving smaller doses of anesthetic. Hypothyroidism, if present, must be ensured *not* to be primary (TSH is elevated in primary hypothyroidism), since such stimulus to TSH secretion frequently causes pituitary hyperplasia severe enough to be mistaken for a pituitary tumor.

Preoperative screening for hypocortisolism is unnecessary, since all patients receive perioperative hydrocortisone as well as eventual postoperative cosyntropin stimulation testing. Baseline prolactin and growth hormone levels should be obtained and the patient should receive at least a 1-mg dexamethasone suppression test preoperatively, even if the patient does not appear clinically cushingoid at that time. Patients with prolactin-secreting macroadenomas of 2 cm or more in diameter should be pretreated with bromocriptine, but preoperative treatment of prolactin microadenomas is inadvisable, since dissection planes are made less distinct, making total selective removal more difficult. There is ongoing controversy over the indications for surgical resection of prolactin-secreting microadenomas. Grossly destructive unresectable prolactin-secreting adenomas are best treated with a trial of bromocriptine plus irradiation. Surgery for grossly destructive adenomas is reserved for failure to respond to this regimen, since surgery does not result in cure and has more associated morbidity because surgical anatomy is disturbed, making hemorrhage, cerebrospinal fluid leak, and cranial nerve palsies more common. Patients with apparently unresectable pituitary tumors or visual field defects often require surgery to reduce tumor size and quickly improve symptoms before radiation treatment.

Proper neuroradiology must be obtained to assess the presence of an empty sella or aneurysm as well as the size and location of the tumor and any sphenoid sinus anomalies.

Patients are all pretreated with nose drops consisting of bacitracin, 1000 U/mL (2–3 drops in each nostril 4 times daily), and phenylephrine hydrochloride 0.25% (2 drops in each nostril 4 times daily) for 1–2 days prior to surgery. The patient is given hydrocortisone, 100 mg intramuscularly immediately preoperatively and 50 mg intramuscularly in postanesthesia recovery, with tapered doses thereafter unless stressful complications arise.

Procedure

The procedure itself involves an incision in the superior gingival line and delicate dissection of the mucous membranes away from the anterior cartilaginous portion of the nasal septum and then away from the vomer bone. Excessive cartilaginous dissection is also avoided to avert olfactory nerve injury. A self-retaining speculum is placed carefully to avoid dental injuries and then advanced. The surgeon uses an operating microscope with image intensifier. The sphenoid sinus is entered and a full view of the anterior sellar floor is attained, except in the 14% of cases involving an only partially pneumatized sinus that requires a high speed air drill for exposure. In the well-pneumatized sphenoid, care must be taken not to mistake a lateral carotid prominence for the sellar floor. Upon entering the sella, dural venous sinuses obstruct the approach in about 10% of cases and can cause troublesome bleeding. These venous sinuses can be carefully retracted with angled bipolar coagulating forceps. Certain patients with high central venous pressure (CVP) may have bleeding that is difficult to control. Therefore, patients suspected to have high CVP (eg, cushingoid with obesity and hypertension) may have a CVP line inserted preoperatively. If venous bleeding occurs intraoperatively, the CVP may be lowered with isofluorane anesthesia or other agents.

In many patients, the anterior lobe or tumor bulges forth upon opening of the dura. In about 80%, the tumor is sharply demarcated, soft, or even gelatinous and may be removed with aspiration or a small rongeur. Some tumors are more fibrotic and difficult to remove.

Patients with tumors having suprasellar extension should have a lumbar subarachnoid catheter inserted preoperatively, which allows the anesthesiologist to adjust the position of the tumor's suprasellar component. Adenomas with mild suprasellar extension (stage A) generally are forced into the sella spontaneously by the increased intracranial pressure caused by general anesthesia. Tumors that do not descend into the surgeon's vision may be forced down into the sella via small injections of normal saline into the subarachnoid catheter. Once the tumor is resected, the saline is withdrawn to elevate the capsule and allow the surgeon to view the posterior-superior aspect of the cavity using a small mirror. The tumor cavity is irrigated with bacitracin solution. Care must be taken not to injure the stalk or unnecessarily remove normal pituitary tissue. If a total hypophysectomy is required, a low stalk section will avert permanent diabetes insipidus.

If the location of the adenoma is not evident on scan or visual inspection of the pituitary, multiple vertical incisions may be made in order to explore the gland, which has not produced detectable endocrine dysfunction in reported series.

Once the adenoma is removed, hemostasis is obtained and the tumor bed is washed with absolute alcohol for 6–10 minutes if the cavity does not have subarachnoid communication. Intrasellar volume is replaced by use of the patient's own subcutaneous fat (usually taken from the low abdomen); this avoids optic nerve herniation, which must be prevented especially in patients requiring postoperative sellar irradiation. The sellar floor is closed with a small piece of nasal cartilage or bone.

Postoperative Evaluation & Management

Postoperatively, the patient has both nasal cavities packed gently with bacitracin-coated petrolatum gauze. The packs are removed after 24–48 hours. Oral decongestants and antihistamines are given to aid sinus drainage. Headache is controlled with mild analgesics. High altitudes, excessive head motion, and nose blowing are best avoided for about 4 weeks postoperatively, to prevent displacement of the sellar floor closure and cerebrospinal fluid rhinorrhea. Cerebrospinal fluid rhinorrhea can be distinguished from nasal secretions by its persistence despite antihistamine administration. The cerebrospinal fluid is usually clear and tests trace-positive for glucose with glucose oxidase test strips. Any cerebrospinal fluid leakage usually corrects itself in 3–4 days with a regimen of head elevation, acetazolamide, and a lumbar drain.

Postoperative body weight and serum electrolytes are measured frequently as are intake and output to screen for diabetes insipidus, SIADH, and cerebral salt wasting. Diuretics are interrupted, if possible, to reduce the incidence of hyponatremia. Serum electrolytes are also obtained 10 days postoperatively. Excessive urination in the first 2 postoperative days (> 2000 mL/d) may be due to DI but is more likely due to excretion of the operative fluid load if the patient's weight is increased, the serum sodium is under 140 mEq/L, and the patient has no complaint of thirst. DI, if it occurs, is managed as described on pp 26–27. Any polyuria must also prompt fractional urine testing for glucose, since diabetes mellitus may often be precipitated by perioperative hydrocortisone and excessive intravenous dextrose. For this reason, intravenous fluid replacement of over 150 mL/h should be with 0.9 N or 0.45 N saline rather than 5% dextrose in these patients.

Postoperatively, hydrocortisone coverage is individualized. Patients with Cushing's disease require a careful reduction in dose. Most patients in whom the postoperative endocrine status of the pituitary is not entirely certain may be discharged on replacement hydrocortisone doses (eg, 20 mg at 7 AM, 10 mg at 6 PM) for 4–6 weeks when adrenal, thyroid, and gonadal functions are reassessed. Hydrocortisone replacement is held for 12 hours, and a morning cosyntropin stimulation test is performed. Thyroid function is also assessed about 4–6 weeks postoperatively by determining a free thyroxine index. Gonadotropin function that has been suppressed by hypercortisolism will ordinarily recover within about 4 months unless the normal pituitary has been damaged by the pituitary adenoma or by therapy. It is assessed with a serum testosterone in men and a menstrual history in women. Nonmenstruating women between the ages of 15 and 50 are further evaluated with a serum β-hCG pregnancy test; if negative, a serum estradiol level is obtained; alternatively, medroxprogesterone acetate (10 mg) may be administered for 5 days to assess the adequacy of estrogen effects on the endometrium. Women having withdrawal menses may be cycled with monthly progestin; otherwise, cyclic estrogen and progestin are prescribed. Children are carefully followed for any deceleration of growth, at which time GH stimulation tests are considered. All children who are short and growing poorly preoperatively are tested for GH deficiency postoperatively. Patients with obvious gross total pituitary resection should be started immediately on replacement therapy. Patients with minimal pituitary trauma usually need no prophylactic hydrocortisone replacement after hospital discharge.

Assessment for resolution of secretory adenomas can be done with PRL or GH on days 3 and 4 postoperatively. Assessment for Cushing's disease resolution is more involved (see p 249).

Patients with obvious incomplete resection of their tumor (owing, for example, to cavernous sinus extension) are usually given radiation therapy beginning no sooner than 4 weeks postoperatively, allowing time for tissue healing. A CT scan or MRI should be repeated before radiation therapy but should not be done in the first month postoperatively since sellar packing, clots, and serum coagulum can be misleading.

Patients with prolactinomas may not need radiation postoperatively, especially if they respond to bromocriptine. Specific postoperative management for secreting tumors is described in appropriate sections elsewhere.

Success of the surgery may often be clinically apparent within 1 day postoperatively. Visual field abnormalities improve immediately in 90% of patients. Those with acromegaly have abrupt cessation of sweating, and women with galactorrhea note immediate improvement.

RADIATION THERAPY

Conventional Radiation

Conventional radiation therapy is ordinarily used as an adjunct to pituitary surgery or bromocriptine (or both); patients with certain hypothalamic tumors and invasive unresectable pituitary tumors may be candidates for radiation without surgery.

Radiation therapy to pituitary tumors should be delivered only by radiation therapists with proper equipment who are experienced in the technique. The patient usually receives radiation from either a 4- or

6-mev linear accelerator or 60 cobalt (preferably the former) in a dose of up to 180 rads* each day, 5 days weekly, up to 4500 rads at the 95% isodose line (maximum about 4750). The target volume should be slightly larger than the tumor volume. If total dose is kept to 4500 rads and daily dosage is 180 rads or less, the incidence of optic nerve damage or brain necrosis is less than 1%. The beam must be carefully aimed to avoid the eyes, using techniques to minimize the dose to the optic nerves and temporal lobes. The patient's head is fixed and exactly positioned with skin marks. Beam verification films are taken before and weekly during radiation therapy. A technique using a linear accelerator in bicornal arc rotations of 110 degrees each with a moving, reversing wedge filter, reduces hair loss and avoids temporal lobe necrosis.

Acute side effects of radiation therapy include malaise and nausea, which is treated with a nonphenothiazine medication if the tumor is prolactin-secreting and PRL levels are being monitored. Radiation therapy presents a mild stress. During treatment any patient with suspected hypoadrenalism should receive hydrocortisone in doses of 20–30 mg, 3 times a day.

Conventional radiation is highly effective in controlling further pituitary tumor growth. Actual cure of hormone excess syndromes is less likely. Therapeutic effect is delayed several months, and a nadir in serum hormone concentrations may not be reached for 3–7 years. The efficacy of radiation therapy is discussed elsewhere for craniopharyngiomas, germinomas, prolactinomas, acromegaly, and Cushing's disease.

Anterior pituitary deficiency of clinical importance probably ultimately occurs in as many as 60% of patients receiving 4500 rads or more of pituitary irradiation. Deficiencies are also common after nasopharyngeal radiation for carcinoma. Deficiencies occur gradually over years and may have subtle clinical manifestations. Growth hormone deficiency occurs in about 69% but is usually not symptomatic in adults. Adrenal insufficiency occurs in about 37% but is often partial. Hypothyroidism is difficult to assess, since mild hypothyroidism may occur with T_4 RIA in the normal range. The incidence of hypothyroidism, if mild symptoms or decrease of T_4 within the normal range are included, probably ultimately exceeds 35%. Hypogonadotropic hypogonadism is also common. These deficiencies may be caused by hypothalamic damage more than by pituitary destruction, since elevations in PRL occur in about 60% of patients (who had normal levels prior to radiation), probably as a result of decreased hypothalamic prolactin-inhibiting factor (PIF, dopamine).

* 1 rad = 0.01 gray (Gy, joule per kilogram).

Complications of conventional radiation therapy are most common in infants and very young children, who may suffer profound deficits in cognitive function. Aside from hypopituitarism, *complications in adults are rare (less than 1%) when the radiation is properly administered*. Virtually all cases have been ones who have received more than 5000 rads or daily fractions of more than 220 rads. Instances of brain necrosis are also caused by excessive total or daily radiation doses. Only 4 fibrosarcomas have been reported among all patients receiving conservative radiation doses. Other second malignancies may ultimately occur, especially in young patients and those receiving large radiation doses.

Heavy-Particle Therapy

Proton beam therapy is currently available in the USA at the Harvard-MIT Cyclotron in Boston. The efficacy of heavy-particle therapy is discussed separately for acromegaly and Cushing's disease.

By imparting exactly enough energy to the proton beam, the particles decelerate within the pituitary; radiation is given off only with deceleration, which produces a very localized dose of radiation (Bragg effect). Only intrasellar tumors can be thus treated, since treatment of suprasellar extension risks optic nerve damage.

The main indication for heavy-particle therapy is Cushing's disease without extrasellar tumor extension, documented by selective venous ACTH sampling or CT scan, and unresponsive to transsphenoidal surgery. The incidence of hypopituitarism may ultimately be less with proton beam therapy than with conventional radiation, since the hypothalamus is not damaged.

REFERENCES

Pituitary Neuroradiology

Ahmadi H et al: Normal pituitary gland: Coronal imaging of infundibulum tilt. *Radiology* 1990;**177:**389.

Brooks BS et al: Frequency and variation of the posterior pituitary bright signal on MR images. *AJNR* 1989;**10:**943.

Chakeres DW et al: Magnetic resonance imaging of pituitary and parasellar abnormalities. *Radiol Clin North Am* 1989;**27:**365.

DeSouza B et al: Pituitary microadenomas: A PET study. *Radiology* 1990; **177:**39.

Newton DR et al: Gd-DTPA enhanced MR imaging of pituitary adenomas. *AJNR* 1989;**10:**949.

Empty Sella

Bjerre P: The empty sella: A reappraisal of etiology and pathogenesis. *Acta Neurol Scand [Suppl]* 1990;**130:**1.

Cybulski GR et al: Intrasellar balloon inflation for treatment of symptomatic empty sella syndrome. *Neurosurgery* 1989;**74**:105.

Ishikama S: Empty sella in control subjects and patients with hypopituitarism. *Endocrinol Jpn* 1988;**35**:665.

Lambert M: Empty sella syndrome associated with diabetes insipidus: Case report and review of the literature. *J Endocrinol Invest* 1989;**12**:433.

Pucecco M et al: High frequency of empty sella syndrome in children with growth hormone deficiency. *Helv Paediatr Acta* 1989;**43**:295.

Hypopituitarism

Abboud CF: Laboratory diagnosis of hypopituitarism. *Mayo Clin Proc* 1986; **61**:35.

Arafah BM et al: Improvement of pituitary function after surgical decompression for pituitary tumor apoplexy. *J Clin Endocrinol Metab* 1990;**71**:323.

Berezon M et al: Successful GnRH treatment in a patient with Kallman's syndrome who previously failed hMG/hCG treatment. *Andrologia* 1988; **20**:285.

Bistritzez T et al: Hormonal therapy and pubertal development in boys with selective hypogonadotropic hypogonadism. *Fertil Steril* 1989;**52**:302.

Conway AJ et al: Randomized clinical trial of testosterone replacement therapy in hypogonadal men. *Int J Androl* 1988;**11**:247.

Cunningham GR et al: Testosterone replacement with transdermal therapeutic systems: Physiological serum testosterone and elevated dihydrotestosterone levels. *JAMA* 1988;**1**:1146.

Diamond T et al: Osteoporosis in hemochromatosis: Iron excess, gonadal deficiency, or other factors? *Ann Intern Med* 1989;**110**:430.

Frisch H et al: Psychological aspects in children and adolescents with hypopituitarism. *Acta Paediatr Scand* 1990;**79**:644.

Libber SM et al: Long-term follow-up of hypopituitary patients treated with human growth hormone. *Medicine* 1990;**69**:46.

Liu L et al: Two-year comparison of testicular responses to pulsatile gonadotropin-releasing hormone and exogenous gonadotropins—in men with isolated hypogonadotropic hypogonadism. *J Clin Endocrinol Metab* 1988;**67**:1140.

Miura M et al: Lymphocytic adenohypophysitis: Report of two cases. *Surg Neurol* 1989;**32**:463.

Root AW: Magnetic resonance imaging in hypopituitarism. *J Clin Endocrinol Metab* 1991;**72**:10.

Rudman D et al: Effects of human growth hormone in men over 60 years old. *N Engl J Med* 1990;**323**:1.

Whitcomb RW, Crowley WF Jr: Diagnosis and treatment of isolated gonadotropin-releasing hormone deficiency in men. *J Clin Endocrinol Metab* 1990; **70**:3.

Diabetes Insipidus

Bayliss P, Gill GV: The investigation of polyuria. *Clin Endocrinol Metab* 1984;**13**:294.

Binzilay Z et al: Diabetes insipidus in severely brain damaged children. *J Med* 1988;**19**:47.

Comtois R et al: Low serum urea level in dehydrated patients with central diabetes insipidus. *Can Med Assoc J* 1988;**139**:965.

Dunger DB et al: The frequency and natural history of diabetes insipidus in children with Langerhans'-cell histiocytosis. *N Engl J Med* 1989;**321**:1157.

Harris AS: Clinical experience with desmopressin efficacy and safety in central diabetes insipidus and other conditions. *J Pediatr* 1989;**114**:711.

Hughes JM et al: Recurrent diabetes insipidus associated with pregnancy: Pathophysiology and therapy. *Obstet Gynecol* 1989;**73**:462.

Iwasaki Y et al: Aggravation of subclinical diabetes insipidus during pregnancy. *N Engl J Med* 1991;**324**:572, 556.

Knoers N, Monnens LA: Amiloride-hydrochlorthiazide versus indomethicin-hydrochlorthiazide in the treatment of nephrogenic diabetes insipidus. *J Pediatr* 1990;**117**:499.

Ralston C, Butt W: Continuous vasopressin replacement in diabetes insipidus. *Arch Dis Child* 1990;**65**:896.

Robertson GL, Harris A: Clinical use of vasopressin analogues. *Hosp Prac* 1989;**24**:114.

Stasior DS et al: Nephrogenic diabetes insipidus responsive to indomethacin plus dDAVP. *N Engl J Med* 1991;**324**:850.

Thompson CJ et al: Vasopressin secretion in the DIDMOAD (Wolfram) syndrome. *Q J Med* 1989;**71**:333.

Craniopharyngiomas & Other CNS Lesions

Backlund EO et al: Treatment of craniopharyngiomas: The stereotactic approach in a ten to twenty-three years' perspective. *1.* Surgical, radiological and ophthalmological aspects. *Acta Neurochir (Wien)* 1989;**99**:11.

Fischer EG et al: Craniopharyngiomas in children: Long-term effects of conservative surgical procedures combined with radiation therapy. *J Neurosurg* 1990;**73**:534.

Jereb B et al: Intracranial germinoma: Report of seven cases. *Pediatr Hematol Oncol* 1990;**7**:183.

Legido A et al: Suprasellar germinomas in childhood: A reappraisal. *Cancer* 1989;**63**:340.

Saaf M et al: Treatment of craniopharyngiomas: The stereotactic approach in a ten to twenty-three years' perspective. Psychosocial situation and pituitary function. *Acta Neurochir (Wien)* 1989;**99**:97.

Shiminski-Mater T, Rosenberg M: Late effects associated with treatment of craniopharyngioma in childhood. *J Neurosci Nurs* 1990;**22**:220.

Wen BC et al: A comparison of the roles of surgery and radiation therapy in the management of craniopharyngiomas. *Int J. Radiat Oncol Biol Phys* 1989;**16**:17.

Prolactinoma

Bevan JS et al: Misinterpretation of prolactin levels leading to management errors in patients with sellar enlargement. *Am J Med* 1987;**82**:29.

Dalkin AC, Marshall JC: Medical therapy of hyperprolactinemia. *Endocrinol Metab Clin North Am* 1989;**18**:259.

Katz E et al: Successful treatment of a prolactin-producing pituitary macroadenoma with intravaginal bromocriptine mesylate: A novel approach to intolerance of oral therapy. *Obstet Gynecol* 1989;**73:**517.

Klibanski A, Zervas NT: Diagnosis and management of hormone-secreting pituitary adenomas. *N Engl J Med* 1991;**324:**822.

Kupersmith MJ et al: Growth of prolactinoma despite lowering of serum prolactin by bromocriptine. *Neurosurgery* 1989;**24:**417.

Maira G et al: Prolactin-secreting adenomas: Surgical results and long-term follow-up. *Neurosurgery* 1989;**24:**736.

Molitch ME: Management of prolactinomas. *Annu Rev Med* 1989;**40:**225.

Moriondo P et al: Bromocriptine treatment of microprolactinomas: Evidence of stable prolactin decrease after drug withdrawal. *J Clin Encocrinol Metab* 1985;**60:**764.

Schlechte J et al: The natural history of untreated hyperprolactinemia: A prospective analysis. *J Clin Endocrinol Metab* 1989;**68:**412.

Vance ML et al: Treatment of hyperprolactinemia. *J Clin Endocrinol Metab* 1989;**68:**336.

Wollesen F, Bendsen BB: Effect rates of different modalities for treatment of prolactin adenomas. *Am J Med* 1985;**78:**114.

Acromegaly

Barkan AL: Acromegaly. Diagnosis and therapy. *Endocrinol Metab Clin North Am* 1989;**18:**277.

Barakat S et al: Reversible shrinkage of a growth hormone–secreting pituitary adenoma by a long-acting somatostatin analogue, octreotide. *Arch Intern Med* 1989;**149:**1443.

Diamond T et al: Spinal and peripheral bone mineral densities in acromegaly: The effects of excess growth hormone and hypogonadism. *Ann Intern Med* 1989;**111:**567.

Daughaday WH: Octreotide is effective in acromegaly but often results in cholelithiasis. *Ann Intern Med* 1990;**112:**159.

Dowsett RJ et al: Results of radiotherapy in the treatment of acromegaly: Lack of ophthalmologic complications. *Int J Radiat Oncol Biol Phys* 1990;**79:**453.

Ezzat S, Melmed S: Are patients with acromegaly at increased risk for neoplasia? *J Clin Endocrinol Metab* 1991;**72:**245.

Frohman LA: Therapeutic options in acromegaly. *J Clin Endocrinol Metab* 1991;**72:**1175.

Halse J: et al: A randomized study of SMS 201-995 versus bromocriptine treatment in acromegaly: Clinical and biochemical effects. *J Clin Endocrinol Metab* 1990;**70:**1254.

Harris PE et al: Successful treatment by chemotherapy for acromegaly associated with ectopic growth hormone releasing hormone secretion from a carcinoid tumor. *Clin Endocrinol* 1990;**32:**315.

Jackson IT et al: Surgical correction of the acromegalic face: A one stage procedure with a team approach. *J Craniomaxillofac Surg* 1989;**17:**2.

Lieberman SA, Hoffman AR: Sequelae to acromegaly: Reversibility with treatment of the primary disease. *Horm Metab Res* 1990;**22:**313.

Littley MD et al: Low dose pituitary irradiation for acromegaly. *Clin Endocrinol* 1990;**32:**261.

Ludecke DK et al: The choice of treatment after incomplete adenomectomy in acromegaly: Proton versus high voltage radiation. *Acta Neurochir (Wien)* 1989;**96**:32.

McCarthy MI et al: Familial acromegaly: studies on three families. *Clinical Endocrinol* 1990;**322**:966.

Melmed S: Acromegaly. *N Engl J Med* 1990;**322**:966.

Moran A et al: Gigantism due to mammosomatotroph hyperplasia. *N Engl J Med* 1990;**323**:322.

Mountcastle RB et al: Pituitary adenocarcinoma in an acromegalic patient: Response to bromocriptine and pituitary testing—A review of the literature on 36 cases of pituitary carcinoma. *Am J Med Sci* 1989;**298**:109.

Octeotride: A synthetic somatostatin. *Med Lett Drugs Ther* 1989;**31**:66.

Pestell RG et al: Familial acromegaly. *Acta Endocrinol (Copenh)* 1989; **121**:286.

Sassolas G et al: Long term effect of incremental doses of somatostatin analog SMS 201-995 in 58 acromegalic patients. *J Clin Endocrinol Metab* 1990; **71**:391.

Serri O: Acromegaly: Biochemical assessment of cure after long term follow-up of transsphenoidal selective adenomectomy. *J Clin Endocrinol Metab* 1985; **61**:1185.

Cushing's Syndrome, Cushing's Disease, and Adrenal Tumors

References for these topics can be found in Chapter 6, beginning on page 284.

Pituitary Tumors (TSH, Gonadotropin, & Nonsecreting)

Beck-Peccoz P et al: Treatment of hyperthyroidism due to inappropriate secretion of thyrotropin with somatostatin analog SMS 201-995. *J Clin Endocrinol Metab* 1989;**68**:208.

Burrow GN et al: Microadenomas of the pituitary and abnormal sellar tomograms in an unselected autopsy series. *N Engl J Med* 1981;**304**:156.

Flickinger JC et al: Radiotherapy of non-functioning adenomas of the pituitary gland. Results with long-term follow-up. *Cancer* 1989;**63**:2409.

Galway AB et al: Gonadotroph adenomas in men produce biologically active follicle-stimulating hormone. *J Clin Endocrinol Metab* 1990;**71**:907.

Gesundheit N et al: Thyrotropin-secreting pituitary adenomas: Clinical and biochemical heterogeneity—Case reports and follow-up of nine patients. *Ann Intern Med* 1989;**111**:827.

Gharib H et al: The spectrum of inappropriate thyrotropin secretion associated with hyperthyroidism. *Mayo Clin Proc* 1982;**57**:556.

McCutcheon IE et al: Surgical treatment of thyrotropin-secreting pituitary adenomas. *J Neurosurg* 1990;**73**:674.

Mclellan AR et al: Clinical response of thyrotropin-secreting macroadenoma to bromocriptine and radiotherapy. *Acta Endocrinol (Copenh)* 1988;**119**:189.

Oppenheim DS et al: Medical therapy of glycoprotein hormone–secreting pituitary tumors. *Endocrinol Metab Clin North Am* 1989;**18**:339.

Transsphenoidal Pituitary Surgery & Pituitary Apoplexy

Ahmed M et al: Classical pituitary apoplexy presentation and follow-up of 13 patients. *Horm Res* 1989;**31**:125.

Pituitary apoplexy. (Case records of the Massachusetts General Hospital.) *N Engl J Med* 1986;**314:**229.

Wilson CB: A decade of pituitary microsurgery: The Herbert Olivecrona Lecture. *J Neurosurg* 1984;**61:**814.

Pituitary Radiation

Al-Mefty O et al: The long-term side effects of radiation therapy for benign brain tumors in adults. *J Neurosurg* 1990;**73:**502.

Grigsby PW et al: Long term results of radiotherapy in the treatment of pituitary adenomas in children and adolescents. *Am J Clin Oncol* 1988;**11:**607.

Kovalic JJ et al: Recurrent pituitary adenomas after surgical resection: The role of radiation therapy. *Radiology* 1990;**177:**273.

Thoren M et al: Stereotactic irradiation for pituitary disease. *Horm Res* 1988;**30:**101.

Hyponatremia

Andrews BT et al: Cerebral salt wasting after pituitary exploration and biopsy: Case report. *Neurosurgery* 1986;**18(4):**469.

Berl T: Treating hyponatremia: Damned if we do and damned if we don't. *Kidney Int* 1990;**37:**1006.

Berry PL, Belsha CW: Hyponatremia. *Pediatr Clin North Am* 1990;**37:**351.

Cheng JC et al: Long-term neurologic outcome in psychogenic water drinkers with severe hyponatremia: The effect of rapid correction. *Am J Med* 1990;**88:**561.

Maesaka JK et al: Hyponatremia and hypouricemia: Differentiation from SIADH. *Clin Nephrol* 1990;**33:**174.

Mitnick PD, Bell S: Rhabdomyolysis associated with severe hyponatremia after prostatic surgery. *Am J Kidney Dis* 1990;**16:**73.

Papadakis MA et al: Hyponatremia in patients with cirrhosis. *Q J Med* 1990;**76:**675.

Schrier RW, Briner VA: The differential diagnosis of hyponatremia. *Hosp Pract* 1990;**25:**29.

Sklar C et al: Chronic syndrome of inappropriate secretion of antidiuretic hormone in childhood. *Am J Dis Child* 1985;**139:**733.

Sterns RH et al: The treatment of hyponatremia: First, do no harm. *Am J Med* 1990;**88:**557.

Weissman JD et al: Pontine myelinolysis and delayed encephalopathy following the rapid correction of acute hyponatremia. *Arch Neurol* 1989;**46:**926.

Wijdicks ER et al: The effect of fludrocortisone acetate on plasma volume and natriuresis in patients with aneurysmal subarachnoid hemorrhage. *Clin Neurol Neurosurg* 1988;**90:**209.

Sexual Differentiation | 2

Dennis M. Styne, MD

NORMAL SEXUAL DIFFERENTIATION

Normal sexual differentiation consists of 4 aspects: (1) chromosomal sex (genotype), which determines (2) gonadal sex, which usually directs (3) phenotypic sexual differentiation; (4) gender identification in human beings seems most dependent upon the social environment but is normally influenced by the first 3 aspects. Phenotypic sexual differentiation in humans proceeds toward a female phenotype unless the fetus is exposed to androgens.

CHROMOSOMAL SEX (GENOTYPE, KARYOTYPE)

The normal human being has 22 paired autosomes and 2 sex chromosomes. The male is 46,XY and the female 46,XX. Although a female has two X chromosomes, the Lyon hypothesis states that all X chromosomes except one must be inactivated so that only a single dose of the genes found on the X chromosome is active in any human being. (The exception is that the distal portion of the short arm of the X chromosome is not inactivated in normal females.) The inactivation process is random early in development, and inactivated X chromosomes can be seen as X chromatin (or Barr) bodies on the nuclear membrane of Giemsa-stained cells collected from a buccal smear. Males and patients with 45,XO karyotypes lack Barr bodies; normal females or patients with Klinefelter's syndrome (47,XXY) have a Barr body in 20–30% of their cells. Patients with 48,XXXY karyotype have 2 Barr bodies, and so on. Unfortunately, the buccal smear test is subject to misinterpretation, and since few laboratories can accurately perform the determination, a karyotype rather than Barr body determination is the test of choice.

Testis-Determining Factor (TDF):

The factors responsible for causing an indifferent fetal gonad to develop into a testis are still unknown. The H-Y antigen was once thought to bind to receptors on the bipotential gonad and cause development into a testis. The long arm of the Y chromosome contains a gene that codes for the H-Y antigen; an X chromosome locus may also be necessary for the expression of H-Y antigen. The H-Y antigen is a histocompatability antigen; it is detected at the 8-cell stage of human embryogenesis and later is disseminated by the primitive Sertoli cell. However, a small region on the distal short arm of the Y chromosome just proximal to the pseudo-autosomal region is critical to testicular development. A gene in this area codes for a DNA binding protein with 13 zinc finger domains and is homologous to an area of the X chromosome that escapes inactivation. The protein was thought to switch on genes leading to testicular development. However, discrepancies in the theory that this protein is the testis-determining factor itself have recently appeared and another gene from near the pseudoautosomal border, SRY, may prove to be the TDF.

Gonadal Development

Ovaries and testes both arise from the same genital primordia during the first 6 weeks of gestation; the early fetal gonad is bipotential.

If TDF is present, the gonad organizes into a testis between 6 and 7 weeks, with seminiferous tubules appearing at 7 weeks and Leydig cells 10 days thereafter. In the absence of TDF, follicles appear and an ovary differentiates after 11–12 weeks of gestation. In the absence of TDF and with only one X chromosome (Turner's syndrome), the ovary starts to develop normally, but in the fourth month of gestation, germ cells decrease in number compared to those of normal individuals and the gonad becomes a streak gonad composed of fibrous tissue by or shortly after birth.

PHENOTYPE

Internal Genital Duct Development

Both female (müllerian) and male (wolffian) ducts are present in all fetuses by the seventh week of gestation. If a normal testis has developed, it produces a protein hormone (müllerian duct inhibitory factor, MIF) from the Sertoli cells and a steroid hormone (testosterone) from the Leydig cells; MIF then causes ipsilateral müllerian duct regression, and testosterone supports ipsilateral wolffian duct development into the epididymis, vas deferens, seminal vesicles, and ejaculatory ducts. If no testis forms or if it is dysgenetic, the absence of MIF allows the ipsilateral müllerian duct to develop into the uterine tube, uterus, cervix, and upper third of the vagina; without local testosterone production, the ipsilateral wolffian duct spontaneously regresses; girls with fetal virilizing syndromes due to adrenal enzyme defects or maternal androgen ingestion develop müllerian-derived organs but do not retain wolffian ducts because the local androgen concentrations are not high enough.

External Genital Development

Until the eighth week of gestation, external genitalia are bipotential. Without testosterone, the genital tubercle remains a clitoris, the urogenital sinus develops into the lower third of the vagina, and the labia remains unfused. In the normal male fetus, the testis produces testosterone, which is converted in genital skin to dihydrotestosterone (DHT) by the enzyme 5α-reductase. DHT binds to a cytosol receptor in genital skin and is translocated to the nucleus for chromatin binding so that masculinization will occur; the genital tubercle grows into a penis, the urogenital slit encloses the penile urethra, and the labial folds fuse to become the scrotum.

The secretion of testosterone from the Leydig cells is stimulated at first by human chorionic gonadotropin (hCG), but as hCG levels fall by mid-gestation, the secretion of LH and FSH by the fetal pituitary gland becomes more important in maintaining testosterone secretion. Without fetal pituitary gonadotropins during the last two-thirds of pregnancy, testosterone levels are inadequate to allow normal growth of the differentiated penis to normal newborn length of about 4 cm.

In a genetic male, if any of the steps toward masculine development are partially or completely defective, a degree of ambiguous genital development will occur. In the absence of any androgen or complete resistance to androgen action, the genital tubercle will become a clitoris, the urogenital slit will widen and urogenital folds will become labia minora, and the labioscrotal swelling will become labia majora. Without testosterone, development of the vesicovaginal septum and differentiation of the lower two-thirds of the vagina will proceed before the 12th week of gestation.

In a genetic female, any degree of intersexuality can be formed by androgen exposure from endogenous or exogenous sources. Before 12 weeks of gestation, androgens will masculinize a fetus to some degree, as described above, with some fusion of the urogenital slit; after 13 weeks of gestation, the major effect will be phallic enlargement without posterior fusion of the vagina.

Gender Development

Sexual identification seems not to be affected by karyotype or sex steroids to as great a degree in humans as in other mammals. The gender in which a child is raised, the clues given the child by those in the family or social sphere, and the similarity of the child's external genitalia to those children of the same gender are the major determinants of sexual identification. In all cultures, gender role is normally established by age 18 months, but exceptions are known. (Gender identity is routinely changed in a village in the Dominican Republic where patients with 5α-reductase deficiency become "men" at puberty after being socially raised as "girls".)

AMBIGUOUS GENITALIA

PSYCHOLOGICAL APPROACH

It is impossible to overemphasize the importance of correct psychological management of parents and patients with ambiguous genitalia. Parents, regardless of educational level or social status, carry a predetermined pattern of thinking concerning a son or daughter, and the process starts as soon as they are informed of the sex of their offspring. The first statement of gender from the physician attending the birth sets in motion a chain of parental assumptions and expectations that cannot easily be reversed. Thus, the suggestion that the newborn with a 2.5-cm penis, a bifid, rugated scrotum, and no palpable testes is a boy will be difficult to counter if the diagnosis is finally made of virilizing congenital adrenal hyperplasia in a potentially fertile phenotypic female. Although it is difficult for all concerned, no gender can be assigned to any baby with ambiguity of genitalia of unknown cause. Testing to determine the nature of the defect may take days to weeks, but no favor is done to parents by a doctor who confides in them a "hunch" that "you are going to have a little boy when all these tests return." Most patients who are appropriately supported from birth do well; their worst psychological prob-

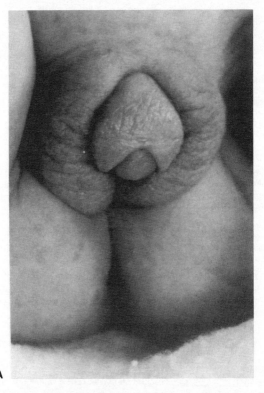

A

Figure 2–1. A. This newborn has a 46,XX genotype, an enlarged clitoris with a dimple on the tip and rugated labia resembling a bifid scrotum. (*continued*)

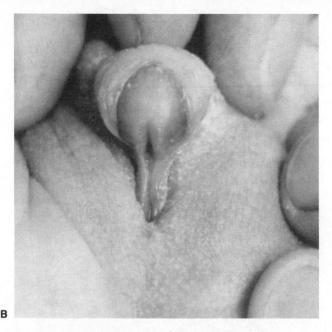

B

Figure 2–1 (cont'd). B. When the clitoris is lifted, a urethra ending below the base of the clitoris (perinoscrotal hypospadias) and a slitlike vagina with posterior fusion become visible. No gonads are palpable. The infant has P-450c 21 deficiency with a phenotype of ambiguous genitalia.

lems may arise from frequent examinations rather than from the actual endocrine disorder.

Even if an error of sex assignment is corrected, parents may retain doubts about the appropriateness of the activities of their child and wonder whether the doctor who changed the sex assignment was not wrong to do so. These problems are avoided if sex is correctly assigned *after* appropriate studies.

The physician can refer to the child as having "unfinished genitalia" and "baby gonads" and assure parents that a sex will be assigned when enough is known about the reason the child has not completely developed. The child should never be referred to as half-male and half-female. Once test results allow assignment of sex, support for the decision must be complete and an unambiguous name given to the baby.

CONSIDERATIONS OF GENDER ASSIGNMENT

The decision to raise a child in a certain gender involves several factors. Retaining fertility, if possible, is a primary goal. However, if a fertile male has inadequate penile tissue that cannot be made to grow with testosterone therapy and if it appears that surgery cannot enlarge the penis, it may be appropriate to raise the child as a female. The presence of hypospadias or unfused labia in a male pseudohermaphrodite with scrotal folds should not in itself prompt a female sex assignment in 46,XY patients, since these defects can be corrected surgically. Similarly, the lack of palpable testes should not prompt a female sex assessment, since undescended testes are common in newborns. A 46,XY pseudohermaphrodite with marked androgen insensitivity cannot look or function as a male and, therefore, should be raised as a female. Conversely, an extremely virilized female pseudohermaphrodite with congenital adrenal hyperplasia will have normal ovarian function if appropriately treated and can be made to exhibit a female phenotype by means of cosmetic surgery; this patient should be raised as a female. Thus, each diagnosis carries its own indication for raising the child in a given gender. Reconstructive surgery is best done during the first 2 years of life, and certainly most major modifications should be completed by school age. In late diagnosed cases, if an error was made in sex assignment at birth and gender change is necessary, it must be carried out before the age of 18 months is reached if the child is to accept its gender and act appropriately; after this age the incidence of psychopathology rises dramatically.

The birth of a patient with ambiguous genitalia is always a psychological emergency and may become a medical emergency. Every newborn with ambiguous genitalia must be observed closely for the salt-losing form of 21-hydroxylase deficiency or 3β-hydroxysteroid dehydrogenase (3β-HSD) deficiency; if salt-losing complicates the picture, shock may develop within days to weeks of birth.

DIAGNOSTIC APPROACH

Rapid diagnosis is the goal when a baby with ambiguous genitalia is born. Fig 2–2 outlines the approach when no testes are palpable and Fig 2–3 when testes are palpable. A detailed history must be elicited from the mother of any drug ingestion during the pregnancy, especially testosterone and similar androgenic steroids or progestins of androgen derivation, such as found in oral contraceptives. The mother should be examined for evidence of any virilization herself, which would provide a clue to a maternal virilizing ovarian or adrenal neo-

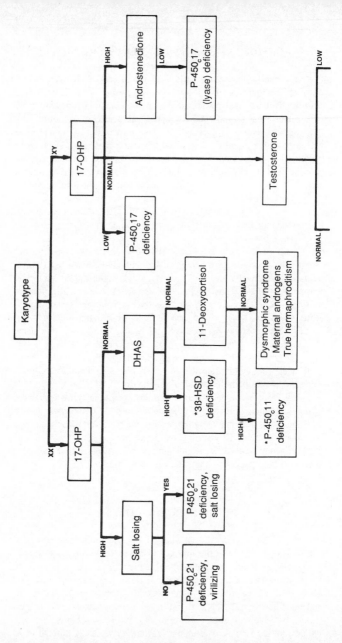

80

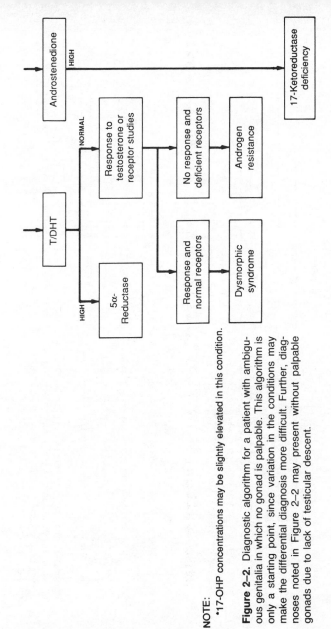

NOTE:

*17-OHP concentrations may be slightly elevated in this condition.

Figure 2–2. Diagnostic algorithm for a patient with ambiguous genitalia in which no gonad is palpable. This algorithm is only a starting point, since variation in the conditions may make the differential diagnosis more difficult. Further, diagnoses noted in Figure 2–2 may present without palpable gonads due to lack of testicular descent.

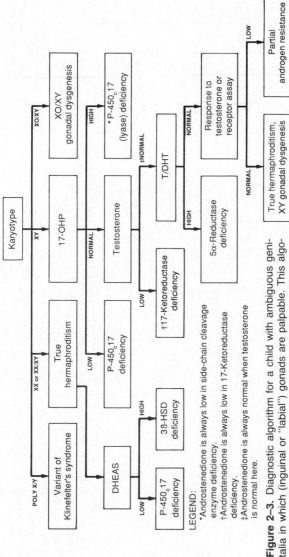

Figure 2–3. Diagnostic algorithm for a child with ambiguous genitalia in which (inguinal or "labial") gonads are palpable. This algorithm is only a starting point, since variation in the conditions may make the differential diagnosis more difficult.

LEGEND:
*Androstenedione is always low in side-chain cleavage enzyme deficiency.
†Androstenedione is always low in 17-Ketoreductase deficiency.
‡Androstenedione is always normal when testosterone is normal here.

82

plasm, a luteoma of pregnancy, or maternal congenital adrenal hyperplasia.

The newborn must have a careful physical examination. Examination should include measurement of the (stretched) phallic structure from pubis to tip. The location of the urethra must be noted as well as the degree of fusion of the labial-scrotal fold. Gonad presence, location, and size must be noted. A digital rectal examination with the smallest digit should reveal the presence or absence of a cervix (which is normally enlarged in the newborn period following fetal exposure to maternal estrogen). A pelvic ultrasound examination will document the presence of a uterus and vagina.

Laboratory Tests

Tests ideally include measurement of serum 17-hydroxyprogesterone, testosterone, androstenedione, and dehydroepiandrosterone and its sulfate. Cord blood is not ideal for 17-hydroxyprogesterone levels, since the values in normal babies within the first 12–24 hours may be misleadingly high. In the unlikely case that serum levels for the above hormones are not available (even from a sendout specialty laboratory), a 24-hour urine is obtained for 17-ketosteroids. 17-Ketosteroid excretion rates are high in normal infants during the first week of life, so values must be related to age and laboratory normals. A urinary collection must be complete over 24 hours, or the results will be misleading.

Other tests should include measurements of sodium and potassium daily until salt-losing is documented if P-450c21, 3β-HSD, or P-450scc (side-chain cleavage enzyme; rare) deficiencies are suspected. In cases of microphallus, periodic serum glucose levels should be obtained to rule out growth hormone or ACTH deficiency associated with hypopituitarism.

The sex chromosomes should be determined by means of a karyotype; the specimen should be 2.5 mL of blood collected in a heparinized tube (without preservative) and transported without delay at room temperature to the genetics laboratory where blood lymphocytes will be cultured. Twenty-four hours may safely elapse between specimen collection and lymphocyte culture. Most newborns with ambiguous genitalia should have a karyotype drawn immediately in order to avoid diagnostic delays. If an exchange transfusion is necessary for hyperbilirubinemia, the karyotype sample must precede the procedure.

In the past when karyotyping was not available, a buccal smear was obtained if the laboratory was adept at its interpretation. A scraping of the inside of the cheek is placed on a slide, immediately submerged into alcohol, and Giemsa stained. Inactivated X chromosomes can be seen as X chromatin (Barr) bodies on the nuclear membrane of these cells. Normal (46,XY) males and patients with Turner's syndrome (45,XO) lack Barr bodies; normal (46,XX) females and patients with Klinefelter's syndrome (47,XXY) have a Barr body in 20–30% of these cells; patients with 48,XXXY karyotype have 2 Barr bodies, and so on. Unfortunately, the buccal smear test is subject to misinterpretation; since few laboratories can accurately perform the determination, a karyotype is the test of choice.

Another rough approximation for inactivated X chromatin may be made by reviewing a patient's peripheral blood polymorphonuclear neutrophils for "drumsticks" (nuclear appendages of inactivated X chromatin attached to the rest of the nuclear chromatin by a thin stalk). In 46,XX females, 1–15% of neutrophils (mean = 2.5%) have a drumstick. Drumsticks are not found in normal 46,XY males or patients with 45,XO Turner's syndrome. This technique cannot replace the definitive results of a Karyotype.

46,XX Karyotype: Female Pseudohermaphroditism (Testes Never Palpable)

Virilization of a genetic female is the most common cause of ambiguous genitalia and is usually due to 21-hydroxylase deficiency. Studies of female fetuses naturally or iatrogenically exposed to androgens have revealed that androgen excess before 12 weeks of gestation can cause some degree of ambiguous genitalia affecting vagina and clitoris, whereas after 13 weeks the sole manifestation is clitoromegaly. Patients with female pseudohermaphroditism usually can be raised as fertile females, since they have normal internal sexual ducts and ovaries.

A. Congenital Adrenal Hyperplasia: When adequate cortisol cannot be produced owing to an enzyme deficiency, ACTH rises and the adrenal gland produces excessive amounts of precursor steroids. If the precursor leads to excessive androgen production, virilizing congenital adrenal hyperplasia results. Steroid hormone enzyme pathways are outlined in Fig 2–4. All these disorders are inherited in an autosomal recessive pattern. Because enzymatic blocks may be partial, there is great variation of expression in these disorders and some patients may reach later childhood or adolescence before symptoms become manifest. These disorders are discussed below in decreasing order of frequency.

B. 21-Hydroxylase (21-OH) P-450c21 Deficiency: This is the most common cause of congenital adrenal hyperplasia (95%) and occurs in 1:14,000 live Caucasian births. It is caused by various mutations or deletion of the gene encoding the enzyme P-450c21. This enzyme is necessary for both cortisol and aldosterone production (Fig 2–4). Different mutations produce varying severities of enzyme dysfunction or deficiency. Severe deficiencies of both cortisol and aldosterone cause shock and virilization (classic salt-losing form). Milder deficiencies afford enough cortisol and aldosterone to avoid shock except occasionally under stress (classical non-salt-losing form). Virilization occurs owing to shunting of the accumulating precursor of the enzyme block (17-hydroxyprogesterone) into androgen production.

Even milder P-450c21 dysfunction may produce nonclassical (''late onset'') 21-OH deficiency that is manifest only as hirsutism during adolesence or adulthood.

Recent studies have closely linked the gene or genes for virilizing classical and nonclassical 21-hydroxylase to the HLA locuses on chromosome 6, close to the locus for complement C4 and between HLA-B and HLA-D. Most patients with 21-OH deficiency have point gene deletions or microgenic conversions, while the remaining 25% have gene deletions or macrogenic conversions. There is an increase in HLA type BW47 in the salt-losing form and in BW51 in the non-salt-losing form of 21-OH deficiency. Affected siblings within a family have identical HLA types while heterozygotes share half of the HLA sites with the homozygotes. Thus, if an affected sibling has already been diagnosed, HLA typing of fetal cells in the amniotic fluid or chorionic villus sample can predict whether the fetus is affected or not. The variable degrees of virilization appear due to the fact that several alleles of the 21-hydroxylase gene control of the appearance of the classical and nonclassical virilizing types. Within a family affected with the salt-losing form, clinical salt loss appears in all affected patients.

Clinical manifestation in a 46,XX newborn may include any aspect of ambiguous genitalia including clitoromegaly, posterior vaginal fusion with pigmentation and rugation of the apparent scrotal sack, and lack of an adequate vesicovaginal septum leading to formation of a urogenital sinus; genetic females have been observed with a penile urethra and a fully male external genital phenotype (except testes). Generally, the salt-losing form has been associated with greater degrees of virilization. Affected males look normal at birth and may go undiagnosed for months or years if salt loss or shock does not occur.

Patients with the salt-losing form demonstrate a decreasing sodium and rising potassium at approximately 5 days after birth. Since a normal-looking child will be discharged and home by this time, many males go undiagnosed for weeks or months and may die owing to hyponatremic crisis. Usually the appearance of a female child's genitalia will assure her evaluation immediately. If no treatment is offered, the patient will develop poor weight gain and vomiting. Children with salt loss will have hyponatremia and hyperkalemia. Some males may be misdiagnosed as having pyloric stenosis because of the severe vomiting. The history of a previous sibling with unexplained death in the newborn period should suggest a possible diagnosis of congenital

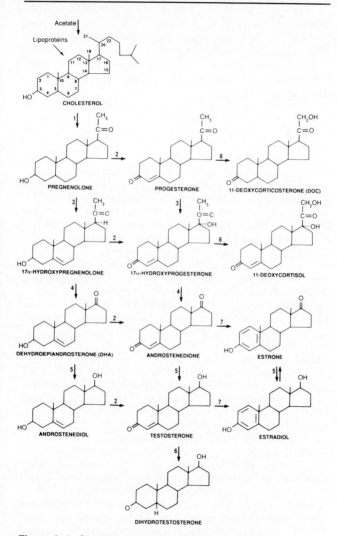

Figure 2–4. Steroid hormone biosynthetic pathways.

adrenal hyperplasia. Mild salt-losing cases may not have life-threatening electrolyte abnormalities but have elevated plasma renin activity. Such patients will do better if treated with a mineralocorticoid; this tends to reduce the glucocorticoid dose required to suppress androgen overproduction.

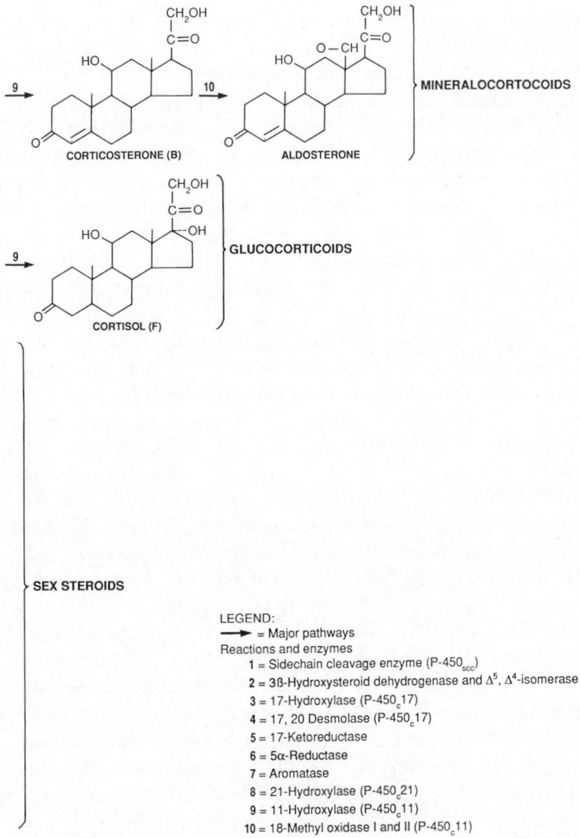

Figure 2–4. (Cont'd.)

LEGEND:
⟶ = Major pathways

Reactions and enzymes
1 = Sidechain cleavage enzyme (P-450$_{scc}$)
2 = 3β-Hydroxysteroid dehydrogenase and Δ^5, Δ^4-isomerase
3 = 17-Hydroxylase (P-450$_c$17)
4 = 17, 20 Desmolase (P-450$_c$17)
5 = 17-Ketoreductase
6 = 5α-Reductase
7 = Aromatase
8 = 21-Hydroxylase (P-450$_c$21)
9 = 11-Hydroxylase (P-450$_c$11)
10 = 18-Methyl oxidase I and II (P-450$_c$11)

Children who are simply virilized without salt loss may live for years without diagnosis or treatment because of parental (or medical) indifference, although they may have hyponatremia and shock when stressed. They may develop pubic hair before the first year, abnormal muscular hyperplasia, lower voice, and excessive linear growth with advanced bone ages. The severe degree of virilization in girls and prepubertal testes in boys with virilization usually distinguishes these patients from children with central precocious puberty. Males with congenital adrenal hyperplasia have small testes, and their condition should not be confused with central precocious puberty, in which testes are greater than 2.5 cm in length. High plasma ACTH concentrations may cause increased pigmentation. Some males may have adrenal rests in the testes that enlarge under ACTH stimulation and present as local masses. These should not be confused with Leydig cell tumors, in which case ACTH is not elevated.

Advanced bone age in patients undiagnosed for years will severely limit final height. Remarkably, after such children have had adrenal androgens suppressed with glucocorticoids (and if necessary, mineralocorticoids), they may enter central precocious puberty because the androgen exposure has matured their hypothalamic-pituitary-gonadal axis. Thus, final height may be further compromised by advancing bone age due to precocious puberty, in addition to the advanced bone age due to the underlying virilizing adrenal hyperplasia.

Nonclassical congenital adrenal hyperplasia may or may not manifest virilization several years after birth or in adult life. This condition is the most common autosomal recessive disease, with a gene incidence of more than 1:50 in Ashkenazic Jews and Hispanics and an incidence of 1:1000 in diverse Caucasian populations. Blood values of testosterone and 17-hydroxyprogesterone in the basal or ACTH-stimulated state are midway between classical cases and normals. Asymptomatic non-classical cases have no physical manifestation of 21-hydroxylase deficiency but reside in the same families as late-onset patients and may have blood steroid values indistinguishable from them. The cause of these variable manifestations may relate to the combination of a severe and a non-severe genetic defect or two non-severe defects.

1. Diagnosis–21-OH deficiency should be suspected in (1) children with ambiguous genitalia and no palpable testes; (2) a phenotypic male without palpable testes; (3) any male baby or child with ambiguous genitalia who has severe vomiting, hypoglycemia, shock, or other sign of adrenal insufficiency; and (4) a boy with premature virilization or a girl with virilization of any degree and at any age.

The sine qua non of this disorder is an elevated plasma 17-hydroxyprogesterone value. Unfortunately, cord blood levels of 17-hydroxyprogesterone (and dehydroepiandrosterone) are high (as is urinary 17-ketosteroid secretion in the first week after birth), and in the first 24 hours of life, 17-hydroxyprogesterone values may be misleadingly elevated in normal children. Thereafter, classical patients are diagnosed by 17-hydroxyprogesterone values of greater than 3000 ng/dL. Twenty-four-hour urinary 17-ketosteroid (or pregnanetriol) is difficult to collect in a neonate, and since values are elevated in the first week of life of normal newborns because of persisting fetal adrenal activity, this test is usually unnecessary if a reliable laboratory can quickly perform a plasma 17-hydroxyprogesterone determination. (Sendout laboratories should always be able to do this.) Sodium and potassium should be monitored daily for the first 2 weeks of life and repetitively, but less frequently, for another 2 weeks if 21-OH deficiency is suspected. A plasma renin activity at 7 days of age is helpful, but values are usually not quickly available from the laboratory. While missing the diagnosis of salt loss can cause fatal complications, extreme difficulties are caused by incorrect assignment of salt-losing status. Because the suppressed adrenal gland may be slow to restore mineralocorticoid secretion, a baby treated for months unnecessarily with mineralocorticoids may require more weeks or months of careful weaning from mineralocorticoids before it can be established that the child does not have a salt-losing disorder. (See pp 59, 180, 465, 467.)

Older patients suspected of having 21-OH deficiency will require plasma 17-hydroxyprogesterone and plasma renin determinations, but suspected late onset or cryptic cases may require ACTH stimulation to demonstrate an elevated response of 17-hydroxyprogesterone in the face of normal resting values. A bone age is also essential. In long-untreated cases, sellar erosion by a pituitary gland secreting excess ACTH may be seen on lateral skull x-ray or CT scan. The sella will usually remineralize as glucocorticoid therapy suppresses ACTH secretion and reduces pituitary size.

2. Treatment–Glucocorticoid replacement sufficient to suppress ACTH secretion but not so high as to suppress growth is the aim of therapy. Intramuscular cortisone acetate ($14 \text{ mg/m}^2/\text{d}$ every 3 days) or oral liquid hydrocortisone ($18 \text{ mg/m}^2/\text{d}$ divided into 3 doses) is a starting point for therapy in newborns, but individual variation in metabolism and absorption of glucocorticoids necessitates fine tuning of dosage by growth rate, bone age advancement, plasma testosterone, and 17-hydroxyprogesterone determinations. Table 2–1 contains suggested dosages of glucocorticoid preparations. There is little justification for the use of any preparation other than cortisone acetate or hydrocortisone during the growing years. After epiphyseal fusion, appropriate doses of longer acting synthetic glucocorticoids may be useful to ensure regular menses in female patients. The serum testosterone should be maintained below 10 ng/dL. Growth rate should be normal and is monitored by plotting height measurements every 3 months on a growth chart. Excessive growth suggests continued androgen secretion, and decreased growth indicates excessive glucocorticoid dosing. Bone age (determined yearly) should advance 1 year for each year of chronological age progression. Urinary 17-ketosteroids

Table 2–1. Dosages of glucocorticoid preparations.*

	Actual dose† in mg/m²/24 hr	Equivalent Dose‡
Dexamethasone§	0.23	1
Methylprednisolone	2.4	10
Prednisone	3.7	16
Hydrocortisone	18.4	80
Cortisone acetate (intramuscular)	13.9	60
Cortisone acetate (by mouth)	22.0	96

* Reproduced with permission from Styne et al in Lee PA et al: *Congenital Adrenal Hyper-*

plasia. University Park Press, 1977.

† *Actual dose* refers to the usual dose required in congenital adrenal hyperplasia to best achieve normal growth.

‡ *Equivalent dose* refers to the dose of glucocorticoid preparations equivalent to 1 mg dexamethasone.

§ Individual variation occurs. Certain drugs (such as phenytoin) accelerate the metabolism of dexamethasone, decreasing its potency.

should be in the high normal range for age, and plasma 17-hydroxyprogesterone should be about 200–300 ng/dL (a bit higher than normal) measured 2 hours after the morning cortisol dose. Overtreatment during puberty may suppress the pubertal growth spurt. The normal secretion of pubertal androgens during adolescence will complicate evaluation of therapy during this period.

Salt losers must receive mineralocorticoid and extra dietary salt. Deoxycorticosterone acetate (DOCA) is given to newborns in doses of 0.5–1 mg/d intramuscularly. (At the time of this writing, DOCA is no longer available.) 9α-Fluorohydrocortisone, 0.05–0.15 mg/d is given orally; the dose varies with age, plasma sodium and potassium levels, and blood pressure. Mineralocorticoid cannot work without adequate salt intake; infants need 1–2 gm/d of extra table salt added to their formula (mark a few test tubes with a line indicating the amount of salt to give), while older children will crave salt and usually add enough to their food. Too little salt impairs the mineralocorticoid effect and too much causes hypertension; hypertensive crisis is possible, and blood pressure must be carefully monitored.

Inadequate sodium or mineralocorticoid in salt-losing patients may be interpreted as stress by the body and result in increased ACTH secretion causing increased androgen secretion. Thus, the patient with poorly controlled androgen production on a given dose of glucocorticoid may require more mineralocorticoid rather than more glucocorticoid; elevated plasma renin activity may be the clue to this situation.

Patients should receive 3 times the normal dose of glucocorticoid if they have a fever (> 37.5°C). If vomiting, they must be given parenteral glucocorticoid, glucose, salt, and mineralocorticoid (if needed). In emergency situations, hydrocortisone sodium succinate should be given subcutaneously, intramuscularly, or preferably intravenously. Intramuscular cortisone acetate will not exert an effect until hours after administration and cannot be used for emergencies. Parents should be instructed in the administration of 50–100 mg of hydrocortisone sodium succinate intramuscularly or subcutaneously for emergencies (auto or sports accidents, sudden shock) and keep several bottles, syringes, and needles at hand. Unnecessary acute glucocorticoid administration is not harmful, but absence of glucocorticoids in the face of shock can lead to death.

A vomiting or shocky patient requires immediate intravenous glucocorticoid and sugar (a 50-mg bolus of hydrocortisone sodium succinate followed by 5% or more dextrose/normal saline with 50–100 mg hydrocortisone sodium succinate in the bottle is an appropriate start). DOCA, 1 mg, or 0.05–0.1 mg orally every 12 hours can be given intramuscularly every 12–24 hours to assist in salt retention. Blood pressure and serum sodium and potassium levels must be watched carefully and the calculated deficit of sodium and water replaced. Too much salt and DOCA will cause hypertension while too little will allow shock to recur. Patients and parents should have a copy of such instructions to give to an emergency room doctor for rapid action if necessary. A medical alert bracelet is also highly recommended.

Patients being prepared for surgery need special care. A bolus of 50 mg of hydrocortisone sodium succinate should be given intravenously before anesthesia and 50 mg/m^2/d given in doses every 4 hours. Normal or half-normal saline with glucose must be given, and if the patient is a salt loser, DOCA or oral fluorohydricortisone is used. If complications ensue, the dosage is kept high. If not, the patient can be quickly tapered to the regular dose of glucocorticoids as soon as oral feeding is resumed.

Patients with other forms of congenital adrenal hyperplasia receive glucocorticoids in a manner similar to treatment of 21-hydroxylase deficiency except that, rather than 17-hydroxyprogesterone, the precursor steroid to the particular enzymatic block is elevated in the untreated state and is suppressed by glucocorticoid therapy.

C. 11β-Hydroxylase (11β-OH) P-450c11 Deficiency: Affected patients cannot convert 11-deoxycortisol to cortisol and have elevated plasma 11-deoxycortisol, androgens, and deoxycorticosterone (DOC) levels, leading to virilization, salt-retention, hypokalemia, and alkalosis. Affected females have ambiguous genitalia and hypertension. Some affected females being raised as males may present with pubic hair or gynecomastia.

Males look normal at birth but virilize soon afterward and develop hypertension. Gynecomastia has been described in affected young boys.

D. 3β-Hydroxysteroid Dehydrogenase (3β-HSD) Deficiency: This form of congenital adrenal hyperplasia occurs with variable manifestations. Complete deficiency precludes the production of glucocorticoids and mineralocorticoids with the resulting build-up of the weak androgen dehydroepiandrosterone (DHA). Affected females have a normal phenotype or clitorimegaly with partial labial fusion. Males have incomplete masculinization, ranging from hypospadias to lack of labioscrotal fusion, and the full appearance of ambiguous genitalia. Salt loss can be life threatening by the first week after birth. Diagnosis is made by evidence of salt losing in the presence of elevated plasma DHA or DHA sulfate and urinary 17-ketosteroids with a normal or low plasma 17-hydroxyprogesterone level.

E. Maternally Ingested Androgens & Dysmorphic Syndromes: Mothers taking androgens (including progestins of androgen derivation, eg, oral contraceptives) run the risk of virilizing their female fetuses. Some dysmorphic syndromes or teratologic agents can cause an appearance of ambiguous genitalia.

True Hermaphrodites (Usually 46,XX)

Hermaphrodites have both testicular and ovarian tissue present. They most frequently have both types of gonadal tissue bilaterally as ovotestes but may have an ovary on one side and a testis on the other or other variations. The testicular tissue has variable production of MIF, and therefore müllerian derivatives may be partially suppressed on one side but not the other; usually a uterus is present, and although it may be hypoplasic, it can exhibit menstrual bleeding if appropriately stimulated at puberty.

Karyotype is usually 46,XX but may be 46,XY (a presumed undetected chimerism with a 46,XX cell line) or 46,XX/46,XY (chimera).

Physical examination usually reveals ambiguous genitalia, although hermaphrodites may have a male or female phenotype. They are distinguished from patients with congenital adrenal hyperplasia by the absence of elevation of precursor steroids. The ovarian portion of the gonads may retain some normal function and cause breast development and menstruation at puberty. The testicular portion may secrete androgens but is usually dysgenetic and may undergo malignant degeneration into gonadoblastoma, dysgerminoma, seminoma, or teratoma; thus, gonadectomy of abnormal testicular tissue is recommended. Patients are usually raised as females because of the greater ability to achieve a good cosmetic effect in genital reconstruction.

46,XY Karyotype: Male Pseudohermaphroditism (Testes Often Palpable)

A child with a 46,XY (male) genotype, testicular but not ovarian tissue, and ambiguous genitalia has male pseudohermaphroditism. It is usually caused by decreased effects of testosterone rather than excess estrogen. This situation may be due to (1) inability to produce testosterone, (2) inability to convert testosterone to dihydrotestosterone, or (3) resistance to androgen action. These disorders are discussed below in order of frequency.

A. Microphallus: A newborn penile stretched length < 2.5 cm is 2 SD below the mean length for age and is classified as a microphallus. Early in gestation, the fetal testes are stimulated by hCG; afterward fetal pituitary luteinizing hormone (LH) secretion is necessary. After sexual differentiation of the male genitalia at 13 weeks, testosterone must be present for normal penis length to occur. In patients with gonadotropin-releasing hormone (GnRH) deficiency, LH secretion does not occur and microphallus results. Often growth hormone (GH) deficiency is present as well as GnRH deficiency in such children; GH deficiency can, by itself, cause microphallus. A fullterm male who has microphallus and hypoglycemic seizures must be considered to have GH deficiency with or without ACTH deficiency until it is proved otherwise. This condition cannot be expected to improve spontaneously, and definitive tests of hypothalamic-pituitary function are necessary in any patient with microphallus and hypoglycemia; hypopituitary patients may have undescended testes as well. Alternatively, isolated microphallus without hypoglycemia may be a dysmorphic event related to partial androgen resistance or may be associated with urologic anomalies such as epispadias.

The first step in diagnosis is assessment of testicular function. Baseline testosterone, 17-hydroxyprogesterone, DHA, and androstenedione are measured, and hCG (3000 U/m² intramuscularly 3 times a week for 6 doses) is given. Repeat serum sex steroid determinations are made at 72 hours after the first injection and 24 hours after the last. In a normal boy, testosterone will rise above 100 ng/dL and other metabolites will rise as well. If certain precursors rise higher than others, an enzymatic block is diagnosed. Undescended testes may descend with this regimen as well, indicating lack of necessity for surgical orchiopexy. Pubic hair growth is a potential side effect.

An abnormally small phallus due to GnRH deficiency will grow in breadth and length with 25-mg doses of testosterone enanthate intramuscularly monthly for 3 months. This treatment will not advance bone age excessively or cause other signs of virilization. Failure to respond suggests androgen resistance or, as is often the case in extrophy of the bladder, inadequate penile tissue to allow increased size with androgen treatment. A patient whose penis increases in size with testosterone can usually be raised as a normal male. Children with isolated GH deficiency and microphallus will have further penile enlargement with GH therapy. Testosterone-resistant patients with microphallus may be candidates for castration and female sex assignment.

B. XY Gonadal Dysgenesis: These patients are phenotypically female (clitorimegaly and even ambiguous genitalia are possible) with normal or tall stature, eunuchoid habitus, and a 46,XY karyotype. The gonads may be streak or dysgenetic testes with the possibility of some testosterone secretory ability. Gonadectomy is indicated if functioning testicular tissue is present to prevent malignant degeneration.

C. Congenital Enzyme Deficiencies: See also Table 2–2.

1. 17α-Hydroxylase (17α-OH) P-450c17 Deficiency– Deficiency of this enzyme impairs the production of cortisol and sex steroids but allows excessive concentrations of corticosterone and DOC; aldosterone is not formed because DOC causes salt retention, hypertension, and therefore suppression of renin. Female patients retain a normal female phenotype, but males have ambiguous genitalia or a female phenotype depending on the degree of block. Diagnosis rests upon the finding of hypertension, hypokalemic alkalosis, elevated plasma progesterone, pregnenolone, corticosterone, and DOC levels, and decreased plasma renin, 17-hydroxyprogesterone, and aldosterone levels in patients with female or ambiguous genitalia. Some patients are not diagnosed until lack of pubertal progession becomes apparent and may present as sexually infantile girls with primary amenorrhea.

2. 17β-Ketosteroid Reductase (17β-HSO) Deficiency–Males with this disorder cannot convert androstenedione to testosterone (or estrone to estradiol) and at birth have female or ambiguous genitalia. MIF is present and müllerian structures absent while wolffian ducts are present; there is a blind vaginal pouch and undescended or inguinal

Table 2–2. Manifestations of steroid enzyme defects.

| Defect | Phenotype | | Post-natal Virili-zation | Salt-losing | Hypo-kalemia | Hyper-tension |
	XY Karyotype	XX Karyotype				
Side-chain cleavage enzyme (20,22 desmolase) deficiency	Infantile female	Infantile female	−	+	−	−
3β-HSD deficiency	Ambiguous	Female or ambiguous	+	+	−	−
17α-OH deficiency	Infantile female	Infantile female	−	−	+	+
11β-OH deficiency	Male	Ambiguous	+	−	+	+
21-OH deficiency	Male	Ambiguous	+	+ in 50%	−	−

testes. At puberty, incomplete virilization and gynecomastia will result.

3. 17,20-Desmolase (Lyase) P-450c17 Deficiency–Affected males produce MIF, which causes regression of müllerian structures; inability to convert 17-hydroxyprogesterone to androstenedione and 17-hydroxypregnenolone to DHA limits testosterone production, and female or ambiguous genitalia result with undescended or inguinal testes. Measurement of the ratio of the metabolites listed above indicates the diagnosis. At puberty, patients may incompletely virilize.

4. Side-Chain Cleavage Enzyme (20,22-Desmolase) P-450scc Deficiency–Deficiency of this enzyme precludes production of any steroid compounds and results in large lipid-laden adrenal glands that may cause inferior displacement of the kidneys on an intravenous pyelogram study. Since no steroids are produced by adrenal glands or gonads, in the full manifestation of the deficiency, regardless of genotype, infants usually have a female phenotype; partial deficiency in a male can cause ambiguous genitalia and partial virilization. Phenotype is female in 46,XX babies. No steroids are measureable in urine or blood. Death may occur owing to glucocorticoid deficiency or salt loss and potassium retention because of mineralocorticoid deficiency. This is a rare autosomal recessive defect. All reported male patients have been raised as girls; replacement estrogen therapy can be given at puberty. The testes in XY babies are usually intra-abdominal and should be resected to prevent malignant degeneration.

5. 5α-Reductase Deficiency–A fascinating family of patients reared as ''girls'' who later became ''men'' was described in the Dominican Republic; similar patients have been found in North America and elsewhere. Ambiguous genitalia with small phallus, hypospadias, cordee, bifid scrotum, and urogenital sinus are seen at birth. Müllerian structures are absent, and wolffian structures are normal. At puberty, the scrotum becomes pigmented, testes descend, the penis enlarges, and spermatogenesis occurs. In addition, muscle mass increases and the voice deepens, but there is no acne, temporal hair recession, or gynecomastia. Gender role changes have been well documented from female to male although the expectations of parents of these abnormal appearing ''girls'' who historically are known to virilize at puberty may be different from those of parents of girls in other environments. Likewise, the privileged social position of males in the village may ease the transition to a male gender role. However, this disorder challenges the hypothesis that gender role is determined in the first 18 months of age.

The defect has been biochemically defined as a deficiency of 5α-reductase and therefore an inability to convert testosterone to dihydrotestosterone in skin. The virilization at puberty is not well explained but may be due to increased testosterone levels causing direct effects on the dihydrotestosterone receptor. The lack of acne, hirsutism, and temporal hair recession indicates that these may be dihydro-testosterone-specific effects that cannot occur even with increased testosterone.

Laboratory evaluation will reveal a high plasma T/DHT ratio postpubertally (ratio greater than 18) or prepubertally before (ratio greater than 17) or after (ratio more than 8 before age 6 months and ratio more than 19 from age 6 months to 14 years) hCG stimulation.

D. Incomplete Androgen Resistance: Phenotypes in these heterogeneous conditions range from infertility in a normal male to hypoplastic male genitalia to frank ambiguity. Müllerian duct development is inhibited by MIF, but wolffian ducts are hypoplastic. Gynecomastia (less than in complete resistance) and pubic and axillary hair development (more than in complete resistance) is usual at puberty. Reifenstein's syndrome fits in this classification.

This disorder is X linked and 2 types are described: (1) decreased androgen receptor levels and (2) normal androgen receptors and a presumptive postreceptor defect. During pubertal years, LH and testosterone levels are high, whereas follicle-stimulating hormone (FSH) levels are usually normal.

E. Testicular Unresponsiveness to hCG and LH: Rare 46,XY males have been described who have no apparent ability to respond to hCG or fetal pituitary LH and therefore have ambiguous genitalia or male phenotype.

F. Defects of Testicular Development: Abnormalities of renal development may be accompanied by dysgenetic testicular development. Defective gonadal development may occur because of XY gonadal dysgenesis or XO/XY mosaicism.

SURGICAL REPAIR

Plastic surgical repair of ambiguous genitalia should occur before 1 year of age. It is best to perform clitoral recession rather than clitorectomy, to preserve sensation in the area. Long-term psychological support by counselors or the treating physician should stress the likelihood of a good psychosocial outcome in these patients to their parents.

POSTNATAL VIRILIZATION IN A PHENOTYPIC FEMALE

A child who has a normal female phenotype at birth but who later develops clitoral enlargement, muscular development, pubic hair, and even a deepening voice has been exposed to excessive androgens.

Ingestion of exogenous sources of androgens is rare unless a member of the household has been prescribed testosterone, but some geriatric vitamins have contained androgens and must be considered as a source. Endogenous androgens may rise in a girl with late-onset congenital adrenal hyperplasia or adrenal carcinoma (which may also produce signs of Cushing's syndrome). An arrhenoblastoma, a lipoid tumor of the ovary, or a gonadoblastoma are rare sources of androgen secretion. Disorders limited to phenotypic females that cause virilization at puberty include 17-oxidoreductase deficiency and 17-20 desmolase deficiency. 5α-Reductase deficiency and incomplete androgen resistance usually present with some degree of ambiguous genitalia, but virilization does occur at puberty.

SHOCK & HYPONATREMIA IN THE NEWBORN WITHOUT AMBIGUOUS GENITALIA

Shock in the Normal Male Infant

A boy with salt-losing 21-hydroxylase deficiency congenital adrenal hyperplasia will be born with a normal male phenotype and may not be suspected of having the disease. Although the family may include siblings that died of unknown causes in infancy, the diagnosis may still be missed. Because weight loss and vomiting leading to shock is the usual presentation, pyloric stenosis is often diagnosed (and sometimes incorrectly surgically treated). An electrolyte determination will indicate hyponatremia and hyperkalemia, and a blood glucose measurement will demonstrate hypoglycemia. A non-salt-losing male with 21-hydroxylase deficiency who has intercurrent illness may go into hypoglycemic shock, but an immediate diagnosis may not be possible due to the time required for steroid determination; if non-salt-losing adrenal hyperplasia is suspected, blood should be drawn for 17-hydroxyprogesterone and 11-deoxycortisol measurements before glucocorticoids are administered.

Shock in the "Normal Female" Infant

Adrenal 3β-HSD deficiency (more common) as well as side-chain cleavage enzyme (20,22-desmolase) deficiency (rare) can produce shock and hyponatremia in a newborn with ambiguous or female genitalia. Glucocorticoid deficiency and shock can occur in 17α-hydroxylase deficiency. Such infants may have female or ambiguous phenotype owing to relative or complete lack of androgens during intrauterine development; the karyotype may be 46,XX or 46,XY.

REFERENCES

Amrhein JA et al: Androgen insensitivity in man: Evidence for genetic heterogeneity. *Proc Natl Acad Sci USA* 1976;**73:**891.

Burstein S, Grumbach MM, Kaplan SL: Androgen responsiveness is important in the management of microphallus. *Lancet* 1979;**2:**983.

Chrousos GP et al: Late-onset 21-hydroxylase deficiency mimicking idiopathic hirsutism or polycystic ovarian disease. *Ann Intern Med* 1982;**96:**143.

Conte FA, Grumbach MM: Pathogenesis, classification, diagnosis, and treatment of anomalies of sex. In: *Endocrinology*, 2nd ed. DeGroot L (editor). Grune & Stratton, 1988.

Ehrhardt AA, Meyer-Bahlberg HFL: Prenatal sex hormones and the developing brain: Effects on psychosexual differentiation and cognitive function. *Annu Rev Med* 1979;**30:**415.

Griffin JE, Wilson JD: The syndromes of androgen resistance. *N Engl J Med* 1980;**302:**198.

Grumbach MM, Conte FA: Disorders of sex differentiation. In: *Endocrinology* Wilson JO, Foster DW (editors). Saunders 1991.

Hochberg Z et al: Growth and pubertal development in patients with cogenital adrenal hyperplasia due to 11β-hydroxylase deficiency. *Am J Dis Child* 1985;**139:**771.

Imperato-McGinley JL et al: Androgens and the evolution of male-gender identity among male pseudohermaphrodites with 5α-reductase deficiency. *N Engl J Med* 1979;**300:**1233.

Josso N: Antimüllerian hormone: New perspectives for a sexist molecule. *Endocr Rev* 1986;**7:**421.

Manual M, Katayama KP, Jones HW Jr: The age of occurrence of gonadal tumors in intersex patients with a Y chromosome. *Am J Obstet Gynecol* 1976;**124:**293.

Money J, Ehrhardt AA: *Man and Woman, Boy and Girl: The Differentiation and Dimorphism of Gender Identity from Conception to Maturity.* Johns Hopkins, 1972.

New MI et al: The adrenal hyperplasias. In: *The Metabolic Basis of Inherited Disease*, 6th ed. Scriver CR, Bendet AL, Sly WS et al (editors). McGraw-Hill, 1989.

Palmer MS et al: Genetic evidence that ZFY is not the testis determining factor. *Nature* 1989;**342:**937.

Page DC et al: The sex-determining region of the human Y chromosome encodes a finger protein. *Cell* 1987;**51:**1091.

Richards GE et al: Plasma sex steroids and gonadotropins in pubertal girls with congenital adrenal hyperplasia: Relationship to menstrual disorders. Pages 287–296 in: *Congenital Adrenal Hyperplasia.* Lee PA et al (editors). University Park Press, 1977.

Saenger P: Abnormal sexual differentiation. *J Pediatr* 1984;**104:**1.

Schneider G et al: Persistent testicular Δ5-isomerase-3β-hydroxysteroid dehydrogenase (Δ5-3βHSD) deficiency in the Δ5-3β-HSD form of congenital adrenal hyperplasia. *J Clin Invest* 1975;**55:**681.

Simpson JL: *Disorders of Sexual Differentiation: Etiology and Clinical Delineation.* Academic Press, 1977.

Styne DM: The Testes: Disorders of the sexual differentiation and puberty. In: *Clinical Peadiatric Endocrinology*, 2nd ed. Kaplan, SA (editor). Saunders, 1989.

Styne DM et al: Growth patterns in congenital adrenal hyperplasia correlation of glucocorticoid therapy with stature. Pages 247–261 in: *Congenital Adrenal Hyperplasia*. Lee PA et al (editors). University Park Press, 1977.

Wachtel SS: The genetics of intersexuality: Clinical and theoretic perspectives. *Obstet Gynecol* 1979;**54:**671.

Wilson JD, et al: The androgen resistance syndromes. In: *The Metabolic Basis of Inherited Disease*, 6th ed. Scriver CR, Beaudet AL, Sly WS (editors). McGraw-Hill, 1989.

Wilson JD, Griffen JE: Disorders of sexual differentiation. In: Braunwald E, et al, eds. *Harrison's Principles of Internal Medicine*, 11th ed. McGraw-Hill, 1989.

Wischusen J, Baker HWG, Hudson B: Reversible male infertility due to congenital adrenal hyperplasia. *Clin Endocrinol* 1981;**14:**571.

Yanase T, et al: 17 alpha-hydroxylase/17, 20-lyase deficiency: from clinical investigation to molecular definition. *Endocr Rev* 1991;**12:**91–108.

Growth Disorders | 3

Dennis M. Styne, MD

PHYSIOLOGY OF NORMAL GROWTH

In utero, the major known stimulant to fetal growth is fetal insulin secretion, although increasing evidence implicates various growth factors. Gender and other genetic factors also influence intrauterine growth. Maternal good health is necessary for optimal fetal development.

Following birth, proper nutrition, emotional support, and good health are important; growth hormone, thyroid hormone, and insulin are all required for proper childhood growth. These hormones are postulated to stimulate growth by stimulating somatomedin production or receptors.

The somatomedins, or insulinlike growth factors, are growth hormone–dependent peptides. IGF-I (somatomedin C) appears to stimulate linear growth in childhood; it is increased by growth hormone, thyroid hormone, insulin, prolactin, and androgen. IGF-I is decreased by poor nutrition, advancing age, and deficiencies of the latter hormones. IGF-II may stimulate fetal growth, but its postnatal role is not yet clear.

Somatomedins were once postulated to be secreted entirely by the liver but are now thought to be secreted by multiple tissues including the proliferating chondrocyte cells at epiphyseal growth areas. In fact, somatomedins may be paracrine factors that cause effects locally in their organs of production. The serum levels of somatomedins may thus only represent 'spillover' into the circulation of somatomedin that is locally produced and locally active. Since circulating somatomedins are bound to proteins, they have an increased plasma half-life compared with the free form. (See Chapter 1.)

RATES OF GROWTH

Genetic, economic, and psychosocial factors and chronic disease as well as endocrine disorders can affect growth rate and ultimate height. Accurate measurements of stature and weight should be taken and plotted on a growth chart every time a child is examined, to detect early or subtle disorders.

MEASUREMENT OF GROWTH

The accurate determination and plotting of height and weight may furnish important information in the diagnosis of a condition; if a patient should develop a chronic disorder, a change in slope in a previously normal growth curve may indicate the onset of the disease.

Although the bars used to measure height on commonly used platform scales are convenient, they are useless for accurate height determination. Height must be measured with the child's back to a flat surface, with *bare feet* together flat on the ground, and with the height at the top of the head indicated by a flat horizontal surface exactly perpendicular to the wall. A Harpenden stadiometer can accurately perform this task but is costly. A simpler device may be made of a square block of wood that slides in a groove or track to keep its lower surface parallel to the floor and perpendicular to the wall. If an accurate metal tape measure is attached to the wall parallel to (or within) the groove, reproducible height determinations can be made between the top of the head and the floor. The Ross and Genentech companies have provided pediatricians in the USA with accurate plastic measuring devices.

Children under 2 years of age are measured supine, and *two people are required for an accurate determination*! An infantometer or similar device should be used so that the infant can be gently stretched to full length with a measurement made from a point perpendicular to the head to another point perpendicular to the feet.

Reproducibility of measurements is more important than absolute accuracy in actual height; growth rate can be calculated from multiple determinations over time on the same device. If measurements are obtained from different devices, systematic errors may be introduced into the determination. Measurements should be made in centimeters, since the gradations are smaller than inches (0.5 in = 1.27 cm, and this represents one-quarter year of normal growth; rounding off by 0.5 in will significantly affect accuracy).

INTERPRETATION OF GROWTH

Height measurements must be interpreted and compared to the mean for age rather than simply recorded in a blank in the patient file. In the USA, height is usually expressed in percentiles (Fig 3–1), and children below the fifth percentile are considered abnormal. However, statistically, 5 of 100 children are normally below the fifth percentile and do not need evaluation. Height velocity, expressed in cm/yr is a better reflection of growth; standards are available and vary with age (Fig 3–2), but as a rule, a growth rate of less than 4.5 cm/yr between age 4 years and the onset of puberty is abnormal. The normal growth curves for refugee oriental children are about 2 SD below US curves. Height can also be interpreted with relation to midparental height (the average of father's and mother's heights) between ages 2 and 9 years; this narrows the range of comparisons from all children of a given age to the expected height of children whose midparental heights are equal to that of the child being evaluated.

A child may be suspected of an abnormality of growth if the height is well below the fifth percentile, if the growth rate is abnormally low, or if the child's height is not appropriate for the parents' heights. If more than one of these three criteria are met, there should be even more suspicion of a problem.

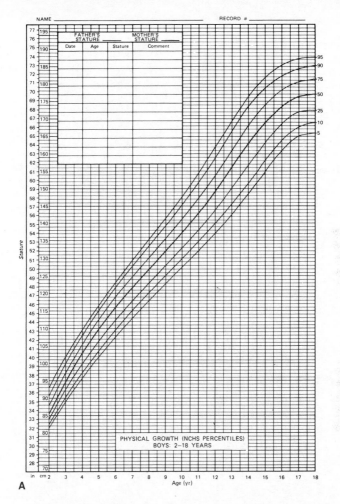

Figure 3–1. A. Growth chart for boys in the USA. [Redrawn and reprinted with permission of Ross Laboratories, Columbus, OH. © 1980 Ross Laboratories. Sources of data: 1976 study of the National Center for Health Statistics (NCHS: Hyattsville, MD); Hamill PVV et al: Physical growth: National Center for Health Statistics percentiles. *Am J Clin Nutr* 1979;**32:**607.] (*continued*)

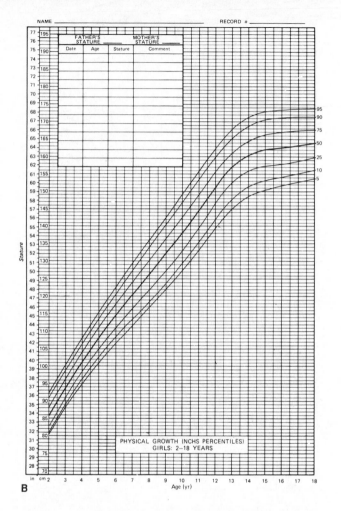

Figure 3–1. (cont'd). B. Growth chart for girls in the USA. [Redrawn and reprinted with permission of Ross Laboratories, Columbus, OH. © 1980 Ross Laboratories. Sources of data: 1976 study of the National Center for Health Statistics (NCHS: Hyattsville, MD); Hamill PVV et al: Physical growth: National Center for Health Statistics percentiles. *Am J Clin Nutr* 1979;**32**:607.]

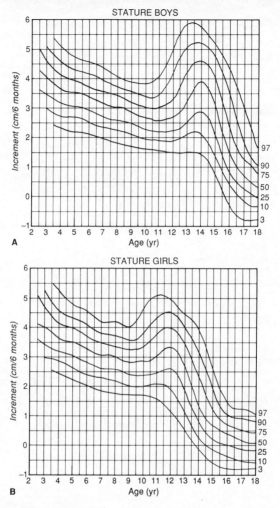

Figure 3–2. Incremental growth charts for boys **A** and girls **B**. Height velocity measured over a period of at least 6 months can be compared with the percentiles on the right axis of the charts. [Redrawn and reprinted with permission of Ross Laboratories, Columbus, OH 43216. © 1981 Ross Laboratories. Sources of data: Longitudinal studies of the Fels Research Laboratories (Yellow Springs, OH); Roche AF, Himes JH: Incremental growth charts. *Am J Clin Nutr* 1980;**33:**2041.]

Table 3–1. The RWT method for predicting adult stature.*

The Roche-Wainer-Thissen (RWT) method estimates adult stature of an individual from data recorded at a single childhood examination. It is considered more accurate than the Bayley-Pinneau method and makes use of Tables 3–4 and 3–5. The following predicts stature (standing height) at age 18 years. After this age, total increase in stature is 0.6 cm in girls and 0.8 cm in boys.

Recumbent length (in cm) of the child should be measured; if only standing height without shoes (stature) is available, 1.25 cm is added to stature to approximate recumbent length. **Nude weight** (kg) should be recorded. **Midparental stature** (cm) is determined by averaging the measured height of each parent without shoes; if a parent's stature is not available, a sex appropriate value for the population may be employed; for the USA these values are 174.5 cm (father) and 162 cm (mother). The **skeletal age** of the left wrist is assessed, bone by bone, using the Greulich-Pyle atlas; if more than half of these bones are adult, the RWT method is not applied. Prior to age 13 in boys and age 8 in girls, chronological age can be substituted for skeletal age for most normal children without endocrine or other disorders, but it is less accurate.

The prediction uses the following steps:
1. Record the child's data below.
2. Consult the appropriate table for either girls or boys (Tables 3–4 and 3–5).
3. For the child's age, record the positive or negative multipliers and adjustment factor.
4. Multiply data by multipliers to get positive or negative products.
5. From the summation of the products (subtotal), add or subtract the adjustment-factor height to predict stature at age 18. For final adult stature, add 0.6 cm for girls and 0.8 cm for boys.

Data		Multipliers		Products
Recumbent length (cm) _____	×	_____	=	_____
Weight (kg) _____	×	_____	=	_____
Midparental stature (cm) _____	×	_____	=	_____
Skeletal age (years) _____	×	_____	=	_____

Subtotal _____

Subtotal ± adjustment factor = Predicted height at age 18 (cm)

Conversions: cm = 2.54 × in.   kg = lb ÷ 2.205

* Reproduced, with permission, from Roche AF, Wainer H, Thissen D: The RWT method for the prediction of adult stature. *Pediatrics* 1975;**56**:1026.

SKELETAL AGE (BONE AGE)

The Greulich and Pyle atlas of radiographic development contains photographs of standard x-rays of hands and wrists at various ages. An average child will have a bone age within 2 SD (read from the atlas) of chronological age. While a delay or advance in bone age does not define a disease, a discrepancy between bone age and chronological age may be found in various disease states. Fusion of epiphyses is effectively complete at a bone age of 15 years in girls and 17 years in boys; the lower a bone age is compared with these limits, the more remaining growth is available to a child. Thus, a moderately delayed bone age in a short child may induce optimism with regard to expected final height and need not suggest a disease.

HEIGHT PREDICTION

The combination of accurate height measurement and bone age can be used to predict adult height by the use of the Bailey-Pinneau tables, which are found at the end of the Greulich and Pyle atlas. Accuracy of prediction improves as a patient reaches the last few years of growth, but estimates can be made after a bone age of 6 years is reached. The Roche-Wainer-Thissen method (Table 3–1) incorporates patient weight and parental heights to improve the accuracy of prediction. The folk method of estimating final height by doubling the height at age 2 years does not take bone age or parental height into consideration and is inaccurate.

CHILDHOOD SHORT STATURE

EVALUATION OF CHILDHOOD SHORT STATURE

A detailed history, including familial heights and patterns of pubertal development, psychosocial history, and nutritional intake, and a physical examination including accurate height, upper to lower segment ratio, and arm span determinations are the essential first steps in diagnosing the cause of short stature. Evaluation for chronic disease or dysmorphology is important. If no diagnosis is suggested by this stage, screening laboratory tests are performed including urinary pH and concentrating ability, Hgb, Hct and sedimentation rate, and an SMA 20 determination with attention to serum bicarbonate, calcium,

Table 3–2. Tables of multipliers for prediction of adult stature in **boys** by RWT method. For use with Table 3–1.

Age (Yr)	(Mo)	Recumbent length	Weight	Midparental stature	Skeletal age	Adjustment factor
1	0	0.966	0.199	0.606	− 0.673	1.632
1	3	1.032	0.086	0.580	− 0.417	− 1.841
1	6	1.086	− 0.016	0.559	− 0.205	− 4.892
1	9	1.130	− 0.106	0.540	− 0.033	− 7.528
2	0	1.163	− 0.186	0.523	0.104	− 9.764
2	3	1.189	− 0.256	0.509	0.211	− 11.618
2	6	1.207	− 0.316	0.496	0.291	− 13.114
2	9	1.219	− 0.369	0.485	0.349	− 14.278
3	0	1.227	− 0.413	0.475	0.388	− 15.139
3	3	1.230	− 0.450	0.466	0.410	− 15.729
3	6	1.229	− 0.481	0.458	0.419	− 16.081
3	9	1.226	− 0.505	0.451	0.417	− 16.228
4	0	1.221	− 0.523	0.444	0.405	− 16.201
4	3	1.214	− 0.537	0.437	0.387	− 16.034
4	6	1.206	− 0.546	0.431	0.363	− 15.758
4	9	1.197	− 0.550	0.424	0.335	− 15.400
5	0	1.188	− 0.551	0.418	0.303	− 14.990
5	3	1.179	− 0.548	0.412	0.269	− 14.551
5	6	1.169	− 0.543	0.406	0.234	− 14.106
5	9	1.160	− 0.535	0.400	0.198	− 13.672
6	0	1.152	− 0.524	0.394	0.161	− 13.267
6	3	1.143	− 0.512	0.389	0.123	− 12.901
6	6	1.135	− 0.499	0.383	0.085	− 12.583
6	9	1.127	− 0.484	0.378	0.046	− 12.318
7	0	1.120	− 0.468	0.373	0.006	− 12.107
7	3	1.113	− 0.451	0.369	− 0.034	− 11.948
7	6	1.106	− 0.434	0.365	− 0.077	− 11.834
7	9	1.100	− 0.417	0.361	− 0.121	− 11.756
8	0	1.093	− 0.400	0.358	− 0.167	− 11.701
8	3	1.086	− 0.382	0.356	− 0.217	− 11.652
8	6	1.079	− 0.365	0.354	− 0.270	− 11.592
8	9	1.071	− 0.349	0.353	− 0.327	− 11.498
9	0	1.063	− 0.333	0.353	− 0.389	− 11.349
9	3	1.054	− 0.317	0.353	− 0.455	− 11.118
9	6	1.044	− 0.303	0.355	− 0.527	− 10.779
9	9	1.033	− 0.289	0.357	− 0.605	− 10.306
10	0	1.021	− 0.276	0.360	− 0.690	− 9.671
10	3	1.008	− 0.263	0.363	− 0.781	− 8.848
10	6	0.993	− 0.252	0.368	− 0.878	− 7.812
10	9	0.977	− 0.241	0.373	− 0.983	− 6.540
11	0	0.960	− 0.231	0.378	− 1.094	− 5.010
11	3	0.942	− 0.222	0.384	− 1.211	− 3.206
11	6	0.923	− 0.213	0.390	− 1.335	− 1.113
11	9	0.902	− 0.206	0.397	− 1.464	1.273

(continued)

Table 3–2. (Continued)

Age (Yr)	(Mo)	Recumbent length	Weight	Midparental stature	Skeletal age	Adjustment factor
12	0	0.881	−0.198	0.403	−1.597	3.958
12	3	0.859	−0.191	0.409	−1.735	6.931
12	6	0.837	−0.184	0.414	−1.875	10.181
12	9	0.815	−0.177	0.418	−2.015	13.684
13	0	0.794	−0.170	0.421	−2.156	17.405
13	3	0.773	−0.163	0.422	−2.294	21.297
13	6	0.755	−0.155	0.422	−2.427	25.304
13	9	0.738	−0.146	0.418	−2.553	29.349
14	0	0.724	−0.136	0.412	−2.668	33.345
14	3	0.714	−0.125	0.401	−2.771	37.183
14	6	0.709	−0.112	0.387	−2.856	40.738
14	9	0.709	−0.098	0.367	−2.922	43.869
15	0	0.717	−0.081	0.342	−2.962	46.403
15	3	0.732	−0.062	0.310	−2.973	48.154
15	6	0.756	−0.040	0.271	−2.949	48.898
15	9	0.792	−0.015	0.223	−2.885	48.402
16	0	0.839	−0.014	0.167	−2.776	46.391

Table 3–3. Tables of multipliers for prediction of adult stature in **girls** by RWT method. For use with Table 3–1.

Age (Yr)	(Mo)	Recumbent length	Weight	Midparental stature	Skeletal age	Adjustment factor
1	0	1.087	−0.271	0.386	0.434	21.729
1	3	1.112	−0.369	0.367	0.094	20.684
1	6	1.134	−0.455	0.349	−0.172	19.957
1	9	1.153	−0.530	0.332	−0.374	19.463
2	0	1.170	−0.594	0.316	−0.523	19.131
2	3	1.183	−0.648	0.301	−0.625	18.905
2	6	1.195	−0.693	0.287	−0.690	18.740
2	9	1.204	−0.729	0.274	−0.725	18.604
3	0	1.210	−0.757	0.262	−0.736	18.474
3	3	1.215	−0.777	0.251	−0.729	18.337
3	6	1.217	−0.791	0.241	−0.711	18.187
3	9	1.217	−0.798	0.232	−0.684	18.024
4	0	1.215	−0.800	0.224	−0.655	17.855
4	3	1.212	−0.797	0.217	−0.626	17.691
4	6	1.206	−0.789	0.210	−0.600	17.548
4	9	1.199	−0.777	0.205	−0.582	17.444
5	0	1.190	−0.761	0.200	−0.571	17.398
5	3	1.180	−0.742	0.197	−0.572	17.431
5	6	1.168	−0.721	0.193	−0.584	17.567
5	9	1.155	−0.697	0.191	−0.609	17.826
6	0	1.140	−0.671	0.190	−0.647	18.229
6	3	1.124	−0.644	0.189	−0.700	18.796
6	6	1.107	−0.616	0.188	−0.766	19.544
6	9	1.089	−0.587	0.189	−0.845	20.489

(continued)

Table 3–3. (Continued)

Age (Yr)	(Mo)	Recumbent length	Weight	Midparental stature	Skeletal age	Adjustment factor
7	0	1.069	−0.557	0.189	−0.938	21.642
7	3	1.049	−0.527	0.191	−1.043	23.011
7	6	1.028	−0.498	0.192	−1.158	24.602
7	9	1.006	−0.468	0.194	−1.284	26.416
8	0	0.938	−0.439	0.196	−1.418	28.448
8	3	0.960	−0.411	0.199	−1.558	30.690
8	6	0.937	−0.384	0.202	−1.704	33.129
8	9	0.914	−0.359	0.204	−1.853	35.747
9	0	0.891	−0.334	0.207	−2.003	38.520
9	3	0.868	−0.311	0.210	−2.154	41.421
9	6	0.845	−0.289	0.212	−2.301	44.415
9	9	0.824	−0.269	0.214	−2.444	47.464
10	0	0.803	−0.250	0.216	−2.581	50.525
10	3	0.783	−0.233	0.217	−2.710	53.548
10	6	0.766	−0.217	0.217	−2.829	56.481
10	9	0.749	−0.203	0.217	−2.936	59.267
11	0	0.736	−0.190	0.216	−3.029	61.841
11	3	0.724	−0.179	0.214	−3.108	84.136
11	6	0.716	−0.169	0.211	−3.171	66.093
11	9	0.711	−0.159	0.206	−3.217	67.627
12	0	0.710	−0.151	0.201	−3.245	68.670
12	3	0.713	−0.143	0.193	−3.254	69.140
12	6	0.720	−0.136	0.184	−3.244	68.966
12	9	0.733	−0.129	0.173	−3.214	68.061
13	0	0.752	−0.121	0.160	−3.166	66.339
13	3	0.777	−0.113	0.144	−3.100	63.728
13	6	0.810	−0.105	0.127	−3.015	60.150
13	9	0.850	−0.085	0.106	−2.915	55.522
14	0	0.898	−0.083	0.083	−2.800	49.781

phosphate, and alkaline phosphatase as well as liver and kidney function tests. Serum folate and carotene may reflect the ability to absorb fats. Antigliadin antibody determinations are suggested as a useful diagnostic technique in celiac disease and may eliminate the need for small-bowel biopsy. In cases still without diagnosis, a lateral skull x-ray may be performed to look for abnormalities including enlargement of the sella turcica or calcifications characteristic of craniopharyngioma. Bone age is not diagnostic but may be useful in estimating height prognosis even in a child under age 6. Short girls with no specific diagnosis should have a karyotype to rule out Turner's syndrome even in the absence of other stigmata of this syndrome.

CAUSES OF CHILDHOOD SHORT STATURE
(See Table 3–4.)

Small Newborns

Infants weighing less than 2500 g at birth are considered to be small. Commonly, such newborns are premature and have a weight that is appropriate for gestational age (AGA). It is essential to distinguish whether a newborn with low birthweight is AGA or small for gestational age (SGA). This is done by careful assessment of physical features and neurologic maturation.

Chronic maternal diseases, other environmental influences, and numerous syndromes can cause a baby to be SGA. Maternal causes include alcohol consumption of even moderate degree during pregnancy, smoking, eclampsia, and preeclampsia. Severe maternal malnutrition has a devastating effect on fetal growth; malnutrition may accompany systemic disease or be self-imposed via dieting. Maternal congestive heart failure, asthma, and other disorders may lead to poor growth even if nutrition is adequate.

Sex chromosomal and autosomal factors may affect fetal growth. Boys are larger than girls by the second trimester, and this sexual dichotomy is greater at birth. Patients with 45,XO gonadal dysgenesis are shorter than average at birth and remain so thereafter. A variety of other karyotypic abnormalities lead to small birth size, poor postnatal growth, and short adult stature.

Many dysmorphic syndromes, with or without karyotypic abnormalities, are associated with small birth size and short postnatal stature. One of the more common SGA syndromes is Russell-Silver syndrome; such infants are small with triangular shaped faces and, frequently, asymmetry of physical features (such as extremities) and clinodactyly (crooked fifth finger because of a triangular shape to the fifth medial phalyngeal bone).

Rubella, toxoplasmosis, and cytomegalovirus infections can cause small size as well as developmental abnormalities. Microcephaly, intracranial calcifications, and retinal pigmentation are characteristic of these infections.

Constitutional Delay in Growth

Constitutional delay in growth refers to the normal, healthy child who has a significant delay in physical maturation (reflected by delayed bone age) but no delay in mental maturation. This condition frequently is present in another family member. Puberty usually will be delayed for chronologic age but not for skeletal age. Short stature generally is moderate rather than severe, and the patient is customarily thin. History reveals a normal birthweight and length but a gradual decrease in percentiles of height compared with the mean between 1

Table 3–4. Causes of short stature.

Variations of normal
  Constitutional (delayed bone age)
  Genetic (short familial heights)

Endocrine disorders
  GH deficiency
    Congenital
      Isolated GH deficiency
      With other pituitary hormone
        deficiencies
      With midline defects
      Pituitary agenesis
    Acquired
      Hypothalamic/pituitary tumors
      Histiocytosis X
      CNS infections and
        granulomas
      Head trauma (birth and later)
      Hypothalamic/pituitary
        radiation
      CNS vascular accidents
      Hydrocephalus
      Psychosocial dwarfism
        (functional GH deficiency)
      Amphetamine treatment for
        hyperactivity
    Biologically inactive GH
    Laron's dwarfism (increased GH
      and decreased IGF-I)
    Pygmies (normal GH and IGF-II
      but decreased IGF-I at
      puberty)
  Hypothyroidism
  Glucocorticoid excess
    Endogenous
    Exogenous
  Diabetes mellitus under poor
    control
  Diabetes insipidus (untreated)
  Virilizing congenital adrenal
    hyperplasia (tall child, short
    adult)
    P450c21, P450c11 deficiencies

Skeletals dysplasias
  Osteogenesis imperfecta
  Osteochondroplasias

Lysosomal storage diseases
  Mucopolysaccharidoses
  Mucolipidoses

Syndromes of short stature
  Turner's syndrome (syndrome
    of gonadal dysgenesis)
  Noonan's syndrome (pseudo–
    Turner's syndrome)
  Prader-Willi syndrome
  Laurence-Moon-Biedl syndrome
  Autosomal abnormalities
  Dysmorphic syndromes
  Pseudohypoparathryoidism

Chronic disease
  Cardiac disorders
    Left-to-right shunt
    Congestive heart failure
  Pulmonary disorders
    Cystic fibrosis
    Asthma
  GI disorders
    Malabsorption (eg, celiac
      disease)
    Disorders of swallowing
  Hepatic disorders
  Hematologic disorders
    Sickle cell anemia
    Thalassemia
  Renal disorders
    Renal tubular acidosis
    Chronic uremia
  Immunologic disorders
    Connective tissue disease
    Juvenile rheumatoid arthritis
    Chronic infection
  Hereditary fructose intolerance

Malnutrition
  Inadequate food availability
  Iron deficiency
  Zinc deficiency
  Anorexia due to chemotherapy
    of neoplasms
  Malabsorption

and 2 years. Growth rate is therefore normal. The prognosis is good for ultimately achieving acceptable adult height; no treatment is indicated. There may be a transient decrease in growth hormone secretion in teenagers with constitutional delay just before they spontaneously undergo puberty.

Familial Short Stature

If a child's parents are short and come from short families (in the absence of malnutrition), it is expected that the child will be short at all ages and have a bone age appropriate for chronologic age. Usually of normal birth length and weight, such children will reach a lower percentile for height by 1–2 years of age. These patients will plot closer to the mean after correction on midparental height charts than on standard growth charts. A child with both constitutional delay in growth and genetic short stature will be more likely to seek evaluation because of the increased severity of the short stature due to 2 factors than a child who has only one of the factors present.

Malnutrition & Chronic Illness

Caloric malnutrition of any cause may result in childhood short stature. The poor nutrition may be due to obvious illness or lack of food ingestion. Intestinal malabsorption also retards growth and may sometimes present with only subtle signs aside from short stature and low weight for chronological age. Celiac disease and regional enteritis may be heralded by changes in a child's growth before gastrointestinal symptoms are noted. Likewise, the onset of chronic renal failure may present with a reduction in growth rate.

Psychosocial Dwarfism

Even in the absence of caloric deprivation, aberrant parent-child interaction can lead to poor growth. A medical history may include strict disciplinary measures by the parents or elaborate rationale for parents confining the child at home, sometimes even locking the child in a room. Physical punishment may or may not occur. Affected children may forage or beg for food from neighbors or classmates and drink from toilet bowls. The patient may have a pot belly and extremely immature appearance. Functional hypopituitarism may be documented in these children with a reversal from growth hormone (GH) deficiency to normal GH secretion on provocative testing within days after removal from the home. Separation from the family and placement into the hospital or a foster home may lead to a striking improvement in growth; growth may decrease again if the child is returned to the home and no change has occurred in the family dynamics.

Growth Hormone Deficiency & Its Variants

Clinical disorders may be caused at every step in the growth hormone–releasing hormone (GHRH)–growth hormone–somatomedin axis: There may be absence of GHRH, absence of pituitary somatotropes, possible production of inactive GH by somatotropes, inability of organs to produce somatomedins, or cartilage resistance to somatomedin action.

A. Congenital GH Deficiency: Birth weight and length are normal in the absence of fetal GH secretion in the intrauterine period, but careful observation of growth in length will indicate decreased height velocity during the first year after birth. Males with congenital GH deficiency may have microphallus (less than 2.5 cm of stretched phallic length excluding the foreskin); this will be more likely to occur with concurrent gonadotropin-releasing hormone (GnRH) deficiency and resulting fetal LH and FSH deficiency. Of more immediate importance is hypoglycemia and even seizures, which can occur with isolated GH deficiency or with concurrent ACTH deficiency. Thus, a full-term baby of normal weight who develops hypoglycemia without explanation may have congenital hypopituitarism: if the child is a male with microphallus, this diagnosis must be considered likely.

Congenital GH deficiency is usually due to a developmental defect of the hypothalamus, causing GHRH deficiency. Other midline defects may be present, such as cleft palate, hypoplasia of the optic discs (possibly with absence of the septum pellucidum), or a single giant central maxillary incisor. Pituitary aplasia is a rare cause of congenital hypopituitarism. Patients have been described who lack the gene for GH production and have profound GH deficiency. Isolated GH deficiency and hypopituitarism may also be caused by birth trauma, and there is an increased frequency in these patients (especially males) of breech deliveries. Hypoglycemia in a full-term normal-weight infant with a breech delivery may be due to GH deficiency.

B. Acquired GH Deficiency: GH deficiency developing later in childhood is ominous, since it indicates the possible presence of a hypothalamic or pituitary tumor. If diabetes insipidus accompanies anterior pituitary dysfunction, the diagnosis of neoplasia becomes even more likely. Irradiation of the hypothalamic-pituitary region for a tumor located near the area (but not necessarily in it) may also lead to GH deficiency 1 or more years after the irradiation. Patients surviving such treatment for tumors must be prospectively evaluated for decreasing growth rate. Other causes of acquired GH deficiency include infection, granuloma, trauma, and vascular accidents of the hypothalamic-pituitary region.

C. Variations of GH Deficiency: Several patients with short stature, poor growth, low somatomedin values, but normal GH secretory dynamics have demonstrated improved growth after exogenous GH therapy. Growth was attributed to the production of GH molecules that are immunoreactive in radioimmunoassay determinations but biologically inactive in the child. This condition of bioinactive GH is probably rare and its existence has been questioned.

Some short patients respond normally to provocative tests of GH secretion but have inadequate baseline secretion of GH when monitored over a 24-hour period. Others have intermediate response to provocative tests or partial GH deficiency. These conditions have responded to GH therapy in clinical trials.

D. GH Resistance: Patients with low somatomedin and elevated GH concentrations who cannot increase their growth rate or raise their somatomedin values to exogenous GH have Laron's dwarfism, an autosomal recessive condition. These subjects have absence of receptors for GH. When IGF-I becomes clinically available, they may benefit from such therapy with IGF-I.

E. Tests for GH Deficiency: Plasma GH is present in low concentration throughout most of the day in normal subjects, so a random GH determination is useless in diagnosing GH deficiency; provocative tests of GH secretion must be used. Classically, if a value of plasma growth hormone over 10 ng/mL is reached after any stimulatory influence, the child is considered normal. (Laboratories may have different standards for the normal peak value after provocation.) However, many children with low 24-hour integrated GH levels may respond to a provocative test. A normal test does not rule out partial GH deficiency. Any single test may fail to raise GH concentrations in up to 20% of normal children (false-positive result), so two or more tests are required to assure GH deficiency. Children receiving cranial irradiation for treatment of a tumor may have barely normal GH peak values but still require GH therapy.

1. Exercise–The easiest and least invasive screening test for GH sufficiency is the exercise stimulation test. The child is made to exercise strenuously for 10 minutes; in most normal children plasma GH rises 10 minutes after cessation of the exercise; a plasma GH level > 10ng/mL obtained at that time can rule out classic GH deficiency; levels below that can occur in normal children and indicate only a need for further testing for GH deficiency.

2. Sleep–Sleep is a physiologic stimulus for GH release. GH rises to a maximum about 60–120 minutes after the onset of sleep during EEG stages III and IV sleep; blood is drawn at that time. This test is usually practical only for hospitalized children.

3. Arginine, Levodopa, Clonidine–Sequential tests combining 2 stimuli may be used to determine GH sufficiency. Arginine HCl is infused intravenously (0.5 g/kg body weight [up to 20 g] over 30 minutes). This test is cumbersome and may be the least effective one. Levodopa is given orally at the end of the infusion (125 mg for less than 15 kg body weight; 250 mg for 16–35 kg; 500 mg for more than 35 kg). Clonidine may also be given orally often at the end of the L-dopa test (0.15 mg/m^2). Blood is drawn for serum GH at 30, 60, and 90 minutes after each stimulus. The side effects of levodopa are nausea and vomiting; clonidine produces drowsiness. Administration of propranolol 90 minutes before stimulus increases the likelihood of response but with clonidine may lead to bradycardia and hypertension.

4. Plasma Insulinlike Growth Factor I (IGF-I; Somatomedin C)–Commercial determinations are available and a low level can, in certain circumstances, provide evidence of GH deficiency. It is useless to perform the test in patients who are under 2 years of age or who have evidence of malnourishment or psychosocial dwarfism, since IGF-I levels are known to be low in such patients. IGF-I levels are also normally low in prepubertal children and rise after the onset of puberty. Patients must, therefore, have their IGF-I values interpreted in terms of pubertal status rather than chronological age; this is mostly important when performing the test in a child with delayed adolescence. Normal IGF-I levels do not eliminate the necessity for GH therapy, since some children with normal IGF-I levels grow with GH therapy. A low IGF-I level for bone age may be a useful indication of the necessity for growth hormone therapy in the absence of malnutrition or psychiatric disorders. The combination of low IGF-I and IGF-II concentrations is suggested to *more* strongly indicate GH deficiency.

5. Growth Hormone–Releasing Hormone (GHRH)–GHRH has just become clinically available for diagnostic testing; it does not appear to have a strong clinical advantage over the other stimuli for GH tests.

6. Insulin-induced Hypoglycemia–This is another good test of GH (and ACTH reserve) but carries a serious risk of hypoglycemic seizures. The physician must stay next to the child throughout the test; the patient's intravenous line (saline) must be maintained for emergency glucose administration; the patient must have no history of hypoglycemia or a seizure disorder. A normal initial blood glucose > 70 mg/dL must be confirmed before regular insulin (≤ 0.1 U/kg) is given in an IV bolus. A 50% drop in glucose is expected 20–40 minutes later, and a rise in ACTH, cortisol, and GH should follow at 30, 60, and 90 minutes. The patient should become sleepy and sweaty, but if it becomes impossible to arouse the patient or if a seizure occurs, dextrose (0.5 mg/kg) should be administered as D25W to reverse the symptoms; excessive dextrose administration can raise plasma glucose sufficiently to cause hyperosmolar complications. Thus, many precau-

logic complications c
Average intelligence
found in sources liste

Mucopolysaccharido
More than 8 typ
identified. They are
usually autosomal or
drome (MPS I-H), H
drome (MPS IV).

Turner's Syndrome
Any short girl m
diagnosis should be
made. Classic 45,XO
nosed on physical exa
of Turner's syndrome
a karyotype for diag
short stature, epicanth
mouth, low-set ears,
bing at the neck, cub
short fourth metacar
nevi, and a tendency
hypoplasia of the nip
disease, usually coar
hypertension. Some
syndrome only after
malities of the kidney
can cause urinary tra
mon.
Newborns with
of the hands and feet
arise. Another mani
hygroma that occurs i
fetal life and leads to
and the webbed neck
syndrome is applied
Patients with a
notype (including no
progress through se
other physical findin
The dysgenetic
ate into streak gona
levels are extremely

tions must surround the performance of an insulin tolerance test, and it is not appropriate for routine testing of children with short stature.

The insulin test may be performed before the arginine, levodopa, clonidine test.

7. Multiple Plasma GH Concentrations–Numerous authors have supported or refuted the use of averaged or pooled plasma GH concentration based on multiple samples drawn overnight or over 24 hours. At present, this laborious study is reserved for the clinical experimental situation.

Hypothyroidism

Congenital hypothyroidism is detected by neonatal screening programs in most states (and countries), and this source of mental retardation and poor growth is expected to be rarely undiagnosed in the future. However, acquired hypothyroidism or more subtle congenital abnormalities may present with growth failure and some increase in weight (rarely severe obesity). Characteristics include immature (high) upper to lower segment ratio because of poor long-bone growth, retarded bone age (with epiphyseal dysgenesis or stippling), and decreased physical activity. Remarkably, children with acquired hypothyroidism may perform well in school because of their increased attention span. Treatment with synthetic levothyroxine (3–8 μg/kg/d up to a usual maximum dose of 0.1 mg) will result in catch-up growth. In neonatal hypothyroidism, the goal of therapy is to replace thyroxine so that serum T_4 is in the normal range for age. Normalization of elevated thyroid-stimulating hormone (TSH) is not necessary in the newborn period but later can be used to assess adequacy of thyroxine therapy in most cases of primary hypothyroidism.

Cushing's Syndrome

Glucocorticoids in excess are potent growth suppressors, and short stature may even precede weight gain in Cushing syndrome. Unexpected sources of glucocorticoids such as topical cream to treat eczema or oral steroids for asthma must be considered in the differential diagnosis, as well as adrenal adenomas, adrenal carcinomas, and bilateral adrenal hyperplasia due to inappropriate secretion of ACTH (Cushing's disease). Because of variation in cortisol secretion, multiple tests are required in children before the diagnosis of Cushing's syndrome is confirmed or denied. Laboratory values must be corrected for a child's size; urinary free cortisol excretion should not exceed 60 μg/m^2/24 h and urinary 17-hydroxysteroids should not exceed 4 mg/m^2/24 h. Elimination of the source of excess cortisol will allow improved growth if the epiphyses of the bones are not fused.

Pseudohypoparathyr

Pseudohypoparath
and round-faced, have
bones, and usually are
calcium, high phosphc
hormone (PTH) levels
strated in the guanyln
ples PTH-occupied re
spond to exogenous P
urinary phosphorus e
nephrogenic cAMP e>
sponse to PTH.

Additional clinic
dentition, subcutaneo
Seizures may occur v
have been described v
Ca, PO$_4$, and PTH le\
thyroidism. Further, p
plus osteitis fibrosa cy

Treatment of ps
parathyroidism; high-
ment and PO$_4$ bindin{
stature remains short

Diabetes Mellitus

Normal growth
litus, but poor contro
be nutritional. Soma
but increase to the
blood sugar.

Diabetes Insipidus

Untreated diabe
without other endoc
interfering with ade<
ments and improve:

Osteochondroplasi

Osteochondror
number of cases of !
with regard to arm
most common type
.ominant syndrome
.tics include extrem.
.e for height, promine.

pubertal years, but lower values of LH and FSH, almost into the normal range, are encountered during ages 4–10 years.

A. X-Chromosome Structural Abnormalities: These abnormalities may cause certain selective elements of classic Turner's syndrome similar to those caused by the complete loss of one X chromosome. Abnormalities or the deletion of certain genes on the short arm of the X chromosome cause the short stature and other physical manifestations of Turner's syndrome; abnormalities or deletion of genes located on both the long and short arms of the X chromosome cause abnormalities of gonadal development. Phenotype depends upon which of these genes are missing. Such patients may have a chromatin-positive buccal smear or a "46(abnormal)X" karyotype; these patients may have some ovarian function (rarely, even fertility) rather than nonfunctioning streak gonads.

B. XO/XX Mosaicism: Such patients may be taller and have some gonadal function and fewer physical stigmata of classic 45,XO Turner's syndrome.

C. 45,XO/46,XY Mosaicism: This abnormality produces clinical features of Turner's syndrome along with some element of virilization. These patients often have ambiguous genitalia. They may have a partially functioning dysgenetic testis rather than a streak gonad and have a chromatin-negative buccal smear. Patients with a Y cell line and dysgenetic undescended testes are at risk for gonadal neoplasm and should have prophylactic gonadectomy. A gonadoblastoma may secrete estrogen; feminization in a patient with 45,XO/46,XY mosaicism does not indicate functioning ovarian tissue but rather a tumor.

D. Conditions Associated with Turner's Syndrome: Associated conditions include diabetes mellitus, Hashimoto's thyroiditis, rheumatoid arthritis, inflammatory bowel disease, and difficulty with spatial orientation (and mathematical reasoning).

Noonan's Syndrome

Short stature and some physical characteristics are shared by Noonan's and Turner's syndromes, but the former is inherited in an autosomal dominant pattern and has no karyotypic abnormalities. In addition, Noonan's patients more frequently have mental retardation. Physical characteristics shared by Noonan's and Turner's syndromes include ptosis, low posterior hairline and webbed neck, low-set ears, cubitus valgus, shield chest, and hypoplastic nipples. Features distinct from Turner's syndrome include hypertelorism, pectus excavatum, and right-sided congenital heart disease. Lymphedema has been described in some patients. Males may have a small penis and cryp-
.hidism.

Prader-Willi Syndrome

Infantile hypotonia (and poor intrauterine activity), acromicria (small hands and feet) mental retardation, almond-shaped eyes with characteristic facies, ravenous appetite, and extreme obesity are found in this syndrome. Puberty is often delayed due to hypogonadotropism. Glucose intolerance can be demonstrated (probably due to obesity). Weight control is extremely difficult in these patients, but behavior modification has led to some success. Over 50% of patients have abnormalities of banding of chromosome 15.

Laurence-Moon-Biedl Syndrome

Retinitis pigmentosa, polydactyly or syndactyly, short stature, obesity, and mental retardation characterize this autosomal recessive disorder. Puberty is often delayed.

Pygmies

The pygmies of Zaire have normal levels of GH and IGF-II during childhood, when their growth velocity is normal. Short stature results from a deficient pubertal growth spurt due to lack of pubertal IGF-I hypersecretion.

TREATMENT OF CHILDHOOD SHORT STATURE

In treatable causes of short stature, growth rate may increase above normal with initial therapy. Thus, patients with hypothyroidism or Cushing's disease will experience catch-up growth upon replacement with thyroxine or removal of the source of excessive cortisol if therapy begins before the epiphyses of the long bones are fused. The same sort of catch-up growth is observed with the reversal of malnutrition or chronic disease. Growth hormone–deficient patients will likewise grow faster than normal during the first year of treatment but slow down to rates approximating those normal for age thereafter.

Growth Hormone Treatment

A. Children with Low GH Levels: A major consideration in treating short stature is to decide which patients will most likely benefit from the expensive treatment with human growth hormone. Patients with a classic deficiency of growth hormone secretion show the most reliable growth results; however, 6 of 15 very short children (height 3 SD below mean; growth rate less than 5 cm/yr) with normal plasma GH levels and normal somatomedin values have also shown improved growth rates with GH therapy. Patients with Laron's dwarfism do not respond to GH but may benefit from IGF-I when it becomes available.

In 1985 in the USA, the FDA ordered all natural pituitary GH to be removed from distribution because of the discovery of Creutzfeld-Jacob disease (a slow, fatal infection of the central nervous system developing in patients 5–15 years after they had received GH prepared from cadaver donors. It was suggested that the GH was contaminated by prions or slow virus. Since then, a few more patients treated with cadaver GH have been diagnosed with Creutzfeld-Jacob disease.

Growth hormone produced by recombinant DNA technology is available for use. The usual dose of GH is 0.1 mg/kg, 3 times per week, subcutaneously or intramuscularly. Using the 0.3 mg/kg dose in a daily or six times per week schedule has proved even more effective than the three time per week schedule. Commercial preparations either have an additional methionyl group on the terminus of the GH molecule, or have no methionyl group and are identical to natural GH.

Recipients of GH must have an appropriate balance of other endocrine factors and good nutrition. GH will not increase growth rate in the presence of hypothyroidism; thus, thyroxine must be given to hypothyroid patients to make them euthyroid before administering GH therapy. Initially euthyroid children may have decreasing T_4 values with GH therapy, and *careful monitoring of thyroid function is essential*. Excess cortisol will likewise decrease growth rate, and patients with ACTH deficiency must not be overtreated with replacement glucocorticoids. Usually 10 mg/m^2 of oral hydrocortisone is adequate and not growth suppressive, but each child must be assessed individually.

B. Children with Normal GH Levels: Patients with normal growth hormone levels and low somatomedin concentrations due to presumptive bioinactive growth hormone have been successfully treated with GH. Extremely short children with abnormally low growth rates and normal peak GH and somatomedin values have also rarely responded to GH. Thus, GH and somatomedin values do not reliably indicate the responsiveness to GH therapy. The question "How do you determine who will respond to GH?" cannot easily be answered. In some cases it may be necessary to treat an ostensibly normal but short patient empirically for several months before it is clear whether GH will improve growth. Only those patients with a severely delayed bone age who are well below the fifth percentile for height and are growing less than 4.5 cm/yr after 4 years of age have been shown to benefit from GH. If GH is present in excess, such as in a pituitary giant or an ᵃomegalic, glucose intolerance or frank diabetes mellitus may result ᵃll as organomegaly and acromegalic physical and skeletal fea- ᵃ̄H therapy has been suggested to increase the risk of slipped ᵃ̄oral epiphyses. Of greatest concern is the report of children who developed leukemia after GH therapy. However, only a few can be said to be unexpected cases of leukemia, and a relationship between GH and leukemia has not been proved. Thus, further studies are necessary before GH can be considered a safe drug for non–GH deficient short children. At present, the only absolute indication for growth hormone therapy is growth hormone deficiency. Growth hormone should not be used because a child or parent wants a boy's final height to be 5 ft 10 in rather than 5 ft 8 in; nor is there any proof that normal doses will accomplish such a goal.

Several studies show improved growth rate in short non-growth hormone deficient children with 1 or more years of treatment with GH doses often higher than those used for classic GH deficiency; long-term follow-up of final height is still lacking. Ongoing studies of patients with **Turner's syndrome** have demonstrated an improved growth rate over 1–3 years of GH therapy. Growth may be further improved with the addition of estrogen or weak androgen. However, this regimen is still experimental, awaiting the final height determination in a large number of treated patients before it can be recommended for routine therapy. It must also be decided whether a final height that improved by a few centimeters is worth the very high cost of several years of GH therapy.

Psychological Management

Psychological management of exceedingly short patients is also of prime importance. Parents, teachers, and peers tend to treat GH-deficient children as younger than their years, and their psychosocial development and body image may be compromised even after therapy restores their height. Supportive therapy or even regular psychotherapy may be necessary to avert long-term psychological problems.

CHILDHOOD TALL STATURE

EVALUATION OF CHILDHOOD TALL STATURE

Historical records of a child's growth and family heights will indicate whether a given patient is out of the range expected for genetic endowment. Midparental height charts may be used to correct for this effect. Rapid increase in growth rate suggests the presence of disease rather than familial pattern. Physical examination should focus upon finding stigmata of the conditions listed above. Bone-age determination will help confirm a diagnosis of constitutional tall stature but will also be advanced in precocious puberty. Thyroid function tests will be used to confirm suspected thyrotoxicosis. Elevated resting growth hormone values or paradoxic release of GH with glucose or thyrotropin-releasing factor (TRF) and high plasma somatomedin values will indicate pituitary gigantism.

CAUSES OF CHILDHOOD TALL STATURE (See Table 3–5.)

Large Newborns

Although all factors controlling normal fetal growth are not yet known, an excess of fetal insulin secretion clearly can cause large size at birth. Thus, infants or diabetic mothers with minimal to moderate hyperglycemia are heavier and longer than average. The effect of maternal diabetes upon the fetus and newborn is discussed in Chapter 10.

Permanent hyperinsulinism and hypoglycemia is seen in the Beckwith-Weidemann syndrome of large neonatal size (due to intrauterine hyperinsulinism), macroglossia, fetal adrenocortical cytomegaly, and large kidneys with medullary dysplasia. Maintenance of blood glucose is critical to avoid seizures and mental retardation, and aggressive therapy is necessary; in some patients, insulin values may be well suppressed with diazoxide, 5–20mg/kg/d, but partial pancreatectomy is often necessary to decrease insulin secretion.

Constitutional Tall Stature

Constitutional tall stature is diagnosed in a child with advanced bone age and tall stature without organic cause.

Genetic Tall Stature

Children from a tall family may have genetic tall stature without bone age advancement. Children with extremely tall height predictions may request therapy to limit their final height; usually this request comes from parents who have not adjusted well to their own tall stature. More girls than boys ask for treatment to reduce final height.

Table 3–5. Causes of tall stature.

Variations of normal	Nonendocrine disorders
Constitutional	Marfan's syndrome
Genetic	Klinefelter's syndrome
	XYY syndrome
Endocrine disorders	Cerebral gigantism
Pituitary gigantism	
Sexual precocity	
Thyrotoxicosis	
Beckwith-Weidemann syndrome	

appeared to decrease g
in one study. Althoug|
mocriptine decreased p
boys and girls.

Ad Hoc Committee on Gro
    Endocrine Society, and
    ment of children with s
August GP, Lippe BM, B
    United States: demogra
    Pediatr 1990;**116**:899.
Aynsley-Green A, Zachm
    effects of growth hormo
    Pediatr 1976;**89**:992.
Ballard FJ, Baxter RC, Bin
    binding proteins. *J Clin*
Baumann G, Shaw MA, V
    binding protein in L:
    1987;**65**:814.
Bierich JR: Treatment by
    cence. *Acta Paediatr Sc*
Borges JLC, et al: Stimul
    idiopathic GH deficient
    synthetic human panc
    (hpGRF)-40. *J Clin End*
Brown P: Human growth |
    drama in three acts. *Pea*
Clayton PE, Price DA, Sha
    treatment with growth h
Conte FA, Grumbach MM
    use in children and adol
Daughaday WH, Rotwein
    messenger ribonucleic ac
    tions. *Edocr Rev* 1989;**1**
Evain-Brion D, et al: Studi
    bromocriptine on growth
    Clin Endocrinol Metab 1
Frasier SD, Lippe BM: The
    Clin Rev II 1990;**71**:269
Frasier SD: Human pituitai
    mone deficiency. *Endocr*
Frazer T et al: Growth hor
    101:12.
Furlanetto RW, Underwoo
    levels in normals and pat
    Clin Invest 1977;**60**:648.
Hall JG et al: Turner's syn

Pituitary Gigantism

A GH-secreting pituitary adenoma will lead to increased growth and tall stature if it occurs before epiphyseal fusion. Organomegaly and diabetes mellitus may occur; acromegalic features begin to occur in late adolescence and early adulthood. Elevated IGF-I and nonsuppressible GH concentrations are customarily found and allow diagnosis (see Chapter 1).

Sexual Precocity

Estrogen or androgen secretion due to any cause of sexual precocity will increase height velocity and bone age advancement. Thus, the child will be tall but will cease growing early due to premature epiphyseal fusion and have short adult stature.

Thyrotoxicosis

Height velocity and bone age will advance in thyrotoxicosis. If the onset is in infancy, craniosynostosis may result as well. Excessive thryoxine dosage can lead to the same effects as endogenous thyrotoxicosis.

Marfan's Syndrome

Characteristic features include tall stature, pectus excavatum, long thin fingers, hyperextension of joints, lens subluxation, and aortic aneurysm. This is an autosomal dominant disease.

Klinefelter's Syndrome

Patients with XXY karyotype tend to be taller than average even during childhood. They may be diagnosed by behavioral abnormalities and decreased upper to lower segment ratio (see Chapter 4).

XYY Syndromes & Variants

The presence of one or more excess Y chromosomes leads to greater than average adult height. Slow mentation and antisocial behavior are described.

Cerebral Gigantism

The Soto syndrome includes rapid growth in infancy, prominent forehead, sharp chin, high arched palate, and hypertelorism. No GH excess can be documented, and growth becomes normal in later childhood.

Beckwith-Weidemann Syndrome

Beckwith-Weidemann syndrome, or the exomphalos-macroglossia-gigantism syndrome, is a sporadic disorder that has been well described. The omphalocele is obvious at birth and requires immediate surgical treatment. However, hypoglycemia due to increased insulin secretion from a hyperplastic pancreas in about one-third to one-half of

cases may lead to brain da
necessary. Kidneys are ofte
and fetal adrenal cortical c
findings include characteri:
diastasis recti in addition t
Wilms's tumor, gonadobla
cryptorchidism, and inters
patients have unusual linea
Mental performance may
glycemia. The tongue is ex
tion may be necessary fo
normal respiration. Affecte
hood, often at the 90th p
healthy if the neonatal con
effort should be taken to :

TREATMENT OF

Therapy for thyrotoxi
in Chapters 4 and 5. Pitu
sphenoidal microadenome

More difficult is the
parents may project their c
due to excessive tall statu
dicted to be over 6 ft ta
considered as potential sub
They should have several y
mined by bone age) to ju
should be made by child
expressing unrealistic expe
child's height, counseling
is in order.

In girls, high-dose es
day) induce pubertal chang
and decrease final height l
years. These doses are ext
limited to nausea, obesity,
effects on reproduction and
dose estrogen therapy mus

Boys rarely request t
limited. Testosterone thera
fuse epiphyses earlier; the
Paradoxic GH secreti
thyrotropin-releasing horn
constitutionally tall childre

Hamill PVV, et al: Physical growth: National Center for Health Statistics percentiles. *Am J Clin Nutr* 1979;**32:**607.

Himes JH, Roche AF, Thissen D: *Parent-Specific Adjustments for Assessment of Recumbent Length and Stature.* Vol. 13 of: Monographs in Paediatrics. Karger, 1981.

Hintz RL et al: Plasma somatomedin and growth hormone values in children with protein-calorie malnutrition. *J Pediatr* 1978;**92:**153.

Hintz RL et al: Biosynthetic methionyl human growth hormone is biologically active in adult man. *Lancet* 1982;**1:**1276.

Horner JM, Throsson AV, Hintz RL: Growth deceleration patterns in children with constitutional short stature: An aid to diagnosis. *Pediatrics* 1978;**62:**529.

Jones KL: *Smith's Recognizable Patterns of Human Malformation.* Saunders, 1988.

Kaplan SL, Grumbach MM: Pathophysiology of GH deficiency and other disorders of GH metabolism. Pages 45–55 in: *Problems in Pediatric Endocrinology.* La Causa C, Root AW (editors). Academic Press, 1980.

Kaplan SL: Normal and abnormal growth. Pages 75–92 in: *Pediatrics,* 19th ed. Rudolph AM, Hoffman JIE (editors). Appleton & Lange, 1991.

Kowarski AJ et al: Growth failure with normal serum RIA-GH and low somatomedin activity: Somatomedin restoration and growth acceleration after exogenous GH. *J Clin Endocrinol Metab* 1978;**47:**461.

Lovinger RD, Kaplan SL, Grumbach MM: Congenital hypopituitarism associated with neonatal hypoglycemia and microphallus: Four cases secondary to hypothalamic hormone deficiencies. *J Pediatr* 1975;**87**(part 2):1171.

Marshall WA: *Human Growth and its Disorders.* Academic Press, 1979.

Merimee TJ et al: Insulin-like growth factors in pygmies. *N Engl J Med* 1987;**316:**906.

Miller WL, Kaplan SL, Grumbach MM: Child abuse as a cause of post-traumatic hypopituitarism. *N Engl J Med* 1980;**302:**724.

Phillips JA, III: Inherited defects in growth hormone synthesis and action. In: *The Metabolic Basis of Inherited Disease,* 6th ed. Scriver CR, Beaudet AL, Sly WS, Valle D (editors). McGraw-Hill, Inc., 1989.

Powell GF, Brasel JA, Blizzard RM: Emotional deprivation and growth retardation simulating idiopathic hypopituitarism. 1. Clinical evaluation of the syndrome. *N Engl J Med* 1967;**276:**1271.

Powell GF et al: Emotional deprivation and growth retardation simulating idiopathic hypopituitarism. 2. Endocrinologic evaluation of the syndrome. *N Engl J Med* 1967;**276:**1279.

Preece MA: The insulinlike growth factors. In: *Current Concepts in Pediatric Endocrinology.* Styne DM, Brook GG (editors). Elsevier, 1987.

Reiter EO, Lovinger RD: The use of a commercially available somatomedin-C radio-immunoassay in patients with disorders of growth. *J Pediatr* 1981; **99:**720.

Reiter EO et al: Variable estimates of serum growth hormone concentrations by different radioassay systems. *J Clin Endocrinol Metab* 1988;**66:**68.

Richards GE et al: Delayed onset of hypopituitarism: Sequelae of therapeutic irradiation of central nervous system, eye, and middle ear tumors. *J Pediatr* 1976;**89:**553.

Roche AF, Himes JH: Incremental growth charts. *Am J Clin Nutr* 1980; **33:**2041.

Rogol AD et al: Growth hormone release in response to human pancreatic tumor growth hormone–releasing hormone–40 in children with short stature. *J Clin Endocrinol Metab* 1984;**59**:580.

Rosenfeld RG, Update on growth hormone therapy for Turner's syndrome. *Acta Paediatr Scand [Suppl]* 1989;**356**:103.

Rosenfeld RG, Kemp SF, Hintz RL: Constancy of somatomedin response to growth hormone treatment of hypopituitary dwarfism, and lack of correlation with growth rate. *J Clin Endocrinol Metab* 1981;**53**:611.

Schwarz HP, Joss EE, Zuppinger KA: Bromocriptine treatment in adolescent boys with familial tall stature: A pair-matched controlled study. *J Clin Endocrinol Metab* 1987;**65**:136.

Sklar CA et al: Hormonal and metabolic abnormalities associated with central nervous system germinoma in children and adolescents and the effect of therapy: Report of 10 patients. *J Clin Endocrinol Metab* 1981;**52**:9.

Smith DW: *Growth and its Disorders.* Saunders, 1977.

Smith DW et al: Shifting linear growth during infancy: Illustration of genetic factors in growth from fetal life through infancy. *J Pediatr* 1976;**89**:225.

Styne DM et al: Treatment of Cushing's disease in childhood and adolescence by transsphenoidal microadenomectomy. *N Engl J Med* 1984;**310**:889.

Styne DM: Growth. Chapter 8 in: *Basic and Clinical Endocrinology,* 3rd ed. Greenspan FS (editor). Appleton & Lange, 1991.

Takano K et al: Plasma growth hormone (GH) response to GH-releasing factor in normal children with short stature and patients with pituitary dwarfism. *J Clin Endocrinol Metab* 1984;**58**:236.

Tanner JM, Whitehouse RH: Clinical longitudinal standards for height, weight, height velocity, weight velocity, and stages of puberty. *Arch Dis Child* 1976;**51**:170.

Thomsett MJ et al: Endocrine and neurologic outcome in childhood craniopharyngioma: Review of effect of treatment in 42 patients. *J Pediatr* 1980;**97**:728.

Unsworth DJ, Walker-Smith JA, Holborow EJ: Gliadin and reticulin antibodies in childhood coeliac disease. *Lancet* 1983;**1**:874.

US Department of Health, Education, and Welfare, Public Health Service: *NHCS Growth Curves for Children: Birth-18 Years, United States.* Publication No. (PHS) 78-1650. Series II, No. 165,1977.

Van Vliet G et al: Growth hormone can increase growth rate in short normal children: evaluation of the somatomedin C generation test in the assessment of children wtih short stature. *N Engl J Med* 1983;**309**:1016.

Wainer H, Thissen D: Two programs for predicting adult stature of individuals. *Pediatrics* 1976;**58**:369.

Witt JM et al: Effects of two years of methionyl growth hormone therapy in two dosage regimens in prepubertal children with short stature, subnormal growth rate, and normal growth hormone response to secretagogues. *J Pediatr* 1989;**115**:720.

Wettenhall HNB, Cahill C, Roche AF: Tall girls: A survey of 15 years of management and treatment. *J Pediatr* 1975;**86**:602.

Zapf J, Walter H, Froesch ER: Radioimmunological determination of insulin-like growth factors I and II in normal subjects and in patients with growth disorders and extra-pancreatic tumor hypoglycemia. *J Clin Invest* 1981; **68**:1321.

Disorders of Puberty | 4

Dennis M. Styne, MD

Puberty is not a single event but a stage in the continuum of growth and development. This chapter focuses on the endocrine and physical changes of puberty rather than the profound psychologic changes that also occur.

PHYSICAL CHANGES OF PUBERTY

The stage of development of a child should be objectively described at the time of each examination so that accurate assessment is made of the rate of progression of secondary sexual development. Standards of physical development described by Marshall and Tanner are widely used and are presented below.

THE FEMALE

Breast development, stimulated mainly by ovarian estrogens, and pubic hair development, caused mainly by ovarian and adrenal androgens, usually proceed in close temporal relationship but may occur separately. Thus, each is staged separately.

Stages of Female Breast Development
See Fig 4–1.

Stages of Female Pubic Hair Development
See Fig 4–2.
Axillary hair usually first appears in stage PH3.
The uterus, as revealed by ultrasonography, enlarges with estrogen stimulation and the fundus becomes relatively larger than the cervix, changing the contour. Clear or whitish vaginal discharge is noted in the 6 months prior to menarch. In the USA, menarche occurs at a mean age of 12.8 years.

THE MALE

Testicular enlargement is the first sign of normal puberty in the male. It is best to stage genital development separately from pubic hair development because they may be unrelated temporally, although they are both mediated by androgens. The penis is always measured stretched from the dorsal base to the end of the glans (without including the prepuce). The length and diameter of the penis are recorded. Testes are measured by their length and width excluding the epididymis; alternatively, their volume may be compared to the ellipsoids of the Prader orchidometer (Chapter 8).

Stages of Male Genital Development
See Fig 4–3.

Stages of Male Pubic Hair Development
See Fig 4–3.

Facial hair in boys usually occurs in stage P3, as does the beginning of axillary hair. "Breaking" of the voice occurs at a mean age of 13.5 years. The first conscious ejaculation occurs at a mean age of 13.5 years with histologic evidence of spermatogenesis occurring between 11 and 15 years. Thus in the male as in the female, fertility may occur prior to reaching adult physical development.

ONSET OF PUBERTY

The age of puberty has decreased 4 months each decade over the last century with improvement of socioeconomic conditions, but this trend has not continued during the last 4 decades in the USA. In the

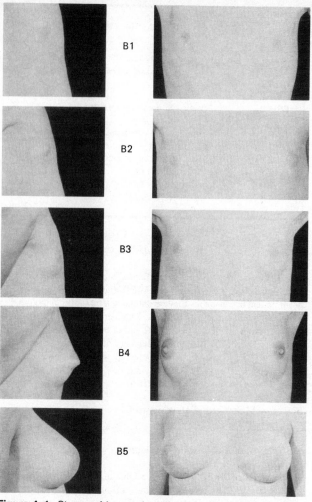

Figure 4–1. Stages of breast development, according to Marshall and Tanner. (Photographs from van Wieringen JC et al, 1971; with permission.) *Stage B1:* Preadolescent; elevation of papilla only. *Stage B2:* Breast bud stage, elevation of breast and papilla as a small mound, and enlargement of areolar diameter. *Stage B3:* Further enlargement of breast and areola, with no separation of their contours. *Stage B4:* Projection of areola and papilla to form a secondary mound above the level of the breast. *Stage B5:* Mature stage; projection of papilla only, owing to recession of the areola to the general contour of the breast. (Reproduced, with permission, from Marshall WA, Tanner JM: *Arch Dis Child* 1969;**44:**291).

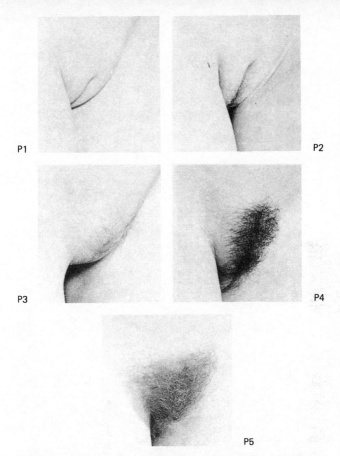

Figure 4–2. Stages of female pubic hair development, according to Marshall and Tanner. (Photographs from van Wierignen JC et al, 1971; with permission.) *Stage P1:* Preadolescent; the vellus over the pubes is no further developed than that over the anterior abdominal wall, ie, no pubic hair. *Stage P2:* Sparse growth of long, slightly pigmented, downy hair, straight or only slightly curled appearing chiefly along the labia. This stage is difficult to see in photographs. *Stage P3:* Hair is considerably darker, coarser, and curlier. The hair spreads sparsely over the junction of the pubes. *Stage P4:* Hair is now adult in type, but the area covered by it is still considerably smaller than in most adults. There is no spread to the medial surface of the thighs. *Stage P5:* Hair is adult in quantity and type, distributed as an inverse triangle of the classic feminine pattern. Spread is to the medial surface of the thighs but not up the linea alba or elsewhere above the base of the inverse triangle. (Reproduced, with permission, from Marshall WA, Tanner JM: *Arch Dis Child* 1969;**44**:291.)

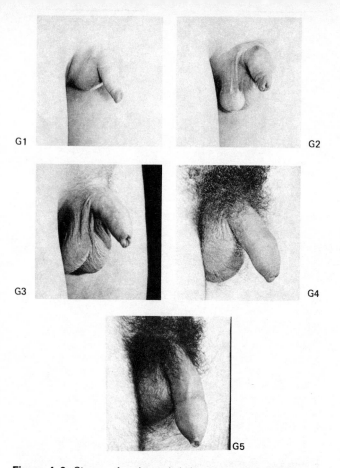

Figure 4–3. Stages of male genital development and pubic hair development, according to Marshall and Tanner. (Photographs from van Wieringen JC et al, 1971; with permission.) Genital: *Stage G1:* Preadolescent. Testes, scrotum, and penis are about the same size and proportion as in early childhood. *Stage G2:* The scrotum and testes have enlarged, and there is a change in the texture and some reddening of the scrotal skin. *Stage G3:* Growth of the penis has occurred, at first mainly in length but with some increase in breadth; further growth of testes and scrotum. *Stage G4:* Penis further enlarged in length and girth with development of glans. Testes and scrotum further enlarged. The scrotal skin has further darkened. *Stage G5:* Genitalia adult in size and shape. No further enlargement takes place after stage G5 is reached. Pubic hair: *Stage P1:* Pre-

USA, the onset of secondary sexual development in over 97% of girls occurs between ages 8 and 13 years (mean = 10.5 years), with enlargement of the breast, and in over 97% of boys between ages 9.5 and 14 years (mean = 11.5 years), with enlargement of the testes. In girls, the progress from onset of breast enlargement to menarche requires 1.5–6 years (mean = 2.3 years). In boys, the progress from onset of testes enlargement to mature genitalia requires 2–4.5 years (mean = 3 years). Any child falling outside these limits (either by age of onset or length of progression) may either have a medical problem or be at the extremes of normal.

PUBERTAL GROWTH SPURT

The marked increase in height velocity during puberty (pubertal growth spurt) occurs on average of 2 years earlier in girls than boys. Growth hormone and sex steroids appear to be of primary importance in causing the pubertal growth spurt. Somatomedin C values rise markedly in pubertal subjects compared with those in younger children as values in midpuberty are higher than adult normal values. However, the rise in somatomedin is more closely temporally related to elevations in sex steroids than to peak height velocity. Somatomedin secretion may be stimulated by sex steroid–induced increases in growth hormone secretion. Since the growth spurt usually occurs before menarche and only 2.5–5 cm of growth remain after menarche, on average a short girl who is menarcheal will usually have a less favorable height prognosis than one of the same height who has not yet reached menarche.

Figure 4–3 (cont'd).
adolescent. The vellus over the pubes is no further developed than that over the abdominal wall, ie, no pubic hair. *Stage P2:* Sparse growth of long, slightly pigmented, downy hair, straight or only slightly curled, appearing chiefly at the base of the penis. *Stage P3:* Hair is considerably darker, coarser, and curlier and spreads sparsely over the junction of the pubes. *Stage P4:* Hair is now adult in type, but the area it covers is still considerably smaller than in most adults. There is no spread to the medial surface of the thighs. *Stage P5:* Hair is adult in quantity and type, distributed as an inverse triangle. Spread is to the medial surface of the thighs but not up the linea alba or elsewhere above the base of the inverse triangle. Most men will have further spread of pubic hair. (Modified and reproduced, with permission, from Marshall WA, Tanner JM: *Arch Dis Child* 1970;**45**:13.)

ENDOCRINE PHYSIOLOGY OF PUBERTY

PREPUBERTAL CHANGES

Gonadotropin and gonadal steroid secretion has been demonstrated in fetal life. Several stages of maturation of gonadotropin secretion occur during infancy and childhood, well before gonadotropin stimulates gonadal steroids to cause the striking physical changes of puberty. By 12 weeks of gestation, gonadotropins are found in the fetal pituitary gland and gonadotropin-releasing hormone (GnRH) is present in the hypothalamus. By midgestation, the hypophyseal portal plexus is fully developed and plasma gonadotropins are at peak values, presumably because hypothalamic GnRH can reach the pituitary gland. Fetal testes secret testosterone during the gonadotropin peak, demonstrating the biologic activity of the fetal pituitary gonadotropins. Thereafter, gonadotropin secretion decreases as inhibitory influences develop in the fetal brain, restraining hypothalamic GnRH secretion. The neonatal period is characterized by episodic secretion of gonadotropins and gonadal steroids; testosterone values characteristic of early puberty can be intermittently demonstrated during the first months after birth in normal males. Thereafter, until the onset of puberty, gonadotropin secretion is restrained and sex steroid values decrease to the low levels characteristic of prepuberty.

ADRENARCHE

Adrenarche refers to the onset of adrenal androgen secretion. This phenomenon normally precedes gonadarche by 2 years. Thus, the adrenal androgen dihydroepiandrosterone (DHA) and its sulfate (DHAS) rise well before the first physical changes of puberty. At present, it is not known what mediates adrenarche. One postulate is that an as yet undiscovered pituitary hormone (other than LH, FSH, or ACTH) is operative in stimulating adrenal androgen secretion, and another is that local intra-adrenal processes cause adrenarche. Adrenarche can occur without gonadarche (in gonadal failure) and vice versa (in adrenal failure). Of note is the fact that DHA and DHAS are reflected in urinary 17-ketosteroids, whereas testosterone only minimally contributes to urinary 17-ketosteroid values. Approximately 2 years after the onset of increasing adrenal androgen secretion, pubic hair will appear and axillary hair development follows. In girls, pubic hair will be sparse if there is no ovarian estrogen and androgen secretion (as in gonadal dysgenesis); thus, adrenal androgens alone do not cause full pubic hair maturation.

GONADARCHE

In the peripubertal period (just before the onset of sexual development), episodic gonadotropin secretion increases in amplitude in response to increased pulsatile GnRH secretion. This can be demonstrated first at night and then throughout the day. Gonadal sex steroids rise in concert with the increasing gonadotropin secretion. This is the first stage of gonadarche, or the awakening of gonadal function. Because of the episodic nature of gonadotropin secretion, individual LH and FSH values cannot easily indicate whether pubertal endocrine development has started; if multiple sequential samples are obtained and pulsatile secretion of LH or FSH demonstrated, the diagnosis of pubertal endocrine activity can be established.

A more convenient demonstration of pubertal endocrine development is the **GnRH test**, which is now widely available. A 100-µg dose of GnRH is infused by intravenous bolus, and gonadotropins are sampled at 0, 15, 30, 60, and 120 minutes. If LH rises more than 15.6 mIU/mL it may be assumed that the pituitary has already experienced endogenous GnRH stimulation, causing an increase in readily releasable LH, and that the pubertal reawakening of GnRH secretion has begun. Physical puberal development will usually follow within 6 months after conversion to a pubertal LH pattern following a dose of GnRH. In the prepubertal period before GnRH secretion increases, the LH rise after GnRH is much lower, indicating a state of relative GnRH deficiency.

Patients with gonadotropin deficiency will either have GnRH test results similar to those of normal prepubertal children or have no rise in LH or FSH after GnRH; lack of conversion of the pattern to a pubertal one by 18 years of age may be the only way to definitively diagnose gonadotropin deficiency. Thus, repetitive testing of gonadal steroid concentrations or even of response to GnRH over a period of years may be necessary to determine which patient has severely constitutionally delayed puberty and which has permanent gonadotropin deficiency. It is rare for a patient who has not spontaneously entered puberty by 18 years of age to do so afterwards, although one reported patient began puberty at 25 years of age.

Gonadal steroids are bound to sex hormone–binding globulin (SHBG) and have a longer plasma half-life than gonadotropins, and individual testosterone (T) or estradiol (E) determinations can better determine the progression, or lack of progression, of puberty. If a GnRH test is performed, increased T or E values 4 hours after administration will indicate recent endogenous gonadotropin stimulation of the gonad; this is a more sensitive test for the beginning of puberty than is a single gonadal steroid determination. Many laboratories do not have adequately sensitive techniques to detect early pubertal values of testosterone (eg, 20–50 ng/dL) or estradiol (eg, 10–30 pg/mL). Unfortunately, some laboratories report values which are at the lower limits of their insensitive assay when they should report the value as less than that limit (eg, a serum sample with 20 ng/dL of testosterone may be reported to contain 100 ng/dL rather than "less than 100 ng/dL"). It is important to know each laboratory's limitations, the sensitivity of its assay, and its method of reporting.

DELAYED PUBERTY

A boy of 14 years or a girl of 13 years who has no signs of puberty may be considered delayed. However, there still will be children who are normal but statistically late. The physician's job is to determine who requires therapy and who needs only watchful waiting.

CONSTITUTIONAL DELAY IN GROWTH & ADOLESCENCE

Children with constitutional delay have slow physiologic development reflected by delayed bone age. They are usually thinner and shorter than average (third to fifth percentile) but grow at a normal rate for their bone age. They may have familial histories of delayed development. They are brought for evaluation when their friends have begun puberty but they have not. Even though they appear prepubertal, at the time of examination they may already have episodic gonadotropin secretion; a pubertal GnRH test or rising sex steroid concentrations indicate the likelihood that sexual development will commence within 6 months. In some patients with no endocrine changes of early pubertal development, the family and physician must engage in watchful waiting by physical examination and gonadal steroid determination for years to differentiate between constitutional delay in puberty and hypogonadotropic hypogonadism. Almost all patients with constitutional delay will spontaneously enter puberty by 18 years of age.

HYPOGONADOTROPIC HYPOGONADISM

The lack of GnRH stimulation of the gonadotropes may be total or partial. Patients may resemble those with constitutional delay in adolescence both physically and endocrinologically, but historical features are often different. If hypogonadotropic hypogonadism is accompanied by growth hormone (GH) deficiency, severe short stature will result. Undescended testes are common in patients lacking gonadotropin secretion. The most common causes of delayed puberty are discussed below (see also Table 4–1).

ISOLATED GONADOTROPIN DEFICIENCY

Kallmann's Syndrome

This syndrome combines impaired olfaction with GnRH deficiency due to a developmental defect of the diencephalon; either feature may be partial, so careful assessment of the sense of smell is necessary

Table 4–1. Causes of delayed puberty.

Constitutional delay in growth and adolescence	Miscellaneous hypogonadotropism
	Prader-Willi syndrome
Hypogonadotropic hypogonadism	Laurence-Moon-Biedl syndrome
Isolated gonadotropin deficiency	Chronic illness (eg, diabetes mellitus)
Kallmann's syndrome	Malnutrition
Congenital adrenal hypoplasia	Anorexia nervosa
Multiple pituitary hormone deficiencies	Dieting
Sporadic	Stress
Genetic	Increased physical activity
Autosomal recessive	Hypothyroidism
Autosomal dominant	Cushing's syndrome
X-linked	
Central nervous system disorders	**Hypergonadotropic hypogonadism**
Brain tumors	Primary testicular failure
Craniopharyngioma	Klinefelter's syndrome and variants
Germinomas	Anorchia
Gliomas	XY gonadal dysgenesis
Astrocytomas	Radiation, chemotherapy; other
Pituitary tumors	Primary ovarian failure
Prolactinomas	Turner's syndrome and variants
Other	XX gonadal dysgenesis
Histiocytosis X	Radiation, chemotherapy; other
Granulomas	P450c17-Hydroxylase deficiency
Infections	Androgen insensitivity (testicular feminization)
Vascular accidents	
Trauma	**Normogonadotropic primary amenorrhea** (phenotypic females with normal thelarche)
Developmental defects	Müllerian discontinuities (imperforate hymen, transverse vaginal septum)
Irradiation	

in anyone suspected of isolated gonadotropin deficiency. Propionic acid is used in logarithmic dilutions as a primary scent, but any mild, nonirritating odor can be used for rough screening of olfaction. Kallmann's syndrome is genetically heterogeneous and can be inherited in an autosomal dominant or recessive pattern (as opposed to the X-linked inheritance initially suggested in this condition). Other developmental defects such as facial dysraphism, cleft palate, cleft lip, and unilateral renal agenesis have accompanied cases of Kallmann's syndrome.

Sporadic isolated gonadotropin deficiency as well as selective absence of the secretion of LH or FSH may occur. Boys who have FSH but lack LH may be fertile but not sexually mature (the fertile eunoch syndrome). Boys who secrete LH but lack FSH may be sexually mature but infertile.

Congenital Adrenal Hypoplasia (X-linked, Cytomegalic)

These patients often have isolated gonadotropin deficiency in addition to primary adrenal insufficiency. The adrenals contain large vacuolated cells.

MULTIPLE PITUITARY HORMONE DEFICIENCIES

The assortment of pituitary hormone deficiencies will dictate the patient's physical presentation, but GH and gonadotropin deficiency will lead to the combination of extremely poor growth and lack of pubertal development. Hypothyroidism may aggravate the problem. If the patient is male, congenital GH and gonadotropin deficiency may manifest with microphallus at birth associated with hypoglycemic seizures. Patients with isolated GH deficiency are delayed in the start of puberty but finally undergo spontaneous pubertal progression when the bone age reaches 12–13 years. Treatment with GH will promote bone-age advancement and pubertal onset. Idiopathic hypopituitarism is usually sporadic but may follow autosomal recessive dominant or X-linked patterns. Midline defects are associated with all types of hypothalamic deficiencies. Birth injury or breech delivery may be found in the history of patients.

Central Nervous System Disorders

Tumors of the hypothalamic-pituitary area may disturb any or all pituitary hormonal function. The combination of acquired anterior and posterior pituitary deficiency points strongly to the presence of a tumor.

A. Craniopharyngiomas: These tumors originate in Rathke's pouch but may develop into a suprasellar tumor by upward extension.

They are the most common tumors affecting pubertal development and have a peak incidence between 6 and 14 years of age. Symptoms include headache, visual disturbance, poor growth, polyuria, and polydipsia. Visual field defects, papilledema or optic atrophy, and signs of gonadotropin, GH, and thyroid deficiency may be found. Four-fifths of craniopharyngiomas are calcified on lateral skull x-ray with even more calcification detected on CT scan. The tumor is often cystic. The critical location of these tumors makes complete removal hazardous. Usually subtotal resection followed by radiotherapy provides the best management of large tumors; small intrasellar tumors can be reached by the transsphenoidal approach.

B. Neoplasms: Neoplasms such as germinomas of the pineal region, gliomas (with neurofibromatosis or isolated) and astrocytomas can affect gonadotropin function. Chromophobe adenomas can interfere with gonadotropic function but are rare in childhood and adolescence. Hyperprolactinemia with or without a pituitary adenoma can delay the onset of puberty.

C. Other Lesions: Histiocytosis X may involve the hypothalamus and can cause hypothalamic defects besides diabetes insipidus. Granulomas due to tuberculosis or sarcoidosis, postinfectious lesions, vascular accidents, and trauma may all affect gonadotropin secretion. Midline developmental defects of the central nervous system may cause hypogonadotropic hypogonadism as well as other pituitary deficiencies.

Prader-Willi Syndrome

This syndrome describes the combination of decreased fetal activity and infantile hypotonia, short stature, obesity, and characteristic facies with almond-shaped eyes, small hands and feet, and developmental delay. Delayed menarche has been noted in females, and microphallus and undescended testes have been noted in males. Hypothalamic GnRH deficiency is usually implicated as the cause of disorders of puberty. Abnormalities of chromosome 15 have been described in 50% of patients. The syndrome occurs sporadically.

Laurence-Moon-Biedl Syndrome

This syndrome includes short stature, obesity, polydactyly, delayed development and retinitis pigmentosa. Hypogonadism has been recorded in males and females, and both hypothalamic GnRH deficiency and gonadal abnormalities have been described. This disorder is inherited in an autosomal recessive pattern.

Chronic Disease & Malnutrition

Chronic disease and malnutrition may lead to delayed puberty. Characteristically, weight loss to less than 80% of ideal weight leads to decreased gonadotropin secretion with resolution following weight gain.

Anorexia Nervosa

This psychiatric disorder is characterized by a distorted body image; patients (usually girls) avoid food or regurgitate if they do eat, exercise to lose more weight, and develop rituals around eating and cooking. Immune function may be compromised, and circulatory collapse may occur if weight loss continues. Secondary sexual development may cease, and in affected girls, amenorrhea (primary or secondary) is a classic finding. Dieting not associated with a psychiatric disorder can also cause hypogonadotropic hypogonadism.

Stress

Women of normal weight, usually with documented psychologic stress, may have functional amenorrhea.

Increased Physical Activity

In girls, athletic activities such as running or dancing may delay pubertal development; delayed menarche or irregular menses are common. The effects are not always related to weight loss because extremely active girls of normal weight may manifest these symptoms. Physical activity in boys has not been shown to delay puberty, but adult male runners can develop hypothalamic hypogonadism.

Hypothyroidism

Decreased thyroxin can delay sexual development as well as growth; menstrual irregularity may occur if pubertal development has already progressed.

Cushing's Syndrome

Excess glucocorticoids due to any cause can interfere with gonadotropin secretion or action.

PHENOTYPIC FEMALES WITH HYPERGONADOTROPIC HYPOGONADISM

Turner's Syndrome (Syndrome of Gonadal Dysgenesis)

Sexually infantile females may have Turner's syndrome. These girls are usually diagnosed before puberty owing to their short stature. If no other signs of Turner's syndrome are found in a sexually infantile girl, a mosaic form may be diagnosed by karyotype.

Complete Androgen Resistance

Maturing pubertal girls who do not manifest menses may have a 46,XY karyotype with complete androgen resistance; they lack pubic and axillary hair but have normal thelarche (breast development) at puberty. They may have an inguinal (testicular) mass. (See p 78).

Other Causes

Premature ovarian failure (possibly due to ovarian antibodies), XX gonadal dysgenesis, ovarian hCG/LH resistance, chemotherapy, and radiation therapy all lead to sexual infantilism and amenorrhea. Complete 17α-hydroxylase deficiency patients likewise manifest sexual infantilism and female phenotype regardless of genotype. (See pp 76 and 77).

PHENOTYPIC FEMALES WITH NORMOGONADOTROPIC PRIMARY AMENORRHEA

Secondary amenorrhea is discussed in Chapter 9. Primary amenorrhea may be due to anatomic defects such as imperforate hymen or vaginal septum. Girls with congenital adrenal hyperplasia frequently have delayed menarche and require readjustment of their therapeutic regime to achieve menstruation.

PHENOTYPIC MALES WITH HYPERGONADOTROPIC HYPOGONADISM

Klinefelter's Syndrome (Syndrome of Seminiferous Tubular Dysgenesis)

This most common form of primary testicular failure has an incidence of 1 in 1000 males. The age of onset of puberty is usually not delayed, but the degree of virilization varies in relation to the amount of Leydig cell function present. The karyotype is 47,XXY classically, but variants include 46,XY/47,XXY mosaicism, XXYY, XXXY, XXXYY, and XXXXY karyotypes, and 46,XX males. All these patients have positive buccal smear chromatin studies, but definitive diagnosis rests on karyotype.

Physical features include small, firm testes measuring less than 3 cm in length in the adult that are not sensitive to palpation. Other features include tall stature with long legs (but normal arm span) and greatly decreased upper to lower segment ratio, subnormal IQ, poor gross motor control, and personality and behavior disorders. All these features present in prepubertal subjects, and the diagnosis can be made in the first decade. After the onset of puberty, progressive destruction of seminiferous tubules leading to azoospermia and decreased Leydig cell function are accompanied by high plasma LH and FSH values. Gynecomastia appears, probably owing to an increased estradiol to testosterone ratio. Cosmetic surgery is often necessary to reduce breast tissue. There is an increased risk for cancer of the breast.

The only etiologic factor identified in Klinefelter's syndrome is advanced maternal age.

Patients with XY/XXY mosaicism may have less prominent features of Klinefelter's syndrome, and some may be fertile. Patients with variants having multiple X and Y chromosomes have more significant mental deficiency and may have other physical features such as clinodactyly and synostosis. Males with 46,XX karyotype are shorter than 47,XXY males and have normal phenotype but testicular changes similar to those with 47,XXY.

Anorchia

Bilateral anorchia ("vanishing testes syndrome") is associated with normal fetal development of the penis and scrotum. Thus, the disappearance of the testes must occur late in gestation or either ambiguous genitalia or microphallus would have occurred. Patients appear as bilaterally cryptorchid males. Administration of hCG, 2000 U every 3 days for 2 weeks, will lead to a rise in plasma testosterone to values over 100 ng/dL in cryptorchid males, and, in many, testes will actually descend into the scrotum, if the condition is retractile testes rather than true cryptorchidism; anorchic individuals will have no rise in testosterone and, of course, no descent of testes. Without a testosterone rise or detectable testes by ultrasound, it is unlikely that much dysgenetic testicular tissue remains to undergo malignant degeneration.

Artificial testes may be implanted in the scrotum and the size increased with advancing age for cosmetic effect. Testosterone should be administered to promote virilization.

Other causes

Male hypergonadotropic hypogonadism can be produced by XY gonadal dysgenesis (usually with ambiguous genitalia), irradiation or chemotherapy for malignancy, viral infection, or rarely autoimmunity.

EVALUATION OF DELAYED PUBERTY

Failure of a boy to begin pubertal development by age 14 or a girl by age 13 is an indication of a potential disorder of puberty. Further, if puberty has begun, failure of a boy to progress to adult development by 4.5 years or a girl to menstruate by 5 years after the onset of puberty may indicate hypogonadism.

Historical assessment of birth trauma, drug or teratogen exposure during pregnancy, general health, symptoms of chronic systemic or neurologic disease, psychiatric disorder, exercise activity, and parental and sib progression through puberty must first be obtained. A full physical examination with particular note of percentile of height, upper to lower segment ratio, weight, and head circumference is intended to rule out chronic systemic disease, endocrine disorders, and the physically diagnosable syndromes noted above. Breast and areolar size and stage in girls, testicular and penile size in boys, and pubic hair stage in boys and girls must be determined and recorded.

The presence of acne, greasiness of hair, moustache, voice change, and muscular development is similarly important. Sense of smell should be investigated. ''Scratch and sniff'' children's stickers may be used if a graded scent kit is unavailable.

In the absence of physical characteristics of syndromes, the first step of diagnosis is to determine gonadotropin levels. If gonadotropins are low, the differential diagnosis is between constitutional delay in adolescence (temporary) or hypothalamic GnRH or pituitary LH and FSH deficiency (permanent). The GnRH test may not differentiate between these 2 possibilities initially, but the test becomes pubertal approximately 6 months before physical pubertal development in constitutionally delayed patients. In the absence of congenital midline defects or neurologic manifestations, observation for signs of puberty in patients with prepubertal GnRH tests may have to continue until the patient is 18 years of age or older; constitutionally delayed patients will usually undergo spontaneous pubertal development by that time.

If a patient with delayed puberty is shown to have low plasma gonadotropins, a brain tumor may be the cause and a decision must be made as to whether an MRI brain scan is indicated. A classic history of constitutional delay in growth and adolescence including familial occurrence and classic physical features usually confirms this diagnosis, but any such patient can still have a craniopharyngioma! Thus, a careful neurologic examination with particular attention to visual fields and optic discs is essential in all patients. A lateral skull x-ray will not detect small or uncalcified hypothalamic pituitary tumors, and if suspicion remains that a patient cannot be completely categorized, an MRI scan of the head is necessary.

TREATMENT OF DELAYED PUBERTY

Psychological support is essential to counteract the patient's feelings of being different and the social stress received from peers. Reassurance in cases expected to spontaneously progress through puberty may be sufficient, but some severely depressed patients may require psychotherapy. Excusal from gym so that the patient will not have to shower or change in front of peers may be indicated.

Sex steroids may safely be offered in low doses and short courses to patients sufficiently disturbed by their immature appearance to not respond to supportive therapy. This treatment is not recommended until boys are 14 years or girls are 13 years of age, since before those ages the patients are not actually out of the average range. Testosterone enanthate, 100 mg intramuscularly every month for 3 months, can cause sufficient maturation to satisfy most patients while they await spontaneous progression. Girls may receive 3 months of oral ethinyl estradiol, 10 μg/d or conjugated estrogens, 0.3 mg/d. In constitutional delay, these short courses will not advance bone age or decrease final height, but resulting physical development will increase self esteem. If the diagnosis of permanent hypogonadism has been established and final height has been achieved, continuous therapy is indicated for boys with testosterone enanthate (start with 100 mg/month and increase dosage to 200 mg/month over 6 months). For girls, give ethinyl estradiol, 10–30 μg/d for the first 21 days of the month, and medroxyprogesterone acetate, 5 mg/d for days 12–21 of the month. Patients with gonadotropin deficiency who have not achieved final height (bone age is not fused) should not be placed on full replacement until height is no longer a concern. Gonadotropin therapy (hCG) given intramuscularly 1–3 times weekly is less convenient than testosterone enanthate given intramuscularly every month for hypogonadotropic hypogonadism, but gonadotropin administration has led to better pubic hair growth than testosterone treatment.

Patients with gonadal dysgenesis present a particular problem because their extreme short stature should not be compromised by early epiphyseal fusion but their psychological development should not be compromised owing to lack of feminization. They can receive ethinyl estradiol, 10 μg/d for days 1–21 of the month starting at age 12–13 years, to allow progressive feminization while not rushing epiphyseal fusion. Later, full replacement can be offered. They, and all girls on replacement estrogens, should have a pelvic examination yearly to determine whether uterine neoplasia has developed as a result of estrogen therapy. Growth hormone therapy is being investigated as a method of increasing final height (see page 123).

PRECOCIOUS PUBERTY

Puberty is considered precocious if it begins in girls before age 8 or in boys before age 9 years. Premature sexual development will cause rapid growth and advance children's bone ages. Thus, untreated children are tall at first but cease growing early and have short adult heights due to premature epiphyseal fusion. Complete precocious puberty indicates premature activation of the hypothalamic-pituitary-gonadal axis. The sine qua non of complete precocious puberty is the presence of a pubertal response of LH and FSH to GnRH. Incomplete (pseudo) precocious puberty denotes ectopic hCG secretion in boys or autonomous sex steroid production in boys or girls; the condition is so named because it is not caused by normal gonadotropin secretion and thus precludes early fertility. The GnRH test is never pubertal in incomplete precocious puberty. Isosexual precocity means that virilization is occurring in a boy or feminization in a girl. Heterosexual precocity indicates feminization in a boy or virilization in a girl. (See Table 4–2.)

Table 4–2. Causes of isosexual precocious puberty.*

Complete (true) precocious puberty	Incomplete (pseudo) precocious puberty
Constitutional	Males
Familial	Gonadotropin-secreting tumors
Idiopathic	HCG-secreting CNS tumors (eg, germinoma, teratoma)
Central nervous system disorders	HCG-secreting non CNS tumors (eg, hepatoma, teratoma, choriocarcinoma)
Hamartomas of the tuber cinereum	LH-secreting pituitary tumor
Other hypothalamic tumors	Excessive androgen secretion
Gliomas	Congenital adrenal hyperplasia
Astrocytomas	Leydig cell tumors
Ependymomas	Adrenal carcinoma
Meningitis/encephalitis	Premature Leydig cell maturation
Granulomas	Exogenous androgens
Brain abscess	Exogenous HCG
Suprasellar cysts	Severe hypothyroidism
Hydrocephalus	Females
Head trauma	Ovarian tumors
Irradiation	Granulosa cell tumor
Prior androgen exposure	Lipoid tumor
	Cystadenoma
Variation in pubertal development	Ovarian carcinoma
Premature thelarche	Gonadoblastoma
Premature adrenarche	Ovarian cysts
Premature isolated menarche	McCune-Albright syndrome
Adolescent gynecomastia	Adrenal tumor
	Exogenous estrogen
	Severe hypothyroidism

*"True" precocious puberty is caused by activation of the hypothalamic LRH (luteinizing hormone releasing hormone) pulse generator. "Pseudo" precocious puberty is independent of hypothalamic LRH.

COMPLETE (TRUE) PRECOCIOUS PUBERTY

Constitutional or Familial Precocious Puberty

Some children will enter puberty before the normal limits because of advanced physiologic maturation. A family tendency may be discovered. Such children usually are age 6–8 years and have no electroencephalographic, MRI or CT brain scan abnormalities.

Idiopathic (Sporadic) Precocious Puberty

Isolated cases of precocious puberty may occur even in children less than 1 year of age in a sporadic manner. Twenty percent of patients are less than 2 years of age. Electroencephalographic abnormalities can be documented in 80%. Endocrine changes are the same as found in normal puberty, and the first physical changes in boys will be testicular enlargement. The clinical course may be similar to normal puberty, or a waxing and waning course may be described. Parents are more prone to worry about early development in girls than in boys. Idiopathic precocious puberty occurs 9 times more commonly in girls than in boys who are brought for examination. Central nervous system lesions are twice as common as the idiopathic form of central precocious puberty in males, whereas in females the latter form is 2.5 times more common than the former.

Central Nervous System Disorders

Children are judged to have organic true precocious puberty (rather than idiopathic) if they have known head trauma, infection, tumors of the hypothalamic area, or another type of central nervous system disorder.

A. Hamartomas of the Tuber Cinereum: These are composed of ectopic hypothalamic tissue containing GnRH granules. These tumors may cause central pituitary gonadotropin secretion and subsequent secondary sexual development by episodically releasing GnRH as does the normal hypothalamus. They are not known to be progressive or invasive.

B. Other Hypothalamic Tumors: Less frequently, optic or hypothalamic gliomas (with or without neurofibromatosis), astrocytomas, and ependymomas may cause precocious puberty by interfering with the normal restraining mechanisms on GnRH secretion.

C. Other Central Nervous System Conditions: Conditions such as meningitis, encephalitis, granulomas (tuberculin, sarcoid), brain abscesses, suprasellar cysts, hydrocephalus, head trauma, and hypothalamic pituitary irradiation have caused precocious puberty. Children with epilepsy and mental retardation have an increased incidence of precocious puberty.

McCune-Albright Syndrome

Irregular café au lait spots, polyostotic fibrous dysplasia of the long bones, and precocious puberty can be associated with autonomous hyperfunction of the thyroid and adrenal gland or ovaries as well as true precocious puberty.

Severe Hypothyroidism

Severe untreated hypothyroidism can cause galactorrhea and sexual precocity in some patients; as previously stated, hypothyroidism can also cause delayed puberty in other children.

Androgen Exposure

Androgen exposure of either exogenous (eg, anabolic steroids) or endogenous (eg, adrenal tumor or hyperplasia) origin causes pseudoprecocious puberty. Androgen exposure can also cause maturation of the hypothalamic-pituitary axis; when the source of androgens is removed, true precocious puberty can result.

INCOMPLETE (PSEUDO) PRECOCIOUS PUBERTY

Males

Virilization may be caused by either (1) tumors secreting hCG, which causes Leydig cells to secrete testosterone, or (2) autonomous androgen secretion.

A. hCG-Secreting Tumors: Hepatomas or hepatoblastomas as well as germinomas of the pineal or hypothalamic region can secrete hCG and cause incomplete sexual precocity in the male. The hCG is identical in action to pituitary LH and stimulates Leydig cells to secrete testosterone. In girls with hCG-secreting tumors, hCG has no effect on granulosa cells, neither estrogen nor androgens is secreted, and no secondary sexual development results.

B. Excessive Androgen Secretion: Excessive androgen secretion can be due to adrenal enzyme defects, virilizing adrenal carcinoma, Leydig cell tumors, and familial premature Leydig cell and germ cell maturation.

Clinical characteristics of incomplete sexual precocity include less testicular enlargement for pubertal stage of development than in true precocious puberty; with hCG stimulation or premature Leydig cell maturation, the testes frequently enlarge to more than 2.5 cm, but with autonomous androgen production from other sites, the testes remain less than 2.5 cm. Premature Leydig cell maturation is inherited as a sex-limited dominant condition. Gonadotropin values are low and do not rise to pubertal levels after GnRH administration, while testosterone values are pubertal.

Females

Autonomous estrogen secretion is the cause of incomplete precocious puberty in girls. This may be due to isolated or recurrent follicular cysts that cause breast development and withdrawal bleeding; plasma estrogen levels in girls with ovarian cysts can reach values in excess of 100 pg/mL and mimic levels found in girls with estrogen-secreting tumors. Alternatively, an estrogen-secreting granulosa cell tumor of the ovary may be the cause of incomplete precocious puberty in girls. Four-fifths of these tumors are palpable on rectal examination, and most can be detected by ultrasonography. Less common estrogen-secreting tumors of the ovary are lipoid tumors, cystadenomas, ovarian carcinomas, and gonadoblastomas. Ovarian cysts leading to feminization and galactorrhea owing to simultaneous elevation of prolactin may occur in severe primary hypothyroidism. Adrenal neoplasms as well as ovarian tumors may secrete estrogen.

Exogenous Sex-Steroid Administration

Boys ingesting testosterone or receiving hCG injections will show virilization; testes will be smaller with exogenous testosterone ingestion. Girls or boys receiving estrogens, either ingested (eg, from oral contraceptives) or absorbed (eg, from skin contact with estrogen-containing cosmetics on mother), will show breast development. An even more disguised source of estrogens may be commercially purchased chicken or beef treated with substances to promote growth. Chicken necks are often the location of the deposit of estrogen. Epidemics of premature breast development in girls and gynecomastia in boys have been thought to be due to estrogen-containing chicken and veal.

EVALUATION OF SEXUAL PRECOCITY

Historical investigation and physical examination should include the same approach as for delayed puberty. Extra attention must be directed to discovering a source of exogenous hormone. During the physical examination, a search for stigmata of McCune-Albright syndrome or neurofibromatosis is important. Laboratory determination starts with plasma gonadotropin and sex steroid determinations performed at a reliable laboratory. If estradiol is greater than 20 pg/mL or testosterone is greater than 20 ng/dL and FSH and LH values are not suppressed to less than 5 mIU, the likely diagnosis is central precocious puberty. Plasma estradiol levels over 100–150 pg/mL may indicate an estrogen-secreting tumor or a cyst of the ovary. Girls with central precocious puberty may have significant variation in estradiol so that undetectable values as well as levels over 60 pg/mL can occur during the same day; boys' testosterone values show less variation and are always above 20 ng/dL. The definitive diagnosis is made with the GnRH test. If LH rises more than 17.6 mIU/mL (pubertal result), central precocious puberty is diagnosed, whereas no rise in LH in the presence of sex-steroid secretion indicates incomplete precocious puberty. If basal LH levels are very high and a specific 6k betaB-hCG test is positive in boys with precocious puberty, the cause is an hCG-secreting tumor, and a search must be instituted for the source (abdomen or central nervous system).

The diagnosis of central precocious puberty mandates CT or MRI scan of the brain, with fine cuts and magnification of the hypothalamic-pituitary area to rule out a brain tumor as the cause.

TREATMENT OF SEXUAL PRECOCITY

Central Precocious Puberty

Criteria for treatment of central precocious puberty include pubertal pattern of spontaneous or GnRH-stimulated LH release; rapid progression of height velocity, bone age, or secondary sexual characteristics; serum testosterone concentration in boys over 100 ng/dL if younger than age 8; and onset of menses in girls less than 9 years of age.

Potent GnRH analogs (GnRHa) are the best treatment of central precocious puberty. These agents briefly stimulate the pituitary, then cause down-regulation of pituitary GnRH receptors, leading to suppression of gonadotropin secretion and then sex-steroid secretion. They are derivatives of the naturally occurring 10-amino-acid GnRH. GnRHa is injected subcutaneously or given intranasally daily. Depot forms that last 1 month are now available. Physical signs of puberty cease to progress or regress, rapid growth and bone-age advancement slow, and patients likely will reach taller adult heights than without therapy. In the USA, GnRHa is available for treatment of prostatic carcinoma and soon should be approved for treatment of precocious puberty.

A progestational agent, medroxyprogesterone acetate, has been used to suppress pubertal development, but it is less effective than GnRHa and has side effects, including adrenal suppression, the induction of Cushingoid features when high doses are used, and the possibility of the development of breast nodules.

Psychological support is of major importance for the child and family. Menstruation and breast development in young girls and frequent erections and aggressive behavior in young boys distresses patients and families. Children who look older are often expected to act older by adults and teachers. Professional counseling is recommended.

Incomplete (Pseudo) Precocious Puberty

The treatment of incomplete precocious puberty involves detecting the cause (Table 4–2) and directing therapy accordingly.

Boys with premature Leydig cell maturation (familial "testotoxicosis"; male-limited autosomal dominant) do not initially respond to GnRHa. Successful treatment of this entity with ketoconazole (200 mg every 8 hours orally) has been reported in 4 boys over a 1-year period. After control is achieved with this agent, central precocious puberty may develop because of long-term exposure to androgens; GnRH then is indicated in addition to ketoconazole. Oral medroxyprogesterone acetate has been effective in some boys, and recent reports have shown successful use of testolactone and spironolactone.

Girls with McCune-Albright syndrome may initially be treated with medroxyprogesterone or testolactone to suppress ovarian cyst formation. In a later stage of gonadotropin-dependent pubertal progression, GnRHa may be invoked. Recurrent ovarian cysts may be responsive to medroxyprogesterone or testolactone. The sexual precocity of hypothyroidism is reversible with thyroxine administration.

VARIATIONS IN PUBERTAL DEVELOPMENT

Premature Thelarche

Premature thelarche is early breast development in girls without other signs of feminization, such as vaginal secretion or nipple enlargement. Characteristically, the affected girl is less than 3 years of age, and breast development can be unilateral or bilateral. The cause is unknown, but it may be due to brief estrogen secretion from transient ovarian cysts. A small uterus and small ovarian cysts by ultrasound, low E_2, and slight increase in FSH after GnRH are usual. Breast development does not proceed past stage II or early stage III and may regress after several months; other aspects of pubertal development occur at the normal age.

Premature Adrenarche

Premature adrenarche is the early appearance of pubic or axillary hair without other signs of virilization. Patients are usually over 6 years of age at onset, but other aspects of pubertal development occur at a normal age. The cause is a premature rise in plasma DHAS and urinary 17-ketosteroid values to early pubertal levels owing to early activation of adrenal androgen secretion. This condition may be confused with late-onset congenital adrenal hyperplasia in which serum

17-hydroxyprogesterone (21-hydroxylase deficiency) or 17-hydroxy-pregnenolone is elevated in the basal state or after ACTH administration.

Adolescent Gynecomastia

Adolescent gynecomastia refers to breast development in boys. Mild gynecomastia is common in normal boys in early puberty, prior to reaching genital stage II, and usually regresses within 2 years. The cause has been attributed to an elevated estrogen/testosterone ratio, although T and E values are each within the normal range. Disorders such as Klinefelter's syndrome, Reifenstein's syndrome, 11-hydroxylase deficiency, and incomplete androgen resistance also produce gynecomastia. In the absence of such disorders, idiopathic gynecomastia is diagnosed. Usually, no therapy is indicated for pubertal gynecomastia and the condition is transient, but severely affected patients may require reduction mammoplasty to alleviate psychological stress.

REFERENCES

Bayley N, Pinneau SF: Tables for predicting adult height from skeletal age: Revised for use with the Greulich-Pyle standards. *J Pediatr* 1952;**40**:423.

Boepple PA et al: Use of a potent, long-acting agonist of gonadotropin-releasing hormone in the treatment of precocious puberty. *Endocr Rev* 1986;**7**:24.

Boyar RM et al: Simultaneous augmented secretion of luteinizing hormone and testosterone during sleep. *J Clin Invest* 1974;**54**:609.

Cacciari E et al: How many cases of true precocious puberty in girls are idiopathic? *J Pediatr* 1983;**102**:357.

Comite F et al: Cyclical ovarian function resistant to treatment with an analogue of luteinizing hormone releasing hormone in McCune-Albright syndrome. *N Engl J Med* 1984;**311**:1032.

Comite F et al: The short-term treatment of idiopathic precocious puberty with a long-acting analogue of luteinizing hormone-releasing hormone. *N Engl J Med* 1981;**305**:1546.

Crowley WF Jr et al: Therapeutic use of pituitary desensitization with a long-acting LHRH agonist: A potential new treatment for idiopathic precocious puberty. *J Clin Endocrinol Metab* 1981;**52**:370.

Egli CA et al: Pituitary gonadtropin-independent male-limited autosomal dominant sexual precocity in nine generations: Familial testotoxicosis. *J Pediatr* 1985;**106**:33.

Feuillan PP et al: Treatment of precocious puberty in the McCune-Albright syndrome with the aromatase inhibitor testolactone. *N Engl J Med* 1986; **315**:1115.

Forest MG, de Peretti E, Bertrand J: Hypothalamic-pituitary-gonadal relationships in man from birth to puberty. *Clin Endocrinol* 1976;**5**:551.

Greulich WW, Pyle SI: *Radiographic Atlas of Skeletal Development of the Hand and Wrist*, 2nd ed. Stanford University Press, 1959.

Grumbach MM et al: Hypothalamic-pituitary regulation of puberty in man: Evidence and concepts derived from clinical research. Pages 115–166 in: *Control of the Onset of Puberty.* Grumbach MM, Grave GD, Mayer FE (editors). Wiley, 1974.

Harlan WR, Harlan EA, Grillo GP: Secondary sex characteristics of girls 12 to 17 years of age: The US Health Examination Survey. *J Pediatr* 1980; **96:**1074.

Harlan WR et al: Secondary sex characteristics of boys 12 to 17 years of age: The US Health Examination Survey. *J Pediatr* 1980;**95:**293.

Harris DA et al: Somatomedin-C in normal puberty and in true precocious puberty before and after treatment with a potent luteinizing hormone-releasing hormone agonist. *J Clin Endocrinol Metab* 1985;**61:**152.

Hoffman AR, Crowley WR: Induction of puberty in men by long-term pulsatile administration of low dose gonadotropin-releasing hormone. *N Engl J Med* 1982;**307:**1237.

Holland FJ, Kirsch SE, Selby R: Gonadotropin-independent precocious puberty ("testotoxicosis"): Influence of maturational status on response to keto-conazole. *J Clin Endocrinol Metab* 1987;**64:**328.

Holland FJ et al: Ketoconazole in the management of precocious puberty not responsive to LHRH-analogue therapy. *N Engl J Med* 1985;**312:**1023.

Judge DM et al: Hypothalamic hamartoma: A source of luteinizing-hormone-releasing factor in precocious puberty. *N Engl J Med* 1977;**296:**7.

Kaplan SL, Grumbach MM, Rosenfield RG, Styne DM: Pathophysiology and treatment of sexual precocity. *J Clin Endocrinol Metab* 1990;**71:**785.

Kaplan SL, Grumbach MM, Aubert ML: The ontogenesis of pituitary hormones and hypothalamic factors in the human fetus: Maturation of central nervous system regulation of anterior pituitary function. *Recent Prog Horm Res* 1976;**32:**161.

Leyendecker G, Wildt L, Hansmann M: Pregnancies following chronic inter-mittent (pulsatile) administration of GnRH by means of a pulsatile pump ('zyklomat'): A new approach to the treatment of infertility in hypothalamic amenorrhea. *J Clin Endocrinol Metab* 1980;**51:**1214.

Mansfield MJ et al: Long-term treatment of central precocious puberty with a long-acting analogue of luteinizing hormone-releasing hormone. *N Engl J Med* 1983;**309:**1286.

Marshall WA, Tanner JM: Variations in the pattern of pubertal changes in boys. *Arch Dis Child* 1970;**45:**13.

Marshall WA, Tanner JM: Variations in the pattern of pubertal changes in girls. *Arch Dis Child* 1969;**44:**291.

Reiter EO, Fuldauer VG, Root AW: Secretion of the adrenal androgen, dehy-droepiandrosterone sulfate, during normal infancy, childhood, and adoles-cence, in sick infants and in children with endocrinologic abnormalities. *J Pediatr* 1977;**90:**766.

Rivkees SA, Crawford JD: The relationship of gonadal activity and chemother-apy-induced gonadal damage. *JAMA* 1988;**259:**2123.

Rohn RD: Nipple (papilla) development in puberty. Longitudinal observations in girls. *Pediatrics* 1987;**79:**745.

Rosenfield RL: Puberty and its disorders in the female. *Endocrin Metab Clin North Am* 1991;**20.**

Rosenfield RL: The ovary and female sexual maturation. In: *Clinical Pediatric Endocrinology*. Kaplan SA (editor). Saunders, 1989;**259**.

Rosenthal SM, Grumbach MM, Kaplan SL: Gonadotropin-independent familial sexual precocity with premature Leydig and germinal cell maturation ('familial testotoxicosis'): Effects of a potent luteinizing hormone-releasing factor agonist and medroxyprogesterone acetate therapy in four cases. *J Clin Endocrinol Metab* 1983;**57**:571.

Sadeghi-Nejad A, Kaplan SL, Grumbach MM: The effect of medroxyprogesterone acetate on adrenocortical function in children with precocious puberty. *J Pediatr* 1971;**78**:616.

Sklar CA, Kaplan SL, Grumbach MM: Evidence for dissociation between adrenarche and gonadarche: Studies in patients with idiopathic precocious puberty, gonadal dysgenesis, isolated gonadotropin deficiency, and constitutionally delayed growth and adolescence. *J Clin Endocrinol Metab* 1980;**51**:548.

Styne DM, Grumbach MM: Puberty in the male and female: Its physiology and disorders. In: *Reproductive Endocrinology*. Yen SCC, Jaffe RB (editors). Saunders, 1991.

Styne DM et al: Treatment of true precocious puberty with a potent luteinizing hormone–releasing factor agonist: Effect on growth, sexual maturation, pelvic sonography, and the hypothalamic-pituitary-gonadal axis. *J Clin Endocrinol Metab* 1985;**61**:142.

Tanner JM et al: The adolescent growth spurt of boys and girls of the Harpenden Growth Study. *Ann Hum Biol* 1976;**3**:109.

Valk TW et al: Hypogonadotropic hypogonadism: Hormonal responses to low dose pulsatile administration of gonadotropin-releasing hormones. *J Clin Endocrinol Metab* 1980;**51**:730.

Van Wierigen JC et al: *Growth Diagrams 1965 Netherlands: Second National Survey on 0-24 years Olds*. Wolters-Noordhoff Publishing 1971.

Wildt L, Marshall G, Knobil E: Experimental induction of puberty in the infantile rhesus monkey. *Science* 1980;**207**:1373.

Wilkins L: *The Diagnosis and Treatment of Endocrine Disorders in Childhood and Adolescence*, 2nd ed. Thomas, 1965.

Wilson DM et al: Effects of testosterone therapy for pubertal delay. *Am J Dis Child* 1988;**142**:96.

Thyroid Disorders | 5

Henry F. Safrit, MD

THYROID ANATOMY & HISTOLOGY

The normal adult thyroid gland weighs 15–20 g. It consists of 2 lobes, one on either side of the trachea. A narrow isthmus crosses the trachea just below the cricoid cartilage, connecting the 2 lobes. Each lobe is 2–3 cm in vertical diameter and 1 cm in width. The pyramidal lobe or remnant of the thyroglossal duct is present in 30% of thyroid glands, rising from the isthmus, usually near the left lobe.

Embryologically, the thyroid gland is formed from the thyroglossal duct, which begins its migration from the pharynx down into the neck. A lingual thyroid develops at the base of the tongue if migration is arrested. In the descent of the thyroglossal duct into the neck, one or both lobes may fail to develop. The thyroid may also follow the pathway of the thymus into the thorax and years later be discovered as a substernal gland. In the few reported cases of agenesis of a lobe, the left lobe is more often absent. All the congenital anomalies are probably very rare; they are usually discovered during the workup for thyroid disease.

The functional unit of the thyroid is the spherical thyroid follicle. Cuboidal cells line the follicle; they become more columnar when active. The lumen of this follicle is filled with colloid, the storage form for thyroglobulin that is secreted by the thyroid cells. Thyroglobulin contains tyrosine residues that are iodinated and ultimately form thyroid hormones. Thyroglobulin molecules in storage will contain monoiodotyrosine (MIT), diiodotyrosine (DIT), as well as thyroxine (T_4), and triiodothyronine (T_3). The thyroid gland is unique among endocrine organs in this capacity to store thyroglobulin. A normal thyroid gland has enough stored thyroid hormone for 100 days of normal secretion.

Physical Examination

Inspection of the neck, both before and during swallowing should precede palpation. In thin necks, normal thyroid glands can often be visualized. Enlargement and nodularity are commonly appreciated.

SOME ACRONYMS USED IN THIS CHAPTER

ACTH	Adrenocorticotropic hormone
CEA	Carcinoembryogenic antigen
DIT	Diiodotyrosine
FTI	Free thyroxine index
FT$_3$	Free T$_3$
FT$_4$	Free T$_4$
hCG	Human chorionic gonadotropin
MEN	Multiple endocrine neoplasia
MIT	Monoiodotyrosine
MTC	Medullary thyroid carcinoma
RAI	Radioactive iodine
RAIU	Radioactive iodine uptake
RIA	Radioimmunoassay
rT$_3$	Reverse T$_3$
T$_3$	Triiodothyronine
T$_4$	Thyroxine
TBG	Thyroid–binding globulin
TBII	TSH–binding inhibitory immunoglobulin
TBP	Thyroid–binding protein
TBPA	Thyroid–binding prealbumin
TRCA	Tanned red cell agglutination assay
TRH	Thyrotropin–releasing hormone
T$_3$RU	T$_3$ resin uptake
TSH	Thyroid–stimulating hormone
TSI	Thyroid–stimulating immunoglobulin

The gland is best palpated with the examiner behind the seated patient. Most normal glands are palpable. The cricoid cartilage is a good landmark to start from. With the first 3 fingers on either side of the trachea at this level, the thyroid gland moves upward with swallowing, and size, consistency, nodularity, and asymmetry may be recorded by the examiner. An outline of any abnormality should be traced on the overlying skin and measured for future comparison.

THYROID PHYSIOLOGY

Thyroid-Stimulating Hormone

Thyroid hormone production within the thyroid gland is stimulated by thyroid-stimulating hormone (TSH; thyrotropin) secreted from the pituitary gland. High thyroid levels cause decreased TSH secretion from the pituitary—a negative feedback system. Thyroid hormone probably has no direct feedback mechanism upon hypothalamic thyrotropin-releasing hormone (TRH), but high thyroid hormone levels may "desensitize" the pituitary to the stimulatory effect of TRH. Low thyroid hormone levels may "sensitize" the pituitary to secrete TSH in response to TRH.

Thyroid Hormonogenesis & Metabolism

TSH is important in all steps of the enzyme-dependent thyroid hormone synthesis, from trapping of iodide to release of thyroid hormone (Fig 5–1).

Most of the thyroid hormone released from the gland is L-thyroxine (T_4) with a much smaller percentage of triiodothyronine (T_3) (Fig 5–2). Both are bound to proteins in the serum (thyroid-binding protein, TBP); 99.975% of T_4 is bound, 75% to thyroid-binding globulin (TBG), 20% to thyroid-binding prealbumin (TBPA), and 5% to albumin. Of T_3 99.7% is bound, 75% to TBG and 25% to albumin. Very small amounts of both T_4 and T_3 are unbound in circulation. The serum half-life for T_4 is long, about 7 days, compared with a 6- to 8-hour half-life for T_3. T_4 is converted in the liver to T_3 and reverse T_3 (rT_3) in roughly equal amounts, by dropping one iodide (5-position) from the T_4 molecule.

Loss of an iodide from the outer ring of the thyroxine molecule results in the formation of T_3. Deiodination from the inner ring results

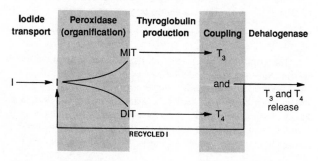

MIT = Monoiodotyrosine
DIT = Diiodotyrosine

Figure 5–1. Steps in thyroid hormonogenesis.

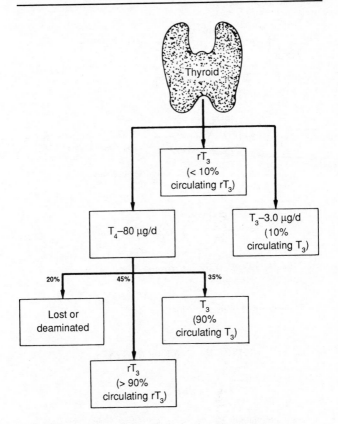

Figure 5–2. Normal thyroid hormone metabolism.

in production of rT_3 (Fig 5–3). T_3 is the most active form of thyroid hormone. T_4 may be thought of as a prohormone. Both T_4 and T_3 can suppress pituitary release of TSH. rT_3 has no biologic activity. In starvation and acute and chronic illness, the equilibrium between T_3 and rT_3 shifts in favor of rT_3.

The very small fraction of free T_4 and T_3 in circulation enters the tissues and exerts metabolic activity. This fraction is controlled by the pituitary gland. The larger bound fractions may vary in certain settings, independent of pituitary control, with changes in levels of TBP and in starvation and illness.

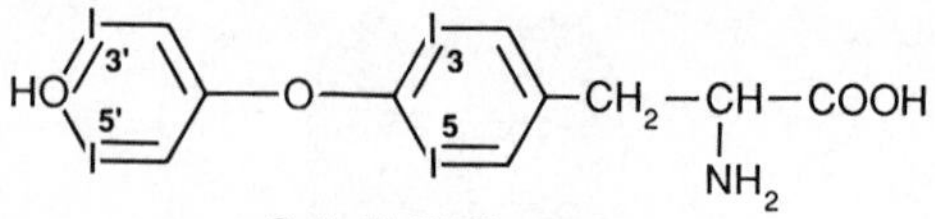

3, 5, 3', 5'-Thyroxine
(T$_4$)

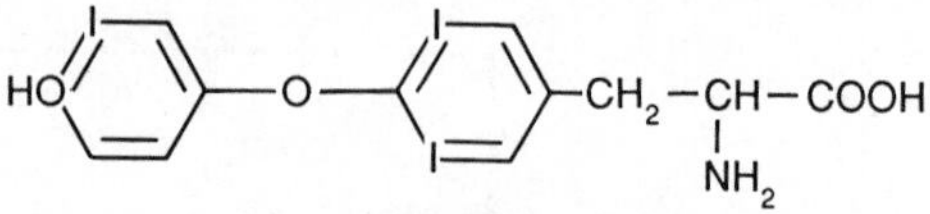

3, 5, 3'-Triiodothyronine
(T$_3$)

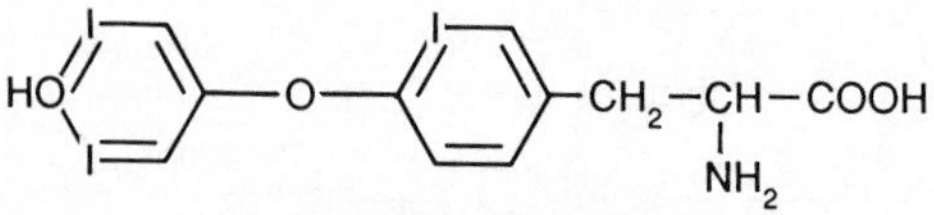

3, 3', 5'-Triiodothyronine
(reverse T$_3$, rT$_3$, T'$_3$)

Figure 5–3. Structural formulas for T$_4$, T$_3$, and rT$_3$.

THYROID FUNCTION TESTS

SERUM T$_4$

Total circulating T$_4$ can be measured accurately by radioimmunoassay (RIA). The normal range is about 5–12 μg/dL. Most of measured T$_4$ is bound to TBP. Only free T$_4$ and T$_3$ are active. An elevated serum T$_4$ is consistent with a clinical diagnosis of hyperthyroidism and a low T$_4$ with a clinical diagnosis of hypothyroidism. Factors that alter serum thyroxine measurements without affecting clinical status are listed in Table 5–1 and discussed below. These factors must always be considered when interpreting a serum thyroxine level.

Factors Increasing Measured T$_4$ Without Affecting Clinical Status

A. Underlying Illness: Certain disease states increase TBP, and T$_4$ and T$_3$ levels in these conditions also tend to be elevated. Such diseases include acute viral hepatitis, chronic active hepatitis, primary

Table 5–1. Factors altering serum thyroxine measurements without affecting clinical status.*

Factors increasing T$_4$	Factors decreasing T$_4$
Acute illness† (eg, viral hepatitis, chronic active hepatitis; primary biliary cirrhosis; acute intermittent porphyria; AIDS)	Severe illness† (eg, chronic renal failure, major surgery, caloric deprivation)
High estrogen states† (may also increase T$_3$)	Acute psychiatric problems†
Oral estrogen-containing contraceptives	Cirrhosis
Pregnancy	Nephrotic syndrome
Estrogen replacement therapy	Hereditary TBG deficiency
Neonatal period	Drugs
Acute psychiatric problems†	Phenobarbital (patients receiving replacement and some normal subjects)
Hyperemesis gravidarum and morning sickness (may also increase T$_3$)	Phenytoin (T$_4$ may be as low as 2 μg/dL)
Familial dysalbuminemic hyperthyroxinemia†	Carbamazepine
Familial X-linked TBG excess (may also increase T$_3$)	Triiodothyronine (T$_3$) therapy
Generalized resistance to thyroid hormone (Refetoff's syndrome)	Androgens
Drugs	5-Fluorouracil
Levothyroxine (T$_4$) replacement therapy	Halofenate (lowers triglycerides and uric acid; not marketed in USA)
Amiodarone†	Mitotane
Heparin, intravenous	Phenylbutazone
Amphetamines	Fenclofenac (nonsteroidal antiinflammatory agent; not marketed in USA)
Methadone (may also increase T$_3$)	Salicylates (large doses)
Heroin	Chloral hydrate
Perphenazine	L-Asparaginase
Clofibrate	

* Symptomatic hyperthyroidism or hypothyroidism may also be present incidentally.
† Discussed in text.

biliary cirrhosis, AIDS, and acute intermittent porphyria. The hypermetabolism and high T$_4$ in an acutely ill patient may be distinguished from true hyperthyroidism by measuring a free T$_4$ that is normal and a free T$_3$ that is low to normal.

B. High Estrogen States: Estrogen increases TBP and, therefore, total T$_4$ and total T$_3$. The distinction between this state and clinical hyperthyroidism may be made as described above.

C. Acute Psychiatric Problems: As many as 30% of recently admitted psychiatric patients may have elevated T$_4$ (hyperthyroxemia); 20% also have high free thyroxine index. Virtually all will return to normal during the hospital course.

D. Drugs: Certain drugs (Table 5–1) may raise total T_4 levels.

Amiodarone is an effective cardiac antiarrhythmic agent usually reserved for resistant arrhythmias owing to its potential adverse effects, eg, its unique effects on serum thyroid hormone levels and thyroid function.

Amiodarone produces a high serum T_4 and free thyroxine index in about 50% of patients receiving it without causing clinical thyrotoxicosis. This effect is due to a partial block in the conversion of T_4 to T_3, with resultant increases in serum T_4 and shunting to inactive rT_3. The following revised serum normal levels have been suggested for patients taking amiodarone: T_4, 5–19 μg/dL; T_3, 36–163 ng/dL; rT_3, 22–131 ng/dL. **Amiodarone may also cause true thyrotoxicosis (p 209) or hypothyroidism (p 217).**

Amiodarone is 37% iodine and is stored in fat and muscle, requiring about 3 months for excretion. The organic iodine floods the body and may cause clinical hypothyroidism (8%) or hyperthyroidism (2.5%) even in patients with otherwise normal thyroid glands. These changes may occur even in the first few months after the drug is stopped.

E. Familial Dysalbuminemic Hyperthyroxinemia: This benign autosomal dominant condition consists of elevations in serum T_4, free thyroxine index, and sometimes T_3 owing to an abnormal albumin molecule that binds T_4 preferentially to T_3. The resin T_3 uptake is not decreased (as in TBG excess), since the T_3 used in the T_3RU assay is not affected greatly. The direct free T_4 level is normal as is TSH.

Factors Decreasing Measured T_4 Without Affecting Clinical Status

A. Severe Illness: With severe illness or caloric deprivation or following major surgery, there is a shift in conversion of T_4 to lesser amounts of T_3 and more rT_3. T_3 is low, free T_3 tends to be low, rT_3 is high, and T_4 is variable, depending on TBP level, which often is low in the same setting.

In severely ill patients there is a circulating inhibitor of thyroid binding to TBP, unrelated to circulating levels of TBP. This inhibitor interferes with thyroid binding to resin as well, so that T_4, T_3, and T_3RU will all be low. The presence of this inhibitor may correlate with severity of illness, and in fact low T_4 has been associated with poor prognosis. In a series of patients with severe nonthyroidal illness and T_4 levels less than 3 μg/dL, the mortality rate was 84%. Low or normal serum TSH helps rule out primary hypothyroidism in this group of patients.

A small percentage of recently admitted psychiatric patients, perhaps 10%, may have a transiently low T_4. This returns to normal with treatment of the underlying psychiatric illness. Very few of these patients are hypothyroid.

B. Drugs: Certain drugs listed in Table 5–1 may decrease total T_4 levels. For example, diphenylhydantoin accelerates the metabolism of T_4 to T_3. Androgens, glucocorticoids, and salicylates cause low TBP. Despite a low T_4, the TSH is normal if the patient is euthyroid.

SERUM T_3 RESIN UPTAKE (T_3RU)*

As long as TBP is normal, T_4 is a reliable test for thyroid function, but changes in TBP are frequent and alter T_4 levels independently of thyroid function. Measuring binding proteins directly is difficult, but T_3RU is an indirect approximation. Radiolabeled T_3 is incubated with a patient's serum and allowed to equilibrate and endogenous hormone. An aliquot is then added to a resin. If there are relatively small amounts of TBP in the serum, relatively more radiolabeled T_3 will be available to bind to the resin. Conversely, with large amounts of TBP, less radiolabeled T_3 binds to resin. T_3RU is expressed as a percentage of the total radiolabeled T_3 that binds to resin, and in most laboratories, normal T_3RU is 25–35%. The test is performed with T_3 rather than T_4 because of the lower affinity of T_3 to the endogenous binding proteins; more T_3 is available for binding to the resin. In the euthyroid state, high TBP is associated with high total T_4 and low T_3RU; low TBP is associated with low T_4 and high T_3RU. A free thyroxine index (FTI) is calculated by multiplying T_4 by T_3RU. The upper limit of FTI is the product of the upper limits of T_4 and T_3RU; the lower limit of FTI is the product of the lower limits of both T_4 and T_3RU. There is a high positive correlation between FTI and free thyroxine. At the extreme ends of the spectrum of circulating binding proteins with resulting abnormal levels of T_4 and T_3RU, the FTI is less reliable. The T_3RU test is unrelated to circulating levels of T_3 in the serum and should not be confused with total T_3. Factors affecting T_3RU are listed in Table 5–2.

Table 5–2. Factors affecting T_3 resin uptake (T_3RU).

Low T_3RU (High TBP*)	High T_3RU (Low TBP*)
Pregnancy	Anabolic steroids
Estrogen therapy	Chronic liver disease
Acute hepatitis	Nephrotic syndrome
Genetic TBP increase	High-dose glucocorticoids
Hypothyroidism	Hyperthyroidism

* TBP = Thyroid binding protein.

* In some assays, radiolabeled T_4 (T_4RU) is used.

SERUM FREE T_4 & FREE T_3

The fraction of free thyroid hormones, the free T_4 and T_3 (FT_4 and FT_3), in circulation is exceedingly small: 0.03% of total T_4 and 0.3% of total T_3. The absolute amounts are 2 ng/dL of FT_4 and 0.4 ng/dL of FT_3. These minute amounts have not been susceptible to direct measurement and as a result have been measured by the very cumbersome dialysis or ultracentrifugation techniques. In the more commonly used dialysis method, a tracer concentration of the hormone being measured (T_3 or T_4) is added to the serum and allowed to distribute between free and bound forms in the same ratio of the endogenous hormone. The free fraction of the tracer then dialyzes through a semipermeable membrane (the bound will not dialyze). This fraction is multiplied by the total endogenous hormone level to get the absolute level of free endogenous hormone level.

More recently, commercial kits for measuring FT_4 and FT_3 have been developed. A good kit produces results that correlate well with results of dialysis measurements and is useful in settings where alteration in standard thyroid function testing is anticipated, such as severe nonthyroidal illness or starvation.

Free T_3 and T_4 levels generally reflect thyroid function accurately regardless of alterations in binding protein and peripheral conversion of T_4 to T_3. Free T_4 may rise transiently in acute nonthyroidal disease if TBP levels fall.

SERUM T_3

Serum T_3 is a radioimmunoassay measurement of total T_3, both bound and free. Normal values are about 80–200 ng/dL. T_3 (as well as T_4) levels vary with changes in TBP. When TBP is high, T_3 tends to be high, and when TBP is low, T_3 is low. A free T_3 index (FT_3I) can be calculated by multiplying T_3 and T_3RU, but this is not as reliable an index of thyroid function as the FTI. Correlation between FT_3I and free T_3 is not as good as that between FTI and free T_4.

Whereas T_4 is variable and unpredictable in nonthyroidal illness, T_3 is more predictably low. With nonthyroidal illness, conversion of T_4 is more toward rT_3 and less toward T_3.

T_3 should be determined only to help diagnose hyperthyroidism. In hypothyroidism it often remains normal after T_4 has dropped and TSH is elevated, since TSH stimulation increases T_3 secretion relative to T_4 secretion. In hyperthyroidism both T_4 and T_3 is elevated. In mild disease, the T_4 and FTI may be normal while T_3 is high, because the increase in T_3 secretion is relatively greater than the increase in T_4

secretion in hyperthyroidism. This state is referred to as T_ and 10% of hyperthyroidism presents as T_3 toxicosis. In p normal T_4 but with clinical pictures consistent with hypert_ T_3 should be run, and a diagnosis of T_3 toxicosis can be made with a normal T_4 and a high T_3.

SERUM TSH

Historically, TSH measurement has been important in investigating hypothyroid states and in titrating replacement hormone in hypothyroid patients. The drawback to the TSH by RIA, however, was relative insensitivity in the lower ranges that could not distinguish between the euthyroid and hyperthyroid states. The development of monoclonal TSH antibodies of high specificity, however, has allowed the development of a sensitive TSH assay that is useful in testing for both hypothyroid and hyperthyroid states. The normal range for this assay is 0.4–4.8 μU/mL. Elevated TSH levels may be seen with low thyroxine levels (primary hypothyroidism) or normal thyroxine levels (subclinical hypothyroidism). Normal TSH levels may be seen in the euthyroid state or with secondary hypothyroidism. Suppressed TSH levels are associated with hyperthyroidism or secondary hypothyroidism. Suppressed levels are commonly seen in euthyroid patients on thyroid replacement with normal FTI and possibly in patients with euthyroid Graves' disease and also in early pregnancy, especially with morning sickness (associated with high hCG levels). TSH levels are generally normal in euthyroid patients with low FTI secondary to underlying nonthryoidal illness. Patients with primary hypothyroidism and nonthyroidal illness may have inappropriately low TSH levels. There have been reports of patients with primary hypothyroidism whose TSH levels drop to normal with prolonged fasting, and also reports of transient elevation in TSH levels during recovery from nonthryoidal illness in euthyroid patients.

This sensitive TSH assay is rapidly replacing both the T_3 suppression test and TRH stimulation test (see below). (See Table 5–3.)

TRH STIMULATION TEST

The sensitive TSH assay has replaced the TRH test, which is used only when the former is unavailable. When TRH is given intravenously as a 500-μg bolus to a normal subject, serum TSH increases 2–5 times from baseline and by at least 6 μU/mL in patients under age 40. Men over age 40 often have less of a TSH response to TRH, and a

Table 5–3. Causes of abnormalities in serum TSH.

Increased	Decreased*
Hypothyroidism	Hyperthyroidism due to—
Primary—clinical or	Autonomous thyroid hypersecretion
subclinical	Exogenous thyroid intake
Pituitary excess TSH	Thyroid hormone replacement
Neoplastic inappropriate	Adequate or excessive
secretion of	Euthyroid Graves' disease
thyrotropin (NIST)	Nonthyroidal illness
Non-neoplastic	Euthyroid
inappropriate	Hypothyroid (primary or pituitary)
secretion of	Acute psychiatric illness
thyrotropin (NNIST)	Hypothyroidism (pituitary insufficiency)
Recovery from	Dopamine—acute or chronic administration
nonthyroidal illness	Glucocorticoids—acute administration
	(several weeks)
	Pregnancy, especially with morning sickness

* By sensitive assay.

rise of 2 μU/mL or more is considered normal for them. Patients who have hyperthyroidism or who are receiving replacement thyroxine will have a blunted or absent response to TRH.

The test is most useful in studying patients with suspected mild hyperthyroidism of any cause where serum T_4 and T_3 levels are not diagnostic. The test is also abnormal in up to 80% of patients with euthyroid Graves' disease presenting with ophthalmopathy.

After a baseline TSH is drawn, a 500-μg bolus of TRH is given intravenously or intramuscularly, and TSH is measured at 30 and 60 minutes.

In the first 2 minutes after administering TRH, up to 50% of patients may experience transient flushing, nausea, and urinary urgency.

SERUM THYROID ANTIBODIES

Two thyroid antibodies are commonly measured in studying patients with goiter. Thyroglobulin or microsomal antibodies are present in virtually all patients with Hashimoto's thyroiditis and most patients with Graves' disease. They are measured principally by one of two methods: the tanned red cell agglutination assay (TRCA) or RIA.

The TRCA is simple. A positive titer is based on the highest dilution of a test serum capable of agglutinating sheep red cells that have been treated with tannic acid and coated with the appropriate antigen. The TRCA is widely used for measuring thyroglobulin antibodies and is relatively sensitive—90% of Hashimoto's patients have measurable thyroglobulin antibodies by TRCA.

By RIA, 100% of patients with Hashimoto's have positive tests. Antibody titers go up early, are high, and often taper off in later years. High titers (1:2000) are strong evidence for Hashimoto's or Graves', where the incidence of positive antibodies also approaches 100%. Lower titers may also be detected in subacute thyroiditis, nontoxic multinodular goiters, and thyroid carcinoma. Fifteen percent of elderly women have detectable thryroglobulin antibodies; they probably have unrecognized Hashimoto's thyroiditis. Detectable but low titers are seen in a large percentage of patients with other autoimmune disease: pernicious anemia, Sjögren's syndrome, arthritis, and diabetes mellitus (type I). The incidence of detectable antithyroid antibodies rises with age and is about 20% in hospitalized patients without clinical thyroid problems.

Microsomal antibodies can be measured by TRCA and RIA. The latter is most sensitive and positive in 100% of patients with Hashimoto's thyroiditis. Close to 100% of Graves' patients are also positive. In Hashimoto's, the titers are high, up to 1:1,000,000, and remain so for the lifetime of the patient. Low titers are present in a small number of patients with nontoxic goiter and thyroid carcinoma. About 20% of hospitalized patients have detectable microsomal antibodies without clinical evidence of thyroid disease.

Antibody titers may drop on suppressive therapy with thyroid hormone and are lower during pregnancy.

THYROID-STIMULATING IMMUNOGLOBULIN (TSI)

The immunoglobulins thought to cause Graves' disease are not measured directly. Assays for these immunoglobulins are employed to detect or measure activity and not a specific compound. Two techniques are most frequently used to detect this activity: (1) The radioreceptor technique tests the ability of a patient's serum IgG to inhibit binding of ^{125} I-labeled bovine TSH to specific binding sites in human thyroid membranes. (2) The adenyl cyclase technique tests the ability of a patient's serum IgG to stimulate adenyl cyclase activity in human thyroid slices.

The term TSI is misleading, since certainly not all the abnormal immunoglobulins in Graves' disease are capable of stimulating thyroid function and causing hyperthyroidism. The IgG antibodies present in autoimmune thyroid disease form a heterogeneous group of antibodies directed at various sites of thyroid cell membranes. Some cause functional stimulation, while others are cytotoxic. TSI is detectable in a small percentage of Hashimoto's thyroiditis without thyrotoxicosis. In Graves' disease the incidence of TSI is close to 100%.

RADIOACTIVE IODINE UPTAKE (RAIU)

RAIU is the percentage of a tracer dose of RAI taken up by the thyroid gland at a given time after the oral ingestion of the isotope. The count over the thyroid gland is usually done at 5 and 24 hours. Normal values in the USA are 5–15% uptake at 5 hours and 10–30% uptake at 24 hours. Normal uptake values have decreased in the past 25 years because of increased iodine ingestion (iodized bread and salt).

[131]I has been the traditional isotope used in this study, but ^{123}I has become the preferred isotope. The half-life of ^{131}I is 8 days compared with the 13-hour half-life of [123]I. For an uptake study, a tracer amount of 20 µCi is given orally. For a rectilinear scan (see below) a tracer amount of 200 µCi is usually given orally. The number of rads delivered to the thyroid varies with the uptake, but ^{123}I delivers only 10% of the radiation of ^{131}I and is preferred. Because of the short half-life of ^{123}I, some nuclear medicine laboratories that do few thyroid studies continue to use [131]I. The various factors affecting thyroidal radioactive iodine uptake are listed in Table 5–4.

Because of the relatively low normal values, RAIU is not a useful study in distinguishing normal from hypothyroid states. It remains useful in diagnosing the various hyperthyroid states: RAIU is generally high in Graves' disease, toxic adenoma (Plummer's disease), and toxic multinodular goiter (Marine-Lenhart syndrome). It is low in

Table 5–4. Factors affecting thyroidal radioactive iodine uptake (RAIU).

Increased RAIU	Decreased RAIU
Graves' disease	Subacute thyroiditis, silent thyroiditis
Toxic nodular goiter	Thyroid gland destruction (surgical;
Recovery from thyroid hormone suppression	RAI; Hashimoto's thyroiditis; external radiation therapy)
Thiourea (antithyroid drugs)	Thiourea (antithyroid) drugs
Recovery from subacute thyroiditis	Thyroid hormone administration
Dietary iodine deficiency	Ectopic functioning thyroid tissue
Chronic malabsorption (diarrhea)	Hypopituitarism
Soybean intake	Excessive iodide intake (kelp; expectorants; amiodarone;
Nephrotic syndrome	radiographic contrast dye)
Pregnancy	Heart failure
Early Hashimoto's thyroiditis	Azotemia
Certain thyroid enzyme deficiencies	Very severe Graves' disease (high turnover)
	Certain thyroid enzyme deficiencies

subacute thyroiditis, silent thyroiditis, factitious hyperthyroidism, excessive iodide intake, and following thyroidectomy in patients with ectopic functioning thyroid tissue (metastatic thyroid carcinoma or struma ovarii).

RAI uptake may be high in early thyroid failure associated with increased TSH stimulation and increased iodide trapping. Hashimoto's thyroiditis with a block in organification of iodine might present in this manner. RAIU at 5 hours might be higher than at 24 hours owing to rapid trapping and release of iodide from the gland.

The 24-hour uptake is used to calculate the therapeutic dose of ^{131}I given to a patient with Graves' disease or toxic nodular goiter.

T_3 SUPPRESSION TEST

If T_3 (Cytomel, 25 μg) is given 3 or 4 times a day for 7 days, a 24-hour RAI uptake should be 50% or less of the baseline uptake in normal subjects. The exogenous T_3 suppresses TSH secretion and results in decreased iodine uptake. Graves' disease, multinodular toxic goiter, and toxic adenomas all function independently of TSH and fail to suppress. Sixty to 80% of euthyroid Graves' patients will not suppress. Abnormal T_3 suppression, then, denotes thyroid autonomy and not necessarily hyperthyroidism.

THYROID SCANS

Scans are useful in detecting anatomic abnormalities, ectopic tissue (lingual thyroid, mediastinal thyroid, struma ovarii) and metastatic disease. ^{123}I is the isotope of choice when both uptake and scanning are needed. Technetium Tc 99m pertechnetate is also concentrated by the thyroid gland and is used for scanning but not uptake.

The rectilinear scan moves back and forth across the patient's neck, and the radioactivity from ^{123}I in the thyroid gland is recorded as dots on paper or x-ray film. This method is slow and resolution is relatively poor, but the scan represents the size of the gland and location of nodules accurately.

The camera scan is done with the pinhole collimated gamma or scintillation camera following administration of technetium Tc 99m pertechnetate. The resolution of this method is high, it is fast, but it is usually recorded on Polaroid film and is not representative of the actual size of the gland. Because technetium Tc 99m pertechnetate is not stored or organified, a scan using this isotope is done 20 minutes after its intravenous injection. Its half-life is 6 hours and delivers 0.1 rad to the adult gland. Since technetium is transported into the gland in the same manner as iodide, a technetium study can be interfered with by iodine contamination, just as studies using ^{131}I and ^{123}I.

Scans are particularly useful in studying thyroid nodules. Most often RAIU is not necessary in studying patients with nodules, but of course the higher the uptake, the better the resolution of the scan. Patients taking iodide-containing drugs should discontinue these drugs for 3–4 weeks before an isotope study. Patients who have had arteriograms, gallbladder studies, intravenous pyelograms, CT scans, and other tests using iodine in contrast media may have uptake suppressed for longer periods of time. Bronchograms and myelograms may result in suppression lasting from months to years.

Pregnant patients should not be studied with radioisotopes.

THE NODULAR THYROID

Most pathologic states of the thyroid gland may present as a palpable goiter or solitary nodule. Thyroid nodules are common; 4–7% of adults in the USA have a nodular thyroid. Ultrasound study of adult thyroids reveals a high incidence of small nodules. Multinodular goiters are generally of less concern than solitary nodules because, in the absence of head-neck radiation exposure, the incidence of cancer with multinodularity is very small.

CAUSES OF THYROID NODULES

Thyroid Carcinoma

Approximately 40 new cases of thyroid carcinoma are diagnosed for each 1 million population each year in the USA. The incidence of carcinoma in patients presenting with a solitary nodule is 5%. Occult carcinoma is present in about 2.3% of random autopsies.

Patients who have been exposed to head or neck radiation have a much higher incidence of carcinoma (papillary)—7% of the whole population and 20–30% of the group who present with thyroid nodularity.

Radiation

Thyroidal exposure to head-neck radiation is an important cause of nodular goiter, both benign and cancerous. The evaluation and treatment of such patients is consequently aggressive and is discussed in a separate section in this chapter.

Hashimoto's Thyroiditis

Goiter formation is common with Hashimoto's thyroiditis but most often presents as a diffuse rather than nodular goiter. One-fifth of Hashimoto's goiters are nodular. The presence of antithyroid antibodies does not eliminate the possibility of concurrent carcinoma. Hashimoto's thyroiditis is the most common cause of hypothyroidism and is discussed later in this chapter.

Reidel's Thyroiditis

Reidel's thyroiditis may be a form of end-stage Hashimoto's thyroiditis. It presents as a stony hard, asymmetric gland in the middle-aged to older woman. The gland is not painful, and the patient is usually euthyroid. Histologically, dense fibrosis is found. There is often local infiltration of neighboring structures. The clinical presentation may suggest carcinoma, but regional nodes are not involved. Symptomatology is related to compression of structures in the neck. Thyroid function tests are normal, infrequently low, and thyroid antibodies are absent. Treatment is directed at relief of compression symptoms, though total thyroidectomy is not possible. Thyroid replacement is given to those patients who are hypothyroid. It is generally unsuccessful in shrinking the gland.

Iodine Deficiency

Iodine deficiency is a common cause of nodular goiters throughout much of the world. It is referred to as endemic goiter in those areas where the soil is iodine-poor and the water and food supply are low in iodine. By definition, endemic goiter is seen in 10% of the population in a given area. The goiter belt around the Great Lakes in the USA disappeared when iodine was added to food, mainly bread and salt. Endemic goiter still occurs in mountain areas in Asia, New Guinea, Africa, and South America and is seen in the USA mainly among immigrants and refugees from these areas.

The daily optimal iodine requirement is 150–300 μg. In endemic goiter areas, daily intake of iodine is below 50 μg, and daily urinary iodine excretion also falls below 50 μg. Prevention of goiter formation due to iodine deficiency is by exogenous iodine. Lugol's solution contains 3000 μg iodine/mL, so that very small volumes are necessary for daily requirements. Once a goiter has formed, iodine is not successful in reducing its size and may even produce hyperthyroidism. The patient is more appropriately treated with long-term thyroid suppression by means of L-thyroxine, 0.15–0.2 mg/d in children and young adults, and 0.10–0.15 mg/d in the elderly.

Sporadic or Nonendemic Goiter

Sporadic, nontoxic multinodular goiter occurs in spite of adequate iodine intake. It is indistinguishable from endemic goiter morphologically and functionally. Rarely is it a cause of hypothyroidism. Characteristically, nodules within the same gland show great heterogeneity; growth and function vary from one nodule to the next, even among follicles within the same nodule. Entirely cold (nonfunctioning) nodules are rare. Nodules of varying size and level of uptake are seen on Tc scan. Some nodules will appear "cold" and others "hot." Thyrotoxicosis occurs when the hot nodules continue to grow and secrete thyroid hormone. This usually happens in older patients with a history of many years of preexisting nontoxic nodular goiter.

The cause of nonendemic goiter is not completely understood, evidence is accumulating that it may be due to a thyroid growth-stimulating immunoglobulin. This might explain why most of these goiters do not respond to thyroid suppression.

Large goiters may cause cosmetic deformity, respiratory difficulty, or dysphagia. Such goiters may be treated with surgery or with ^{131}I. With ^{131}I, the goiter is maximally reduced in size within 6–12 months, with neck circumference reduced in 87% of patients by at least 1.5 cm. The usual dose of ^{131}I is 20–30 mCi. Any hyperthyroidism is treated with pranolol. Hypothyroidism must be treated promptly.

Iodine Administration

Iodine in certain settings becomes an important goitrogen. It can cause a number of alterations in thyroid hormone synthesis, but these changes occur only in a preexisting abnormal thyroid gland. An iodine load given to a normal subject will result in a transient block in organification of iodide, the Wolff-Chiakoff effect, which is usually of no clinical significance. In a patient who has a subtle defect in organification, however, as a result of Hashimoto's thyroiditis, the same iodine load will provoke a prolonged block, resulting in goiter formation and hypothyroidism. A patient with Hashimoto's thyroiditis may go undiagnosed until given iodine-containing medicine such as saturated solution of potassium iodide (SSKI) or an x-ray contrast agent and then suddenly develop a goiter. Because of the high prevalence of Hashimoto's thyroiditis, this possibility must be kept in mind in patients receiving therapeutic iodine.

Lithium Carbonate

Lithium is another important goitrogen because of its wide use in the treatment of manic depressive states. Its main action on the thyroid gland is inhibition of thyroid hormone release. Twenty to 30% of patients on lithium may manifest some evidence of goiter formation and thyroid decompensation. It is important to follow patients on lithium with periodic examination and thyroid function tests.

Other Goitrogens

Certain drugs and foods may produce goiter and hypothyroidism (see Table 5–13).

Dyshormonogenesis

Patients with enzymatic deficiencies resulting in poor, inefficient thyroid hormone production and goiter formation are grouped together as having genetic dyshormonogenesis. These defects are rare and generally autosomal recessive. The homozygote is clinically evident early in life, and cretinism and thyromegaly occur if not treated. The heterozygote state manifests itself with a small goiter. Five separate abnormalities have been described. The most common is **peroxidase deficiency**; iodine is trapped but not organified, and relatively less thyroid hormone is synthesized. This causes increased TSH production, hyperplasia, and ultimately nodularity of the gland.

Many patients with dyshormonogenesis present with goiters with or without hypothyroidism and are empirically placed on long-term suppressive thyroid therapy without a specific diagnosis.

Spontaneous Benign Nodules

Most thyroid nodules have no known underlying cause. They are frequently colloid nodules, cysts, or benign follicular adenomas.

Cowden's Disease

Cowden's disease, or multiple hamartoma syndrome, is a rare disorder of automosomal dominant inheritance. Two-thirds of patients have nodular hyperplasia or follicular adenoma of the thyroid, and 10% of this group develop well-differentiated carcinoma. Two-thirds of women with this syndrome also have breast disease, most often fibrocystic although 30% have carcinoma of the breast.

Acute Pyogenic Thyroiditis (Suppurative)

Acute pyogenic thyroiditis is a rare, life-threatening disease of bacterial origin. Streptococci, staphylococci and pneumococci have been identified as a cause. Clinically, the patient presents with fever, malaise, and severe pain and tenderness of the thyroid gland. Thyroid function tests are normal, and the white blood cell count is high. Diagnosis is made by fine needle aspiration (FNA) biopsy. Appropriate treatment includes drainage of the abscess that is almost always present and antimicrobial treatment.

EVALUATION OF THYROID NODULES

The evaluation of thyroid nodules must take into consideration the relative risk of thyroid carcinoma (Table 5–5).

Patients with nodules having an especially high risk of carcinoma should have the nodule resected surgically. A frozen section should be done at surgery. Patients having a lower risk of thyroid carcinoma should have an evaluation consisting initially of either an FNA biopsy or a thyroid scan (see below). All patients should have serum T_4, T_3RU, TSH, and T_3 measurements. Antimicrosomal and antithyroglobulin antibodies are also helpful.

Fine-needle Aspiration (FNA)

FNA is performed with the patient supine (Fig 5–4). Hyperextension of the neck frequently allows easier palpation of the nodule to be aspirated. The skin is cleaned with an alcohol sponge. A 23-gauge needle and 10-mL syringe are attached to a syringe holder (Cameo syringe holder, Precision Dynamics Corporation, 3031 Thornton Avenue, Burbank, CA 94594) that allows the physician to palpate and stabilize the nodule with one hand and pass the needle into the nodule and draw back on the syringe with the other at the same time. An alternative technique entails using a butterfly 23-gauge needle with an

Table 5–5. Risk factors for thyroid carcinoma.

	High risk	Low risk
History	Family history of medullary cancer or MEN II Head-neck radiation	Family history of goiter
Physical examination	Hard nodule Large nodule (> 2.5 cm) Regional nodes enlarged Evidence of distant metastasis Hoarseness with vocal cord paralysis	Multinodular goiter Soft nodule Hypothyroidism
Age/sex	Young women, children, and all men	Women over 40
Scanning technique Technetium Ultrasound	Nonfunctioning, or "cold" Solid	Functioning, or "hot" Cystic
Response to thyroxine therapy 0.2 mg/d for 3–6 months	Continues to enlarge	Regresses

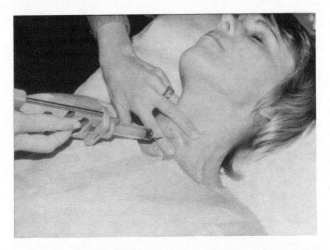

Figure 5–4. The technique used in FNA. The nodule is held steady between 2 fingers of the left hand as the needle is guided by the right hand. The syringe holder enables the operator to aspirate using only one hand.

assistant withdrawing the plunger of the attached syringe. The needle enters the nodule at a 45- to 90-degree angle. Suction is maintained in the syringe as the needle is moved back and forth quickly in different directions inside the nodule. As soon as material is seen in the needle hub, the suction is released and the needle withdrawn. The needle is detached and the syringe is filled with air; the needle is reattached and the contents in the needle expelled onto one or 2 glass slides. A thin smear is then obtained by placing a second slide over the material and pulling them apart. One slide is placed in 95% ethyl alcohol; the other is air dried.

Two or more aspirations are obtained for adequate sampling. No anesthesia is necessary. The procedure is remarkably free of morbidity. Small hematomas are rare.

The air-dried smear is dyed with Wright's stain and the smear fixed in 95% alcohol is stained by the Papanicolaou method. For suspected medullary carcinoma, Congo red dye will show amyloid. If the number of cells is inadequate, a repeat aspiration biopsy is recommended.

Reading the aspiration smears requires special training and experience, and the potential value and usefulness of FNA as a diagnostic tool is limited by the skill of the cytologist.

If the sample is benign, place the patient on suppressive T_4 therapy. Regression of the nodule is reassuring but happens relatively infrequently. Failure to regress should not be interpreted as a bad sign. Growth of the nodule on suppression therapy is an indication for surgical removal.

If the sample shows or suggests papillary, medullary, or anaplastic carcinoma, the nodule must be removed surgically.

If the sample shows follicular neoplasm there is a 20% chance of carcinoma. Technetium scan will identify the functioning nodules, and the nonfunctioning ones are surgically removed. Patients with functioning nodules may be observed.

Fluid will be obtained from cysts at the time of FNA. Patients with fluid-filled cysts should also be suppressed with T_4. There is a tendency for cysts to refill, in spite of suppression.

Thyroid Scan

Fine need aspiration has largely replaced scanning for the evaluation of thyroid nodules.

The preferred scanning technique is the 99m technetium camera scan. The scan helps determine whether a nodule is solitary or part of a multinodular goiter. It also separates functioning from nonfunctioning nodules.

Functioning (hot) nodules are infrequently toxic and usually benign (less than 6% incidence of follicular carcinoma). FNA is usually performed; if FNA cytology is not available, the patient may be followed closely for nodule growth or thyrotoxicosis.

Nonfunctioning (cold) nodules that are solitary have a 5% (up to 22% at certain referral centers) chance of being carcinomas. An FNA biopsy is indicated. If FNA cytology is not available, ultrasound may be done to determine if a cold nodule is cystic. About 20% of cold nodules are cystic. Pure cysts are rarely carcinomas. Solid lesions and those with internal echos may be benign or malignant. With increasing use of FNA biopsy, ultrasound is less often necessary in the diagnostic workup. An optimal study is achieved with a small parts scanner using a proper transducer.

EVALUATION OF MEDIASTINAL MASSES

Superior mediastinal masses may be intrathoracic goiters, usually multinodular colloid type. Rupture of follicles may cause hemorrhage, inflammation, and calcification. A radioactive iodine scan is positive in 50%. CT scan may help distinguish other masses from goiter. The incidence of cancer is about 1%, and most cases are incidental within the goiter.

Substernal nodular goiters are best left alone. In the event of compressive symptoms, they can usually be removed through a neck incision, since the blood supply is from the superior thyroid arteries. However, patients who have had neck surgery may have developed collateral feeder vessels from the innominate artery.

TREATMENT OF BENIGN THYROID NODULES

If a nodule is benign or fits low-risk criteria, a medical approach may be taken, with thyroid suppression.

Most thyroid lesions are TSH-dependent. Even cold nodules trap some iodine, but amounts are smaller relative to normal thyroid tissue. Suppressing TSH with exogenous thyroid might prevent further growth of the nodule and even lead to regression. In practice, regression of the nodule occurs in only about 40% of patients. Most nodules do not change. A small number may grow in spite of suppression, and such nodules should be removed surgically. Similarly, nodular glands, which are large and cause local pressure or cosmetic deformity, should be removed. Those patients whose nodules regress or do not change can remain on suppressive therapy with careful follow-up examinations. Colloid nodules do not shrink in size.

Multinodular goiters are often autonomous and respond poorly to suppression with thyroxine, which may produce thyrotoxicosis.

The usual suppression dose of L-thyroxine in adults is 0.125–0.2 mg/d. In adjusting the dose, the free thyroxine index should be in the upper half of the normal range.

THYROID MALIGNANCIES

WELL-DIFFERENTIATED THYROID CARCINOMA

Papillary Carcinoma

This is by far the most common and least aggressive thyroid malignancy (Fig 5–5). It occurs as pure papillary or mixed papillary follicular and accounts for 60–80% of all thyroid carcinomas. In about 40% of cases, small calcifications called psammoma bodies are present on histologic or cytologic examination that are pathognomonic for this form of cancer. It frequently occurs or spreads in a multicentric fashion throughout the thyroid. Its incidence and multicentric presentation is greatly increased in patients who have been exposed to head-neck irradiation.

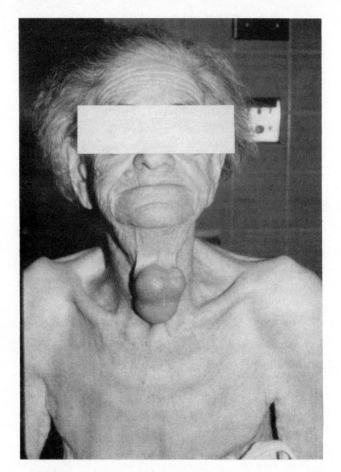

Figure 5–5. Papillary carcinoma in an elderly patient. A large lobu-lated nodule grew slowly over 5 years from within a preexisting small multinodular gland of many years' duration.

Papillary thyroid carcinoma is generally slow growing, having metastasis to regional lymph nodes. It may produce pressure locally or injure the recurrent laryngeal nerve, producing hoarseness. It is unusu-al for a purely papillary thyroid carcinoma to metastasize distally. Mixed papillary follicular carcinoma is somewhat more aggressive and prone to distant metastasis.

Follicular Carcinoma

Follicular carcinoma is more likely to have distant metastasis, especially to lungs and bone. It accounts for about 15% of thyroid carcinomas. Most, but not all, follicular carcinomas take up iodine.

Treatment

A. Surgery: For **papillary thyroid carcinoma**, total lobectomy on the affected side and total or near-total on the opposite side is desirable. At some medical centers, small (< 1 cm diameter) isolated intrathyroidal papillary carcinomas without metastases or prior radiation exposure are treated with simple lobectomy. Patients are not subjected to RIA study but are placed on thyroxine suppression for life.

For **follicular thyroid carcinoma**, there is more general agreement that the initial surgery should be total or near-total thyroidectomy. This is due to the increased possibility of distant metastases that may later require ^{131}I for treatment (see below), requiring ablation of normal thyroid tissue that competes with the malignant tissue for ^{131}I.

The surgical treatment of well-differentiated thyroid carcinoma involves the removal of involved lymph nodes. However, extensive lymph node dissection or radical neck dissection is not appropriate. Neck muscles should not be resected.

Surgical complications of total thyroidectomy include recurrent laryngeal nerve damage with vocal cord paralysis (at least 1.7%) and hypoparathyroid hypocalcemia (at least 2%). Any devascularized parathyroid tissue may be transplanted into neck muscles.

B. Radioactive Iodine (RAI): Patients with larger carcinomas or with evidence of opposite lobe or lymph node involvement are candidates for postoperative radiation therapy with ^{131}I. Here, one advantage of having had a total or near-total thyroidectomy becomes apparent. Many well-differentiated tumors will take up enough iodide to enable further treatment with ^{131}I, but the uptake into metastatic tissue is generally higher if there is no residual normal thyroid tissue that avidly competes to trap ^{131}I. Any residual normal thyroid tissue must be ablated before adequate doses of ^{131}I are taken up by metastases.

In patients who will require further study and possible treatment with ^{131}I, suppressive therapy is begun immediately postoperatively, only with T_3 (12.5 μg three times a day, increasing to 25 μg three times a day after about 1 week) rather than with L-thyroxine because of the shorter half-life of T_3 and shorter delay period between stopping suppression and studying the patient. After 8 weeks, T_3 is stopped, a low iodine diet is begun (Table 5–6), and a ^{131}I uptake and whole body scan are performed using a large tracer dose of 1 mCi 2–3 weeks later. TSH is usually high at this time and optimizes uptake. If a remnant of thyroid tissue is detected, the patient is treated with a dose of ^{131}I

Table 5–6. Iodine diet.* Select from foods with less than 4 μg/serving.

Food	Iodine Content (μg/serving)
Meat	
Pizza	15.0
Chili	9.3
Pork, lean, 3 oz	7.1
Egg, 1 hardboiled	6.4
Spaghetti, ½ cup, and meatball	5.5
Beef, chuck, 3 oz	4.2
Hamburger, 3 oz	4.2
Turkey, 3 oz	4.2
Veal, 3 oz	4.2
Bacon, cured	3.6
Frankfurter	3.0
Cooking fat, 1 tsp	3.0
Pork sausage, 2 links	2.7
Lamb leg, 3 oz	2.1
Liver, 3 oz	2.1
Salami, 1 oz	1.7
Gravy	0.6
Seafood	
Clams, ½ cup	90.0
Shrimp, 3 oz	55.0
Oysters, 5–8	48.0
Halibut, 3 oz	39.0
Salmon, 3 oz	31.0
Sardines, 2	10.0
Tuna, canned, 2 oz	10.0
Dairy products, shortening	
Milk, 8 oz	14.2
Ice cream, ½ cup	9.0
Cottage cheese, 4 oz	5.7
Mayonnaise, 1 tsp	3.4
Cheese, American	2.6
Cheese, blue or Roquefort, 1 oz	2.6
Cheese, Cheddar, 1 oz	2.6
Cheese sauce, 2 tbs	2.5
Milk, dry nonfat solids, instant, 4 tsp	2.0
Sherbet	1.6
Cream cheese, 1 oz	0.9
Olive oil, 1 tsp	0.9
Half and Half, 1 tsp	0.9
Cream, light	0.7
Oil, 1 tsp	0.5
Butter, 1 tbs	0.4
Whipped cream, 1 tsp	0.3
Margarine, 1 tsp	0.3

(continued)

*Adapted, with permission, from Nuclear Medicine Consultants, San Francisco.

Table 5–6. (Continued)

Food	Iodine Content (µg/serving)
Vegetables & fruits	
Peach, canned	16.0
Applesauce	14.1
Pineapple, 3 cups	10.7
Canned spinach	9.9
Banana, 1 small	7.0
Peach	5.0
French fries, 10	4.6
Potato with skin	3.3
Squash, small	3.3
Lettuce, ½ cup	3.1
Mashed potato	2.5
Beans, red	2.1
Broccoli, ½ cup	2.1
Peas, ½ cup	2.1
Apple, raw, small	2.0
Apple juice	2.0
Raw spinach	2.0
Avocado, medium	1.7
Cantaloupe	1.7
Split pea soup	1.7
Cucumber	1.7
Potato, boiled	1.7
Corn, creamed, 3 oz	1.4
Peanuts with skin	1.4
Peas, canned, ½ cup	1.4
Raw cabbage	1.1
Onions, ¼ cup	1.1
Orange juice	1.0
Mixed vegetables, ½ cup	0.7
Raisins	0.7
Cashews, 6–8	0.4
Walnuts, 8 halves	0.4
Cucumber, ¼ medium	0.4
Mushrooms	0.0
Orange	0.0
Starch, breads	
Pancake, 2	4.5
Rye bread	4.2
Apple pie	3.2
Bisquik	2.6
Whole wheat bread	1.7
Cornbread	1.7
Pound cake	1.7
Dough cake	1.7
French bread	1.5
Angel food cake	1.1
Egg noodles	0.7

(continued)

Table 5–6. (Continued)

Food	Iodine Content (μg/serving)
Rice, whole, ½ cup	0.6
Spaghetti, ½ cup	0.6
Graham cracker	0.1
Other	
Tea, 1 cup	32.0
Lemonade, 8 oz	13.2
Pudding, ½ cup	7.6
Coffee, instant	6.7
Cream of chicken soup	6.6
White sauce, 2 tsp	1.9
Chicken noodle soup	1.6
Catsup, 1 tsp	0.8
Maple syrup	0.7
Gin	0.4
Sugar, 1 tsp	0.3
Honey, 1 tsp	0.3
Jelly, 1 tsp	0.2
Soy sauce, 2 tsp	0.2
Specifically avoid	
Fish and shellfish	
Canned fruits & vegetables	
Cured meats	
Bakery bread	
Iodized salt	
Presalted foods (chips, nuts)	
Watercress and parsley	
Tea, instant coffee	
Red food dye (also in red tablets or capsules)	
Vitamins (with minerals)	
X-ray contrast dye	
Iodine-containing skin disinfectant	

calculated to ablate it, about 30–50 mCi. After this initial step is completed, the patient is put back on T_3 for another 4 weeks, is taken off for 2 weeks, and is restudied. If there is residual thyroid tissue or metastatic tissue, another ablative dose of ^{131}I is given. Higher doses of ^{131}I (up to 150 mCi) are generally used for treating metastatic disease with an uptake of more than 0.05%. This procedure can be repeated every 6–12 months until there is no residual metastatic tissue. Further study and treatment with ^{131}I beyond this point is dictated by the clinical course and levels of serum thyroglobulin. The appearance of palpable cervical lymph nodes is suggestive evidence of recurring metastatic disease, and an FNA is confirmative. Such nodes are best removed surgically.

Follicular carcinoma metastasis takes up ^{131}I more readily than papillary metastasis, and functioning follicular metastasis often responds well to ^{131}I, especially soft tissue such as lung and mediastinum. Bone metastasis does not respond so well. Because of the occurrence of distant metastasis in follicular carcinoma, whole body imaging is indicated when the patient is studied. This is optimally done using a gamma scintillation camera. In treating pulmonary metastasis, the dose of ^{131}I may have to be lowered, so as to deliver no more than 50 mCi to lungs at one time. The dose is adjusted to the uptake of ^{131}I into the pulmonary metastasis. Radiation injury to the lungs can cause pulmonary fibrosis.

Follow-up

Patients with follicular carcinoma should have chest x-rays every 1–2 years. Following total thyroidectomy (by surgery or ^{131}I ablation) serum thyroglobulin should be undetectable. It is elevated in patients with metastatic disease, and a rise is indicative of recurring disease.

Without evidence of recurring metastatic disease, restudy of RAI need not be done, and routine restudy is not indicated. Patients are uncomfortable during the preparation and study period because they become clinically hypothyroid.

Patients with metastatic disease also should be on T_4 suppression for life at a dose that suppresses TSH and keeps the serum T_4 high normal or slightly elevated.

Repeat RAI and whole body scans are done about 1 year following initial ^{131}I treatment. Persistent extrathyroidal disease may be retreated at yearly intervals. Bone scans using Tc 99m or thallium-201 may detect bone metastasis but are not specific for it.

The approach to treatment of patients with differentiated thyroid carcinoma must be guided by the fact that this disease is relatively benign.

Prognosis

Overall mortality is low but varies with age and sex. When cancer is discovered before age 20, mortality after 15 years is less than 2%. After age 50, however, cancer-related mortality at 15 years jumps to 34%. Prognosis is better with papillary than with follicular carcinoma. Mortality rates in patients diagnosed after age 50 are 20% for papillary carcinoma and 42% for follicular carcinoma after 15 years. Mortality rates worsen significantly in women diagnosed after age 50 and in men diagnosed after age 40. With aging, there is less female predominance, especially with follicular carcinoma. Table 5–7 presents the conditions in which well-differentiated thyroid carcinoma is likely to

Table 5–7. Risk factors associated with greater aggressiveness of well-differentiated thyroid carcinoma.

Children, men, and patients over 50
Large tumors greater than 3 cm in diameter
Rapid growth, pain, and hoarseness
Distant metastasis

be more aggressive. Such patients should be treated more aggressively, ie, by total thyroidectomy, postoperative study with ^{131}I, and treatment with ^{131}I if residual uptake remains. Interestingly, local node involvement with papillary carcinoma is not associated with greater morbidity and mortality.

MEDULLARY THYROID CARCINOMA (MTC)

Medullary thyroid carcinomas are not derived from thyroid follicular cells but rather from parafollicular (C) cells that are normally distributed between thyroid follicles within the gland. MTC is generally of intermediate aggressiveness, being more malignant than papillary-follicular but less malignant than anaplastic carcinomas. These carcinomas account for fewer than 5% of thyroid malignancies.

Occurrence

About one-third of patients have **sporadic MTC** that generally occurs in the fifth or sixth decade.

About one-third of cases have multiple endocrine neoplasia type II (MEN II), usually an autosomal dominant trait. Patients with MEN IIa (Sipple's syndrome) have MTC (95%), pheochromocytomas (35%), and hyperparathyroidism (20%). The hyperparathyroidism is caused by adenomas in about 15% and hyperplasia in 85% of cases. The MTC generally occurs in the third or fourth decade. Patients with MEN IIb are those having multiple mucosal and gastrointestinal ganglioneuromas and a marfanoid appearance associated with MTC (85%) and pheochromocytomas (45%). The MTC generally presents in the third or fourth decade. Pheochromocytomas are bilateral in two-thirds of such cases and are discussed in Chapter 6.

Another one-third of patients have **isolated familial MTC**. This is also an autosomal dominant trait. Patients tend to present in the third or fourth decade.

Secretions

Medullary thyroid carcinomas secrete **calcitonin** (see below) and some other peptides. Calcitonin excess does not produce hypocalcemia but does serve as a useful tumor marker. Excess calcitonin in the cancer tissue stains for amyloid with Congo red stain; however, this amyloid is distinct from fibrillar immunoglobulin amyloid found in other conditions. **Serotonin** and **prostaglandins** may be responsible for flushing and diarrhea that occurs in up to 30% of patients. Carcinoembryogenic antigen (CEA) is elevated in 70% of patients and can be used as a tumor marker, although it is not specific for MTC. **ACTH** or **corticotropin-releasing hormone** is secreted in about 5% of patients with MTC in amounts sufficient to cause Cushing's syndrome.

Metastases

Metastasis of MTC occurs early to regional and mediastinal lymph nodes; it involves local neck structures. Distant metastases may appear late in the bones, lungs, adrenals, or liver. MTC in the thyroid, lymph nodes, and liver may calcify. Metastasis to the lung does not frequently calcify.

Genetic Predisposition to MTC

Any patient with a first-degree relative having MEN II or familial MTC has a strong genetic predisposition.

A. FNA Biopsy: FNA biopsy should be performed on any thyroid nodule occurring in an individual with a prior pheochromocytoma or with a family history of MTC or MEN II.

B. Serum Calcitonin: Calcitonin is a 32-amino-acid polypeptide that is secreted by normal thyroid parafollicular cells. Serum calcitonin is usually elevated in patients with MTC, and the radioimmunoassay for calcitonin is therefore useful for both the diagnosis and follow-up of MTC.

A patient with an elevated serum calcitonin may have MTC. The differential diagnosis must include other conditions causing increased serum calcitonin (Table 5–8).

Table 5–8. Causes of increased serum calcitonin.

Medullary thyroid carcinoma (MTC)	**Associated with non-MTC malignancies***
Neonatal period	Carcinoma of lung (45%)
Pregnancy	Pancreatic cancer (42%)
Pernicious anemia	Breast cancer (38%)
Chronic renal failure	Colon cancer (24%)
Hypercalcemia	Carcinoid tumors
Thyroiditis	Pancreatic islet cell tumors
	Pheochromocytoma
	Many others

*In such cases, the serum calcitonin may be secreted ectopically or from the thyroid gland itself.

C. Pentagastrin Stimulation Test: Patients with a genetic predisposition to MTC may have a normal thyroid examination and a normal baseline serum calcitonin. They may nevertheless have a microscopic focus of MTC or C-cell hyperplasia, which is considered a premalignant lesion. Such patients should have a periodic pentagastrin stimulation test (see the Appendix). An excessive calcitonin response indicates probable occult MTC.

Young patients having a sibling or parent with MEN IIa or familial MTC are at almost a 50% risk for developing MTC. However, the MTC seen in these conditions tends to be less aggressive than sporadic MTC or MTC associated with MEN IIb, so that prophylactic thyroidectomy is rarely performed in this group. They are ordinarily followed very closely and have pentagastrin stimulation tests either yearly or biannually.

D. Prophylactic Thyroidectomy: Young patients having a sibling or parent with definitive MEN IIb are at extremely high risk for developing MTC of an aggressive variety. For this small group, a prophylactic thyroidectomy should be considered even without a positive pentagastrin stimulation test.

Treatment

Once the presence of MTC is suspected, the patient must be screened for pheochromocytoma. Screening for hyperparathyroidism is also indicated before neck surgery. Pheochromocytomas must be resected first. Then the patient should be reevaluated for MTC if the diagnosis was based on biochemical parameters alone, since the pheochromocytoma may have secreted calcitonin.

MTC tends to be a relatively indolent cancer that is refractory to radiation therapy or chemotherapy. Care must therefore be taken not to treat metastatic disease over-aggressively with therapy that may do more harm than the MTC itself. Recurrences of MTC are best dealt with surgically.

Prognosis

The prognosis for patients with MTC depends on the setting in which it presents. Patients with sporadic MTC usually have lymph node metastasis noted at the time of diagnosis. Distal metastases become apparent years later. Their 10-year survival rate is 46%. Patients with MTC associated with MEN IIb also have an aggressive form. However, patients with MEN IIa and familial MTC tend to have a less aggressive variety and their 10-year survival rate is high. Survival is also better in women under age 40. Tumors with marked reactivity for the myelomonocytic antigen Leu-M1 have been associated with 3 times the local recurrence rate and 4.5 times the death rate of tumors with absent or slight immunoreactivity.

In patients with MTC, primary or metastatic tumor tissue should be stained for calcitonin using the immunoperoxidase method. Calcitonin-rich metastases are compatible with long-term survival even if vital organs are affected. Calcitonin-poor MTC is more virulent.

Preoperatively, calcitonin and CEA levels should be obtained. CEA is elevated in about 70% of patients with MTC and provides a useful second marker, although it is not specific for this type of carcinoma. Serum calcitonin levels often remain elevated postoperatively in patients with apparently complete resections and long-term remission. Therefore, it is a rising level of calcitonin or CEA postoperatively that is cause for concern.

ANAPLASTIC THYROID CARCINOMA

Anaplastic carcinoma is rare, accounting for 1% or less of all thyroid carcinomas. It is locally aggressive, and the prognosis is dismal regardless of treatment. One-year survival is less than 10%. Five-year survival is less than 5%. Treatment involves local resection and radiation for palliation only.

OTHER THYROID MALIGNANCIES

Lymphoma of the thyroid may be increasing in incidence, though it is still rare. Women patients predominate. They present with a nodule, diffuse goiter, or multinodular goiter. Clues to diagnosis include (1) an 80% incidence of positive thyroid antibodies, (2) a 20% incidence of hypothyroidism, (3) painful swelling and rapid growth of the mass, (4) a modest elevation in sedimentation rate, and (5) significant RAIU. Patients who undergo thyroidectomy do poorly, but those treated with external radiation therapy do well.

Hürthle cell tumor, possibly a variant of follicular carcinoma, occurs predominantly in older patients. Hürthle cells, which are eosinophilic with cytoplasmic mitochondria, may be found in benign disease, including Hashimoto's thyroiditis. These carinomas are more aggressive and have a poorer prognosis than papillary or follicular cell carcinomas.

Metastatic cancers may involve the thyroid gland. Among the many types reported to spread to the thyroid are melanomas and renal, breast, and bronchogenic carcinomas.

THYROID RADIATION EXPOSURE

An important risk factor for thyroid nodularity and thyroid cancer is exposure to ionizing radiation. In past years, especially in the 1940s to 1960s, it was standard and acceptable practice to use radiation as treatment for tonsillitis and acne as well as for ''thymic tumors'' in newborns. In these patients, the incidence of thyroid abnormalities varies with the dosage and field of prior radiation. Patients who received thymic radiation in childhood, usually about 200 rads, have about 1% incidence of carcinoma. Patients with prior facial radiation have up to a 7% incidence of carcinoma and 25% overall chance of developing some clinically evident thyroid abnormality. More cancers occurred in the radiation-induced multinodular goiter group than in the nonirradiated group.

There is generally a 10- to 20-year latency period between exposure and discovery of nodularity, although thyroid pathology has been discovered as late as 40 years following exposure. Thyroid exposure to as little as 50 rads has been associated with increased thyroid disease, and there is a direct dose-response relationship up to about 1200 rads.

The thyroid receives doses of 100–400 rads during thymic radiation; it receives 200–1500 rads during radiation therapy for tonsillitis, otitis media, and acne. The higher dose of 10,000 rads used in treating Graves' disease is not carcinogenic, possibly because of its lethal effect on the gland.

Cancer in this group of radiation-exposed patients has been well-differentiated papillary and is probably no more aggressive than the same cancer type in patients not exposed to radiation. It tends to be more multicentric in the radiated group and more often associated with multinodularity. There is no female predominance, in contrast to a 3:1 ratio in nonradiated patients. Radiation exposure is not associated with an increased incidence of follicular, medullary, or anaplastic thyroid carcinoma.

Surgical approach to carcinoma in this group of patients probably should be aggressive, with total or near-total thyroidectomy, because of the multicentric nature of the cancer.

EVALUATION FOLLOWING RADIATION EXPOSURE

The diagnostic approach to the patient with radiation exposure must include a careful physical examination. If the thyroid gland is multinodular, a total thyroidectomy is indicated. If regional nodes are enlarged, they may be studied by FNA and metastatic disease sought. A solitary nodule might also be biopsied by FNA, but a benign nodule does not rule out the possibility of a nonpalpable cancer elsewhere in the gland, considering the multicentricity of cancer in radiation-exposed thyroids. For this reason, a nonfunctioning, solitary nodule is probably best treated with total thyroidectomy. To minimize further radiation exposure, scanning is best done using technetium and gamma camera with pinhole collimator. ^{131}I uptake is not needed.

Patients with normal glands on physical examination do not need scanning but should have an annual examination for possible changes in the thyroid gland. Some physicians suppress such thyroid glands prophylactically with thyroxine.

Reduction of ^{131}I Exposure Following Nuclear Disaster

To reduce ^{131}I exposure after a nuclear disaster, iodide, 30 mg, is administered orally, followed by 15 mg/d. Iodide itself may cause hypothyroidism, goiter, hyperthyroidism, skin rash, and salivary gland tenderness.

HYPERTHYROIDISM

Hyperthyroidism usually presents with classical manifestations (Table 5–9). Documenting hyperthyroidism requires obtaining thyroid function tests discussed earlier in this chapter. Most patients have an elevated serum T_4 and T_3; factors that may increase serum T_4 without affecting clinical status (Table 5–1) must always be considered.

The sensitive TSH assay has proved useful in the diagnosis of hyperthyroidism, being suppressed when manifestations are mild and serum T_4 or T_3 levels are not diagnostic.

Patients with hyperthyroidism must have an RAIU to distinguish the causes listed in Table 5–10, which are grouped according to whether the RAIU is increased or not. Factors affecting thyroid RAIU must be considered (Table 5–3). Each cause of hyperthyroidism discussed below has distinctive distinguishing characteristics. Besides RAIU, the presence and character of goiter and eye findings are important features in making a diagnosis.

GRAVES' DISEASE

Graves' disease is the most common cause of hyperthyroidism and is an autoimmune disease. Abnormal immunoglobulins, among them thyroid-stimulating immunoglobulin (TSI), appear in the serum of all patients with Graves' disease. TSI binds at the TSH receptor site

Table 5–9. Manifestations of hyperthyroidism.*

Symptoms

Restlessness; irritability, emotional instability; poor sleep; fatigue; muscle weakness or cramps; increased appetite; palpitations; heat intolerance; increased sweating; increased bowel movements; dyspnea on exertion; weight change (usually loss in 50–60%); periodic paralysis with hypokalemia (especially males who are Oriental, Filipino, or native American); oligomenorrhea (or any menstrual irregularity); angina pectoris.

Signs

Lid lag and stare; tachycardia, artial fibrillation, wide pulse pressure; heart failure (unusual); finger tremor; hyperreflexia; muscle wasting; onycholysis; smooth, warm, and moist skin; fine hair.

Seen with Graves' disease: Goiter, often with bruit; exophthalmos; pretibial myxedema (rare). Laboratory abnormalities: Antimicrosomal or antithyroglobulin antibodies; thyroid-stimulating immunoglobulin (TSI); antidoublestranded DNA antibody (> 80%).

Nonthyroid laboratory abnormalities: Increased alkaline phosphatase; increased calcium; increased sex hormone–binding globulin; increased ferritin; decreased hematocrit; decreased granulocytes; decreased catecholamines.

* A hyperthyroid patient may have only a few of these manifestations.

Table 5–10. Causes of hyperthyroidism.

Increased thyroid RAI uptake	Decreased thyroid RAI uptake
Graves' disease	Subacute thyroiditis (tender, moderately enlarged thyroid)
Toxic multinodular goiter	
Toxic solitary nodule	Exogenous thyroid hormone ingestion (may be occult or due to ingestion of ground meat contaminated with thyroid during gullet trimming)
Functioning thyroid carcinoma	
Inorganic iodide–induced (eg, SSKI, Lugol's)	
TSH-secreting pituitary adenoma*	
TSH hyperplasia	Silent thyroiditis (nontender, moderately enlarged thyroid)
Struma ovarii* (hyperplasia); increased RAIU also in ovary	Organic iodide–induced (eg, kelp, amiodarone, x-ray contrast)
hCG-secreting trophoblastic tumor* of ovary or testis	Metastatic thyroid carcinoma (tumors take up RAI)
	Struma ovarii* (adenoma); increased RAIU in ovary only

Differential diagnosis: Factors causing increased serum thyroxine without affecting clinical status (Table 5–1)

* Rare.

in the thyroid cell membrane and stimulates increased cellular function. About 70% of Graves' patients have antimicrosomal and antithyroglobulin antibodies as well. A family history of thyroid disease, most often Graves' disease, Hashimoto's thyroiditis, or myxedema can frequently be elicited from patients with Graves' disease. Fifteen percent of patients have relatives with Graves' disease; 50% of relatives have antithyroid antibodies.

With human leukocyte antigen (HLA) typing, HLA-B8 is found in approximately 50% of Caucasians with Graves' disease. HLA-Bw35 is found in greater than expected incidence in Oriental patients with Graves' disease. Relatives of these patients also have a high incidence of these specific tissue antigens. These findings suggest a genetic factor in the pathogenesis of Graves' disease.

Graves' disease occurs 5–6 times more often in females than males. It most commonly occurs in the fourth and fifth decades of life. There is no proven link between emotional crises and Graves' disease.

Graves' disease and Hashimoto's thyroiditis are part of the spectrum of autoimmune thyroid disease. Both occur more commonly in females than males.

Pathologically, glands may show changes of both thyrotoxicosis and chronic thyroiditis. Both Graves' disease and Hashimoto's thyroiditis are associated with other autoimmune processes including pernicious anemia, rheumatoid arthritis, diabetes mellitus, Sjögren's syndrome, idiopathic adrenal insufficiency, primary gonadal failure, hypoparathyroidism, vitiligo, and alopecia. There is also a slightly increased incidence of leukemia and lymphoma.

Clinical Features

In its full clinical presentation, Graves' disease consists of the classic triad of (1) hyperthyroidism with diffuse goiter; (2) ophthalmopathy; and (3) dermopathy, eg, pretibial myxedema. A patient may present with any one or a combination of 2 parts of the triad, and frequently the full triad never develops. Pretibial myxedema is the least common of the 3 and rarely occurs in the absence of exophthalmos. Because the hyperthyroidism is most common, the other two are often thought of as complications of Graves' disease.

A. Hyperthyroidism: The typical patient with Graves' disease is a young woman who presents with nervousness, weight loss, increased sweating, and heat intolerance. On physical examination the patient is hyperkinetic and restless, is hyperreflexic, and has a goiter. The goiter may vary in size from 30 to 120 g, and a bruit is often heard over the goiter. Tachycardia and a wide pulse pressure are invariably present. The stare and lid lag seen in almost all patients with hyperthyroidism are due to spasm of the superior palpebral muscle. This condition is benign.

B. Ophthalmopathy: Although clinically detectable infiltrative ophthalmopathy occurs in 40% of Graves' patients, only 5–10% will manifest severe eye involvement. In addition to protrusion of the globe due to inflammatory changes of the extraocular muscles and fatty infiltration of the oribit, there may be paralysis of the muscles with resulting diplopia, severe chemosis, and damage to the optic nerve, retina, and cornea. The standard classification of Graves' ophthalmopathy, based on severity and structures involved, follows:

Class	Definition
0	No physical signs or symptoms
1	Only signs (noninfiltrative)
2	Soft tissue involvement (edema, chemosis)
3	Proptosis
4	Extraocular muscle involvement
5	Corneal involvement
6	Sight loss (optic nerve involvement)

The first letter of each definition spells the mnemonic "no specs."

Class 1 is the lid-lag and stare associated with spasm of the upper lid.

Classes 2 through 6 are associated with infiltrative ophthalmopathy.

Class 2 represents periorbital edema and redness and swelling of the conjunctiva (chemosis).

Class 3 represents proptosis. Proptosis is measured with a Hertel exophthalmometer. This instrument consists of 2 prisms and a scale mounted on a bar in such a way that the distance between the lateral orbital ridges and the anterior corner can be measured on the scale.

Class 4 represents extraocular muscle involvement. The muscles involved earliest and most commonly are the inferior recti. This results in diplopia and impairment of upward gaze.

Class 5 represents corneal involvement (keratitis) usually related to corneal damage due to inability to close the eye.

Class 6 represents loss of vision due to compression of the optic nerve by swollen muscles in the orbit.

In the initial evaluation of a patient with Graves' disease it is important to measure baseline proptosis. This may be done with an exophthalmometer. Protrusion of the eye beyond the lateral orbital ridge should not exceed 18 mm for Orientals, 20 mm for Caucasians, and 22 mm for blacks. Severe exophthalmos may measure 28 mm or more.

Although ophthalmopathy usually accompanies hyperthyroidism, it may precede it or occur years after successful treatment. It may occur in patients who never develop hyperthyroidism. Four-fifths of patients develop it within 18 months of the onset of hyperthyroidism. The ophthalmopathy tends to stabilize following treatment of the hyperthyroidism. The severe form correlates poorly with the severity of the Graves' disease; it occurs relatively less frequently, but tends to be more severe in males than females, and it rarely occurs in children. Treatment is discussed later in this section.

C. Dermopathy: Pretibial myxedema is less common than infiltrative ophthalmopathy and rarely occurs in its absence. Overall incidence in Graves' disease is 2–3%. Even less common is the associated clubbing, osteoarthropathy, or thyroid acropathy associated with Graves' disease. Treatment is not often necessary for pretibial myxedema, and treatment of hyperthyroidism probably has no effect on its course.

Diagnosis

Early in the course of Graves' disease and early in recurrences, T_3 is secreted from the gland in large amounts, and in such settings T_3 levels in the serum may be high before T_4 levels are. Thus, serum T_3 by RIA is elevated, serum T_4 and RAIU are normal in T_3 toxicosis, and the clinical presentation is one of mild hyperthyroidism. In most patients, the T_3RIA is the single most sensitive serum test for Graves' disease. However, patients with amiodarone- and iodide-induced goiter, as well as some patients with acute illness, may not have an elevated T_3RIA despite being thyrotoxic.

The diagnosis of Graves' disease is usually straightforward. In addition to classic signs and symptoms, circulating thyroid hormones, both T_4 and T_3, are usually elevated and RAIU is high. Many factors increase T_4 measurement without affecting clinical status, and other causes of thyrotoxicosis must also be considered.

Euthyroid Graves' disease may be more difficult to diagnose. Euthyroid Graves' with exophthalmos will have normal T_4 and T_3 levels and normal RAIU. TSI, if positive, is helpful in the diagnosis, as are the presence of antithyroglobulin and antimicrosomal antibodies. Fifty to 80% of euthyroid Graves' patients will have an abnormal T_3 suppression test and a blunted TSH response to TRH stimulation. A significant number of these patients will have an abnormally low TSH (sensitive assay). Any abnormal test is strong support for the presence of Graves' disease in the euthyroid state.

These diagnostic procedures are often necessary and important in investigating the patient who presents with exophthalmos without goiter. CT scanning, ultrasound, or magnetic resonance imaging can be used to help identify orbital tumors, arteriovenous anomalies, and mucoceles. Graves' disease shows the characteristic swollen extraocular muscles on scanning. Even though the exophthalmos may be unilateral clinically, CT scanning will confirm bilateral muscle involvement in Graves' disease.

The older the patient with Graves' disease, the less typical the presentation may be. A prominent goiter may be absent in up to 40% of patients over age 60. Tachycardia is less frequent—40% of patients age 60 or over have rates of less than 100. In ''apathetic hyperthyroidism'' atrial fibrillation may be the initial recognized abnormality. Spontaneous atrial fibrillation in patients over age 60 is caused by hyperthyroidism in 17% of cases. Many such patients have serum T_3 levels that are minimally elevated or even in the upper normal range. A TSH test is useful in such patients to diagnose subtle hyperthyroidism. Older patients may present with anorexia, depression, nausea, vomiting and abdominal pain, cardiac decompensation, or apathy. Graves' disease, thought to be less common in the aging population than toxic multinodular goiter, probably is at least as common. It is important to make the diagnosis in this group of patients. Older patients with unexplained weight loss, atrial fibrillation or congestive heart failure, sudden onset of angina, or depression should be screened with thyroid function tests.

Thyrotoxic periodic paralysis occurs mainly in Asian males with Graves' disease. It is not familial and tends to subside as the hyperthyroidism is brought under control. Propranolol has been used successfully during the acute phase.

Treatment

Since Graves' hyperthyroidism is due to abnormal stimulation of the thyroid gland by the abnormal immunoglobulin, ideally treatment should be directed toward this abnormal stimulation; however, this treatment has not yet been developed.

Acute treatment utilizes propranolol. Long-term treatment may use several approaches: (1) radioactive iodine, (2) surgery, and (3) antithyroid drugs (propylthiouracil or methimazole, ipodate, propranolol). Advantages and disadvantages are associated with each treatment method.

Factors influencing treatment of hyperthyroidism are shown in Table 5–11.

A. Radioactive Iodine: ^{131}I is currently the most popular and most frequently used method of therapy. It is easy to administer, less costly than surgery, can be given to outpatients, has no associated morbidity except for permanent hypothyroidism, and is 100% effective when given in adequate dosage. The ^{131}I dose is computed on the basis of delivering a selected (usually about 0.1 mCi) dose per gram of tissue.

$$\text{Dose} = (\text{mCi/g}) \times \text{thyroid weight (g)/RAI uptake}$$

Radioactive iodine treatment is associated with a high incidence of hypothyroidism: 15–20% in the first year and 70–80% by 20 years after treatment. This was first thought to be a major drawback to its use, but data show an incidence of hypothyroidism following surgery approaching that following RAI, and a 2–3% incidence per year of hypothyroidism following drug therapy. Indeed, the natural history of Graves' disease may be one of the hyperthyroid phase followed eventually by hypothyroidism. Some thyroid clinics give large doses of RAI, attempting to ablate the gland, and place patients on thyroid hormone within a month or 2 of treatment. Following ablative therapy, a high percentage of patients lose their positive TSI titers. Eye complications may be fewer with this approach. More study is required in this area.

A theoretical concern about RAI has been late radiation side effects. However, extensive studies have failed to show ^{131}I-related neoplasm or birth defects. There has been an increasing tendency to treat younger patients, though many physicians hesitate to use ^{131}I in patients under 30–35 years of age. Its use during pregnancy is absolutely contraindicated. A careful history and possibly a pregnancy test should be obtained before study and treatment with radioactive iodine.

Young, otherwise healthy patients may be prepared with propranolol alone before RAI treatment. However, older patients and those with cardiovascular disease should be prepared with propylthiouracil, 100 mg 4 times daily, or methimazole, 40 mg once daily, as well as propranolol so that they are euthyroid before RAI is given. This preparation usually takes 6–12 weeks. The propylthiouracil or methimazole can be stopped 4–5 days before RAI is given, whereas propranolol is continued until the patient is euthyroid. RAI uptake usually remains high in spite of the drug therapy, so therapeutic dosages of RAI do not need to be adjusted. The preparation of the patient with propylthiouracil or methimazole eliminates the possibility of exacerbating the hyperthyroidism as a result of acute radiation injury to the unprepared gland with release of any stored hormone in the gland. Low dose oral drugs are resumed 4 days after RAI treatment and slowly tapered over 6–12 weeks until ablation by the RAI is effective. Rarely is a second RAI treatment necessary.

B. Surgery: Surgery is safe, effective treatment. It renders the patient euthyroid quickly, as compared with the RAI-treated patient. It may be the preferred treatment in the following circumstances: (1) for unusually large goiters that might not shrink with ^{131}I; (2) during pregnancy if the disease is not controlled with low doses of antithyroid drugs (surgery should be done in the middle trimester); (3) in children; (4) in patients who also have a coexisting nonfunctioning thyroid nodule; and (5) in patients who refuse ^{131}I therapy and who are not candidates for antithyroidal drugs. Disadvantages are increased cost,

Table 5-11. Factors influencing treatment of hyperthyroidism.

Factors	Thionamides	^{131}I	Surgery	Propranolol	Ipodate
Graves' disease					
1. Degree of severity	More effective in mild disease	May not be indicated in mild disease	Effective with any severity	Useful adjunct with any severity	Indicated for more severe disease to decrease T_3 quickly
2. Size of gland	Higher percentage of cures with small glands; generally not curative with large gland	Best treatment for moderate to large size gland	Avoid in small glands; may be indicated with very large glands	Useful adjunct with any size	Effective with any size
3. Age	Children, teenagers	Adults—prepare first with propranolol (along with thionamide in elderly)	Children	Useful adjunct with any age	Any age
4. Pregnancy	Low dose usually effective	Contraindicated	Middle trimester	Avoid	Avoid
5. Recurrent disease	Generally not curative	Most effective	Rarely necessary	Useful adjunct to ^{131}I	Rarely necessary

6. Morbidity	Rare drug reaction; 0.2% incidence of agranulocytosis	High incidence of post-treatment hypothyroidism; ?genetic damage	Surgical complications; hypoparathyroidism; severed recurrent laryngeal nerve in less than 1%	Low	Low
7. Long-term remission	20–50% in unselected patients; 50–80% in selected patients	High	High	Low	Probably low, possibly 20%
Nodular goiter	Ineffective as definitive therapy, useful in preparing patient for RAI or surgery	May require large dose for multinodular goiter	Effective, may be preferred treatment for large glands	Useful adjunct to ^{131}I or surgery	Useful adjunct to surgery
Subacute thyroiditis	Ineffective	Ineffective	Not indicated	Best treatment	Acutely useful adjunct to propranolol in severe thyrotoxicosis
Silent thyroiditis (Hashitoxicosis)	Ineffective	Ineffective	Not indicated	Best treatment	Acutely useful adjunct to propranolol in severe thyrotoxicosis
Solitary toxic thyroid nodule	Relatively ineffective	Effective but recurrence or hypothyroidism may occur	Best treatment	Useful adjunct to surgery or ^{131}I	Useful adjunct to surgery

requiring hospitalization, and increased morbidity. Morbidity most often involves damage and destruction to the parathyroid glands and destruction to the recurrent laryngeal nerve. Surgery performed by competent neck surgeons is associated with a morbidity of less than 1%. All patients must be prepared and made euthyroid with thiourea, ipodate, or both. Propranolol is given to diminish symptoms of hyperthyroidism until the T_3 is normal. Iodine is given for 10 days before surgery to reduce vascularity of the gland. Lugol's solution, 2–3 drops a day, is adequate treatment.

C. Antithyroid Drugs:

1. Thiourea drugs–Propylthiouracil and **methimazole** interfere with thyroid hormone synthesis by blocking the organification of iodide. Propylthiouracil has a weak blocking effect on peripheral conversion of T_4 to T_3. The drugs cause no intrinsic damage to the thyroid gland, which is an advantage of their use. There is less posttherapy hypothyroidism than with surgery or RAI. In patients with long-term remission, the incidence of hypothyroidism is about 20% owing to ongoing thyroiditis or TSH-binding inhibitory immunoglobulin (TBII). Unfortunately, there is a high rate of recurrence (50–80%). These rates are probably lower when patients are carefully selected (those with relatively mild disease, small glands, and minimal eye involvement). The rate of relapse in selected patients treated with methimazole or propylthiouracil depends on the presence of antithyroid antibodies. Relapse rate is only 11% if levels of both thyroglobulin antibody (TGA) and microsomal antibodies (MCA) are elevated; 27% if only MCA is elevated; 39% if TGA and MCA are both low after a 2-year treatment period. Drugs are effective treatment during pregnancy and offer an alternative to surgery in this group of patients. They are also important in preparing the patient for surgery. It is advisable to use these drugs in preparing older patients and patients with cardiovascular disease for RAI treatment.

It is recommended that a high dose be given initially (30–60 mg of methimazole daily in 1–2 doses or 300–600 mg of propylthiouracil a day in 4 divided doses); this dose is gradually tapered as the patient returns to the euthyroid state. Eventually most patients can be maintained on methimazole, 10 mg/d or propylthiouracil, 100 mg in 1 daily dose, for a total treatment course of 1–2 years. Recent studies suggest that treatment courses of 1–2 years are more effective than shorter ones of 6 months.

Agranulocytosis is a rare but serious complication of propylthiouracil and methimazole treatment, reported in 0.4% of patients taking propylthiouracil and in 0.1% taking methimazole. It is usually manifested as fever and sore throat and is reversible when the drug is stopped. Before treatment is begun, a baseline blood count should be done because mild leukopenia is common in patients with Graves' disease. If fever or sore throat develops during treatment, the drug is stopped until a blood count is obtained for comparison. Patients must be forewarned of this reaction. It is idiosyncratic, so periodic blood counts are not usually helpful. Less serious but more common side effects are mild rash and pruritus. Antihistamines may control these effects without discontinuance of the drug. Less common toxic reactions include serum sickness, cholestatic jaundice (methimazole), hepatitis and acute hepatic necrosis (propylthiouracil), arthritis, lupus erythematosus, aplastic anemia, thrombocytopenia, hypoprothrombinemia (propylthiouracil), nephrotic syndrome (methimazole), loss of taste (methimazole), and an insulin autoimmune syndrome with hypoglycemia (methimazole). Propylthiouracil and methimazole cross-react; patients who have had a major toxic reaction to one drug should not be given the other.

The choice between propylthiouracil and methimazole can be difficult. Propylthiouracil has the theoretical advantage of blocking T_4 to T_3 and has some immunosuppressant properties. Methimazole has the advantages of less frequent dosing and a seemingly lower incidence of acute hepatic necrosis, making it increasingly favored at some medical centers.

2. Propranolol–As a beta-adrenergic antagonist, propranolol is effective in reversing the effects of catecholamine-induced action that are so prominent in Graves' disease: tachycardia, tremor, and diaphoresis. It has no effect on thyroid hormone synthesis or secretion. It has been used as adjunctive therapy with propylthiouracil or methimazole in preparing patients for surgery and in pre- and post-RAI therapy periods. It is one of the drugs used in thyroid storm, and it has been used successfully in surgical patients who cannot take propylthiouracil or methimazole. Finally, it is the drug of choice for periodic paralysis, commonly associated with Graves' disease among Asian males. Dose range is from 10 mg twice daily to 80 mg 4 times daily. It is also available as a long acting preparation.

3. Iodine–Iodine is also used in treating some cases of Graves' disease. It blocks the release of thyroid hormone from the Graves' gland. Because this therapeutic iodine may be organified and used in hormone production, it is important to start propylthiouracil or methimazole at least 1 hour earlier. The gland may escape the block of hormone release after 14 days, so its usefulness is during that initial period of treatment. It is mostly used to prepare patients for thyroidectomy. It is not used routinely.

4. Ipodate and iopanoic acid–Ipodate sodium (Bilivist, Oragrafin) and iopanoic acid (Telepaque) are iodinated contrast agents that may be given orally to block peripheral conversion of T_4 to T_3 in the liver and produce a drop in serum T_3 within 24 hours; they are sometimes useful in short-term treatment of severe thyrotoxicosis and thyroid storm. Ipodate may be given in a dose of 500 mg orally once daily. It works faster than thiourea. T_3 falls an average of 62% at one day after the first dose of ipodate; T_4 falls an average of 20% at 1 day and 43% at 14 days. However, this improvement in thyroid function is not usually sustained over time, and these preparations should not be used for much longer than 1 month. Patients with larger goiters and more severe thyrotoxicosis are more likely to escape the effect of ipodate and iopanoic acid. They are most effective when used simultaneously with thiourea. The latter should be continued after they have been stopped.

In neonatal Graves' disease, ipodate may be given as 500 mg orally every 3 days for about 5 weeks.

Thyroid Storm

Thyroid storm, a rare complication of Graves' disease, is a life-threatening medical emergency. It presents as a sudden exacerbation of hyperthyroidism, most often associated with intercurrent illness, especially infections. In addition to the heightened signs and symptoms of hyperthyroidism, a fever is present and is considered the distinguishing feature between severe hyperthyroidism and storm. Thyroid function tests are no higher in patients in storm than in those with hyperthyroidism without storm. Psychosis, delirium, and coma may also occur. Diagnosis is made clinically. A careful search for infection is imperative.

Treatment is instituted with large doses of propylthiouracil, 150–250 mg every 6 hours, or methimazole, 15 mg every 6 hours, followed within 1 hour by iodide. Lugol's solution may be used, 30 drops/d in divided doses, or a slow intravenous infusion of sodium iodide, 1 g/d. Ipodate or iopanoic acid, 500 mg/d orally, is useful. Propranolol as an adjunctive drug has replaced reserpine and guanethidine in recent years. The dose of propranolol is 20–80 mg every 6 hours orally, or 0.5–2 mg every 4 hours intravenously. Propranolol may improve thyrotoxic heart failure. If the patient has preexisting congestive heart failure, reserpine, 1 mg every 6 hours, is preferred over propranolol. If there is any suspicion of hypoadrenalism, adrenocorticosteriods should be used in high doses during the first day or so, but rapidly tapered when the acute phase of the disease has subsided. In addition, the patient should be cooled and treated for any intercurrent illness. The patient should be out of storm within a day, but definitive treatment of the hyperthyroidism should be delayed until the patient is in a euthyroid state. The use of aspirin as an antipyretic in this setting should be avoided, since it binds to TBG, displacing thyroxine, making more available in the free state.

Graves' Disease in Pregnancy

Graves' disease in pregnancy presents unique problems because (1) its presentation may be subtle, (2) diagnosis is more difficult, and (3) RAI treatment is contraindicated.

The pregnant woman has features that may simulate hyperthyroidism. The presence of a small goiter is not unusual; tachycardia, nausea and vomiting, and hyperkinesis also occur. T_4RIA and T_3RIA are high because of the increased binding protein seen with pregnancy. FT_4I is reliable but does not rule out T_3 toxicosis. FT_3I is less reliable. RAIU and the T_3 suppression test are contraindicated, but the response of serum T_4 to administered T_3 may sometimes be helpful. A blunted TSH response to TRH stimulation would give strong support to a diagnosis of Graves' disease, as would an abnormally low TSH. Positive tests for thyroid antibodies, especially TSI, would provide further support.

Treatment of Graves' disease during pregnancy is with either thiourea or surgery. As a rule, Graves' disease during pregnancy is relatively mild and easily managed. Severe eye involvement is unusual.

Propylthiouracil is the drug of choice for pregnant women, since it blocks conversion of T_4 to T_3, whereas methimazole does not; methimazole also has been associated with aplasia cutis. Propylthiouracil crosses the placenta, but if doses can be maintained below 200 mg/d, amounts reaching the fetus will result in only a 10% incidence of goiter in the newborn; these infants need brief treatment for hypothyroidism. Serum thyroxine levels are slightly lower in newborns following exposure to antithyroid drugs. These drugs should not be administered to pregnant women unless absolutely indicated and then at the lowest effective dose. The mother should remain mildly thyrotoxic to keep the drug dose as low as possible.

Thyroid hormone does not cross the placenta in significant amounts, so giving the patient exogenous thyroid has no protective effect for the fetus against possible goitrogenic effects of these drugs.

If the patient cannot be controlled on low doses of propylthiouracil or methimazole or if she develops agranulocytosis or other major drug reaction, surgery becomes necessary. Ideally, this is done in the middle trimester. *Iodine should never be given to a pregnant woman, since this may produce massive fetal goiter and neonatal airway obstruction.*

Hyperthyroidism that was mild and easily treated during pregnancy may worsen or relapse during or following labor and delivery. There is a high incidence of postpartum autoimmune thyroid disease. Postpartum hyperthyroidism is usually a transient silent thyroiditis and is treated with propranolol. Hypothyroidism also occurs.

Graves' Disease in the Neonate

Neonatal hyperthyroidism may present in one of 2 ways. The first is associated with current or recent history of Graves' disease in the mother. TSI is present in both the mother and the infant, and the condition has a relatively short, self-limited course of 4–6 months. The infant is small, with goiter, tachycardia, and fever. The eyes may be prominent. Serum T_4 is elevated (>14 µg/dL). Serum T_3 is especially elevated (>125 ng/dL). TSH is low. Recovery coincides with a fall in the child's TSI level. Therapy includes (1) propylthiouracil, 5–10 mg/kg/d in divided doses every 8 hours; (2) SSKI, 1 drop every 8 hours; (3) propranolol, 2 mg/kg/d in divided doses every 8 hours; (4) ipodate, 500 mg orally every 3 days, may be substituted for propylthiouracil. With severe toxicity, prednisone, 2 mg/kg/d is added. Therapy can be slowly tapered and usually stopped by the fourth month.

The second form of neonatal hyperthyroidism is usually more severe and longer lasting. There is a positive family history of Graves' disease among these infants, and they are thought to have true Graves' disease independent of the mother's course. The hyperthyroidism may not develop until the third or fourth month of life but is often severe and resistant to treatment. There is a 20% mortality rate, and survivors may have premature fusion of the cranial sutures and microcephaly, short stature, and mental retardation.

Graves' Ophthalmopathy

(See Figs. 5–6, 5–7, & 5–8.)

Therapy for Graves' ophthalmopathy is only partially successful. Local therapy includes the following: elevation of the head of the bed to minimize periorbital edema, and the use of artificial tears, antibiotic

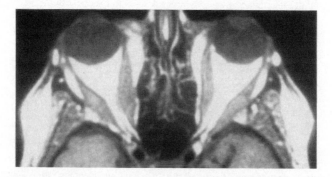

Figure 5–6. MRI scan of the orbit demonstrating the enlarged extra-occular muscles seen in Graves' infiltrative ophthalmopathy. (Courtesy of D. Char, MD.)

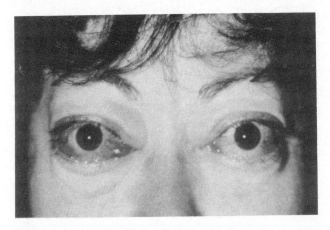

Figure 5–7. Severe ophthalmopathy occurs in 5–10% of patients. Severe edema and chemosis are demonstrated in this patient. (Courtesy of D. Char, MD.)

ointment, shaded glasses, and eyeshields or patches at night to protect the proptotic eye, especially the cornea, from exposure damage. Diuretics have been disappointing.

Ablative thyroid therapy (either surgical or by ^{131}I), followed by replacement thyroxine, is commonly performed for patients with severe, progressive ophthalmopathy, but it is controversial.

If exophthalmos is progressive, especially with decreased visual acuity, high doses of glucocorticoids are given (prednisone, 40–100 mg/d) and tapered slowly over 1–3 months after a therapeutic response is obtained. There is a tendency to recurrence after prednisone therapy.

X-ray therapy to the orbits may also reverse the progression of eye disease and should be considered if glucocorticoids are ineffective. Radiation therapy consists of 200 rads to each orbit for 10 days (directed to avoid the cornea and lens).

Surgical orbital decompression has been refined and is increasingly used as first-line treatment for severe ophthalmopathy. It should certainly be considered when glucocorticoid or radiation therapy fails. The most effective procedure allowing maximum decompression involves opening the floor and medial wall of the orbit. Lateral wall decompression is less effective but has a lower incidence of secondary strabismus.

The above maneuvers often save vision. However, they may not be indicated for less severe disease and usually do not give optimal cosmetic results. Appearance can be improved with eyelid surgery

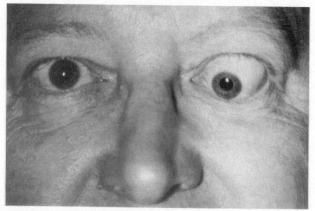

A

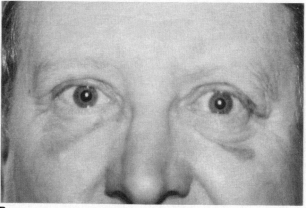

B

Figure 5–8. Unilateral Graves' exophthalmos before (**A**) and after (**B**) decompressive surgery. (Courtesy of D. Char, MD.)

(tarsorrhaphy, canthoplasty). The patient should be absolutely euthyroid to avoid the eyelid retraction of hyperthyroidism or the periorbital puffiness of myxedema.

Pretibial Myxedema

Pretibial myxedema presents as thickening of the skin of the lower legs over the pretibial area. Thickening is due to accumulation of glycosaminoglycans. Occasionally this lesion extends down to involve the dorsum of the foot. Occlusive dressings with fluocinolone is generally effective treatment. Fluocinolone is applied nightly and covered with plastic wrap until the following morning.

SUBACUTE (DE QUERVAIN'S) THYROIDITIS

Subacute thyroiditis is an uncommon, self-limited disease of the thyroid, probably related to viral infection. It occurs twice as frequently in females as males and most often between the ages of 20 and 60. Histologic findings include infiltration of polymorphonucleocytes, macrophages, and giant cells, with destruction of the thyroid follicles.

Clinically, there may be a 2-week prodromal viral illness with fever and malaise before the sudden onset of a tender goiter. Thyroid tenderness is the hallmark of this disease. The tenderness varies from mild to severe, often radiating into the jaws. The gland is usually 2–3 times normal size and firm. The hyperthyroidism is usually mild.

Thyroid function tests are elevated in the early stage owing to release of thyroid hormone into the circulation from the injured gland. RAIU is low, both because of injury with inability to take up iodine and because of TSH suppression secondary to high circulating levels of thyroid hormone. White blood count is often slightly high, and sedimentation rate is elevated. The disease has 3 phases:

The first phase may last 3–4 weeks, followed by the second phase of mild hypothyroidism due to incomplete recovery of the injured gland and exhaustion of stored thyroid hormone. Patients seem most likely to relapse during this phase, with recurrent tenderness, fever, and malaise. Hypothyroidism is rarely permanent, and subsequent thyroid dysfunction is uncommon. The third phase is one of recovery, usually occurring 2–4 months after onset.

Differential Diagnosis

Consider all the hyperthyroid states. The presentation of malaise, mild hyperthyroidism, and a tender goiter will make the diagnosis straightforward in the majority of cases. An elevated sedimentation rate is helpful in distinguishing subacute thyroiditis from other causes of hyperthyroidism with low RAIU, such as silent thyroiditis and factitious hyperthyroidism.

Ninety percent of patients with subacute thyroiditis will ultimately experience return to normal thyroid function; 10% develop permanent hypothyroidism.

Treatment

Treatment in the early phase is usually limited to control of pain. Mild manifestations of hyperthyroidism do not require specific therapy, but if pronounced, a short, 3–4 week course of propranolol, 10–40 mg 2–4 times a day, is indicated. Aspirin is most often adequate for pain control. In more severe cases, prednisone, 40–50 mg/d with tapering after 2 weeks, may be helpful in controlling the inflammatory aspects of the disease acutely, although it does not alter its natural course. Treatment with L-thyroxine, 0.1–0.2 mg/d during the hypothyroid phase may result in less relapse—if the recovering gland is not subjected to TSH drive during this time; given a longer rest period, it is not so likely to become reinflamed.

SILENT THYROIDITIS

Silent thyroiditis is thought to be a variant of Hashimoto's thyroiditis, and its incidence has increased in the past 10 years. In one series, 20% of new hyperthyroid cases were due to silent thyroiditis.

Histologically, there is lymphocytic infiltration, usually less severe than but similar to that seen in Hashimoto's thyroiditis. Giant cells and granulomatous changes of subacute thyroiditis are not found.

The female to male ratio is 2:1 (lower than that seen in Hashimoto's). It frequently occurs in the postpartum period up to 8 months following delivery.

The natural history of silent thyroiditis is similar in some ways to that of subacute thyroiditis. The initial phase of the disease is characterized by sudden-onset but generally mild hyperthyroidism, lasting from 2 weeks to 3 or 4 months. During this phase the thyroid gland may be moderately enlarged or normal but nontender. The second phase is of clinical euthyroidism. About 30% of patients will have a transient hypothyroid period before returning to euthyroidism. About 10–20% of patients remain hypothyroid. In the first phase, thyroid function tests are elevated, but RAIU is low. The sedimentation rate and white blood count, however, are normal. Many patients are left with small, firm goiters, even among the euthyroid group; in neither phase is the gland tender or painful, an important distinguishing feature of subacute thyroiditis. Fever and lassitude are also absent in silent thyroiditis.

Silent thyroiditis can usually be distinguished from factitious hyperthyroidism by the presence of an elevated serum thyroglobulin (but not in most patients furtively ingesting thyroid hormone).

Thyroid antibodies are present in a high percentage of patients with silent thyroiditis in contrast to subacute thyroiditis, where they occur infrequently and in low titers.

The presence of thyroid antibodies, lymphocytic infiltration seen histologically, and common postpartum occurrence all suggest an autoimmune etiology and close relationship to the other autoimmune thyroid diseases—Graves' disease and Hashimoto's thyroiditis.

Differentiating silent thyroiditis from Graves' disease is an important and practical matter, because treatment for silent thyroiditis is so different. High RAIU is characteristic of Graves' disease, whereas it is low in silent thyroiditis. Patients with silent thyroiditis do not have ophthalmopathy or dermopathy.

Because of the self-limited nature of silent thyroiditis, it is inappropriate to ablate the thyroid gland. Usually, it is adequate to treat the mild symptoms of hyperthyroidism seen in the early phase of silent thyroiditis with a beta-blocker, such as propranolol, 10–40 mg 2–4 times a day. L-thyroxine may be given during the transient hypothyroid phase and continued in the small group of patients who remain hypothyroid.

Patients with silent thyroiditis may have recurring disease, especially postpartum, and they have a high incidence of thyroid dysfunction in later years. For this reason, follow-up examinations and screening are important.

TOXIC NODULAR GOITER

The cause of toxic multinodular goiter is unknown, but it usually occurs in patients who have had nontoxic multinodular goiters for many years before developing hyperthyroidism. An abnormal immunoglobulin, thyroid growth-stimulating immunoglobulin, may cause the multinodularity and ultimately the hyperthyroidism. Toxic nodular goiter occurs much less commonly than Graves' disease. Patients are usually over age 50. Exophthalmos and pretibial myxedema are absent.

The hyperthyroidism of toxic nodular goiter is generally milder than that of Graves' disease. Thyroid function tests and RAIU are lower. Because the disease is more commonly seen in an older population, manifestations may not be typical or severe. Cardiovascular symptoms may predominate. Toxic nodular goiter may present as T_3 toxicosis.

Treatment is with either surgery or RAI. The latter is not as effective as it is in Graves' disease. The glands are often large and do not always shrink after RAI. Because RAIU is lower and glands are larger, treatment dose is larger, and patients more frequently require retreatment.

Indications for surgery include local pressure symptoms such as tracheal or esophageal obstruction, a rapidly enlarging nodular goiter, or cosmetic considerations. The patient must be prepared for surgery or RAI just as the Graves' patient.

SOLITARY TOXIC NODULES

Solitary toxic nodules function autonomously. Most functioning nodules are not toxic, but the larger the nodule, the more likely it will be toxic. Most toxic nodules are 2.5 cm or more in size. Whether they grow slowly over many years is unclear, but nontoxic functioning nodules tend to be seen in young to middle-aged patients, whereas toxic nodules are seen in older patients, which suggests a slow evolution toward toxicity.

With nontoxic nodules there is a female predominance of greater than 10:1. It is lower with toxic nodules, around 4:1.

Diagnosis

Diagnosis is based on signs and symptoms, elevated thyroid function tests, RAIU, and a characteristic RAI scan. The functioning nodule will pick up iodide in contrast to a nonfunctioning nodule. If there is little iodine pick-up in surrounding tissue and the RAI concentrates in the nodule, it is more likely toxic. Physiologically, there is enough activity and hormone secretion from the toxic nodule to suppress TSH; the normal thyroid tissue is relatively inactive, trapping only about 8% of the administered iodide.

Treatment

Treatment is with surgery or RAI. Patients under age 40 probably should have surgery; by 6 years postoperatively, 14% have become hypothyroid. Over age 40, RAI is the treatment of choice; by 8 years following RAI, 36% of patients become hypothyroid and 54% of nodules are still palpable. In 9%, the nodule may increase in size.

JODBASEDOW

Iodide-induced thyrotoxicosis is called jodbasedow. Iodine is the only nonhormonal substance known to cause hyperthyroidism. Jodbasedow occurs when iodine is added to the diet, after SSKI use, following injection of iodinated contrast media, and with amiodarone treatment. This phenomenon occurs most frequently in patients who are iodide deficient, who have developed unrecognized thyroid autonomy in nodular goiters. However, it has also been described in patients with nodular goiters who are not iodide deficient. In this latter group, the hyperthyroid state is not necessarily self-limited. Patients treated with amiodarone (for resistant cardiac arrhythmias) are especially prone to develop goiter and hyperthyroidism with previously normal glands. Because of the large body iodide stores, 3 months are required for the thyrotoxicosis to subside. In the meantime, beta-blockers may be used to control symptoms. RAIU is almost universally low in such patients with organic iodide excess, so ^{131}I treatment is not indicated. These patients are also relatively resistant to thionamide treatment, since up to 100 mg (normal-10 mg) of organified iodide may be already stored in the gland.

AMIODARONE-INDUCED HYPERTHYROIDISM

Patients receiving amiodarone usually have asymptomatic elevation of serum T_4 and free T_4. Symptomatic hyperthyroidism occurs in about 2.5% of patients, with onset at 4 months to 3 years after amiodarone therapy is begun. The incidence is higher in areas of the world where iodine intake is low (eg, central Europe and endemic goiter areas). Hyperthyroidism may fatally exacerbate a patient's arrythmia or myocardial ischemia.

Patients may not have the usual catecholamine-like effects of hyperthyroidism, especially when beta-blockers are being used simultaneously. Instead, weakness, weight loss, restlessness, tremor, goiter, or worsening of cardiac disease may predominate.

Such symptoms should prompt the measurement of serum T_4, T_3, and TSH. In hyperthyroidism, TSH (sensitive assay) is suppressed; usually, T_4 is > 20 µg/dL or T_3 is > 200 ng/dL. TSI is frequently present in serum.

Treatment of thyrotoxicosis in these patients can be a problem. If amiodarone can be discontinued, hyperthyroidism may persist for up to 3 months. Beta-blockers may be increased or initiated in the interim if cardiac output is adequate.

RAIU and scan should be performed. Despite massive body stores of iodine, many patients have sufficient RAIU to allow ^{131}I treatment. Thiourea antithyroid drugs (propylthiouracil, methimazole) also cause improvement despite continued amiodarone treatment. Propylthiouracil is usually used, since it blocks T_4 to T_3 conversion. Ipodate or iopanoic acid may also be added following ^{131}I treatment and after the thiourea is begun.

OTHER CAUSES OF THYROTOXICOSIS

Struma Ovarii

As many as 3% of ovarian teratomas and dermoid tumors contain thyroid tissue. Usually of no clinical significance, it rarely produces thyrotoxicosis. Ascites and a palpable ovarian mass in a patient with hyperthyroidism may signal the possibility of this diagnosis. Most patients with struma ovarii and hyperthyroidism have Graves' disease or a multinodular goiter; the struma ovarii contributes to systemic thyroid tissue overactivity. The ectopic thyroid tissue is the sole source of the hyperthyroidism only when it contains an autonomous functioning adenoma. Patients are not relieved of the hyperthyroidism until the teratoma is removed. RAIU in the ovary is diagnostic. Thyroidal uptake may not be suppressed, since some of the nodular goiters may be autonomous.

TSH-Secreting Tumors

TSH-secreting tumors (neoplastic inappropriate secretion of thyrotropin, NIST) is very rare. It may present with visual field cuts, amenorrhea, and elevated TSH, T_4, and T_3. Treatment includes controlling the usually mild hyperthyroidism with antithyroid drugs and removing the tumor by transsphenoidal resection.

TSH Hyperplasia

TSH hyperplasia (non-neoplastic inappropriate secretion of thyrotropin, NNIST) is rare. It is caused by a high pituitary "set point." Serum TSH is increased in the presence of thyrotoxicosis; a normal serum TSH also suggests this diagnosis, but only when a sensitive assay is used. The pituitary may be enlarged. TSH hyperplasia is frequently familial or associated with myasthenia gravis. The pituitary thyrotrophes are resistant to suppression by T_4 but may sometimes respond to T_3. Ironically, T_3 has been used as treatment.

Factitious Hyperthyroidism

Factitious hyperthyroidism is often difficult to ferret out, but it characteristically is associated with a small thyroid gland, high thyroid function tests, and low RAIU in an otherwise healthy patient. In this group of patients it is often possible to obtain a history of emotional instability, overriding concern and fear of obesity, and a possible source for obtaining thyroid hormone surreptitiously. Low serum thyroglobulin levels are helpful in distinguishing this entity from silent thyroiditis.

Metastatic Thyroid Carcinoma

Metastatic thyroid carcinoma has rarely been reported as causing hyperthyroidism. It usually presents along with a thyroid nodule. The diagnosis is made by body scanning, and the carcinoma is usually follicular, demonstrating high uptake levels, usually in the lungs and bone. Treatment with ^{131}I is moderately successful but often results in post-treatment pulmonary fibrosis.

Tumors of Trophoblastic Origin

These tumors may secrete huge quantities of hCG having mild TSH-like activity. Rarely, patients with choriocarcinoma, hydatidiform mole, or testicular embryonal carcinoma have elevated levels of serum T_3 and T_4. The associated hyperthyroidism is usually mild, with small goiters. Treatment consists of removal of the carcinoma or mole. The patient may be prepared for surgery with beta-blockade.

HYPOTHYROIDISM

CLINICAL FEATURES

Infants

Untreated hypothyroidism of any cause during infancy leads to cretinism (Table 5–12). Irreversible retardation of mental development occurs in cretinism during this critical period. Worldwide, cretinism is due most commonly to iodine deficiency, but this is rare in the USA.

Table 5–12. Manifestations of hypothyroidism.*

Signs

Goiter frequently palpable depending upon cause; apathetic countenance; ptosis; slow movements; ataxia; bradycardia; dyslalia; slow reflex relaxation phase; myxedema; dry, scaly skin with hyperkeratosis of elbows and legs; coarse hair; brittle nails; hypothermia; heart failure; muscle hypertrophy (adults—Hoffman's syndrome; children—Kocher-Debré-Sémélaigne syndrome); myxedema coma; facial edema (especially periorbital); nonpitting peripheral edema; hypertension; x-ray changes (pleural or pericardial effusion).

Nonthyroid laboratory abnormalities: Increased cholesterol; increased SGOT, LDH, CPK; increased P_{CO_2}; increased prolactin; increased CSF protein; decreased sodium; decreased hematocrit (increased or normal mean corpuscular volume); decreased glucose; decreased ECG voltage.

Symptoms

Fatigue and lethargy; weakness; headache; weight change (usually gain in 60%); cold intolerance; menstrual irregularity (usually menorrhagia); galactorrhea; dry skin; hair loss; constipation; hoarseness; decreased sweating; paresthesias; neuropathy; carpal tunnel syndrome; diminished hearing; arthralgias and myalgias; memory impairment; psychiatric disturbance.

Neonatal: Persistent physiologic jaundice; somnolence; feeding problems; constipation; protruberant abdomen; umbilical hernia; hoarse cry.

Untreated neonatal: (Cretinism); mental retardation; deaf-mutism; delayed eruption of teeth; incoordination; delayed closure of fontanelles; large head; epiphyseal dysgenesis.

Children: Slow linear growth with delayed bone age; delayed (rarely precocious) puberty.

* A hypothyroid patient may have only a few of these manifestations.

Other causes include congenital absence of thyroid tissue, dyshormonogenesis (hormozygote), and an isolated pituitary TSH deficiency. A delay of 3 months in treating the newborn is associated with significant retardation.

Hypothyroidism developing after the first 18 months of life will affect only physical growth. The associated mental sluggishness occurring with hypothyroidism after this critical time period is reversible.

The disease may be difficult to recognize in infancy. Suggestive, but nonspecific, signs and symptoms of congenital hypothyroid are constipation, hoarse cry, feeding problems, hypothermia, failure to thrive, umbilical hernia, and large tongue. As the undiagnosed infant grows older, a more typical cretin picture develops: large head, flat nose, widely set eyes, protuberant abdomen, protruding tongue, sparse hair, hypotonic muscles, waddling gait, rough skin, mental retardation, and increased trunk/limb ratio. With neonatal screening, a T_4 under 6 μg/dL or TSH over 30 μU/mL is consistent with neonatal or congenital hypothyroidism. The diagnosis can be confirmed by retarded bone age on x-ray. Congenital hypothyroidism occurs once in 4000 births. Goiter is absent in cases of thyroid dysgenesis or pituitary hypothyroidism. Goiter is usually present in cases of defective hormone synthesis, ingestion of a goitrogen by the mother (especially iodide), and iodide deficiency.

Children

Hypothyroidism diagnosed between ages 1 and 5 is usually due to maldeveloped or ectopic thyroid gland (lingual thyroid). Usually no goiter is palpable. Impaired growth during these years is the prominent feature of hypothyroidism. Isosexual precocity with breast development and vaginal bleeding in severe hypothyroidism is due to increased TSH levels and possible overlapping function of TSH with gonadotropins. Pseudomuscular hypertrophy (Kocher-Debré-Sémélaigne syndrome) also occurs.

Hypothyroidism in older children and adolescents is usually associated with goiter, most often due to Hashimoto's thyroiditis. As with adults, the onset is insidious. Signs and symptoms are also similar, except for the prominent retardation of growth and development seen in juvenile hypothyroidism. With treatment, there is a return to normal physical and intellectual levels.

Adults

Manifestations of adult hypothyroidism result from multisystem involvement. Goiter is common. Symptoms occurring in 90% or more of patients include weakness, coarse dry skin, lethargy, slow speech, eyelid edema, and cold intolerance. Less common manifestations are constipation, hair loss, coarse hair, peripheral edema, hoarseness, anorexia, thick tongue, memory impairment, skin pallor, bradycardia, and slow relaxation of deep tendon areas. Patients frequently note sleeping longer. True psychosis is a rare complication of severe myxedema; this has been referred to as myxedema madness.

Weight gain is not a constant finding in hypothyroid patients, and when it does occur, is associated with excessive caloric intake, just as in the euthyroid patient.

Menstrual irregularities vary from menorrhagia to amenorrhea. Infertility is common in advanced hypothyroidism.

Elderly

Hypothyroidism in the elderly is often less typical in its presentation. It is more commonly diagnosed in the elderly than in younger adults, probably owing to a rise in prevalence of Hashimoto's thyroiditis and increased use of RAI therapy for Graves' disease during young adult life. Signs and symptoms of hypothyroidism in the elderly are often overlooked as part of the natural aging process (Fig. 5–9). Presentation may be dominated by abnormalities related to a single organ system, eg, constipation, anorexia, and weight loss; depression and mental dullness; arthritis; and deafness, dizziness, or vertigo.

A. Secondary Hypothyroidism: Secondary hypothyroidism is usually milder than primary. Goiter is absent. The myxedematous changes of primary hypothyroidism are absent. Pericardial or pleural effusion often is associated with long-standing primary hypothyroidism but not seen with secondary hypothyroidism. The skin, rather than being coarse, is smooth, thin, and wrinkly.

B. Myxedema Heart: The myxedema heart is of special interest. It occurs most often in more severe, long-standing hypothyroidism and is frequently associated with underlying heart disease, especially in the elderly. Coronary arteriosclerosis is increased in hypothyroidism. Since with hypothyroidism there is decreased oxygen consumption, bradycardia, and decreased cardiac output, the underlying heart disease may not be manifested until treatment for the hypothyroidism is instituted and oxygen consumption and cardiac output increase, placing a greater work load on the heart.

The myxedema heart is often enlarged, in part because of pericardial effusion. Congestive heart failure with myxedema is rare, although the physical findings of an enlarged heart and coarse, wet breath sounds may lead erroneously to that diagnosis. The absence of pulmonary vascular congestion on x-ray will rule out congestive heart failure in this setting. Angina pectoris is usually minor until the myxedematous patient is treated with thyroid replacement; then it may become severe and unstable.

C. Subclinical Hypothyroidism: Subclinical hypothyroidism is

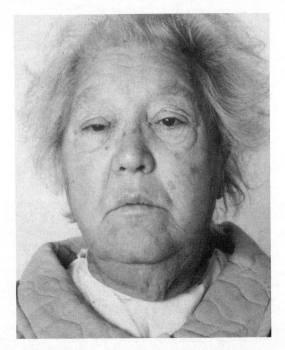

Figure 5–9. Myxedema of the elderly, as demonstrated here with the dull facial expression and periorbital edema, is often mistaken for natural aging. (From Greenspan, F: *Basic and Clinical Endocrinology*, 3rd ed. Appleton & Lange, 1991.)

a relatively asymptomatic state in which serum thyroxine is maintained in the normal range only by increased TSH secretion. A high percentage of patients have detectable antithyroid antibodies.

Many such patients have hyperlipidemia or, upon close questioning, mild nonspecific complaints that sometimes improve with low-dose thyroxine treatment. Truly asymptomatic patients with goiter or TSH levels greater than 20 μg/dL are likely to become clinically hypothyroid and are usually treated. Thyroxine doses are kept low, especially in the elderly, to avoid apathetic hyperthyroidism or exacerbation of underlying myocardial ischemia.

Asymptomatic patients without goiter and with TSH levels less than 20 μg/dL are less likely to become clinically hypothyroid and are not treated. All patients with subclinical hypothyroidism, whether treated or not, require close monitoring.

CAUSES OF HYPOTHYROIDISM

Hashimoto's Thyroiditis

Hashimoto's thyroiditis is the most common cause of hypothyroidism. Subclinical thyroiditis is common at unselected autopsies, with about 25% showing focal thyroiditis and about 3–4% Hashimoto's thyroiditis. The natural history of clinical Hashimoto's is one of slow destruction of the gland. The incidence of hypothyroidism among Hashimoto's patients of 20 years' duration is high, probably greater than 50%. This group of patients most often presents with firm, diffuse, lobular goiters.

Hashimoto's thyroiditis, an autoimmune disease, is chronic and progressive. Histologically, it is characterized by areas of lymphocytic infiltration with germinal centers interspersed with fibrosis. Other areas show follicular cell hypertrophy and oxyphilia (Hürthle cells).

Its incidence has increased dramatically in recent years, possibly owing to growing recognition and improved techniques in diagnosis of the disease. Increased use of dietary iodine may be unmasking previously unrecognized disease. The subtle defect in organification of iodine in Hashimoto's glands is due to decreased peroxidase activity. It becomes clinically evident with increased iodine intake, resulting in decreased thyroid hormone synthesis and increased TSH secretion and ultimately goiter formation and hypothyroidism.

Female predominance is strong, as high as 10:1, and patients with Hashimoto's thyroiditis have a high family incidence of thyroid dysfunction.

Hashimoto's thyroiditis is seen in patients with other autoimmune diseases such as Graves' disease, Addison's disease, type I insulin-dependent diabetes mellitus, hypoparathyroidisim, pernicious anemia, rheumatoid arthritis, and Sjögren's syndrome. The occurrence of hypothyroidism due to Hashimoto's thyroiditis and Addison's disease is known as Schmidt's syndrome. Diabetes mellitus may also be present.

Thyroid antimicrosomal and antithyroglobulin antibodies are seen in virtually all patients with Hashimoto's thyroiditis, in 70% or more of patients with Graves' disease, and in a higher than expected incidence in patients with diabetes mellitus, Addison's disease, pernicious anemia, and rheumatoid arthritis and in family members of patients with Hashimoto's.

The close relationship between Hashimoto's and Graves' disease is particularly striking, and indeed, each may represent a different aspect of the same disease. Both may occur within the same patient, and antibodies occur with high frequency in both. Within a single family, some members may have Hashimoto's, while others have Graves' disease. A small percentage of Hashimoto's patients have thyroid ophthalmopathy without Graves' hyperthyroidism.

The typical Hashimoto patient will present with a euthyroid goiter, which is diffuse or lobular, firm, and nontender. It is usually 2–3 times normal size. One-fifth of patients may present with a multinodular goiter. Fewer may present with hypothyroidism, with or without a goiter. Small subgroups present with variant atrophic myxedema or atropic asymmetry. These variants are usually seen in older patients.

The peak age of diagnosis is in the fourth and fifth decades of life, although it is also a common diagnosis in childhood and adolescence and is the most common cause of hypothyroidism in this age group. It may be noticed first during pregnancy.

The natural history is difficult to establish because most patients are placed on exogenous thyroid hormone for suppression of the goiter. Still, it is probable that with time a large percentage of the patients become hypothyroid. For this reason suppressive therapy is justified once a definite diagnosis is made.

A. Diagnosis: Diagnosis is made on the basis of the goiter and positive antibodies present in high titers. Thyroid function tests are usually normal or low. TSH is normal or high. The combination of normal thyroid function tests and high TSH reflects a failing thyroid gland or subclinical hypothyroidism. RAIU is generally not necessary as part of the diagnostic workup. Uptake is usually normal in the euthyroid patient and low in the hypothyroid patient. It may, however, be high in the setting of a failing gland and increased TSH drive. A small percentage of patients may present initially with mild hyperthyroidism **Hashitoxicosis**. This may be due to either concurrently present Graves' disease or thyroid gland destruction. Hyperthyroidism from the latter is usually short-lived and responds to a short course of propylthiouracil or methimazole. It is not usually necessary to ablate the gland with RAI.

If a patient with Hashimoto's thyroiditis is not suppressed with L-thyroxine, it is important to watch closely for impending hypothyroidism. This is especially important in the aging patient in whom the onset of hypothyroidism may be insidious and is more likely to go unrecognized. Usual and adequate suppressive doses of thyroxine range between 0.12 and 0.20 mg/d. The dose may be adjusted downward with increasing age or in patients with cardiovascular disease who will not tolerate the higher level. The younger the patient at the onset of treatment, the more likely the gland will regress on suppressive therapy. In older patients with long-standing or multinodular goiters, there may be little shrinking.

B. Prognosis: No increased incidence of papillary follicular or anaplastic carcinoma occurs with Hashimoto's thyroiditis. These neoplasms probably occur in the Hashimoto's gland at the same rate as in the non-Hashimoto's gland. Therefore, a solitary nodule in a Hashimoto's gland should be investigated in the same manner as it would be in an otherwise normal gland. Because Hashimoto's thyroiditis is so common, the occurrence of both diseases in the same patient is frequently seen.

Patients with Hashimoto's thyroiditis appear to have a slightly increased risk of systemic myeloproliferative and lymphoproliferative neoplasms as well as thyroid lymphoma. Lymphoma of the thyroid is often seen in the elderly with probable long-standing Hashimoto's. In one large series of patients with chronic lymphocytic thyroiditis, the incidence of myeloproliferative and lymphoproliferative neoplasms was increased (1.4% versus expected 0.4%); the risk of malignant thyroid lymphoma was also increased (0.5% versus expected 0.007%).

Other Causes

   A. Surgery or RAI Treatment of Hyperthyroidism: There is a 20–30% incidence of hypothyroidism in the first 2 years after RAI treatment, and a 2–3% occurrence per year after that; a conservative calculation at 20 years would yield 60% incidence of hypothyroidism. In the 2 years following surgery, the incidence is somewhat lower, but subsequently, onset of hypothyroidism is at 2–3% a year. Both groups of hypothyroid patients usually present without goiters. Thiourea-treated patients do not have the early high occurrence rate, but they also develop hypothyroidism at a rate of 2–3% a year. This represents a large and growing population, and it is significant that it is an aging population by the time hypothyroidism develops.

   B. Amiodarone Administration: Clinically significant hypothyroidism occurs in about 8% of patients receiving amiodarone. It can occur as early as 2 weeks after amiodarone is begun or at any time thereafter. The T_4 level may be normal or low, but the TSH is elevated and generally over 20 ng/dL. Another 17% of patients have less severe elevations in TSH with minimal or no symptoms of hypothyroidism. Such patients frequently tolerate this condition well without progression of symptoms, but they still require close monitoring. Patients over age 60 are especially prone to develop hypothyroidism. Patients with symptomatic hypothyroidism are treated with L-thyroxine at the minimum dose that reverses symptoms.

   C. Dyshormonogenesis: Enzyme deficiencies causing decreased or defective synthesis of thyroid hormone are an unusual cause of goitrous hypothyroidism. These disorders are familial, usually autosomal recessive. The homozygote is often hypothyroid at birth and may develop cretinism if not treated. The heterozygote may be euthyroid with a small goiter, or hypothyroid. In the heterozygote, the goiter may develop during adolescence and need not be present at infancy. The most common defect in this group is peroxidase deficiency, resulting in a block in organification of iodide. When associated with nerve deafness, the peroxidase deficiency is known as Pendred's syndrome.

D. Secondary Hypothyroidism: Secondary hypothyroidism is due to a deficiency of TSH secretion by the pituitary. It may be caused by any of the factors listed in Table 5–13 and is described in Chapter 1. Serum levels of thyroxine are low or low-normal, while the TSH level is not elevated.

LABORATORY FINDINGS

Laboratory findings include low FTI, elevated cholesterol and triglycerides, and very often elevated CPK, LDH, SGOT, and hyponatremia. There is often a mild to moderate anemia, which may be due

Table 5–13. Causes of hypothyroidism.

Goiter present	Goiter absent
Hashimoto's thyroiditis	Secondary hypothyroidism
Iodide deficiency	(deficient pituitary TSH secretion;
Drug goitrogens: lithium, iodide,	includes prolonged dopamine
amiodarone, ethionamide,	infusion)
propylthiouracil, methimazole,	Thyroid gland dysgenesis
aminoglutethimide, prolonged	Malabsorption of replacement oral
nitroprusside, phenylbutazone,	thyroxine[†]: malabsorption,
oxyphenbutazone, topical	cholestyramine, cholestipol,
resorcinol in large amounts	soybean flour (infant formulas)
sulfonamides, p-aminosalicylic	may increase T_4 requirements
acid, perchlorate, interleukin-2,	Postablative ^{131}I or surgery
lymphokine-activated killer cells	Radiation therapy including thyroid
Food goitrogens (only in iodide-	in field
deficient areas): cassava,	Idiopathic
sorghum, maize, millet, almond	Any condition causing goiter can
seeds, cabbage, turnips,	sometimes have unpalpable
rutabaga, mustard, kale,	goiter
cauliflower, brussels sprouts	
Genetic defects in thyroid hormone	**Differential diagnosis**
biosynthesis	Factors causing decreased
Impaired peripheral sensitivity to	thyroxine without affecting clinical
thyroid hormone[*]	status (Table 5–1)
Infiltrating disease[†]: lymphoma,	
sarcoid, amyloid	

[*] Rare
[†] Patients may or may not have a palpable goiter.

to decreased erythropoiesis, folate deficiency (nutritional), or iron deficiency (menorrhagia).

ECG may show bradycardia and low voltage; chest x-ray often reveals an enlarged cardiac silhouette and pleural effusions but not pulmonary vascular congestion.

An elevated TSH with low FTI confirms a diagnosis of primary hypothyroidism. The combination of normal FTI with modest elevation in TSH is considered diagnostic of subclinical hypothyroidism and consistent with a failing thyroid gland. Serum T_3 may be normal in subclinical or mild hypothyroidism, so it is not useful as a diagnostic screening test.

In the absence of obvious factors that decrease the FTI and with a low TSH, a CT scan of the pituitary and hypothalamus is usually done, and the patient is evaluated for other pituitary hormone deficiencies. The TRH test is not of practical value in these patients.

TREATMENT

With a firm diagnosis of hypothyroidism or subclinical hypothyroidism, treatment should be instituted (Table 5–14). The preferred preparation is synthetic L-thyroxine. Synthroid and Levothroid have reliably accurate amounts of bioavailable hormone and are therefore superior to generic preparations. L-thyroxine is stable and inexpensive. Both Synthroid and Levothroid are available in a wide range of doses. Dessicated thyroid extract is of animal origin and is standardized on the basis of iodide content; bioavailable hormone varies from batch to batch, and even pills within the same batch may vary in potency. Because of its much shorter half-life, triiodothyronine produces a spiking, uneven blood hormone level, and is not used in the long-term treatment of hypothyroidism. Combination synthetic T_4 and T_3 preparations are more expensive and are unnecessary because synthetic T_4 is converted to T_3, as is T_4 secreted from the thyroid gland. The T_3 in the synthetic combination also produces an uneven blood level.

Full replacement doses may be begun immediately in infants and children. A full replacement dose in an infant 0–12 months old is around 0.05 mg/d. For a child 1–2 years old, 0.1 mg is the usual replacement dose. Between ages 2 and 4, the dose goes up to 0.1–0.15 mg, and from age 4 to 12, it varies from 0.10 to 0.30 mg/d. Because T_4 degradation rate is greater in children than adults, replacement doses in children are higher on a weight basis than in adults. Also because of the faster degradation rate, children who are not compliant in taking their thyroxine are more likely to develop hypothyroidism. Careful monitoring of blood levels is suggested to keep the T_4 in the upper range of normal values in children.

Table 5–14. Thyroid replacement therapy.

Preparation	Content	Equivalent Dose	Maintenance Dose
Levothyroxine (Synthroid, Levothroid)	Synthetic T_4	0.1 mg	0.12–0.2 mg
Desiccated thyroid (Armour thyroid)	T_4 and T_3 in animal thyroid extract in a 3:1 ratio	1.5 grains	2–3 grains
Thyroglobulin (Proloid)	T_4 and T_3 in hog thyroid extract	1.5 grains	2–3 grains
Liothyronine sodium (Cytomel)	Synthetic T_3	25 μg	50–75 μg/d in divided doses
Liotrix (Thyrolar, Euthroid)	Synthetic T_4 and T_3 in a 4:1 ratio (Thyrolar 1, Euthroid 1)	50–60 μg T_4 12.5–15 μg T_3 (Thyrolar 2, Euthroid 2)	100–200 μg T_4 25–30 μg T_3

Different tablet sizes of each preparation

L-Thyroxine

Synthroid: 0.025 mg (orange); 0.05 mg (white); 0.075 mg (violet); 0.1 mg (yellow); 0.112 (rose); 0.125 mg (brown); 0.15 mg (blue); 0.175 mg (lilac); 0.2 mg (pink); 0.3 mg (green).

Levothroid: 0.025 (orange); 0.05 (white); 0.175 mg (gray); 0.1 mg (yellow); 0.125 mg (purple); 0.15 mg (blue); 0.175 mg (turquoise); 0.2 mg (pink); 0.3 mg (green).

Desiccated thyroid

Armour Thyroid: 15 mg (¼ grain); 30 mg; 60 mg; 90 mg; 120 mg; 180 mg; 240 mg; 300 mg (all tablets are white).

Thyroglobulin

Proloid: 32 mg (½ grain); 65 mg; 100 mg; 130 mg; 200 mg (all tablets are gray).

Liothyronine

Cytomel: 5 μg; 25 μg; 50 μg (all tablets are white).

Liotrix

Euthroid: ½ (0.03 mg T_4/7.5 mg T_3 (orange); 1 (0.6 mg T_4/15 mg T_3 (brown); 2 (0.12 mg T_4 mg T_3 (violet); 3 (0.18 mg T_4/45 mg T_3 (gray).

Thyrolar: ¼ (0.0125 mg T_4/3.1 mg T_3 (violet); ½ (0.25 mg T_4/6.25 mg T_3 (peach); 1 (0.05 mg T_4/12.5 mg T_3 (pink); 2 (0.10 mg T_4/25 mg T_3 (green); 3 (0.15 mg T_4/37 mg T_3 (yellow).

In adults, if the hypothyroidism is long-standing and severe, the starting dose should be low and titrated slowly upward. The usual starting dose is 0.05 mg/d, increased to 0.1 mg after 2–4 weeks. Young adults can be started directly on 0.1 mg/d. Some patients are overly sensitive to thyroid replacement initially, becoming tense, restless, or tachycardic. In these patients, the titration schedule can be slowed as necessary.

In patients with underlying preexisting nonmyxedematous cardiovascular disease, 0.025 mg is a more appropriate starting dose. Even with slow gradual increase, patients may develop increasing or unstable angina or signs of congestive heart failure. The dose in such an event should be dropped back to the previous level. It is sometimes not possible to reach full replacement dosage in this group of patients, and a compromise is made between maintaining stable cardiovascular function and a suboptimal thyroid replacement dose. Myxedematous patients undergoing coronary artery bypass surgery do better if thyroid replacement is begun in the immediate postoperative period rather than preoperatively.

Older patients often do not need as high a maintenance dose of thyroxine as younger ones; 0.075–0.125 mg/d is adequate in many older patients. Usually, suppressed TSH levels can be demonstrated at these lower levels of maintenance T_4 (approximately 10% lower than in younger adults).

Following thyroidectomy, the full replacement dose can be started immediately. Titrating and fixing the long-term replacement dose in best done on clinical grounds. TSH may also be used to titrate dosage both up and down. A persistently elevated TSH indicates lack of adequate thyroxine replacement except in rare patients with long-standing primary hypothyroidism or TSH-secreting pituitary tumors who may still secrete TSH despite becoming euthyroid. TSH determinations may also be falsely elevated in rate patients exposed to rabbits who develop antibodies to the rabbit immunoglobulin used in the RIA. The dosage level at which TSH returns to normal (usually 0.125–0.2 mg in young adults) can usually be maintained. Some patients may remain clinically mildly hypothyroid on replacement despite normal T_4 and TSH serum levels. Often, T_4 blood levels are slightly elevated in patients taking L-thyroxine replacement when they are clinically euthyroid. Periodic monitoring of adult patients is advisable when clinical signs of hypothyroidism and hyperthyroidism occur. Routine monitoring of serum thyroxine levels in adults is not often necessary.

Certain substances interfere with T_4 absorption from the gut. **Cholestyramine** decreases T_4 absorption markedly when the two are given simultaneously and by 30% when they are given 5 hours apart. Other interfering substances include diphenylhydantoin, propranolol, activated charcoal, soybean infant formula, liver residue, cottonseed meal, and walnuts. In such settings, thyroxine doses may need to be increased.

COMPLICATIONS

Myxedema Coma

The incidence of myxedema coma is increasing, probably owing to the growing number of patients with long-standing, untreated hypothyroidism and to the use of tranquilizers and sedatives and increased surgical anesthesia in this enlarging geriatric population. Superimposed infection is a predisposing cause.

Myxedema coma is characteristically seen in elderly women and among the indigent. Characteristic signs and symptoms are hypothermia, hypoventilation, and hypotension. Often a surgical neck scar or goiter will signal the possibility of this diagnosis in a comatose patient. Hyponatremia and hypoglycemia are frequently seen.

This is a medical emergency, and mortality is high, greater than 50%. Treatment is based on clinical presentation and should be started immediately. It is not advisable to delay treatment waiting for thyroid function test and TSH results. L-Thyroxine is given intravenously in an initial dose of 0.4–0.5 mg. This is the estimated amount required to saturate circulating binding sites. Subsequently the dose is lowered to 0.05–0.1 mg/d intravenously. Intestinal absorption may be diminished owing to myxedema at this stage of treatment, so intravenous therapy should be used during this time.

Almost all patients will require assisted respiration, either by endotracheal tube or tracheotomy. Intravenous fluids must be monitored carefully because of hypovolemia and the tendency of myxedema patients to become water intoxicated. They are hyponatremic, probably owing to increased secretion of antidiuretic hormone (ADH). Blood glucose levels should be monitored to prevent hypoglycemia. Although body temperature is low, active rewarming should be avoided. Peripheral vasodilatation will only accentuate the hypovolemia and hypotension and lead to circulatory collapse. Vasopressors are generally avoided because they may precipitate ventricular arrhythmias.

Intercurrent illness and infection must be suspected, but the empirical use of antibiotics is not indicated. Adrenal glucocorticoids, in the form of Solu-Cortef, 200 mg/d intravenously, may be used if hypopituitarism or concurrent adrenal insufficiency (Schmidt's syndrome) is suspected.

Once the patient has improved, replacement therapy should continue at low doses and gradually be increased in the same manner as for any hypothyroid patient.

Evaluation of Patients Already Taking T₄

Many patients take thyroid hormone for many years without prior documentation of hypothyroidism, goiter, or other indications. To accurately evaluate thyroid function in these patients it is necessary to stop the treatment for 6 weeks and then measure thyroid function. Because of the long half-life of thyroxine, 3 weeks may pass after discontinuing thyroid hormone before the patient notices any change consistent with hypothyroidism. Around the fourth to fifth week, thyroid function tests are low, and shortly after this, TSH levels rise and with this, the normal thyroid gland will resume function. By 6 weeks, TSH and T_4 will be normal in a patient on long-term T_4 without thyroid disease. If the patient does have primary hypothyroidism, TSH would be high and T_4 low at 6 weeks, and if the patient has secondary hypothyroidism, TSH and T_4 would remain low at 6 weeks.

REFERENCES

Thyroid Function Tests

Borst GC et al: Euthyroid hyperthyroxinemia. *Ann Intern Med* 1983;**98**:366.

Caldwell G et al: A new strategy for thyroid function testing. *Lancet* 1985; **1**:1117.

Cavalieri RR et al: Serum thyroxine, free T_4, triiodothyronine, and reverse T_3 in diphenylhydantoin-treated patients. *Metabolism* 1979;**28**:1161.

Chopra IJ et al: Serum thyrotropin in hospitalized psychiatric patients: Evidence for hyperthyrotropinemia as measured by an ultrasensitive thyrotropin assay. *Metabolism* 1990;**39**:538.

Chopra IJ et al: Thyroid function in non-thyroid illness. *Ann Intern Med* 1983;**98**:946.

Kaplan MM: Interactions between drugs and thyroid hormones. *Thyroid Today* 1981;**4**:1.

Klee GG: Assessment of sensitive thyrotropin assays for the expanded role in thyroid function testing: Proposed criteria for analytical performance and clinical utility. *J Clin Endocrinol Metab* 1987;**64**:461.

Levy RP et al: Serum thyroid hormone abnormalities in psychiatric disease. *Metabolism* 1981;**30**:1060.

Nicoloff JT, Spencer CA: The use and misuse of sensitive thyrotropin assays. *J Clin Endocrinol Metab* 1990;**71**:553.

Ruiz M et al: Familial dysalbuminemic hyperthyroxinemia: A syndrome that can be confused with thyrotoxicosis. *N Engl J Med* 1982;**306**:635.

Seth J et al: A sensitive immunoradiometric assay for serum thyroid-stimulating hormone: A replacement for the thyrotropin-releasing hormone test? *Br Med J* 1984;**289**:1334.

Spratt DI et al: Hyperthyroxinemia in patients with acute psychiatric disorders. *Am J Med* 1982;**73**:41.

Wehmann RE et al: Suppression of TSH in the low thyroxine state of severe nonthyroidal illness. *N Engl J Med* 1985;**312**:546.

Thyroid Nodules & Cancer

Bashist B, Ellis K, Gold RP: Computer tomography of intrathoracic goiters. *Am J Radiol* 1983;**140**:455.

Bell RM: Thyroid cancer. *Surg Clin North Am* 1986;**66**:13.

Bisi H et al: Unsuspected thyroid pathology in 300 sequential autopsies. *Cancer* 1989;**64**:1888.

Cady B et al: Changing clinical, pathologic, therapeutic, and survival patterns in differentiated thyroid carcinoma. *Ann Surg* 1976;**184**:541.

DeGroot LJ: Diagnostic approach and management of patients exposed to irradiation to the thyroid. *J Clin Endocrinol Metab* 1989;**69**:925.

Ferrucci JT Jr: Multiple hamartoma syndrome (Cowden's disease). *N Engl J Med* 1987;**316**:1531.

Geerdsen JP, Frolund L: Recurrence of nontoxic goiter with and without postoperative thyroxine medication. *Clin Endocrinol* 1984;**21**:529.

Gharib H et al: Suppressive therapy with levothyroxin for solitary thyroid nodules. *N Engl J Med* 1987;**317**:701.

Greenspan FS: Radiation exposure in thyroid cancer. *JAMA* 1986;**237**:2089.

Hamburger JI, Miller JM, Kini SR: Lymphoma of the thyroid. *Ann Intern Med* 1983;**99**:685.

Katlic MR et al: Substernal goiter: Analysis of 80 patients from Massachusetts General Hospital. *Am J Surg* 1985;**149**:283.

Kay TWH et al: Treatment of nontoxic multinodular goiter with radioactive iodine. *Am J Med* 1988;**84**:19.

McConahey WM et al: Papillary thyroid cancer treated at the Mayo Clinic, 1946 through 1970: Initial manifestations, pathologic findings, therapy and outcome. *Mayo Clin Proc* 1985;**60**:51.

Miller, TR, Abele JS, Greenspan FS: Fine-needle aspiration biopsy in the management of thyroid nodules. *West J Med* 1981;**134**:198.

Nel CJC et al: Anaplastic carcinoma of the thyroid: A clinicopathologic study of 82 cases. *Mayo Clin Proc* 1985;**60**:51.

Peter JJ et al: Pathogenesis of heterogeneity in human multinodular goiter. *J Clin Invest* 1985;**16**:1992.

Rojeski MI, Gharib H: Nodular thyroid disease: Evaluation and management. *N Engl J Med* 1985;**313**:428.

Samman NA et al: Impact of therapy for differentiated carcinoma of the thyroid: An analysis of 706 cases. *J Clin Endocrinol Metab* 1983;**56**:1131.

Schlumberger M et al: Long-term results of treatment of 283 patients with lung and bone metastases from differentiated thyroid carcinoma. *J Clin Endocrinol Metab* 1986;**63**:960.

Schroder S et al: Prognostic factors in medullary thyroid carcinomas. *Horm Metab Res [Suppl]* 1989;**21**:26.

Van Herle AJ, Rich P, Ljing BE: The thyroid nodule. *Ann Intern Med* 1982; **96**:221.

Wells SA et al: Early diagnosis and treatment of medullary thyroid carcinoma. *Arch Intern Med* 1985;**145**:1248.

Hyperthyroidism

Allanic H et al: Antithyroid drugs and Graves' disease: A prospective randomized evaluation of the efficacy of treatment duration. *J Clin Endocrinol Metab* 1990;**70**:675.

Bahn RS, Garrity JA, Gorman CA: Diagnosis and management of Graves' ophthalmopathy. *J Clin Endocrinol Metab* 1990;**71**:559.

Bartalena L et al: Use of corticosteroids to prevent progression of Graves' ophthalmopathy after radioiodine therapy for hyperthyroidism. *N Engl J Med* 1989;**321**:1349.

Burrow GN: The management of thyrotoxicosis during pregnancy. *N Engl J Med* 1985;**313**:562.

Cooper DS: Antithyroid drugs. *N Engl J Med* 1984;**311**:1353.

Davis PJ, Davis FB: Hyperthyroidism in patients over the age of 60 years. *Medicine* 1974;**53**:161.

Dobyns BW et al: Malignant and benign neoplasms of the thyroid in patients treated for hyperthyroidism. *J Clin Endocrinol Metab* 1974;**38**:976.

Goette GK: Thyroid acropathy. *Arch Dermatol* 1980;**116**:205.

Goldstein R, Hart IR: Follow-up of solitary autonomous thyroid nodules treated with ^{131}I. *N Engl J Med* 1983;**309**:1473.

Gwinup G, Elias AN, Ascher MS: Effect on exophthalmos of various methods of treatment of Graves' disease. *JAMA* 1982;**247**:2135.

Hamburger J: The autonomously functioning thyroid adenoma: Clinical considerations. *N Engl J Med* 1983;**309**:1512.

Jacobsen DH, Gorman CA: Endocrine ophthalmopathy: Current ideas concerning etiology, pathogenesis and treatment. *Endocr Rev* 1984;**5**:200.

Karpman BA et al: Treatment of neonatal hyperthyroidism due to Graves' disease with sodium ipodate. *J Clin Endocrinol Metab* 1987;**64**:119.

Lamberg BA, Valimaki M (Eds): Advances in endocrine ophthalmopathy of Graves' disease. *Acta Endocrinol [Suppl] (Copenh)* 1989;**121(2)**:1.

Lum SM, Kaptein EM, Nicoloff JT: Influence of nonthyroidal illness on serum thyroid hormone indices in hyperthyroidism. *West J Med* 1983;**138**:670.

Nicoloff JT: Thyroid storm and myxedema coma. *Med Clin North Am* 1985; **69**:106.

Rapaport B: The ophthalmopathy of Graves' disease. *West J Med* 1985; **142**:532.

Robertson JS, Gorman CA: Gonadal radiation dose and its genetic significance in radioiodine therapy of hyperthyroidism. *J Nucl Med* 1976;**17**:826.

Safa AM, Schumacher OP, Rodriguez-Atunez A: Long-term follow-up results in children and adolescents treated with radioactive iodine (^{131}I) for hyperthyroidism. *N Engl J Med* 1975;**292**:167.

Shen DC et al: Long term treatment of Graves' hyperthyroidism with sodium ipodate. *J Clin Endocrinol Metab* 1985;**61**:723.

Spaulding SW: Age and the thyroid. *Endocrinol Metab Clin* 1987;**16**:1013.

Strakosch CR et al: Immunology of autoimmune thyroid disease. *N Engl J Med* 1982;**307**:1499.

Tolis G et al: Pituitary hyperthyroidism. *Am J Med* 1978;**64**:177.

Wang Y-S et al: Long-term treatment of Graves' disease with iopanoic acid (Telepaque). *J Clin Endocrinol Metab* 1987;**65**:679.

Wu SY et al: Comparison of sodium ipodate (Oragrafin) and propylthiouracil in early treatment of hyperthyroidism. *J Clin Endocrinol Metab* 1982;**54**:630.

Thyroiditis

Amino N, et al: High prevalence of transient post-partum thyrotoxicosis and hypothyroidism. *N Engl J Med* 1982;**306**:849.

Dorjman SG, et al: Painless thyroiditis and transient hyperthyroidism without goiter. *Ann Intern Med* 1977;**86**:24.

Holm L, Blomgren H, Lowhagen T: Cancer risks in patients with chronic lymphocytic thyroiditis. *N Engl J Med* 1985;**312**:601.

Kidd A, et al: Immunologic aspects of Graves' and Hashimoto's diseases. *Metabolism* 1980;**29**:80.

Klein I, Levey GS: Silent thyroiditis. *Ann Intern Med* 1982;**96**:242.

Levine SN: Current concepts of thyroiditis. *Arch Intern Med* 1983;**143**:1952.

Hypothyroidism

Coindre JM et al: Bone loss in hypothyroidism with hormone reprlacement: A histomorphometric study. *Arch Intern Med* 1988;**146**:48.

Cooper DS et al: L-thyroxine therapy in subclinical hypothyroidism. *Ann Intern Med* 1984;**101**:18.

Cygan R, Rucker L: Thyroid hormone replacement. *West J Med* 1983;**139**:232.

Fish LH et al: Replacement dose, metabolism, and bioavailability of levothyroxine in the treatment of hypothyroidism. *N Engl J Med* 1987;**316**:764.

Hennessey JV et al: L-Thyroxine dosage: A reevaluation of therapy with contemporary preparations. *Ann Intern Med* 1986;**105**:11.

Robuschi G et al: Hypothyroidism in the elderly. *Endocr Rev* 1987;**8**:142.

Rosenbaum RL, Barzel US: Levothyroxine replacement dose for primary hypothyroidism decreases with age. *Ann Intern Med* 1982;**96**:53.

Rosenthal MJ et al: Thyroid failure in the elderly: Microsomal antibodies as discriminant for therapy. *JAMA* 1987;**258**:209.

Iodide & Thyroid Function

Amico JA, et al: Clinical and chemical assessment of thyroid function during therapy with amiodarone. *Arch Intern Med* 1984;**144**:487.

Block SH: Thyroid function abnormalities from the use of topical betadine solution in intact skin of children. *Cutis* 1980;**26**:88.

Borowski GD, et al: Effect of long-term amiodarone therapy on thyroid hormone levels and thyroid function. *Am J Med* 1985;**78**:443.

Nademanee K et al: Amiodarone and thyroid function. *Prog Cardiovasc Dis* 1989;**31**:427.

Prager EM, Gardner RE: Iatrogenic hypothyroidism from topical iodine-containing medications. *West J Med* 1979;**130**:553.

Rajatanavin R et al: Five patients with iodine-induced hyperthyroidism. *Am J Surg* 1984;**77**:378.

Silva JE: Effects of iodine and iodine-containing compounds on thyroid function. *Med Clin North Am* 1985;**69**:881.

Smyrk TC et al: Pathology of the thyroid in amiodarone-associated thyrotoxicosis. *Am J Surg Pathol* 1987;**11**:197.

*Support and membership is encouraged for the *American Thyroid Association*. c/o Colum Gorman, MD, Mayo Clinic, 200 First Street SW, Rochester, MN 55905.

Adrenal Disorders | 6

Paul A. Fitzgerald, MD, & Paul M. Copeland, MD

ANATOMY & PHYSIOLOGY OF THE ADRENALS

In the fetus, the 2 adrenal glands are relatively large, surpassing the kidneys in size. Adult adrenals are relatively smaller; each normally weighs only 3–5 g but rapidly increases in size during stress.

The relative anatomy of the adrenals is depicted on axial CT scan (Fig 6–1). Both adrenals receive generous arterial blood from both the aorta and renal arteries. The venous drainage is different: the right adrenal vein drains medially directly into the inferior vena cava, whereas the left adrenal drains inferiorly into the left renal vein.

The human adrenal consists of an outer cortex, which secretes steroid hormones and surrounds the smaller adrenal medulla, which secretes catecholamines. These hormones act in a variety of ways to maintain homeostasis and to aid survival in the face of fight-or-flight situations, fasting, injuries, shock, and other stresses.

ADRENAL CORTEX

In the fetus, a unique fetal zone makes up the bulk of the adrenal cortex and secretes steroid precursors necessary for placental estrogen synthesis; this zone regresses quickly postpartum.

The adult adrenal cortex secretes numerous different steroid hormones. Some steroid hormones are still known by the letters (eg, F = cortisol, S = 11-deoxycortisol) arbitrarily assigned when adrenal steroids were being first extracted and characterized. The enzyme pathways involved in adrenal steroid hormone synthesis are depicted in Fig 2–4. The only adrenal hormones necessary to sustain life are aldosterone and cortisol. The adrenal cortex consists of 3 zones: the outer zona glomerulosa, the middle zona fasciculata, and the inner zona reticularis.

227

Zona Glomerulosa; Aldosterone Physiology

Only the zona glomerulosa expresses the enzyme 18-oxidase and can thus secrete aldosterone, the most potent mineralocorticoid. Aldosterone secretion is stimulated mainly by renin (via angiostensin II) and hyperkalemia (to a lesser extent) rather than by ACTH. Secretion is inhibited by atrial natriuretic factor and dopamine.

Mineralocorticoids cause secretory organs to absorb Na^+ and excrete K^+; they thus protect against hypovolemia and hyperkalemia. Their main effect is on the renal tubule to absorb Na^+ from the tubule and transport it to extracellular fluid. The resulting preponderance of anions in the renal tubule causes passive transfer of K^+ and H^+ into the tubule for excretion in the urine. Mineralocorticoids also act in the same fashion on other secretory glands, ie, sweat glands, salivary glands, and the intestinal tract. Aldosterone is the major mineralocorticoid although deoxycorticosterone (DOC), corticosterone (compound B), and high concentrations of cortisol (compound F) also have mineralocorticoid activity. Mineralocorticoid effects are antagonized by progesterone.

Zona Fasciculata & Zona Reticularis

The middle zona fasciculata and inner zona reticularis express the enzyme 17α-hydroxylase and therefore secrete not only cortisol but also a wide range of other glucocorticoids, androgens, and estrogens in

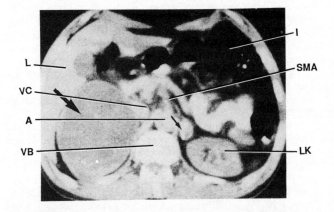

Figure 6–1. CT scan of the abdomen. Axial view at level of adrenals. Apparent normal adrenal shapes vary; the *left adrenal* may appear like an arrowhead (44%), inverted Y (16%), or triangle (40%). The *right adrenal* may appear like an arrowhead (52%) or triangle (3%); it may appear linear between the liver and crus of the diaphragm (36%) or along the vena cava (9%). I = intestines; **SMA** = superior mesenteric artery; **A** = aorta; **LK** = left kidney; **VB** = vertebral body; **L** = liver; **VC** = vena cava. (Courtesy of Henry Goldberg, MD, Department of Radiology, UCSF.)

addition to weak mineralocorticoids. Pituitary ACTH stimulates the secretion of cortisol in a diurnal manner and in response to stress. Normally, plasma cortisol levels are highest at about 7 AM and lowest at about 11 PM.

A. Corticol Physiology: Cortisol exerts its influence via cytoplasmic receptors found in virtually every nucleated cell in the body. Cortisol is considered a glucocorticoid but has effects extending far beyond glucose metabolism and has some effect on mineralocorticoid receptors as well.

Cortisol counterbalances insulin by inhibiting its secretion and by enhancing hepatic gluconeogenesis. It increases the substrate necessary for gluconeogenesis; amino acids are made available by cortisol's inhibition of protein synthesis in muscle, and glycerol is made available by cortisol's stimulation of lipolysis in fat cells. Serum glucose and fatty acid levels are thus increased.

During acute trauma, infection, exercise, and other stresses, cortisol secretion makes increased amounts of glucose and fatty acids available for energy; it also dampens defense mechanisms, thereby protecting against their potentially dangerous overactivity. For example, glucocorticoids inhibit the production or action of many mediators of immunity and inflammation (eg, interleukin-1, lymphokines, prostaglandins, collagenase, leukotrienes, thromboxanes, serotonin, bradykinin, histamine, and plasminogen activator). Glucocorticoids thereby decrease concentrations of lymphocytes, monocytes, and eosinophils; blood neutrophil concentrations are increased. They inhibit fibroblasts in skin and bone.

Cortisol is required for the production of angiotensin II and adequate vascular tone; during stress, increased cortisol levels cause vasodilation and protect against potentially dangerous vasoconstriction.

Glucocorticoids have other effects: they enhance renal free water clearance and decrease vasopressin secretion. They lower serum calcium levels by redistributing calcium intracellularly as well as by inhibiting calcium absorption by the gut and renal tubule. Glucocorticoids also have pervasive effects upon the brain; an excess or deficiency produces extensive mental changes. In excess they cause **Cushing's syndrome.**

B. Adrenal Androgen Physiology: Dehydroepiandrosterone (DHEA) and its sulfated ester (DHEAS) are the most abundantly secreted adrenal steroids. The placenta (as well as other tissues) contains sulfatases that enable it to convert DHEAS to estrogens. The role of DHEAS in nonpregnant individuals is not known. Levels of DHEAS peak around age 25 years and diminish by 95% by age 85–90 years.

ADRENAL MEDULLA

The adrenal medulla is part of the sympathetic autonomic nervous system that receives nerve innervation from the thoracolumbar spinal cord. The cells synthesize catecholamines:

Tyrosine → Dihydroxyphenylanine (dopa) → Dopamine →

$$\text{Norepinephrine} \xrightarrow{\text{PNMT}} \text{Epinephrine}$$

Unlike other postsynaptic sympathetic neurons that secrete mostly norepinephrine, the cells of the adrenal medulla secrete mostly epinephrine, since the enzyme phenylethanolamine-N-methyltransferase

(PNMT) is induced by very high concentrations of cortisol found in the adrenal portal veins. Like polypeptide hormones, catecholamines exert their action via cell-surface receptors. There are 3 types of receptors peripherally: (1) α-Receptor stimulation generally produces skin and visceral arteriole constriction; it produces smooth muscle contraction especially involved with sphincters and pilomotor constriction, mydriasis, and male ejaculation. It also causes sweating and salivation; it inhibits pancreatic insulin release. (2) β_1-Receptor stimulation increases heart rate and contractility. (3) β_2-Receptor stimulation produces muscle arteriole dilatation and relaxation of bronchial muscles and the bladder detrussor. It stimulates secretion of renin, gastrin, parathyroid hormone, and calcitonin. It inhibits gastrointestinal motility. It increases the metabolic rate by increasing glycolysis, lipolysis, and oxygen consumption.

In addition, these and dopamine receptors are present in the central nervous system and mediate brain neurotransmission. Although norepinephrine stimulates mostly α- and β_1-receptors, considerable overlap exists; a stressful stimulus generally produces many of the effects noted above.

Epinephrine is secreted solely by the adrenal medulla and is about 5–10 times as potent as norepinephrine. Serum norepinephrine is derived from both peripheral neurons as well as the adrenal medulla. Epinephrine and norepinephrine are metabolized peripherally to metanephrine and normetanephrine, respectively, which are then excreted in the urine. They are also further metabolized by the enzyme monoamine oxidase (MAO) to vanillylmandelic acid (VMA), which is also found in the urine.

ADDISON'S DISEASE

The term Addison's disease refers to primary hypoadrenalism caused by destruction of both adrenal cortices by any process, producing a deficiency of aldosterone, cortisol, and adrenal androgens.

Secondary hypoadrenalism caused by a deficiency of ACTH is discussed in Chapter 1.

CLINICAL FEATURES

Addison's disease is an uncommon disorder that usually occurs between the ages of 20 and 50; it is slightly more common in women, having a female:male incidence of about 2.6:1.

The clinical features of adrenal insufficiency are listed in approximate order of frequency in Table 6–1. Weakness, fatigue, anorexia, and weight loss are uniformly present. Hypotension is common and is often associated with postural dizziness. Gastrointestinal symptoms are nausea, vomiting, and abdominal pain; occasionally, diarrhea may be a presenting complaint.

Other symptoms may also be prominent. Muscle or joint pains may mimic or accentuate arthritis. Emotional instability may masquerade as a primary psychiatric problem. Salt craving is present in up to 20% of patients; it is especially prominent in hot weather. Increased salt intake can compensate for mineralocorticoid lack.

Symptomatic fasting hypoglycemia can occur but is unusual. It may be seen in settings of fasting, fever or infection, and nausea and vomiting. Hypoglycemia worsens the patient's weakness and produces decreased mentation, which can rarely lead to coma.

Hyperpigmentation is usually present in chronic primary adrenal insufficiency and is due to melanocyte stimulation by compensatory increased levels of ACTH and other melanocyte-stimulating peptides co-secreted with ACTH. The hyperpigmentation may be diffuse but is

Table 6–1. Clinical manifestations of Addison's disease.

Symptoms	Clinical laboratory tests
Weakness and fatigue	Neutropenia
Anorexia and weight loss	Relative lymphocytosis
Nausea, vomiting, diarrhea	Eosinophilia
Abdominal pain	Hyperkalemia
Postural dizziness	Mild anemia
Muscle and joint pains	Increased blood urea
Emotional instability	nitrogen and creatinine
Salt craving	Hypoglycemia
	Hyponatremia
Signs	Hypercalcemia
Hypotension (may →	Acidosis
shock)	
Hyperpigmentation	**Associated autoimmune**
Fever	**disorders**
Women	Hypoparathyroidism ⎤ *PGA I
Decreased axillary and	Mucocutaneous candidiasis ⎦
pubic hair	Hypothyroidism ⎤ *PGA II
Amenorrhea	Hyperthyroidism ⎟
	Diabetes mellitus ⎦
	Primary ovarian failure
	Primary testicular failure
	Vitiligo
	Pernicious anemia

*PGA = polyglandular autoimmune (syndrome).

especially prominent over extensor surfaces such as elbows, knees, posterior neck, and finger and toe joints. Other areas of increased pigmentation include palmar creases, nail beds, nipples, areolae, and perivaginal and perianal mucosa. The buccal mucosa and gingiva may have patchy areas of bluish pigmentation. Pigmentation is often more apparent in areas of pressure such as belt or bra lines. Scar tissue formed since the development of Addison's disease will be hyperpigmented. Hyperpigmentation may be absent in some individuals, especially during the early course of the disease.

Axillary and pubic hair is decreased in many women owing to a deficiency of adrenal androgens. Amenorrhea is common in Addison's disease; it may result from weight loss and chronic illness. In patients with polyglandular autoimmunity, amenorrhea may be due to primary ovarian failure.

Polyglandular Autoimmune Syndrome

Autoimmune adrenal insufficiency can be isolated or be part of a polyglandular autoimmune (PGA) syndrome. Type I PGA includes at least 2 of the triad of Addison's disease, hypoparathyroidism, and chronic mucocutaneous candidiasis. It usually begins in childhood with candidiasis at age 3–6 years, followed by hypoparathyroidism at age 5–8 years, and Addison's disease at age 8–11 years. Patients with PGA I may also have alopecia universalis, cataract, and uveitis. Hypothyroidism and vitiligo may follow in adolescence or adulthood.

Type II PGA includes Addison's disease with either autoimmune thyroid disease (hypothyroidism, 9%; hyperthyroidism, 5%; euthyroid goiter, 2%) or insulin-dependent diabetes mellitus (12%).

The combination of Addison's disease and hypothyroidism is known as Schmidt's syndrome. Primary ovarian failure (40% of women age 15–50) may also occur with Addison's disease and is more common than primary testicular failure (5%), vitiligo (9%), or pernicious anemia (4%). Autoimmune hypophysitis may also occur, producing isolated hypogonadotropic hypogonadism. Hypothyroidism occasionally resolves with glucocorticoid replacement.

LABORATORY FEATURES

The laboratory findings of adrenal insufficiency are listed in Table 6–1. Not all these abnormalities are usually present. Hyponatremia is caused by mineralocorticoid deficiency and a reduced ability to excrete a water load; it may be obscured by severe dehydration. Hyperkalemia is caused by chronic mineralocorticoid deficiency, but in acute adrenal insufficiency there may not be adequate time for hyperkalemia to develop; it may be obscured if a metabolic alkalosis has been caused by vomiting or nasogastric suctioning. Increased blood urea nitrogen and creatinine are consequences of volume depletion. Hypercalcemia, noted in about 6% of cases, is an artifact of an increased albumin concentration; the ionized calcium is usually normal.

The most common hematologic change is eosinophilia. A mild anemia may be present, but dehydration and attendant hemoconcentration may obscure it. Neutropenia and relative lymphocytosis, like the eosinophilia, are a consequence of low cortisol levels. TSH may be increased even in the absence of thyroid disease. In one series of 10 patients with Addison's disease, 3 had increased TSH (2 had decreased T_4I) that normalized with glucocorticoid treatment; one had true primary hypothyroidism.

Radiologic Findings

Chest x-ray may show a small, vertical heart, which probably reflects volume depletion. It may also show evidence of the underlying cause of Addison's disease if due to tuberculosis, sarcoidosis, fungal infection, or cancer. Although CT scanning is the best way to detect adrenal calcification, plain film of the abdomen may also demonstrate adrenal calcification. Such calcification may be the result of chronic granulomatous disease or old hemorrhage. The most common cause of idiopathic adrenal calcification in the general population appears to be hemorrhage into the large fetal adrenal during parturition. Other more unusual causes of adrenal calcification include histoplasmosis, blastomycosis, metastatic melanoma, adrenal carcinoma, pheochromocytoma, and hemorrhage. Nevertheless, in the setting of Addison's disease, adrenal calcification most strongly suggests tuberculosis, since such calcification is present in about 50% of tuberculous cases.

CT scan of the adrenals usually shows adrenals of about normal size in cases of autoimmune adrenal destruction. Enlarged and hyperdense adrenals are characteristic of adrenal hemorrhage. Adrenals are usually irregularly enlarged, and there is usually extra-adrenal evidence of disease in cases of cancer, sarcoidosis, or fungal infection; up to 24% (4 of 17 patients in one series) of patients with tuberculous Addison's disease do not have detectable extra-adrenal tuberculosis.

Diagnostic Tests

The diagnosis of adrenal insufficiency is based on subnormal secretion of cortisol by the adrenal glands in response to the administration of ACTH. A subnormal response is present in all cases of Addison's disease and in most cases of secondary insufficiency, since the adrenal cortex atrophies in the absence of ACTH from the pituitary.

The most practical screening test for Addison's disease is the brief **ACTH stimulation test,** which is performed as follows:

(1) A morning plasma cortisol is drawn.

(2) $ACTH_{1-24}$ (cosyntropin), 250 μg, is given intramuscularly or intravenously.

(3) A second plasma cortisol level is drawn 30–60 minutes after the injection (various protocols use time points from 30 to 120 minutes; 60 minutes is the most reliable). A post-ACTH cortisol value of less than 18 μg/dL is consistent with adrenal insufficiency. In general, a cortisol increment of less than 8 μg/dL is also abnormal; the exception would be for baseline cortisol values that are already maximally stimulated (ie, > 25 μg/dL). The diagnosis is made by either criterion (post-ACTH level or increment) unless there is cortisol-binding globulin (CBG) deficiency. CBG deficiency may occur in liver disease, multiple myeloma, and nephrotic syndrome.

Other tests for adrenal insufficiency (eg, insulin tolerance test and metyrapone test) are available but unnecessary.

If the ACTH stimulation test is abnormal, or if the diagnosis is strongly suspected from the first, a plasma ACTH should be drawn prior to administration of ACTH and at least 12 hours after any hydrocortisone. The specimen must be collected in an iced, plastic heparinized tube and separated within 1 hour. The assay must be performed in a laboratory with a demonstrated good ACTH assay. Most patients with Addison's disease have ACTH levels higher than 200 pg/mL, whereas patients with secondary adrenal insufficiency have plasma ACTH levels below 50 pg/mL. Intermediate levels require further investigation.

If an ACTH assay is unavailable, a 3-day ACTH infusion differentiates primary and secondary adrenal insufficiency. Obtain a baseline 24-hour urine for 17-hydroxycorticosteroids and creatinine. Give consyntropin (25 IU, 250 μg) intravenously in 500 mL normal saline from 8 AM to 4 PM each day for 3 days. Measure plasma cortisol at 4 PM each day, and continue 24-hour urine collections for 17-hydroxycorticosteroids each day. Normal subjects and patients with secondary adrenal insufficiency increase their 24-hour urinary 17-hydroxycorticosteroid levels by 10 mg or more over baseline and have a 4 PM plasma cortisol of at least 25 μg/dL on day 3. Levels less than these are consistent with primary adrenal insufficiency. Maintain dexamethasone coverage (0.5 mg orally at 8 AM and 4 PM in the unstressed patient).

ETIOLOGY

Once Addison's disease is documented to be present, it is necessary to determine its cause (Table 6–2) in order not to miss underlying treatable systemic disease. In adults, autoimmune adrenal destruction accounts for at least 80% of spontaneous cases in the USA and in other areas with a low incidence of tuberculosis. Therefore, the evaluation should check for associated autoimmune diseases (Table 6–2). In their presence, the disease probably is autoimmune. If there is any doubt about the cause of the Addison's disease, a chest x-ray, purified protein derivative (PPD) test, and abdominal CT scan are done to screen for tuberculosis as well as sarcoidosis, fungal disorders, and cancer.

If the chest x-ray shows evidence of tuberculosis, evaluation and a full course of treatment for that disease should be instituted. Tuberculous adrenal destruction without pulmonary disease is rare. Adrenal calcification is present in about 50% of patients with tuberculous Addison's disease, whereas adrenal calcification is rarely present in patients with autoimmune or other destructive disease processes. Adrenal enlargement is present in 87% of cases of adrenal destruction due to neoplasms and granulomatous disease. Studies for serum adrenal autoantibodies may be obtained, but this test is usually unnecessary. Such antibodies are detectable in about 50% of autoimmune cases. Serum adrenal autoantibody studies are not entirely sensitive and require time for completion.

Alternatively, serum may be assayed for thyroid antimicrosomal and antithyroglobulin antibodies; elevation is present in about 45% of

Table 6–2. Causes of adrenal insufficiency.

**PRIMARY ADRENAL INSUFFICIENCY (Addison's disease)—
ACTH elevated**
  Autoimmunity*
  Tuberculosis*
  Surgical bilateral adrenalectomy
  Fungal disorders: Coccidioidomycosis, histoplasmosis, blastomycosis.
  Acquired immunodeficiency syndrome (AIDS): cytomegalovirus
    adrenalitis.
  Congenital disorders: Enzyme deficiencies, aplasia, syphilis,
    unresponsiveness to ACTH.
  Drugs: Enzyme inhibitors (metyrapone, aminoglutethimide); o,p'-DDD
    (mitotane); heparin (aldosterone deficiency); ketoconazole; rifampin
    (increases glucocorticoid requirement); busulfan; methadone; suramin;
    interleukin-2.
  Adrenal hemorrhage: Septicemia, Waterhouse-Friderichsen syndrome,
    anticoagulant therapy, bleeding disorders, birth trauma, other trauma
    (eg, postoperative).
  Other disorders: Metastatic carcinoma, parasites, amyloidosis,
    hemochromatosis, sarcoidosis, radiation therapy, adrenoleukodystrophy
    (in males, X-linked in childhood usually; female carriers have fatigue
    only).
SECONDARY ADRENAL INSUFFICIENCY—ACTH not elevated. See
  Chapter 1.

*Most common causes of primary adrenal insufficiency.

cases and implicates an autoimmune process in the adrenal as well. Antibodies may also be present in other organs without clinical signs of their dysfunction (eg, antigastric parietal cell Ab).

A serum ferritin level should be obtained in most adult-onset cases to screen for hemochromatosis. Although this is an extremely rare cause of Addison's disease, it is treatable and may produce other endocrine gland failure, thus mimicking autoimmune polyendocrine failure.

In cases of Addison's disease of obscure origin, a CT scan of the adrenals may be helpful. Enlarged adrenals implicate a granulo-matous, malignant, parasitic, or hemorrhagic process. Adrenals that are enlarged owing to hemorrhage may be identified by their increased density on CT scan and usually by the clinical situation as well; acute adrenal hemorrhage is usually associated with sepsis or anticoagulant therapy and may produce abdominal or flank pain. Metastatic disease often involves the adrenals but only occasionally produces Addison's disease.

TREATMENT

Acute Adrenal Insufficiency (Adrenal Crisis)

Adrenal crisis occurs during superimposed physiologic stress in patients with chronic adrenal insufficiency. It may also be the initial presentation of adrenal insufficiency following rapid destruction of the adrenal glands or pituitary by hemorrhage or infarction.

The main clinical features of untreated adrenal crisis are hypoten-sion and tachycardia. The hypotension may lead to profound shock that is not fully responsive to intravenous fluid administration and can progress to death. Patients usually also have nausea, vomiting, ab-dominal pain, and fever, which can mimic an acute abdomen with septic shock. In acute adrenal insufficiency, pigment changes are absent. The fever that is usually present may be due to cortisol deficiency itself but may also be due to a precipitating infection.

Treatment should be aggressive and consist of intravenous 5% dextrose in 0.9N saline to prevent hypoglycemia and to replace vol-ume. In adults, glucocorticoid is given either as hydrocortisone, 200 mg intravenously if the patient has known adrenal insufficiency, or dexamethasone, 6 mg intravenously if the diagnosis is yet to be made. Hydrocortisone, 100 mg, is then administered every 6 hours by intra-venous bolus or infusion. Precipitating causes must be detected and treated simultaneously. The dosage must be tapered 50% every 1–2 days as recovery progresses, until physiologic replacement doses are reached. Once the hydrocortisone dose is tapered to below 75 mg/d, mineralocorticoid is usually added as fludrocortisone (Florinef; 0.1-mg tablets available), 0.05–0.1 mg orally once daily.

Chronic Adrenal Replacement Therapy

Glucocorticoid replacement must be individualized and is most safely given to adults as hydrocortisone. An average replacement dose consists of hydrocortisone, 20 mg orally in the morning and 10 mg orally in the evening. The dosage is reduced if excessive weight gain or other signs of hypercortisolism occur. The daily dose ranges from 15 mg to 40 mg. During stressful minor illnesses, such as bronchitis or tooth extraction, the dose may be tripled for 1–2 days, then tapered quickly over 2–3 days as recovery occurs. All patients must wear medical identification that reads "Adrenal Insufficiency. Takes Hydrocortisone." Patients should be instructed to seek medical attention immediately for a major illness or if nausea or vomiting precludes taking the oral medication.

Patients who are away from medical centers or hike into remote areas should be given injectable hydrocortisone (Solu-Cortef, 100 mg) and syringes for self-administration in case they are unable to take oral medication in an emergency.

Patients are advised to take their morning hydrocortisone immediately upon arising. Some patients feel that an additional 5–10 mg of hydrocortisone taken before particularly strenuous physical activity increases endurance. Patients who become especially fatigued in the afternoon may divide the hydrocortisone into 3 daily doses. The last dose of hydrocortisone is usually taken at about 6 PM or with dinner.

Alternative glucocorticoid compounds are available for chronic replacement therapy but have generally proved less satisfactory than hydrocortisone and are reserved for special circumstances. Cortisone acetate is preferred for children by many pediatricians owing to its longer half-life; it should not be given intramuscularly, since intramuscular absorption is erratic. Dexamethasone (0.5 mg $\cong$ 20–50 mg hydrocortisone) or prednisone (5 mg $\cong$ 20 mg hydrocortisone) may be used for patients who have fluctuating symptoms on hydrocortisone or who have coexisting hypertension.

In adults, fludrocortisone (Florinef) is first given in doses of 0.05 mg/d. Some patients do well without this medication if they take extra salt and do not live in very hot climates. Some patients will present without electrolyte imbalance and respond dramatically to hydrocortisone alone; most ultimately develop hyperkalemia or hyponatremia. It is safest to prescribe at least a small dose daily or on alternate days to help ensure electrolyte balance. The dose often may need to be increased in hot seasons or climates. Patients must be warned of signs of overdosage (eg, edema, weakness), in which case the serum electrolytes should be checked and the dose of fludrocortisone usually reduced. Mineralocorticoid may also be replaced parenterally with deoxycortisone, 25 mg intramuscularly weekly. It is generally not required if the patient is being given large doses of parenteral hydrocortisone while unable to ingest oral medication.

DHEA (400 mg orally 4 times a day) in clinical studies of older men has decreased body fat, increased muscle mass, and decreased LDL cholesterol levels. It is not an accepted treatment for obesity.

HYPERKALEMIA & SELECTIVE HYPOALDOSTERONISM

Hyperkalemia generally presents with muscle weakness; flaccid paralysis may occur if the hyperkalemia is severe. It is cardiotoxic, especially when hyponatremia, hypocalcemia, or acidosis is also present. Its effect is noted on the ECG: T waves become peaked, the QT interval shortens, the QRS complex widens; P waves flatten when serum potassium rises above 7 mEq/L and disappear with levels over 8 mEq/L; ST segments rise, suggesting pericarditis or ischemic injury. At that point, bradycardia, ventricular fibrillation, heart block, or asystole may occur. Mild hyperkalemia allows thoughtful evaluation, but severe hyperkalemia, especially to levels of 6.5 mEq/L or more, requires immediate treatment.

CAUSES OF HYPERKALEMIA

The many causes of hyperkalemia are listed in Table 6–3. Despite the key role of aldosterone in potassium secretion, isolated hypoaldosteronism and Addison's disease are infrequent causes of hyperkalemia and are usually considered only after more likely causes have been excluded.

The most common cause for a report of hyperkalemia is artifactual **pseudohyperkalemia.** This happens when a clot of blood is allowed to hemolyze before separation of the serum, thus allowing release of intracellular potassium. Pseudohyperkalemia may also occur in the presence of marked thrombocytosis or leukocytosis. It may also occur owing to muscle ischemia during blood drawing. Misleading high potassium levels may also be reported when the blood is drawn from a vein proximal to an intravenous infusion of potassium or from the line itself. Thus, when unsuspected hyperkalemia is reported, the test should be repeated without delay on a properly drawn plasma specimen to substantiate the diagnosis.

DIAGNOSIS OF SELECTIVE HYPOALDOSTERONISM

After nonendocrine causes of hyperkalemia have been excluded, screening for hypoaldosteronism should begin with an ACTH stimulation test for Addison's disease. If this test is normal, selective hypo-

Table 6–3. Causes of hyperkalemia.

Artifacts
  Hemolysis of blood clot in serum specimen.
  Drawing specimen from arm with potassium infusion.
  Muscle ischemia during blood drawing.
  Marked thrombocytosis. (Plasma K^+ not affected.)
  Marked leukocytosis.
  Rheumatoid arthritis.
Increased potassium input
  Diet, salt substitutes, potassium administration.
  Hemolysis (blood transfusions, hemolytic anemia); gastrointestinal
    bleeding; crush injuries; rhabdomyolysis; severe infection.
Decreased renal potassium secretion
  Renal failure
  Decreased plasma volume (dehydration, hypotension, congestive heart
    failure, cirrhosis, nephrotic syndrome).
  Impaired renin-aldosterone axis (hyporeninemic hypoaldosteronism,
    often with long-term diabetes; selective hypoaldosteronism;
    pseudohypoaldosteronism types I and II; Addison's disease; adrenal
    enzyme deficiencies; drugs [heparin, β-blockers, nonsteroidal
    antiinflammatory agents, captopril and other angiotensin-converting
    enzyme (ACE) inhibitors]; AIDS).
  Aldosterone antagonists (spironolactone, triamterene, amiloride).
  Primary renal secretory defects (sickle cell disease, systemic lupus
    erythematosus, renal transplant, obstructive uropathy, interstitial
    nephritis, congenital or familial primary secretory defect, amyloidosis).
Abnormal potassium distribution
  Acidosis, hypertonicity, hyperkalemic periodic paralysis, succinylcholine,
    insulin deficiency, exercise, digitalis overdosage.

aldosteronism may be considered, and the diagnosis is usually clinically apparent. It is usually seen as hyperkalemia in the presence of
mild or moderate renal disease most often due to diabetes mellitus. It
also occurs in acquired immunodeficiency syndrome (AIDS). If the
diagnosis is obscure, a serum renin and aldosterone may be drawn
following either (1) 4 hours of upright posture and/or (2) 3 days of
sodium restricted diet (< 20 mEq/d). The results may be used to
categorize the causative factors, as follows:

A. Low Aldosterone, Low Renin: Hyporeninemic hypoaldosteronism is most commonly seen in patients with diabetes mellitus or
interstitial nephritis. Hyperkalemia is seen that is disproportionate to
the mild to moderate azotemia. The hyperkalemia is symptomatic in
only about 25% of patients. About half of these patients have an
associated hyperchloremic acidosis (also known as type 4 renal tubular
acidosis). The hyperkalemia is thought to arise from the renal disease
that destroys the juxtaglomerular apparatus; this, together with volume
expansion and autonomic neuropathy, causes loss of renin secretion,

which decreases the generation of angiotensin II, the major stimulus for aldosterone secretion.

Hyperkalemia may also be due to increased renal tubular chloride reabsorption **(pseudohypoaldosteronism type II)** that may be inherited as an autosomal dominant trait. Patients have hyperchloremic metabolic acidosis, normal adrenal and renal function, and aldosterone levels (urine or plasma) that are low or inappropriately normal in the presence of hyperkalemia. Treatment is with hydrochlorothiazide.

B. Low Aldosterone, High Renin: This profile may be seen with any cause of primary adrenal insufficiency. Patients with AIDS, hypotension, and hyperkalemia frequently have this abnormality. The rare congenital deficiencies of 18-hydroxylation or 18-dehydrogenation produce this condition. These isolated enzyme deficiencies produce mineralocorticoid deficiency without cortisol deficiency. It may be diagnosed by obtaining plasma aldosterone levels during a standard ACTH screening test. Plasma aldosterone shows an increment of less than 4 ng/dL, but cortisol rises normally.

C. High Aldosterone, High Renin: This profile for hyperkalemia is usually due to **pseudohypoaldosteronism type I,** a condition that is usually congenital and seen in children who present with salt-wasting and hyponatremia, hyperkalemia, and hyperchloremic acidosis. The distal renal tubule is poorly responsive to mineralocorticoids, but the syndrome usually resolves spontaneously by age 3. Treatment is with oral sodium chloride.

D. Other Conditions: Certain patients have hyperkalemia due to a renal tubule defect in potassium secretion but without salt-wasting. Such patients have mineralocorticoid-resistant hyperkalemia. It has been reported to occur with the interstitial nephritis found after renal transplantation and in the renal disease seen with lupus erythematosus and sickle cell anemia. It may also occur as an inherited resistance to mineralocorticoids associated with hyperkalemia.

MEDICAL TREATMENT

Acute Hyperkalemia

Acute hyperkalemia is defined as an acute rise of serum potassium to 6.5 mEq/L or higher or hyperkalemia associated with changes on the ECG.

Treatment must begin quickly with intravenous therapy, constant electrocardiographic monitoring, and frequent serum potassium measurements. Provocative factors or drugs must be stopped.

A. Sodium Chloride: Sodium chloride 0.9% should be given intravenously to the patients with hyponatremia and hypovolemia; this dilutes the hyperkalemia, aids potassium entry into cells, and promotes potassium excretion by the kidney.

B. Sodium Bicarbonate: Sodium bicarbonate 7.5% may be given intravenously with care, beginning with 50 mL over 10–15 minutes. Within 10 minutes it promotes potassium entry into cells and excretion by the kidney. Another infusion of 50–100 mL may be given if no effect is seen within 15 minutes; its hypokalemic effect wanes after 2 hours. It is effective in correcting hyperkalemia regardless of whether the patient is acidotic. In fact, bicarbonate should be given *with the greatest care* to seriously acidotic patients, since it may decrease compensatory respiratory drive without crossing into the central nervous system, thus producing coma from paradoxical central nervous system acidosis (Plum-Posner effect). Other side effects of intravenous sodium bicarbonate include seizures from hypocalcemia or hyperosmolality; serum calcium and sodium levels must be followed carefully.

C. Calcium Gluconate: Calcium gluconate 10% is given over 5 minutes in doses of 10–30 mL in adults; its effect lasts only 1 hour. Calcium should not be given if the patient is receiving a digitalis preparation or is already hypercalcemic.

D. Insulin: Insulin must be given to diabetics with ketoacidosis and hyperkalemia, along with volume expansion with normal saline 0.9%. Insulin promptly reverses the hyperkalemia by allowing potassium entry into cells.

Insulin is also effective in treating hyperkalemia in nondiabetic patients. It is given as 10 U Regular human insulin in 500 mL of 10% dextrose and infused over 1 hour or constantly at a lower rate.

E. Loop Diuretics: Furosemide and other loop diuretics stimulate renal excretion of potassium in patients with intact renal function. Furosemide may be given in an initial dose at 20–40 mg intravenously and the dose and frequency adjusted according to the patient's response.

F. Sodium Polystyrene Sulfonate: Sodium polystyrene sulfonate (Kayexalate) is an exchange resin containing sodium that binds potassium in exchange for sodium in the gut. It also binds calcium and magnesium; these ions should be monitored and, if low, replaced intravenously or orally (eg, as Dolomite, at alternate times from the resin if the latter is given orally). Kayexalate can be given orally in a dose of 25 g as often as every 4–6 hours; it may also be given as a retention enema in a dose of 50 g every 4–6 hours. Care must be taken to not overload patients with sodium.

G. Hemodialysis: Hemodialysis or peritoneal dialysis should be reserved for hyperkalemia associated with renal failure or if other methods have been unsuccessful. Renal transplant may be used for irreversible renal failure.

H. Pacemaker: Cardiac pacemaker implantation may be necessary temporarily if serious bradycardia or heart block occurs.

Chronic Hyperkalemia

Treatment emphasizes correction of any underlying problem, if possible. Addison's disease is treated with replacement therapy; hypovolemia or acidosis must be corrected; implicated drugs are discontinued. The treatment of selective hypoaldosteronism depends on its cause. It is usually seen in renal disease that produces fluid retention and hypertension; therefore, furosemide rather than mineralocorticoid replacement is the treatment of choice in this setting. Patients with hypoaldosteronism due to adrenal enzyme defects or classic pseudohypoaldosteronism generally present during infancy. Oral fludrocortisone may be used. Chronic hyperkalemia is ordinarily due to impaired renal excretion. Patients with renal tubule defects are ordinarily treated with a loop diuretic such as furosemide. The dose is begun as 40 mg/d and adjusted according to response; larger doses may be required. If these maneuvers fail to reverse hyperkalemia, the patient must restrict dietary potassium to 60 mEq or less daily. Some patients may require dialysis or renal transplant.

Hyperkalemic periodic paralysis has been reported to respond to thiazide diuretics or inhaled albuterol.

HYPERTENSION

GENERAL DIAGNOSTIC APPROACH

History

The patient must be questioned about ingestion of an excess of any drug known to cause hypertension, eg, real licorice, chewing tobacco containing licorice; large doses of topical skin creams, nasal decongestants, or inhalants containing potent fluorinated steroids; carbenoxolone (antacid drug), thyroid hormone, glucocorticoids, mineralocorticoids, appetite suppressants, estrogens, progestins (eg, oral contraceptives), tricyclic anti-depressants, or nonsteroidal anti-inflammatory agents. The patient should also be questioned about weight changes, increase in ring or shoe size (acromegaly); headache, diaphoresis, or palpitations (pheochromocytoma); kidney stones or bone problems (hyperparathyroidism); fatigue or nocturia (hypokalemia).

Physical Examination

Sustained hypertension must be properly documented. Remember that up to 20% of patients have blood pressure that rises in medical facilities. Blood pressure and heart rate should be measured both lying and standing. The definition of hypertension is arbitrary and age-dependent but may be considered to be present in adults if blood pressure is 160/95 or higher. Diabetics are especially prone to hypertensive complications, so lower limits (150/90) may be set for them. Particular attention should be paid to looking for signs of thyroid abnormalities, acromegaly, or Cushing's syndrome. The abdomen and flanks should be auscultated for bruits suggesting renal artery stenosis. The abdomen and flanks should be palpated for masses (polycystic kidneys). Young patients especially must be examined for signs of aortic coarctation.

Screening Laboratory Testing

Initial screening laboratory determinations should be performed in any patient with documented spontaneous hypertension. They should include measurement of plasma potassium, sodium, calcium, blood urea nitrogen, creatinine, hematocrit, T_4, and blood glucose and urinalysis. Measurement of potassium is best performed in plasma rather than serum, since hemolysis during clot formation may increase the potassium level in resultant serum. More specific tests for endocrine disorders are performed if there are indications for their presence from the history, physical, or screening laboratory testing.

EVALUATION OF HYPOKALEMIA & MINERALOCORTICOID EXCESS

Mineralocorticoid excess generally presents with hypertension with or without weakness. Hypertension is due to sodium retention, ranges from mild to moderate, and rarely becomes malignant. Owing to a proximal tubule "escape," edema does not occur. Actual serum levels of sodium are usually normal but may become elevated during a sodium load or in cases of rare aldosterone-producing adrenal carcinomas. Serum potassium may be low or low-normal, but frank hypokalemia can usually be induced with a sodium load (see below). Hypomagnesemia may also be present in primary hypoaldosteronism. Serum renin activity is low. The hematocrit is usually low (owing to dilution) in severe hyperaldosteronism due to an adrenal neoplasm but is usually normal with milder forms of mineralocorticoid excess.

Symptoms

The symptoms of hypokalemia are mainly those of muscle weakness and cramps. Patients may also have polyuria, enuresis, and even some degree of renal failure. Patients may have carpopedal spasm and positive Chvostek's and Trousseau's signs. Some patients may have an ileus and present with nausea, constipation, or abdominal pain. Children may suffer from growth retardation if hypokalemia is chronic. Potassium levels which are less than 2 mEq/L or which fall acutely cause profound muscle weakness that may progress to paralysis and respiratory insufficiency. Severe potassium depletion in skeletal muscle may cause rhabdomyolysis with myoglobinuria. Effects on intestinal muscle may cause paralytic ileus.

Electrocardiographic changes include elevation of the U wave and depression of the ST segment and T wave. Serious arrhythmias ordinarily do not occur except in the presence of digitalis.

Causes of Hypokalemia

The many causes of hypokalemia are listed in Table 6–4. In adults, hypermineralocorticoidism produces hypertension and a low or low-normal serum potassium. Despite the key role of aldosterone in the maintenance of blood pressure, it accounts for only about 0.5% of hypertensive cases. Hypermineralocorticoidism in adults is 3 times more common in women than men and is usually due to an aldosterone-producing adrenal neoplasm (Conn's syndrome) in about 70% of cases; of these adrenal neoplasms presenting with mineralocorticoid excess, only about 2% are malignant. The other 30% of patients have idiopathic adrenal hyperplasia, possibly owing to an aldosterone-stimulating glycoprotein from the pituitary.

In children, mineralocorticoid hypertension is usually due to excessive DOC due to congenital adrenal enzyme deficiency of 11β-hydroxylase or 17α-hydroxylase.

Diagnosis of Mineralocorticoid Excess

In the absence of other causes of hypokalemia, a plasma potassium of less than 3.5 mEq/L raises the suspicion for (1) diuretic or cathartic abuse, surreptitious vomiting, or (2) mineralocorticoid excess. Since diuretic or cathartic abuse is more common, the patient must be closely questioned. If diuretic or cathartic use is denied, it is wisest to still suspect occult use and query family members and former physicians about furtive abuse. Diuretic abuse may be documented with serum or urine assays for common diuretics; cathartic abuse is suggested by melanosis coli on colonoscopy or by loss of colonic haustral markings on barium enema. If the patient has been taking a diuretic (even combined with a potassium-sparing diuretic such as

Table 6–4. Causes of hypokalemia.

Gastrointestinal loss
Diarrhea, cathartics, villous adenoma of colon.

Decreased oral intake
Malnutrition, strict diet for weight loss.

Medications
Diuretics (proximal or loop); institution of insulin treatment; vitamin B_{12} for megaloblastic anemia; gentamicin; carbenicillin; amphotericin B; alkali; barium salt; real licorice ingestion (glycyrrhizinic acid); ACTH; mineralocorticoids; hydrocortisone; prednisone; potent fluorinated corticosteroids (topical, nasal, inhaled); inhaled bronchodilators.

Mineralocorticoid effects
Primary hyperaldosteronism (adrenal adenoma or hyperplasia).
Secondary hyperaldosteronism (high renin) without hypertension:
  Congestive heart failure, vasodilator drugs, hypoalbuminemia, severe salt depletion and dehydration due to excessive sweating, vomiting, diarrhea, diuretics.
Secondary hyperaldosteronism with hypertension:
  Renal artery stenosis, malignant nephrosclerosis, renin-secreting tumors.
Cushing's syndrome due to ectopic ACTH secretion from a neoplasm, adrenal carcinoma.

Primary renal disease
Renal tubular acidosis (type I or II).
Bartter's syndrome: normotensive, hypokalemia, urine potassium > 20 mEq/L, increased renin, increased aldosterone (mostly seen in children).
Liddle's syndrome: hypertension, hypokalemia, alkalosis, low renin, low or normal aldosterone (rule out excess glucocorticoid, DOC, or licorice).

Other conditions
Ureterojejunostomy; acute leukemia; metabolic alkalosis (eg, nasogastric suctioning, vomiting); hypokalemic periodic paralysis.

---

triamterene or spironolactone), a potassium supplement is given until the level is normal, and the diuretic and potassium are discontinued for more than 3 weeks before the plasma potassium level is again measured.

Patients with a spontaneous low-normal plasma potassium (ie, 3.5–3.9 mEq/L) may be masking hyperaldosteronism, since little sodium may be reaching the renal tubule for exchange with potassium. Such patients should receive a 5-day salt load prior to a repeat plasma potassium determination, ie, an unrestricted diet supplemented with sodium chloride at mealtimes (one-fifth teaspoon salt or a 1-g sodium chloride tablet). In addition, any drugs affecting serum potassium should be discontinued for 6 weeks.

Once a low plasma potassium has been documented (either spontaneously or during a sodium load), a potassium supplement is begun and *the high sodium intake (> 120 mEq/d) is continued during the evaluation for mineralocorticoid excess.* A diagnostic approach for evaluating hypokalemic hypertension is presented in Fig 6–2. Once Cushing's syndrome has been eliminated, a plasma renin activity (PRA) is ideally obtained to help distinguish primary from secondary hypermineralocorticoidism (Table 6–4). The assay is expensive and usually requires time for completion; therefore, if the patient has no evidence of any condition causing secondary hyperaldosteronism it is reasonable to proceed directly to measuring aldosterone. A low PRA prompts the 24-hour urine collection for potassium, aldosterone, and creatinine. A 24-hour urine potassium of more than 40 mmol with hypokalemia documents inappropriate kaliuresis consistent with mineralocorticoid excess. Normal urinary excretion of aldosterone is 5–20 μg/24 h. Plasma aldosterone levels may also be measured; levels in normal individuals and those with hyperplasia are usually less than 20 ng/dL, whereas patients with an adrenal adenoma have levels greater than 20 ng/dL.

Patients with a low 24-hour urinary aldosterone excretion are evaluated for DOC excess (11β-hydroxylase and 17α-hydroxylase

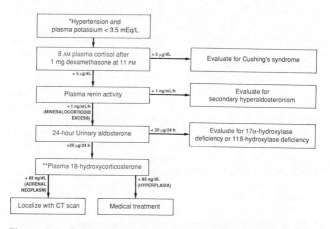

Figure 6–2. Evaluation of hypokalemic hypertension. *Studies are performed during high sodium intake. **In addition, plasma aldosterone may be measured at 8 AM supine after overnight recumbency and after 4 hours upright posture.

deficiency). Patients with 11β-hydroxylase deficiency usually are virilized in childhood; plasma 17-hydroxyprogesterone is increased. Patients with 17α-hydroxylase deficiency are hypogonadal; plasma 17-hydroxyprogesterone is undetectable.

Distinguishing Adrenal Adenomas & Hyperplasia

A. Plasma 18-Hydroxycorticosterone: Patients with low plasma potassium and renin and a high 24-hour urinary aldosterone excretion need further evaluation to distinguish whether they have an adrenal adenoma or hyperplasia. This discrimination is made most accurately by obtaining both plasma 18-hydroxycorticosterone and aldosterone levels: a single plasma level of 18-hydroxycorticosterone is obtained; levels higher than 85 ng/dL are diagnostic of an adrenal neoplasm. Accurate 18-hydroxycorticosterone determinations are now available. Plasma may be frozen and sent to Endocrine Science, Tarzana, California. A plasma aldosterone level of greater than 20 ng/dL is additional evidence of an adrenal neoplasm.

B. Orthostatic Aldosterone Level: An orthostatic study of aldosterone levels also helps distinguish an adenoma from hyperplasia. After the patient has received a high sodium intake (more than 120 mEq/d) for at least 4 days, an 8 AM supine plasma aldosterone level is obtained following overnight constant recumbency of at least 6 hours. A second plasma aldosterone level is then obtained at 12 noon following 4 hours of upright posture. Patients with adrenal aldosterone-secreting adenomas generally have baseline plasma aldosterone levels higher than 20 ng/dL, but the level does not rise with upright posture and may even fall; patients with hyperplasia generally have baseline plasma aldosterone levels lower than 20 ng/dL that usually increase during upright posture.

C. Saline Infusion Test: For adults on a 120 mEq sodium diet, 1.25 L of isotonic saline is infused between 8 and 10 AM while the patient is supine following at least 6 hours of recumbency. Plasma is obtained for 18-hydroxycorticosterone, cortisol, and aldosterone at both 8 AM and 10 AM. The ratio of 18-hydroxycorticosterone to cortisol increases in aldosterone-producing adrenal neoplasms; a ratio of less than 3 is diagnostic of idiopathic hyperaldosteronism. The ratio of aldosterone to cortisol also increases in aldosterone-producing adrenal neoplasms; a ratio of less than 2.2 is diagnostic of idiopathic hyperaldosteronism.

Lateralization & Treatment of Adrenal Adenomas

Once an adrenal adenoma is diagnosed by the above tests, it can be lateralized by CT scan in 80% of cases. In the 20% of patients in whom the CT scan fails to find the adenoma, adrenal vein catheterization is the next step. Alternatively, an adrenal iodocholesterol scan may be done; the patient must be given dexamethasone to reduce uptake by the normal adrenal. Once the adenoma is localized, the patient is given spironolactone in doses of 200–400 mg/d to normalize the serum potassium and improve the blood pressure. Once the serum potassium is normal, the dose of spironolactone may usually be reduced by 50%. If the patient is not prepared for surgery, postoperative hypotension and hyperkalemia may occur owing to prior suppression of the renin-angiotensin system. Surgery consists of unilateral adrenalectomy via flank approach.

Treatment of Adrenal Hyperplasia

A certain rare form of familial hyperaldosteronism due to hyperplasia is glucocorticoid-suppressible; a partial 17α-hydroxylase defect is speculated to be responsible. Nevertheless, it is usually safest to treat all forms with a diuretic (spironolactone or amiloride) rather than 1–2 mg of dexamethasone daily, since that amount of glucocorticoid may cause Cushing's syndrome.

CUSHING'S SYNDROME

The symptoms and signs of glucocorticoid excess are known as Cushing's syndrome (Table 6–5). Cushing's ''disease'' refers to the manifestations of adrenal hypersecretion when caused by pituitary ACTH secretion.

In *adults*, spontaneous hypercortisolism may be due to Cushing's disease (68%) ectopic ACTH-producing tumor (15%) adrenal tumor (15%) or bilateral adrenal hyperplasia without ACTH (1%).

In *children*, spontaneous hypercortisolism may be due to Cushing's disease (50–70%) adrenal neoplasm (30–50%), ectopic ACTH (2%) or bilateral micronodular adrenal hyperplasia without ACTH (1%).

Cushing's disease is caused by a pituitary adenoma (90%) or hyperplasia (10%).

CLINICAL FEATURES

Cushing's disease affects women about 5 times more frequently than men. It may present at any age, but generally affects young adults (mean age 33 years). Each patient may have different manifestations which are especially prominent. (See Figs 6–3 and 6–4.)

Table 6–5. Manifestations of Cushing's syndrome.*

Effects of glucocorticoid excess

Central obesity
  Rounded moon face with
    plethora
  Dorsocervical fat pad (buffalo
    hump)
  Supraclavicular fat pad
Muscle wasting
  Weakness
  Fatigue
Childhood
  Slow growth
  Delay of true (central)
    precocious puberty
Psychiatric/brain changes
  Emotional lability
  Depression
  Hallucinations
  Impaired memory (dementia)
  Cerebral hemispheric atrophy
    on MRI
Opportunistic infection
  Fungal or candidal infections
    of skin, nails, mucosa
  Osteomyelitis

Skin changes
  Thin, papery skin
  Ecchymosis
  Violaceous striae of abdomen,
    thighs, axillae
Poor wound healing
Polyuria and polydipsia (may be
  nonglycosuric)
Renal calculi
Hypogonadism (hypogonadotropic)
  Amenorrhea
  Decreased libido
Eye changes
  Glaucoma
  Cataracts
Laboratory abnormalities
  Hyperglycemia (diabetes mellitus)
  Leukocytosis
  Thrombocytosis
  Lymphopenia
Osteoporosis
  Vertebral compression fractures
  Fractures of long bones or
    ribs

Effects of androgen excess (if present)

Hirsutism, acne, or virilization in
  females
Pseudoprecocious puberty in
  male children
Pseudohermaphroditism in female
  newborns

Effects of ACTH excess (if present)

Hyperpigmentation

Effects of pituitary tumor (if present)

Headache
Visual field abnormalities
Hypopituitarism

Effects of mineralocorticoid excess (if present)

Hypertension
Hypokalemia

*Most patients have only a few of these manifestations.

DIAGNOSTIC APPROACH

Since Cushing's syndrome takes such protean forms, it enters into the differential diagnosis of many conditions. Misleading laboratory or radiologic results occur in 30% of cases.

The following sequential diagnostic approach must be followed for patients presenting with manifestations possibly due to hypercortisolism:

1. Establish the diagnosis of hypercortisolism; then—

2. Distinguish ACTH-induced hypercortisolism from an adrenal neoplasm; then—

3. Distinguish Cushing's disease from an ectopic ACTH-producing tumor.

DIAGNOSIS OF HYPERCORTISOLISM

Laboratory Tests

Tests that help establish the diagnosis of hypercortisolism are described below. Unfortunately, a random plasma cortisol determination is of little value unless a late afternoon or evening plasma cortisol is greater than 30 μg/dL in a nonstressed but suspicious patient. Even then, further confirmation is indicated.

A. The 1-mg Dexamethasone Suppression Test: This is the best screening test for endogenous hypercortisolism of any cause: 1 mg dexamethasone (in children, 20 μg/kg) is taken at 11 PM and blood is drawn at 8 AM the next morning for plasma cortisol. In adults, if the plasma cortisol is less than 5 μg/dL, the diagnosis of hypercortisolism is excluded with 98% certainty. In children with Cushing's disease, suppressibility with overnight low-dose dexamethasone is more common. About 15% of normal individuals will have a supposed plasma control level over 5 μg/dL.

B. Urinary Free Cortisol: If a patient has an abnormal 1-mg dexamethasone suppression test, a 24-hour urine is then obtained and measured for free cortisol and creatinine; 17-hydroxycorticosteroids and 17-ketosteroids are also usually measured. The 24-hour urine free cortisol is increased ($>$ 100 μg/24 h in adults; 60 μg/m^2/d in children) in about 90% of patients with Cushing's syndrome. If the urine free cortisol is also high or if there is a high clinical index of suspicion for Cushing's syndrome, the work-up should proceed.

C. Low-Dose Dexamethasone Suppression Test: If the above tests are abnormal or borderline, this test is performed as follows: dexamethasone, 0.5 mg, is administered orally every 6 hours for 2 days (5 μg/kg every 6 hours in children). A 24-hour urine collection is obtained daily. In normal individuals, the excretion rate of 17-hydroxycorticosteroid drops to below 3 mg/24 h during low-dose dexamethasone administration and the free cortisol excretion drops to below 20 μg/24 h; plasma cortisol falls to below 5 μg/dL.

D. Diurnal Variation of Plasma Cortisol: This may be measured to help determine the presence of hypercortisolism in patients over age 3 years, the time at which diurnal rhythm becomes established. A plasma cortisol is drawn at 8 AM and 11 PM. Normally, plasma cortisol falls to less than 50% of the 8 AM value, except in patients with hypercortisolism.

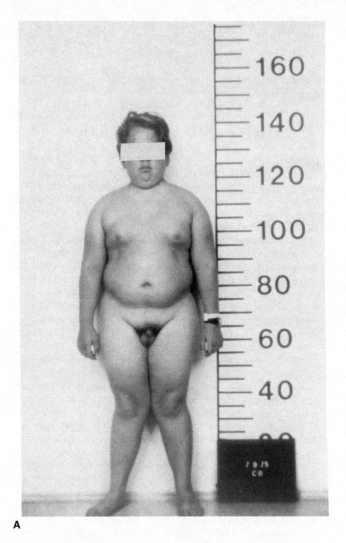

Figure 6–3. Cushing's Disease in childhood. **A.** Patient preoperatively presenting with short stature and obesity.

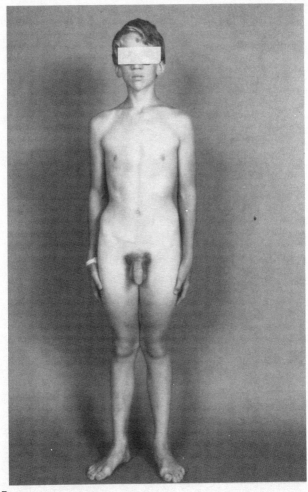

B

Figure 6–3. (*cont'd.*) **B.** Same patient, 18 months following transsphenoidal selective resection of an ACTH-secreting pituitary microadenoma. (Courtesy of JB Tyrrell.)

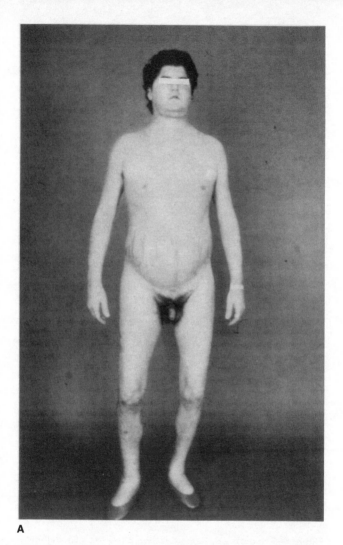

Figure 6–4. Patient with adult-onset Cushing's disease presenting with obesity, psychosis, abdominal striae, muscle wasting, and salmonella osteomyelitis. **A.** Preoperative.

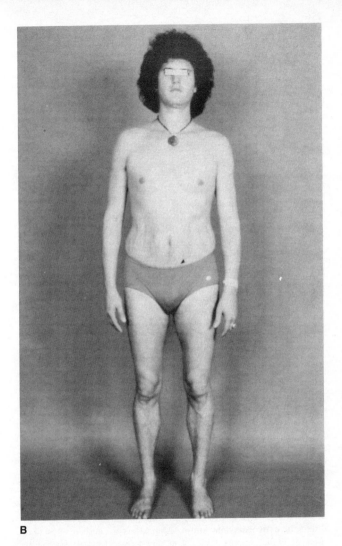

B

Figure 6–4. (*cont'd.*) **B.** Postoperatively, 12 months following selective transsphenoidal resection of a pituitary microadenoma. (Courtesy of JB Tyrrell.)

E. False-Positive Tests: Patients may have false-positive tests for hypercortisolism for the following reasons:

1. Stress–False-positive dexamethasone suppression tests (ie, lack of suppression of 8 AM cortisol to < 5 μg/dL in patients without Cushing's syndrome) may be caused by any acute stress or illness. The test should be repeated following recovery from that stress, if possible.

Hospitalization itself is an emotional stress to many patients; the 1-mg overnight dexamethasone suppression test has a lower false-positive rate when performed on outpatients.

2. Drugs–If a fluorometric rather than specific RIA procedure is used to measure plasma cortisol levels, any 11-hydroxysteroid or other drug the patient is taking that fluoresce at the same wavelength will result in falsely elevated cortisol determinations. Such drugs include spironolactone, niacin, quinidine, quinacrine, fusidic acid, and benzoyl alcohol (found in heparin). These should be discontinued for at least 1 week prior to testing with a fluorometric cortisol assay, or else a more specific assay should be employed. The normal range for plasma cortisol using the fluorometric assay is about 2 μg/dL higher than that using other assays, since normal plasma has some background fluorescence; such background plasma fluorescence is increased in renal and hepatic failure.

A competitive protein-binding assay for cortisol uses cortisol-binding globulin (CBG) rather than an immunoglobulin to bind cortisol. Hence, a falsely elevated cortisol using the CBG assay may be caused by certain other hormones or drugs (eg, prednisolone, methylprednisolone) that also bind to CBG.

Certain anticonvulsant drugs such as phenobarbital, phenytoin, carbamazepine, and primidone cause false-positive low-dose dexamethasone suppression testing by accelerating the hepatic degradation of dexamethasone. The 24-hour urine-free cortisol and plasma cortisol diurnal variation is usually normal in noncushingoid patients taking these drugs; however, some patients taking phenytoin have slightly elevated urine free cortisol excretion. Among patients taking these medications, there is an increased incidence of stress, depression, and alcoholism, which can cause the latter tests to be abnormal. Since the degradation of hydrocortisone is not significantly affected by these drugs, the **hydrocortisone suppression test** is an alternative test to be used in these patients taking anticonvulsants. It is performed by drawing a baseline 8 AM plasma corticosterone (compound B) level and then administering hydrocortisone 50 mg orally at midnight; that morning, an 8 AM plasma corticosterone level is measured. In patients with Cushing's syndrome, the suppressed morning plasma corticosterone level will be greater than 50% of baseline and above 120 ng/dL.

The insulin tolerance test (ITT) cannot be used in patients taking anticonvulsants owing to the danger of inducing a hypoglycemic seizure.

3. High-estrogen states–Estrogen enhances the synthesis of CBG by the liver and thus increases the total plasma cortisol concentration. Plasma cortisol concentrations rise in women who are pregnant or are taking estrogen-containing oral contraceptives or oral estrogen replacement.

The 1-mg dexamethasone suppression test results in lack of suppression of morning cortisol to less than 5 μg/dL in about 50% of normal women taking oral contraceptives. However, false positive tests occur in only about 15% of women taking 0.625 or 1.25 mg of conjugated equine estrogen daily. For the 1-mg dexamethasone suppression test to accurately reflect cortisol suppressibility, oral contraceptives must be discontinued for about 6 weeks and the test repeated. An alternative is to check for diurnal variation of plasma cortisol, which is not affected by high estrogen states. During pregnancy or treatment with oral contraceptives, the urinary 24-hour free cortisol excretion rate rises while the urinary 17-hydroxycorticosteriod excretion rate falls.

4. Obesity–Patients with Cushing's syndrome usually have increased adiposity in the face, neck, and trunk. Unlike noncushingoid obese patients, patients with hypercortisolism most often have thin extremities owing to muscle wasting and lack of fat deposition. However, obese patients often have hypertension and diabetes mellitus; this frequently makes obesity difficult to distinguish from Cushing's syndrome. About 50% of very obese individuals have 8 AM plasma cortisols that are not suppressed to less than 5 μg/dL following 1 mg of dexamethasone. Baseline urinary 17-hydroxycorticosteroid excretion is often increased as well. In obese patients, urinary free cortisol excretion is usually normal, and normal diurnal variation of plasma cortisol is maintained. In addition, the 2-day low dose dexamethasone suppression test is normal in obese patients.

5. Alcoholism–Certain alcoholic patients may look cushingoid (alcoholic pseudo-Cushing's syndrome). Their plasma cortisol may be increased and not suppressed by dexamethasone, and diurnal variation of plasma cortisol is often lost as well. The urinary 24-hour free cortisol excretion is usually normal in these patients, thus helping to exclude Cushing's syndrome with about 94% certainty. Urinary 17-hydroxycorticosteroid excretion is not useful in these patients, since it is diminished by concomitant liver disease.

Testing for Cushing's syndrome should be delayed until alcohol has been entirely withdrawn and the patient has recovered from any withdrawal symptoms. Such patients usually require hospitalization to document abstinence and for reliable collection of urine specimens. Alcoholic patients may not be compliant with abstinence, in which case endocrine testing for Cushing's syndrome may still be carried out. A normal test eliminates the diagnosis of Cushing's syndrome. However, lack of normal cortisol suppressibility by dexamethasone is meaningless.

6. Depression–Endogenous depression often causes abnormalities of cortisol secretion that can closely mimic those of hypercortisolism. These abnormal cortisol dynamics usually occur in patients with unipolar depression but may also be present in patients with bipolar depression or mania. Patients with other psychiatric conditions such as schizophrenia or anxiety states rarely have such abnormal cortisol secretion.

When the distinction between hypercortisolism and depression cannot be made on clinical grounds alone and endocrine testing is abnormal, an insulin tolerance test helps distinguish them. With adequate and symptomatic hypoglycemia (plasma glucose < 40 mg/dL), plasma cortisol usually rises at least an additional 8 μg/dL over the baseline level. Failure of cortisol response to hypoglycemia is rare in depressed patients but is found with hypercortisolism in which high cortisol levels have suppressed the normal hypothalamic-pituitary axis, making it unresponsive to central nervous system stimulation. Children and adolescents with hypercortisolism frequently maintain their cortisol response to hypoglycemia, however.

7. Glucocorticoid Resistance Syndrome—Some people have end-organ resistance to cortisol. They are not cushingoid, but some are hypertensive. Serum ACTH, cortisol, and urine free cortisol are increased and not suppressed by dexamethasone. The adrenals are hypertrophic.

F. False-Negative Tests: False-negative 1-mg overnight dexamethasone suppression tests for hypercortisolism are very uncommon (ie, suppressed 8 AM plasma cortisol < 5 μg/dL in patients with Cushing's syndrome), occurring in about 2% of cases. This may happen in rare cases of periodic hormonogenesis or in patients who metabolize dexamethasone slowly. Falsely low baseline urine 17-hydroxycorticosteroids have been found in 11% and falsely low urine free cortisol in 6% of patients with Cushing's syndrome. Normal suppression of urinary 17-hydroxycorticosteroids to less than 3 mg/24 h with the 2-day low-dose dexamethasone suppression test occurs in 6% of patients with Cushing's syndrome.

Since false-negative tests do sometimes occur, as does laboratory error, patients strongly suspected of having Cushing's syndrome who have negative tests should have tests repeated at a later date.

DISTINGUISHING ACTH-INDUCED HYPERCORTISOLISM FROM ADRENAL NEOPLASM

Plasma ACTH Levels

An undetectable or very low-normal baseline plasma ACTH level in the presence of hypercortisolism is strong evidence for an adrenal tumor. The assay is difficult, however, and falsely low levels may be reported, especially if the blood specimen was not properly collected in a plastic anticoagulated iced tube.

A high or high-normal baseline plasma ACTH level in the presence of hypercortisolism is strong evidence for either pituitary or ectopic production of excessive ACTH. As a group, patients with Cushing's disease have significantly lower ACTH levels than do patients with ectopic ACTH production. However, so much overlap exists that the ACTH level cannot reliably distinguish between the 2 conditions in a given case. If the ACTH level is low, a high-dose dexamethasone test should be done to confirm the presence of an adrenal neoplasm.

High-Dose Dexamethasone Suppression Test

The main value of this test is to confirm the diagnosis of autonomous adrenal neoplasia once hypercortisolism with a low or low-normal plasma ACTH has been confirmed. Lack of suppression confirms the diagnosis.

A. Overnight 8-mg Test: The most convenient way to do the high-dose dexamethasone suppression test is to obtain a baseline 8 AM plasma cortisol determination. Administer 8 mg of dexamethasone at 11 PM, and obtain a 6–8 AM plasma cortisol the next morning. A reduction of plasma cortisol to less than 50% of the baseline value is considered significant suppression.

B. Two-Day Test: The alternative test is the 2-day high-dose dexamethasone suppression test. It is less convenient than the overnight test and no more accurate; its use can be confined to difficult diagnostic cases when more data may be helpful. A baseline 24-hour urine is collected for 17-hydroxycorticosteroids, free cortisol, and creatinine. Then dexamethasone is administered, 2 mg orally every 6 hours for 2 days (20 μg/kg every 6 hours for children). On the second day, a repeat 24-hour urine collection is obtained; a reduction of 17-hydroxycorticosteroids and free cortisol excretion to less than 50% of the baseline value is considered significant suppression.

The high-dose dexamethasone suppression test cannot reliably distinguish between ectopic and pituitary sources of ACTH secretion. About 15% of ectopic tumors are suppressible, especially carcinoid tumors of the lung; about 90% of pituitary tumors are suppressible. Thus, significant cortisol suppression with high-dose dexamethasone favors pituitary Cushing's disease but cannot establish the diagnosis without further testing (see below).

IDENTIFYING THE SOURCE OF ACTH-INDUCED HYPERCORTISOLISM

Once the diagnosis of spontaneous hypercortisolism (Cushing's syndrome) has been established and an adrenal neoplasm has been excluded by the presence of normal or high levels of plasma ACTH, the source of the ACTH must be located, ie, ectopic ACTH from a carcinoma versus ACTH from the pituitary (Cushing's disease), with the latter being about 8 times more common.

Patients with ectopic ACTH production (especially bronchial carcinoid) may sometimes present in a fashion very similar to that of pituitary Cushing's disease. In only 30% of cases of bronchial carcinoid does chest x-ray accurately demonstrate the lesion, whereas CT shows 89% of these lesions. In such cases, it is important not to miss the diagnosis; otherwise unnecessary pituitary surgery may be performed, and the diagnosis of a possibly curable malignancy will be delayed. Most patients with ectopic ACTH production have known malignancies. With ectopic ACTH, hypercortisolism is ordinarily more abrupt in onset and spontaneous hypokalemia is common (69% versus 10% in pituitary-dependent Cushing's disease). Men are affected as often as women. The more common sources of ectopic ACTH secretion are lung, pancreas, thymus, and medullary thyroid carcinoma; however, many other neoplasms can secrete ACTH or corticotropin releasing hormone. Since lung malignancies are most common, a chest x-ray or CT scan must be carefully reviewed. If a suspicious pulmonary lesion is found, a needle biopsy or open lung biopsy is performed.

Ectopic ACTH in childhood is rare but has been reported in children with pheochromocytoma, neuroblastoma, islet cell tumor, and Wilms' tumor.

CT Versus MRI

MRI scanning using high-field (1.5 tesla) thin-section coronal imaging has a sensitivity of 71% and a specificity of 87% for pituitary microadenomas in Cushing's disease. Only about 56% of patients with Cushing's disease have an abnormal pituitary CT scan.

In the absence of a detected malignancy, a pituitary CT scan or MRI should be performed. A minimal pituitary abnormality on the scan may be an artifact or incidental cyst. A definite pituitary abnormality confirms the diagnosis of Cushing's disease, and treatment is directed accordingly. A probable pituitary abnormality in the presence of high-dose dexamethasone suppressibility is also highly suggestive of a pituitary adenoma. Patients with minimal pituitary abnormalities on CT scan or MRI, especially patients not having high-dose dexamethasone suppressibility, must be approached most cautiously, since an occult ectopic ACTH source may be present. In such cases, selective venous ACTH sampling bilaterally from the inferior petrosal sinus is performed, and the CRH stimulation test may also be helpful.

ACTH Sampling from the Inferior Petrosal Sinus

Only an experienced neuroradiologist can catheterize both inferior petrosal sinuses with regularity. Ideally, both sinuses are catheterized simultaneously, and plasma for ACTH is drawn from a peripheral vein simultaneously. A sinus ACTH of 2.5 or more times the peripheral level is strong indication for a pituitary source. A higher level of ACTH in one sinus versus the other during simultaneous bilateral catheterization may help to lateralize the pituitary microadenoma but is not entirely reliable. Administration of CRH may help make this discrimination during the study. Selective ACTH sampling is usually not performed in children, since their risk of ectopic ACTH is much lower than in adults.

Corticotropin-Releasing Hormone Stimulation Test

This test may also help distinguish pituitary Cushing's disease from an occult ectopic ACTH source. CRH is given in a dose of $1\mu g/$ kg body weight intravenously. Plasma ACTH values are measured at -15, 0, 15, 30, 60, 90, and 120 minutes. A rise in ACTH to at least double the baseline value implicates a pituitary ACTH source, although responsive ectopic tumors have been reported. A lack of rise is nonspecific and can be seen with both pituitary and ectopic ACTH-secreting tumors. Therefore, this test is rarely helpful.

Other Tests

Adults with a pituitary ACTH source but normal CT scan or MRI of the pituitary should have serum alpha-fetoprotein and calcitonin determinations to screen for a CRH-secreting hepatoma or medullary thyroid carcinoma.

TREATMENT

Pituitary Surgery for Cushing's Disease

Transsphenoidal pituitary surgery is the treatment of choice for Cushing's disease. The pituitary adenomas found in patients with Cushing's disease tend to be smaller than other adenomas. Discovering and selectively resecting the adenoma is often difficult.

Patients in whom no adenoma is found may therefore have a total hypophysectomy if the diagnosis of a pituitary source of ACTH is secure. Alternatively, patients with negative exploration may have their pituitary left intact, in which case a bilateral adrenalectomy is required, although radiation therapy is an alternative (see below). Since radiation therapy is not usually successful in adults, requires about 6–18 months for an effect, and often causes hypopituitarism, bilateral adrenalectomy or a trial of ketoconazole is usually preferred.

Patients with macroadenomas who do not have complete resection must have postoperative pituitary irradiation and may also require bilateral adrenalectomy or a ketoconazole trial.

Patients who have had successful pituitary surgery for Cushing's disease develop ACTH-cortisol deficiency immediately postoperatively, since the normal pituitary corticotrope cells have been suppressed by hypercortisolism. Adrenal insufficiency persists for 6–36 (median 14) months postoperatively. During that time, hydrocortisone replacement is required. Therefore, hydrocortisone is tapered postoperatively to normal replacement levels (20 mg at 8 AM, 10 mg at 5 PM), and more is given if the patient develops intolerable manifestations of cortisol withdrawal at higher hydrocortisone doses.

About 1 week following transsphenoidal selective resection of a pituitary adenoma, hydrocortisone is held after 6 PM and a 6–8 AM plasma cortisol is drawn: if it is below 5 μg/dL, a remission is expected and hydrocortisone replacement is continued; if it is above 5 μg/dL, a remission is unlikely, hydrocortisone is stopped, and the patient is reassessed.

Hydrocortisone is continued at the minimum tolerated dose for about 6 weeks postoperatively, at which time the hydrocortisone is held after 6 PM and a cosyntropin stimulation test is performed the next morning. A 1-mg dexamethasone suppression test is also performed. Most patients with successful transsphenoidal surgery for Cushing's disease develop isolated ACTH-cortisol insufficiency. Hydrocortisone replacement alone is adequate, since mineralocorticoid secretion remains intact.

Since some patients with Cushing's disease develop autonomous adrenal nodules that may nevertheless involute, a high postoperative cortisol level should prompt a repeat determination 4 weeks postoperatively. Persistent hypercortisolism indicates the need for a repeat plasma ACTH level prior to further therapy directed at the pituitary.

Patients having a remission from Cushing's disease not only have transient adrenal insufficiency but also usually experience a **cortisol withdrawal syndrome.** Symptoms may include pruritus, dry skin, arthralgias, depression, and edema. Symptoms of adrenal insufficiency such as nausea, fatigue, and hypotension also may occur at usual hydrocortisone doses. Many patients cannot tolerate initial postoperative hydrocortisone doses below 20 mg 3 times daily. The minimum tolerated dose of hydrocortisone must be found for each individual patient and further dose reduction accomplished gradually over several months.

Signs of hypercortisolism resolve gradually following successful treatment. The most striking improvement in body habitus occurs in younger patients. Diabetes mellitus and hypertension improve but sometimes do not entirely resolve. Psychiatric changes resolve slowly; hallucinations and other psychotic manifestations may persist for a year or longer and may recur. Muscle strength gradually improves, and an exercise program emphasizing proximal muscle groups may hasten recovery.

Pituitary Radiation Therapy for Cushing's Disease

Conventional radiation therapy for Cushing's disease is not optimal owing to its low remission rate in adults (23% cured; 30% improved) and delayed remission in those who do not respond. Cushing's disease has such life-threatening effects that it is generally best not to delay definitive therapy by radiating and then waiting for an unlikely remission. Conventional radiation for Cushing's disease appeared to be more successful in one series of 15 children and adolescents (80% remission rate) but risks hypopituitarism.

Heavy-particle radiation of the pituitary produces a higher remission rate (65% cured; 20% improved) in patients with microadenomas but cannot be used in patients with suprasellar extension owing to the danger of damage to the optic chiasm. The remission requires 4–6 months, and hypopituitarism of some degree probably occurs in about 60% of cases.

Medical Therapy for Cushing's Disease

Medical treatment for Cushing's disease is inadequate. Treatment with ketoconazole, metyrapone, aminoglutethimide, RU 486, or mitotane (o,p'DDD) is fraught with side effects. However, among these drugs, ketoconazole has become favored (see p 267). Delaying pituitary or adrenal surgery to prepare the patient medically is usually not worth the risk of side effects and the possibility of stimulating pituitary tumor growth. Treatment with one or a combination of these drugs may be given to patients having had pituitary radiation, awaiting the radiation effect, or requiring adrenal surgery and who have inordinate surgical risk.

Cyproheptadine has not proved successful in treating patients chronically and produces sedation and weight gain. Bromocriptine, while producing acute suppression of cortisol in certain patients with Cushing's disease, has not been successful in chronic treatment.

Adrenal Surgery for Cushing's Disease

Since transsphenoidal surgery is the treatment of choice for Cushing's disease, adrenal surgery is reserved for those patients who do not have a surgical remission. Bilateral adrenalectomy results in permanent Addison's disease and frequent complications. An incidental appendectomy may result in peritonitis. Recurrences sometimes occur in adrenal remnants. Furthermore, hyperpigmentation as well as growth of the pituitary adenoma often occurs following bilateral adrenalectomy (Nelson's syndrome).

Treatment for Nelson's Syndrome

Nelson's syndrome consists of the clinical progression of an ACTH-secreting pituitary adenoma following bilateral adrenalectomy for Cushing's disease. Approximately 30% of the latter patients develop significant hyperpigmentation and pituitary tumor growth. These tumors may become particularly aggressive, causing headache, visual field defects, extraocular muscle palsies, and hypopituitarism. Some of these tumors may become frankly malignant, invading local structures and exhibiting intracranial and even extracranial metastases. ACTH levels usually range from 1000 pg/mL to over 10,000 pg/mL. Pituitary apoplexy frequently occurs.

About 50% of patients with Cushing's disease treated with bilateral adrenalectomy develop modest hyperpigmentation (ACTH levels between about 500 pg/mL and 4000 pg/mL) without progressive enlargement of their pituitary microadenoma. Another 20% of patients never develop a pituitary adenoma detectable on CT scan and are not hyperpigmented, having ACTH levels only modestly elevated in the range of 100 pg/mL to 500 pg/mL.

The treatment of Nelson's syndrome consists of pituitary surgery. Radiation therapy is given to unresectable tumors in maximal dosage using techniques to minimize damage to surrounding structures. Pituitary hormone replacement should be prescribed as needed. However, supraphysiologic glucocorticoid administration should not be given in an attempt to suppress the tumor; such treatment is ordinarily ineffective and produces a recurrence of Cushing's syndrome.

Treatment for Ectopic ACTH

In patients with hypercortisolism due to ectopic ACTH, the underlying malignancy must first be discovered and treated, if possible. Meanwhile, the patient's hypercortisolism, hypokalemia, hypertension, and virilization may be treated with trilostane, metyrapone, ketoconazole, or a combination of these drugs (see p 266). This treatment will be effective for most patients, since ectopic ACTH sources are usually autonomous; the compensatory ACTH hypersecretion that would be seen in Cushing's disease will ordinarily not occur.

Occult ectopic ACTH-producing tumors occur in certain patients, sometimes eluding localization for years. Such patients must receive a CT scan of the chest and thorough ongoing evaluation. Patients with autonomous tumors (cortisol not suppressible with high-dose dexamethasone) may be treated as above. Bilateral adrenalectomy is reserved for patients with reactive ACTH hypersecretion in whom rising ACTH levels overcome medical treatment, or for patients who are intolerant or resistant to drug treatment.

ADRENOCORTICAL NEOPLASMS

Adrenal neoplasms are lateralized by abdominal CT scan. If a mass is not localized, surreptitious glucocorticoid intake must be considered; an iodocholesterol scan may localize a small or rare ectopic benign neoplasm. Adrenal carcinoma does not take up iodocholesterol but is usually seen by CT.

Adrenal adenomas causing Cushing's syndrome occur somewhat more frequently in women than in men. They usually secrete mainly cortisol; serum levels of adrenal androgens (eg, DHEAS) are usually low.

Adrenal cortical carcinomas producing Cushing's syndrome are usually large (6 cm or more in diameter) and rapidly growing. Unlike a benign adenoma, a carcinoma commonly produces a variety of adrenal hormones and hormone precursors. A carcinoma may be a source of cortisol, corticosterone, aldosterone, androgens, and estrogens. In addition, relative enzyme deficiencies may lead to production of inactive precursors. Clinically nonfunctioning carcinomas may be sources of excess 11-deoxycortisol or pregnenolone secretion. Urinary excretion of 17-ketogenic steroids and 17-ketosteroids may be especially high. Presumed nonfunctioning tumors make up about one-third of all adrenal cortical carcinomas. Overall, carcinomas are an uncommon cause of Cushing's syndrome in adults but account for 50% of cases of spontaneous Cushing's syndrome in children. Nonfunctioning carcinomas are uncommon in children.

Metastases generally occur to lung (42%), retroperitoneal lymph nodes (68%), liver (42%), bone (26%), and the contralateral adrenal (12%). A second primary cancer has been noted in 22% of cases, most commonly breast carcinoma and lymphoma.

Surgical Treatment

Aggressive surgical resection is the treatment for benign adenomas and the initial treatment for carcinomas, even those with metastases. CT scan can be used to determine the extent of a carcinoma. Metastases or invasion into the vena cava makes the full tumor unresectable, but partial resection may be indicated to reduce steroid secretion.

Perioperative management of cortisol-secreting tumors should include the expectation of adrenal insufficiency, since the remaining adrenal cortex will be atrophic. Patients with tumors that secrete mineralocorticoids as well as cortisol should be treated preoperatively with spironolactone (Aldactone and others, 25-, 50-, and 100-mg tablets available; use 50–100 mg, 2–4 times a day) to restore normal serum potassium and to reduce suppression of the uninvolved zona glomerulosa. Alternatively, if surgery is desired sooner, observe post-operatively for hyperkalemia, and supplement temporarily with increased sodium intake or fludrocortisone (Florinef, 0.1-mg tablets available; use 0.05 mg/d). Corticosteroid supplements may be gradually tapered. Anticipate that the patient will require doses and duration of therapy similar to those used in withdrawal from long-term glucocorticoid therapy.

Medical Treatment

Elevated cortisol levels (and/or androgen, estrogen, or mineralocorticoid levels, depending on the enzyme deficiencies found in each neoplasm) will persist after incomplete resection of a carcinoma. Excess steroid secretion from residual, recurrent, or inoperable carcinomas may be treated with o,p'-$\overline{\text{DDD}}$ (mitotane, Lysodren), aminoglutethimide (Cytadren), metyrapone (Metopirone), ketoconazole (Nizoral), and trilostane (Modrastane).

To maximize effectiveness of a drug regimen and minimize adverse reactions, combinations of these drugs may be used at submaximal doses of each.

A. o,p'-$\overline{\text{DDD}}$: Reduction in tumor size occurs in 35% of patients treated with the adrenolytic o,p'-$\overline{\text{DDD}}$. Cures, however, are very rare. Beginning dose is 1 g/d. The aim is to achieve the maximum tolerated dose. o,p'-$\overline{\text{DDD}}$ has a plasma half-life of 55–60 days, making cumulative toxicity a problem; it may need to be discontinued if severe toxicity occurs and then restarted at a lower dose if indicated. Plasma levels of o,p'-$\overline{\text{DDD}}$ of about 15–20 μg/mL may be required. Chronic administration of o,p'-$\overline{\text{DDD}}$ at doses of 3 g/d or more result in adrenal cortical atrophy. Replacement of both glucocorticoids and mineralocorticoids is necessary early in therapy. Doses of glucocorticoid (hydrocortisone) often need to be greater than usually given for adrenal insufficiency, since o,p'-$\overline{\text{DDD}}$ accelerates the extrarenal metabolism of cortisol to 6β-hydrocortisol. o,p'-$\overline{\text{DDD}}$ is indicated for most patients with functioning or nonfunctioning adrenocortical carcinoma, since it prolongs life expectancy to 8.4 months from time of diagnosis (versus 2.9 months in untreated patients); complete responses have been reported but are unusual. About 70% of patients achieve a satisfactory reduction in steroid secretion. Side effects are common (87%) and include nausea, vomiting, or diarrhea (79%), central nervous system depression (49%), and skin rash (15%); they may necessitate reduction in dosage.

B. Aminoglutethimide: Aminoglutethimide inhibits the conversion of cholesterol to Δ^5-pregnenolone. Inhibition of steroid synthesis can be achieved with 250–500 mg, 2–4 times a day. Since aminoglutethimide is not adrenolytic, there is no regression of tumor size. The most prominent side effects are rash, nausea, dizziness, depression, and severe drowsiness. Somnolence is a major factor limiting its use.

C. Metyrapone: Metyrapone inhibits the final step of cortisol synthesis, the conversion of 11-deoxycortisol to cortisol. Cortisol synthesis can be inhibited by 2–4 g/d divided into 2–4 doses. Since adrenal androgen synthesis is not inhibited, hirsutism in women would not be ameliorated. Mineralocorticoid synthesis also continues. Metyrapone is expensive for use in long-term therapy.

D. Ketoconazole: Ketoconazole inhibits at least 3 cytochrome P-450–dependent adrenal enzymes: cholesterol desmolase, 11β-hydroxylase, and 17,20-lyase. Cortisol and adrenal androgen synthesis can be inhibited by doses of 200 mg every 6 hours. Ketoconazole is being used increasingly and has produced some long-term remissions. The level of hepatic enzymes may rise, and patients require surveillance for hepatotoxicity.

E. Trilostane: Trilostane (Modrastane) inhibits the adrenal enzyme 3β-hydroxysteroid dehydrogenase (3β-HSD). Therapy is started with 30 mg orally, 4 times daily, and increased to 50 mg after 4 days. Individual responsiveness varies, and doses up to 250 mg, 4 times daily, may be required. Improvement in cortisol secretion and hypertension is usually seen. Hypokalemia improves. Hirsutism and acne improves although urinary 17-ketosteroids and serum DHEAS levels increase. Side effects include gastrointestinal symptoms (5–17%), a burning sensation in the mouth and other mucous membranes (5–10%), flushing, and headache.

FRU 486 (mifepristone) is a steroid receptor blocker that is used outside the USA to induce abortion because of its antiprogesterone activity. It also blocks cortisol activity. Patients need careful clinical surveillance, since cortisol levels do not fall with adrenal neoplasms and may rise with responsive ACTH-secreting tumors, despite a salutary clinical response leading to effective adrenal insufficiency. Expense limits its use.

CUSHING'S SYNDROME CAUSED BY BILATERAL ADRENAL NODULAR HYPERPLASIA

During the evaluation of Cushing's syndrome, some patients are found to have bilateral nodular adrenals and poor cortisol suppressibility with dexamethasone but detectable plasma levels of ACTH. Such patients have Cushing's disease, which has produced variable degrees of adrenal autonomy. These patients may have therapy directed at the pituitary. The nodular adrenals ordinarily regress.

Some rare patients with the onset of Cushing's syndrome in childhood or adolescence have bilateral micronodular adrenals with undetectable plasma levels of ACTH. The condition appears to be due to adrenal-stimulating immunoglobulins. This condition, known as primary pigmented nodular adrenocortical disease, can occur sporadically or as part of a familial autosomal dominant syndrome called the **Carney syndrome.** Carney syndrome manifestations also include blue nevi and facial lentigines; myxomas occur in the breast, skin, and heart. Schwannomas (peripheral nerve tumors) also occur. Bilateral testicular tumors (Leydig cell, Sertoli cell, or adrenal rest) may cause sexual precocity in boys. Pituitary growth hormone–secreting tumors may cause gigantism or acromegaly. The condition may be familial. Care must be taken to ensure that the plasma ACTH assay is accurate. Then, bilateral adrenalectomy is performed.

Other rare patients have bilateral macronodular hyperplasia (nodules 1 cm or more in diameter) with undetectable plasma levels of ACTH. There is inadequate suppression with high-dose dexamethasone. The absence of a pituitary tumor must be documented by undetectable levels of ACTH from inferior petrosal sinus sampling and by CT scanning or magnetic resonance imaging (MRI). Then, bilateral adrenalectomy is performed.

EXOGENOUS GLUCOCORTICOIDS

The therapeutic administration of glucocorticoids or ACTH is by far the most common cause of Cushing's syndrome. Cushing's syndrome may also be caused by topical, nasal, or inhaled glucocorticoids. In an effort to reduce the morbidity associated with administration of pharmacologic doses of prednisone, dexamethasone, and other glucocorticoids, the regimen listed in Table 6–6 is recommended for patients who are to receive glucocorticoids in above-replacement doses.

Table 6–6. Management of patients receiving glucocorticoids.

1. Do not administer glucocorticoids unless absolutely indicated and more conservative measures have failed.

2. Keep dosage and length of administration to the minimum required for adequate treatment. Consider alternate-day or local therapy for certain conditions. Asthmatics who are prednisone-dependent may be able to reduce their systemic dosage of glucocorticoids if inhaled beclomethasone is added to the regimen; systemic absorption and oral moniliasis caused by beclomethasone may be reduced by using a spacer device to catch large droplets prior to inhalation.

3. Obtain a pretreatment chest x-ray, and apply a PPD (purified protein derivative). Treat any latent tuberculosis as indicated to avoid reactivation. Repeat the chest x-ray periodically.

4. Screen for diabetes mellitus before treatment and at each physician's visit. Train the patient to test urine weekly with Tes-Tape, Diastix, Chemstrip uG strips, or Clinistix.

5. Screen for hypertension before treatment and at each physician's visit.

6. Screen for glaucoma and cataracts before treatment, 3 months after treatment, and then at least yearly.

7. Prepare the patient and family for possible adverse effects on mood, memory, and cognitive function. Inform them about other possible side effects.

8. Institute a vigorous physical exercise and isometric regimen tailored to each patient's disabilities.

9. Avoid prolonged bed rest that will accelerate muscle weakness and bone mineral loss. Ambulate early after fractures.

10. Treat hypogonadism in women or men.

11. Administer calcium (1 g elemental calcium) orally daily. Check spot morning urines, and alter dosage to keep urine calcium concentration below 30 mg/dL. If the patient is receiving thiazide diuretics, check for hypercalcemia, and administer only 500 mg elemental calcium daily.

12. Avoid elective surgery, if possible. Vitamin A in a daily dose of 20,000 U orally for 1 week may improve wound healing.

13. Avoid activities that could cause falls or other trauma.

14. Watch for fungal or yeast infections of skin, nails, mouth, vagina, and rectum, and treat properly. Prophylaxis or treatment of nail mycoses with ciclopirox olamine cream (Loprox 1%, 15- and 30-g tubes) may be done by applying cream around nail edges twice daily.

15. Ulcer prophylaxis: Administer oral glucocorticoids with meals. Consider prophylaxis with sucralfate, 1 g, an hour before meals or at bedtime. Ranitidine may also be used. Avoid large doses of antacids containing aluminum hydroxide (many popular brands) unless the patient is azotemic; aluminum hydroxide binds phosphate and may cause a hypophosphatemic osteomalacia that can compound glucocorticoid osteoporosis. If calcium carbonate is used (eg, Tums, Titralac), the total calcium dose must be monitored and screening done for hypercalciuria and hypercalcemia.

16. Treat any infections agressively. Consider unusual pathogens.

17. Weigh daily. Use dietary measures to avoid obesity and optimize nutrition.

18. Measure height frequently. In children, this serves to document the degree of growth retardation. In adults, this serves to document the degree of axial spine demineralization and compression.

(continued)

Table 6–6. (cont'd.)

19. Treat edema as indicated.
20. Monitor plasma potassium for hypokalemia. Treat as indicated.
21. With dosage reduction, watch for signs of adrenal insufficiency or glu-
    cocorticoid withdrawal syndrome.

GLUCOCORTICOID WITHDRAWAL SYNDROME

When pharmacologic glucocorticoid treatment is withdrawn, patients usually experience a glucocorticoid withdrawal syndrome similar to that experienced by patients who have been treated for Cushing's
disease (p 262). Subgroups of this syndrome include (1) Symptoms of
adrenal insufficiency with biochemical evidence of hypothalamic-
pituitary-adrenocortical suppression. Symptoms are relieved by replacement doses of glucocorticoids. (2) Symptoms of the disease for
which the glucocorticoids were originally prescribed. (3) Symptoms of
withdrawal that persist despite replacement doses of glucocorticoids.
These symptoms often include anorexia, nausea, weight loss, fatigue,
weakness, fever, arthralgias, pruritus, and desquamation of the skin.
Any combination of types may coexist. Some patients have no symptoms.

PHEOCHROMOCYTOMA

Pheochromocytomas are uncommon tumors that arise from cells
of the sympathetic nervous system and secrete catecholamines. These
cells are called chromaffin cells, since fixatives containing chromium
salts stain them amber. Most occur in the adrenal medulla; tumors
outside the adrenal medulla are usually within sympathetic ganglia and
are called paragangliomas. Generally, the occurrence of pheochromocytoma can be remembered by the *rough rule of 10*. About 10% are
malignant; 10% are familial; they usually produce hypertension but
account for only about 0.01% of hypertensive cases; about 10% of
cases do not have hypertension; 10% are extra-adrenal and of those
about 10% are extra-abdominal; about 10% are bilateral; and 10%
occur in children.

In children, tumors are much more likely to be bilateral or extra-
adrenal (30%). Bilateral tumors are also more common in patients
with familial (70%) or sporadic multiple endocrine neoplasia (MEN II
or III). Pheochromocytomas occur in both sexes and at any age but are
most common in the fourth and fifth decades.

Neuroblastomas are similar to pheochromocytomas in that they may secrete catecholamines. They are, however, found almost entirely in children under age 18 years. About 85% of neuroblastomas are adrenal and 15% extra-adrenal; the latter are usually found in the posterior mediastinum or are "dumbbell" tumors of the spinal cord neuroforamina. Extra-adrenal pheochromocytomas are most commonly found in the aortic bifurcation, mediastinum, urinary bladder, or carotid body, but they may be found elsewhere.

The pathophysiology of pheochromocytomas is due to the large quantities of catecholamines released. Pheochromocytomas synthesize primarily norepinephrine. Some also synthesize large quantities of dopamine or epinephrine (especially intra-adrenal tumors and occasionally those of the aortic bifurcation arising from the organs of Zuckerkandl). Norepinephrine secretion causes hypertension, tachycardia, and a progressive cardiomyopathy. Epinephrine and enkephalin secretion may produce orthostatic hypotension.

SYMPTOMS & SIGNS

The clinical manifestations of pheochromocytomas are listed in Table 6–7 and are quite variable depending on the relative amounts, ratios, and pattern of norepinephrine and epinephrine.

About 90% of patients have hypertension which may be *intermittent, remittent* (sustained hypertension with episodic increases), or *persistent;* patients with persistent hypertension sometimes lack paroxysmal symptoms.

Hypertension during a paroxysm may achieve severe levels. Patients may develop hypertensive encephalopathy. The blood pressure may paradoxically increase in response to some antihypertensive drugs (ganglionic blocking agents, β-blockers, guanethidine). It may also increase in response to general anesthetics. An unusually exquisite sensitivity to the hypotensive effect of prazosin (Minipress), an α-blocker, should raise the suspicion of pheochromocytoma.

Orthostatic hypotension can occur even in the untreated patient. The orthostatic hypotension has been variously ascribed to decreased plasma volume, to the desensitization of sympathetic reflexes by high circulating catecholamine levels, and to the hypotensive effects of epinephrine or enkephalins released by the tumor.

Paroxysmal symptoms are expressed by most patients. Paroxysms commonly include headache, perspiration, and palpitations; patients may also have anxiety, dread, chest discomfort, paresthesias, or tremor. Such symptoms are also seen with typical anxiety attacks; however, the latter patients ordinarily are not hypertensive. Attacks last minutes to hours. The frequency of episodes varies from every few

Table 6–7. Clinical manifestations of pheochromocytoma.

Symptom or sign:	Approximate frequency
Hypertension (sustained or paroxysmal)	90%
Headache*	80%
Perspiration*	70%
Palpitation*	60%
Anxiety	50%
Tremor	40%
Hyperglycemia	35%
Nausea	35%
Thoracic or abdominal pain	35%
Weakness	25%
Weight loss (> 10%)	15%
Dyspnea	15%
Visual disturbance	10%
Hot flushes or heat intolerance	10%

Other manifestations: Raynaud's phenomenon, confusion, psychosis, constipation, paresthesias, seizures, bradycardia, hypotension, palpable mass, neurofibromatosis, erythrocytosis, neutrophilia.

Associated features
　　Multiple endocrine neoplasia (MEN) type II (Sipple's syndrome):
　　　　Medullary thyroid carcinoma, parathyroid hyperplasia, or adenomas.
　　Multiple endocrine neoplasia (MEN) type III:
　　　　Medullary thyroid carcinoma, marfanoid body type (without aortic or lens abnormalities); mucosal neuromas of lips, tongue, eyelids, and gastrointestinal tract.

*At least one of these symptoms is present at some time in at least 95% of patients with pheochromocytoma.

months to as often as 25 times a day. A particular pattern often develops in a given patient with some worsening of the severity or frequency of symptoms over time. Attacks usually begin abruptly and subside gradually. During an episode, physical signs include hypertension, which may be accompanied by tachycardia or reflex bradycardia, arrhythmia, pallor of face and upper body, and dilated pupils. Some patients have paroxysms following lifting, straining, bending, exertion, or micturition (see below). Often, paroxysms do not have a discernible provocation.

　　Persistent catecholamine excess can contribute to constipation caused by decreased gut motility. Cholelithiasis occurs in 15–20% of patients. Catecholamine-induced cardiomyopathy is an effect of prolonged elevated levels of catecholamines.

　　Hypermetabolism results from the stimulatory effects of catecholamines. Heat intolerance and weight loss are common. Glucose intolerance may result from stimulation of glycogenolysis, inhibition of glucose disposition, and blockade of insulin release.

Although pheochromocytoma of the urinary bladder is rare, it may be considered if paroxysms occur during the initiation of micturition or with a distended bladder. Painless hematuria is noted in 65% of these patients. The tumors can generally be visualized with cystoscopy.

EVALUATION

Pheochromocytoma should be suspected in any child or young adult with hypertension. Adults with hypertension, especially with paroxysms, should also be evaluated if they have one of the major symptoms: headache, perspiration, or palpitation, one of which is present in at least 95% of pheochromocytoma patients. Patients should also be screened if they have a history of severe hypertension or unexplained shock (which may occur with anesthesia, childbirth, or certain antihypertensive drugs). Patients with severe or unresponsive hypertension should also be screened, as should hypertensive patients about to undergo anesthesia (if the diagnosis is at all suspected). Patients with an undiagnosed suprarenal or paraaortic mass should be evaluated for pheochromocytoma. Patients with a personal or family history of pheochromocytoma, mucosal neuromas, or medullary thyroid carcinoma (eg, MEN II or III) should be screened for pheochromocytoma with a high index of suspicion.

Untreated pheochromocytoma may cause stroke owing to cerebrovascular hemorrhage or ischemia; myocardial infarction and heart failure are common. It is difficult to screen patients for pheochromocytoma immediately after such events, since falsely elevated tests are usual.

BIOCHEMICAL TESTS

Urinary Catecholamines, VMA, Metanephrine

Before screening for pheochromocytoma, be sure the patient does not have any drug, food, or condition that will affect the tests (Table 6–8). Interfering medications should generally be withdrawn for at least 5 days before testing. Diet should also be specified for at least 48 hours if a fluorometric VMA assay is used. Certain factors universally affect testing for urinary catecholamines, metanephrine, and VMA no matter how specific the assay. Fluorescent substances cause falsely elevated readings for any substance when fluorometric assay methods

Table 6–8. Drugs, food and conditions affecting chemical tests for pheochromocytoma.

Test	Increase	Decrease
Universally affecting catecholamines, metanephrines, and VMA	Sympathomimetics (amphetamines, ephedrine, nasal decongestants, bronchodilators) L-Dopa Rapid clonidine withdrawal Excess ingestion of bananas Vasodilators (nitroprusside, nitroglycerine) Methylxanthines (theophylline, aminophylline) Severe stress (emotion, exercise, pain, myocardial infarct) Certain diseases (intracranial lesions, acute psychosis, Guillain-Barré syndrome, lead poisoning, eclampsia, hypoglycemia, carcinoid, acute porphyria, acrodynia, quadriplegia, amyotrophic lateral sclerosis) Fluorescent substances (fluorometric method*): quinidine, chloral hydrate, tetracyclines, methenamine, methocarbamol, nicotinic acid, erythromycin, quinine, riboflavin, bretylium, sulfobromophthalein, phenolsulfonphthalein	Large doses of ganglionic blockers: guanethidine, reserpine (with chronic administration; acute administration causes initial increases). Fenfluramine (anorectic). Renal insufficiency. Certain diseases— malnutrition, dysautonomia, quadriplegia (quiescent).
Catecholamines	Ethanol, isoproterenol, methyldopa, MAO inhibitors, phenothiazines, α-methyl-p-tyrosine, methenamine, urine bilirubin, labetalol	
Metanephrines	Ethanol, methyldopa, MAO inhibitors, benzodiazepines, phenothiazines	Radiopaque media (methylgluca-mine): Renografin, Hypaque-M, Renovisit, Cardiografin, Urografin, Conray. *(continued)*

Table 6–8. *(cont'd.)*

Test	Increase	Decrease
Metanephrines *(cont'd.)*		(Hypaque as diatrizoate sodium is all right.)
VMA	Lithium, nalidixic acid, methocarbamol, glycerol guaiacolate, *p*-aminosalicylic acid, salicylates, mephenesin, sulfa drugs, excess ingestion of (fluorometric method*) chocolate, citrus, tea, vanilla, coffee	Ethanol, MAO inhibitors, phenothiazines, disulfiram, clofibrate, mandelamine, salicylates (Pisano method).

*Fluorometric assay methods are subject to most types of interference. The most specific assays use chromatographic and spectrophotometric methods. Drugs should be stopped for 1 week before testing.

are used without proper preliminary chromatographic separation. Even chromatography may not entirely separate substances having molecular structures similar to catecholamines. A common culprit is methyldopa, a commonly used antihypertensive drug that, even after chromatography, causes increased fluorometric determinations for catecholamines and metanephrines; it does not affect VMA testing, however.

Diet preparation should always include avoidance of bananas for about 48 hours prior to testing. Other foods increase urinary VMA measurements in nonspecific fluorometric assays but do not usually affect determinations using chromatographic and spectrophotometric (eg, Pisano) methods.

The most practical screening test for patients with a low probability of pheochromocytoma is a random (spot) urine collection for metanephrine, VMA, and creatinine concentrations. The container does not require acid preservative. Patients with pheochromocytomas generally have urinary levels on spot collections of more than 2.2 μg metanephrine/mg creatinine and more than 5.5 μg VMA/mg creatinine; this test is especially sensitive when collected after a typical paroxysm.

To further investigate the diagnosis, a 24-hour urine specimen for total catecholamines, metanephrine, VMA, and creatinine may be collected (in a container containing 10 mL of 6N hydrochloric acid to preserve the catecholamines; VMA and metanephrines may be collected with acid preservative but do not require it). The results are still best expressed in terms of μg/mg creatinine, since timed urine collections are often inaccurate. Patients with pheochromocytomas usually have high urinary excretion rates: total catecholamines > 0.12 μg/mg creatinine (or > 18 μg/dL); metanephrine > 0.7 μg/mg creatinine; VMA > 10 μg/mg creatinine. If expressed as mg/24 h, high excretion rates are considered to be the following: total catecholamines > 115 μg/24 h; metanephrine > 0.7 mg/24 h; VMA > 10 mg/24 h.

Such urine collection studies usually are adequate to make the diagnosis. If these tests are normal in the face of rather typical but infrequent attacks, then a 2-hour timed urine specimen immediately following an attack may document increased catecholamine/metabolite excretion.

Plasma Catecholamines

Tests for plasma catecholamines usually are not required to make a diagnosis of pheochromocytoma. They are more sensitive than the measurement of urinary catecholamines and metabolites; however, false-positive tests are more common (to 20%) owing to even minimal physical or mental stress. Illness and azotemia increase plasma levels. Falsely elevated plasma catecholamine levels can be minimized but not eliminated if the following precautions are followed: The test should be performed in the morning on a fasting, nonstressed patient who has been supine for at least 30 minutes prior to testing. An intravenous line (19 or 20 gauge) should be inserted in a large vein at least 30 minutes prior to blood collection and run slowly. Efforts should be made to reduce pain and anxiety, which can raise the level of plasma catecholamines and result in false positives. Ideally, the blood should be collected quietly without a tourniquet and placed in iced heparinized tubes. The blood should be centrifuged and separated immediately. The test should be scheduled in advance with the laboratory.

The upper limit of normal for plasma total catecholamines (norepinephrine and epinephrine) in patients with essential hypertension is 950 pg/mL. Values between 950 and 2000 ng/L are equivocal. Total plasma catecholamine levels greater than 2000 ng/L are indicative of pheochromocytoma. Measurement of urine metanephrine, catecholamines, and VMA, especially when combined with plasma catecholamine determinations, have a sensitivity of about 98% for pheochromocytoma. The real problem is with specificity, since false-positive tests are not unusual.

Glucagon Stimulation Test

In the unusual case with equivocal testing and diastolic blood pressure not higher than 100 mm Hg, a provocative test with glucagon may be employed if the patient has no condition that would make a hypertensive response dangerous. This test entails 2 steps: (1) The cold pressor test, in which the blood pressure is measured before and after immersion of one hand in ice water for 5 minutes. (2) The following day an intravenous line is begun as outlined above for plasma cate-cholamines. A baseline plasma total catecholamine level is obtained; then glucagon, 2 mg, is given as an intravenous bolus. Between 1 and 3 minutes later, another total plasma catecholamine level is obtained. A positive response is (1) any level over 2000 pg/mL or (2) an increase to over 3 times basal level. The blood pressure is measured immediately after the blood is drawn; an increase of more than 20/15 mm Hg above the cold pressor blood pressure increase is also considered positive but is insensitive.

Clonidine Suppression Test

In the unusual case with equivocal testing and diastolic blood pressure higher than 100 mm Hg or a condition contraindicating a provocative test, the clonidine suppression test may be employed.

The patient should have any β-adrenergic blocking agent stopped for at least 48–72 hours prior to testing. Good hydration should be assured. The patient must be supine for at least 30 minutes with an intravenous line as described above. Clonidine, 0.3 mg, is adminis-tered orally. Blood is collected 2 and 3 hours afterward and assayed for *free catecholamines*. Most assays for plasma catecholamines mea-sure both conjugated and free hormone; the longer half-life of conju-gated catecholamines can cause a misleading appearance of nonsup-pressibility (a false-positive test). Following clonidine administration, patients with a pheochromocytoma ordinarily have plasma levels of total free catecholamines above 500 pg/mL.

LOCALIZATION

After the presence of a pheochromocytoma has been established biochemically, the patient is prepared for surgery (see Treatment, below), and preoperative localization studies are performed.

CT Scan

Preoperative localization is quite helpful; it is of course absolutely essential to exclude a neck, pelvic, or chest tumor. All patients suspected of harboring a pheochromocytoma must have a careful neck palpation as well as abdominal palpation and a rectal/pelvic examina-tion. Patients should also have a chest x-ray with oblique as well as routine views; CT or MRI of the thoracic spine for paraganglioma are done when indicated. Since 90% of pheochromocytomas are adrenal in origin, the adrenal CT scan ordinarily detects the tumor. If the initial

CT imaging of the adrenals fails to demonstrate a mass, the CT field should be widened to include the rest of the abdomen. In the event a tumor is still not found, pelvic ultrasound may disclose it.

Epinephrine

In the event no tumor is localized, a suggestion of its location can be derived from the urinary or plasma-fractionated catecholamine data: a high production of epinephrine indicates an adrenal origin, since extra-adrenal pheochromocytomas generally produce mainly norepinephrine.

^{131}I-MIBG

Scintigraphy using ^{123}I or ^{131}I-metaiodobenzylguanidine (^{131}I-MIBG) may be useful for finding an occult pheochromocytoma or confirming that a mass found by CT scan, routine x-ray, or palpation is a pheochromocytoma. ^{131}I-MIBG selectively accumulates in tissues that store catecholamines. To reduce thyroid uptake of free ^{131}I, 5 drops of Lugol's solution are given 3 times daily on the day before, the day of, and for 7 days following the injection of ^{131}I-MIBG. ^{123}I or ^{131}I-MIBG (0.5 mCi/1.7 m^2 body surface area) is given intravenously and gamma camera scanning performed 1, 2, 3, and occasionally 5 days afterwards. The isotope is taken up preferentially by about 85% of both benign and malignant pheochromocytomas.

False extra-adrenal positives are unusual. Uptake in the normal adrenal and renal pelvis is common on day 1. When this occurs, the scan is repeated after 3 and 5 days. False negatives are more common in patients taking tricyclic antidepressants (within 6 weeks prior to test). Reserpine, phenothiazines, haloperidol, thiothixene, cocaine, amphetamines, nasal decongestants, and phenylpropanolamine HCl (anorexiant) may also cause decreased uptake (if taken within 2 weeks prior to test). Labetalol may cause some decreased uptake but is not an absolute contraindication to the test.

Consider ^{131}I-MIBG for screening in MEN IIa and MEN IIb (15% positive), von Recklinghausen's disease (10% positive, of which 75% are extra-adrenal), medullary thyroid carcinoma (15% positive), and paragangliomas. Unresectable tumors may be treated with ^{131}I-MIBG, 300 mCi.

Selective venous sampling for plasma catecholamines is seldom necessary for localization and should only be done in a patient under good medical treatment in whom the diagnosis is secure and all other localization steps have failed. If the tumor is in the abdomen and has not been further localized preoperatively, exploration at surgery can identify its location. In addition, the possibility of multiple tumors makes abdominal exploration (rather than flank approach) imperative.

INCIDENTALLY DISCOVERED ADRENAL MASS

Adrenal nodularity is common. Small (1–6 cm in diameter) benign nodules are found in up to 9% of unselected autopsies. They are also common in the general population. Routine CT scans of the abdomen run for other purposes demonstrate an adrenal nodule in about 0.7% of cases; most are benign. Larger nodules (larger than 6 cm) are less likely benign. An adrenal mass discovered incidentally during another radiologic procedure must therefore be approached with caution in order to avoid unnecessary surgery. Adrenal masses in patients with known cancer are most likely metastases. A mass discovered after major trauma is most likely hemorrhagic. Such posttrauma patients require evaluation for adrenal insufficiency or excess secretion, but exploratory surgery is usually not required. A repeat CT scan can be performed in 2, 6, and 18 months to detect any growth.

A suggested approach in a nontrauma patient is diagrammed in Fig 6–5. Biochemical assessment should consist of screening for (1) pheochromocytoma: 24-hour urine for total catecholamines, VMA, metanephrine, and creatinine; (2) Cushing's syndrome: 1-mg overnight dexamethasone at 11 PM with an 8 AM plasma cortisol; (3) hyperaldosteronism in hypertensive patients, with a plasma potassium drawn while the patient is receiving no diuretics and a diet containing more than 200 mEq sodium and less than 100 mEq potassium daily. Also obtain a chest x-ray to screen for cancer, systemic tuberculosis, and fungal infections.

MRI may assist the diagnosis in certain cases. Venous varicosities from high portal pressures have a low-intensity signal.

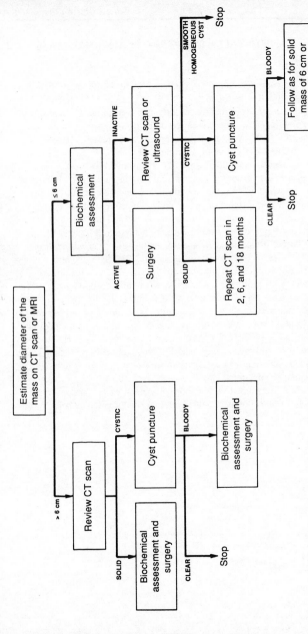

Figure 6–5. Approach to the nontrauma patient with an adrenal mass.

REFERENCES

Adrenal Anatomy & Imaging

Boechat MI: Magnetic resonance imaging of abdominal and pelvic masses in children. *Top Magn Reson Imaging* 1990;**3**:25.

Bretan PN Jr et al: Adrenal imaging: Computed tomographic scanning and magnetic resonance imaging. *Urol Clin North Am* 1989;**16**:505.

Egglin TK et al: MRI of the adrenal glands. *Semin Roentgenol* 1988;**23**:280.

Newhouse JH: MRI of the adrenal gland. *Urol Radiol* 1990;**12**:1.

Silverman ML et al: Anatomy and pathology of the adrenal glands. *Urol Clin North Am* 1989;**16**:417.

Addison's Disease

Ahonen P et al: Clinical variation of autoimmune polyendocrinopathy-candidiasis-ectodermal dystrophy (APECED) in a series of 68 patients. *N Engl J Med* 1990;**322**:1829.

Biglieri EG: Adrenocortical function in AIDS. *West J. Med* 1988;**145**:70.

Burke BA et al: Congenital adrenal hypoplasia and selected absence of luteinizing hormone: A new autosomal recessive syndrome. *Am J Med Genet* 1988;**31**:75.

Dahlberg PJ et al: Adrenal insufficiency secondary to adrenal hemorrhage: Two case reports and review of cases confirmed by CT. *Arch Intern Med* 1990;**150**:905.

Fitzpatrick PM et al: Report of an unusual case of postpartum adrenal hemorrhage in a young woman. *Am J Med 1989*;**86**:487. Comment in *Am J Med* 1989;**87**:4.

Groves RW et al: Corticosteroid replacement therapy: Twice or thrice daily? *J R Soc Med* 1988;**81**:514.

Heij HA et al: Diagnosis and management of neonatal adrenal hemorrhage. *Pediatr Radiol* 1989;**19**:391.

Inman K: Alopecia universalis as a feature of polyglandular autoimmunity type I. *West J Med* 1988;**149**:338.

Mier A: Respiratory muscle weakness in Addison's disease. *Br Med J* 1988;**297**:457.

Neufield M et al: Two types of Addison's disease associated with different polyglandular autoimmune (PGA) syndromes. *Medicine* 1981;**60**:355.

Osborne TM et al: Disseminated tuberculosis causing acute adrenal failure: CT findings with post mortem correlation. *Australas Radiol* 1988;**32**:394.

Rao RH et al: Bilateral massive adrenal hemorrhage: Early recognition and treatment. Ann Intern Med 1989;**110**:227. Comment in *Ann Intern Med* 1989;**111**:185.

Sadeghi-Nejad A. Senior B. Adrenomyeloneuropathy presenting as Addison's disease in childhood. *N Engl J Med* 1990;**322**:13.

Seidenwurm DJ et al: Metastases to the adrenal glands and the development of Addison's Disease. *Cancer* 1984;**54**:552.

Shapiro MS et al: Myalgias and muscle contractions as the presenting sign of Addison's disease. *Postgrad Med J* 1988;**64**:953.

Stewart PM et al: The medical treatment of adrenal disease. *Br J Hosp Med* 1989;**42**:20.

Tobin MV et al: Addison's disease presenting as anorexia nervosa in a young man. *Postgrad Med J* 1988;**64**:953.

Vita JA et al: Clinical clues to the cause of Addison's disease. *Am J Med* 1985;**78**:461.

Woeber KA: Adrenal apoplexy revisited. *West J Med* 1989;**150**:582.

Hyperkalemia & Selective Hypoaldosteronism

Aldo M, Warnock, DG: Hyperkalemia. (Medical Staff Conference.) *West J Med* 1984;**141**:666.

Almeida OD Jr et al: Maternal Bartter's syndrome and pregnancy. *Am J. Obstet Gynecol* 1989;**160**:1225.

Armanini D et al: Aldosterone-receptor deficiency in pseudohypoaldosteronism. *N Engl J Med* 1985;**313**:1178.

Edelman S et al: Hyperkalemia during treatment with HMG-CoA reductase inhibitor. (Letter.) *N Engl J Med* 1989;**320**:1219.

Grande Villoria J et al: Hyporeninemic hypoaldosteronism in diabetic patients with chronic renal failure. *Am J Nephrol* 1988;**8**:127.

Ralston SH et al: Rheumatoid arthritis: An unrecognized cause of pseudo-hyperkalemia. *Br Med J* 1988;**297**: 523.

Take C et al: Increased chloride reabsorption as an inherited renal tubular defect in familial type II pseudohypoaldosteronism. *N Engl J Med* 1991;**324**:472. [Editorial, p. 488.]

Hypokalemia, Hypertension, & Mineralocorticoid Excess

Arteaga E et al: Aldosterone-producing adrenocortical carcinoma: Preoperative recognition and course in three cases. *Ann Intern Med* 1984;**101**:316.

Biglieri EG: Spectrum of mineralocorticoid hypertension. *Hypertension* 1991;**17**:251.

Bravo EL: Primary aldosteronism. *Urol Clin North Am* 1989;**16**:481.

Clementsen P et al: Bartter's syndrome treatment with potassium, spironolactone and ACE inhibitor. *J Intern Med* 1989;**225**:107.

Gelmont DM: Hypokalemia induced by inhaled bronchodilators. *Chest* 1988;**94**:763.

Gordon RD et al: Unexpected incidence of low blood pressure 2 years after unilateral adrenalectomy for primary aldosteronism. *Clin Exp Pharmacol Physiol* 1989;**16**:281.

Horky K et al: Long-term results of surgical and conservative treatment of patients with primary aldosteronism. *Exp Clin Endocrinol* 1987;**90**:337.

Ikeda DM et al: The detection of adrenal tumors and hyperplasia in patients with primary aldosteronism: Comparison of scintigraphy, CT and MRI imaging. *Am J Roentgenol* 1989;**153**:301.

Lapworth R et al: 18-Hydroxycorticosterone as a marker for primary hyper-aldosteronism. *Ann Clin Biochem* 1989;**26**:227.

Ma JT et al: Fifty cases of primary hyperaldosteronism in Hong Kong Chinese with a high frequency of periodic paralysis: Evaluation of techniques for tumour localisation. *Q J Med* 1986;**61**:1021.

Matsumoto J et al: Hypercalciuric Bartter's syndrome: Resolution of neph-rocalcinosis with indomethicin. *Am J Roentgenol* 1989;**152**:1251.

Melby JC: Endocrine hypertension. *J Clin Endocrinol Metab* 1989;**69**:697.

Morales JM: Long-term enalapril therapy in Bartter's syndrome. (Letter.) *Nephron* 1988;**48**:327.

Noth RH et al: Primary hyperaldosteronism. *Med Clin North Am* 1988;**72**:1117.

Takeuchi K et al: Plasma aldosterone level in a female case of pseudohyper-aldosteronism (Liddle's syndrome). *Endocrinol Jpn* 1989;**36**:167.

Young WF Jr et al: Primary aldosteronism: Diagnosis and treatment. *Mayo Clin Proc* 1990;**65**:96.

Young WF Jr et al: Primary aldosteronism: Diagnostic evaluation. *Endocrinol Metab Clin North Am* 1988;**17**:367.

Cushing's Syndrome
Cushing's Disease

Amado JA et al: Successful treatment with ketoconazole of Cushing's syndrome in pregnancy. *Postgrad Med J* 1990;**66**:221.

Carpenter PC: Diagnostic evaluation of Cushing's syndrome. *Endocrinol Metab Clin North Am* 1988;**17**:445.

Cook DM et al: Failure of hypophysectomy to correct pituitary-dependent Cushing's disease in two patients. *Arch Intern Med* 1988;**148**:2498.

Fitzgerald PA et al: Cushing's disease: Transient secondary adrenal insufficiency after selective removal of pituitary adenomas; evidence for a pituitary origin. *J Clin Endocrinol Metab* 1982;**54**:413.

Freidberg SR: Transsphenoidal pituitary surgery in the treatment of patients with Cushing's disease. *Urol Clin North Am* 1989;**16**:589.

Gardner DF et al: Cushing's disease in two sisters. *Am J Med Sci* 1989;**297**:387.

Gorden P et al: Somatostatin and somatostatin analogue (SMS 201-995) in treatment of hormone-secreting tumors of the pituitary and gastrointestinal tract and non-neoplastic diseases of the gut. *Ann Intern Med* 1989;**110**:35.

Hale AC: A bromocriptine-responsive corticotroph adenoma secreting alpa-MSH in a patient with Cushing's disease. *Clin Endocrinol (Oxf)* 1988;**28**:215.

Hearn PR et al: Lung carcinoid with Cushing's syndrome: Control of serum ACTH and cortisol levels using SMS 201-995 (Sandostatin). *Clin Endocrinol (Oxf)* 1988;**28**:181.

Invitti C et al: Treatment of Cushing's syndrome with the long-acting somatostatin analogue SMS 201-995 (Sandostatin). *Clin Endocrinol* 1990;**32**:275.

Kaye TB, Crapo L: The Cushing syndrome: An update on diagnostic tests. *Ann Intern Med* 1990;**112**:434.

Kelly W et al: Long-term treatment of Nelson's syndrome with sodium valproate. *Clin Endocrinol (Oxf)* 1988;**28**:195.

Lamberts SW et al: The effect of the long-acting somatostatin analogue SMS 201-995 on ACTH secretion in Nelson's syndrome and Cushing's disease. *Acta Endocrinol (Copenh)* 1989;**120**:760.

Leinung MC et al: Diagnosis of corticotropin-producing bronchial carcinoid tumors causing Cushing's syndrome. *Mayo Clinic Proc* 1990;**65**:1314.

Pass HI et al: Management of the ectopic ACTH syndrome due to thoracic carcinoids. *Ann Thorac Surg* 1990;**50**:52.

Peck WW et al: High resolution MR imaging of pituitary microadenomas at 1.5 T: experience with Cushing diseases. *AJNR* 1988;**9**:1085.

Tindall GT: Cushing's disease: Results of transsphenoidal microsurgery with emphasis on surgical failures. *J Neurosurg* 1990;**72**:363.

Adrenal Tumors

Adrenal carcinoma. (Case Records of the Massachusetts General Hospital.) *N Engl J Med* 1991;**324**:400.

Bertagna C, Orth DN: Clinical and laboratory findings and results of therapy in 58 patients with adrenocortical tumors admitted to a single medical center (1951–1978). *Am J Med* 1981;**71:**855.

Boven E et al: Complete response of metastasized adrenal carcinoma with *o,p'*DDD: Case report and literature review. *Cancer* 1984;**53:**26.

Didolkar MS: et al: Natural history of adrenal cortical carcinoma: A clinicopathologic study of 42 patients. *Cancer* 1981;**47:**2153.

Dunnick NR et al: Percutaneous biopsy of the kidney and adrenal gland. *Urol Radiol* 1990;**12:**125.

Hughes S et al: The surgical treatment of adrenal disease. *Br J Hosp Med* 1989;**41:**350.

Huiras CM et al: Adrenal insufficiency after operative removal of apparently nonfunctioning adrenal adenomas. *JAMA* 1989;**261:**894.

Libertino JA: Surgery of adrenal disorders. *Surg Clin North Am* 1988;**68:**1027.

Luton J-P et al: Clinical features of adrenocortical carcinoma, prognostic factors, and the effect of mitotane therapy. *N Engl J Med* 1990;**322:**1195.

Moriyama N et al: The appearance of adrenal myelolipoma as seen on nuclear magnetic resonance imaging. *Br J Urol* 1988;**62:**3874.

Novick AC et al: Posterior transthoracic approach for adrenal surgery. *J Urol* 1989;**141:**254.

Paivansalo M et al: Ultrasound in the detection of adrenal tumours. *Eur J Radiol* 1988;**8:**183.

Nodular Adrenal Hyperplasia

Aron DC et al: Pituitary ACTH dependency of nodular adrenal hyperplasia in Cushing's syndrome. *Am J Med* 1981;**71:**302.

Cheitlin R et al: Cushing's syndrome due to macronodular adrenal hyperplasia without ACTH: Culture of cells on extracellular matrix. *Horm Res* 1988;**29:**162.

McArthur RG et al: Primary adrenocortical nodular dysplasia as a cause of Cushing's syndrome in infants and children. *Mayo Clin Proc* 1982;**57:**58.

Smals AGH et al: Macronodular adrenocortical hyperplasia in long-standing Cushing's disease. *J Clin Endocrinol Metab* 1984;**58:**25.

Young WF Jr et al: Familial Cushing's syndrome due to primary pigmented nodular adrenocortical disease: Reinvestigation 50 years later. *N Engl J Med* 1989;**321:**1659.

Glucocorticoid Therapy

Dixon RB, Christy NP: On the various forms of corticosteroid withdrawal syndrome. *Am J Med* 1980;**68:**224.

Horber FF et al: Evidence that prednisone-induced myopathy is reversed by physical training. *J Clin Endocrinol Metab* 1985;**61:**83.

Pheochromocytoma

Averbuch SD et al: Malignant pheochromocytoma: Effective treatment with a combination of cyclosphosphamide, vincristine and dacarbazine. *Ann Intern Med* 1988;**109:**267.

Benowitz NL: Pheochromocytoma. *Adv Intern Med* 1990;**35:**195.

Brendel AJ et al: Radionuclide therapy of pheochromocytomas and neuroblastomas using iodine-131 metaiodobenzylguanidine (MIBG). *Clin Nucl Med* 1989;**14:**19.

Calhoun DA, Oparil S: Treatment of hypertensive crisis. *N Engl J Med* 1990;**323:**1171.

Connor CS et al: Pitfalls in the diagnosis of pheochromocytoma. *Ann Surg* 1988;**54:**634.

Greene JP et al: New perspectives in pheochromocytoma. *Urol Clin North Am* 1989;**16:**487.

Guo JC et al: Malignant pheochromocytoma: Diagnosis and treatment in fifteen cases. *J Hypertens* 1989;**7:**261.

Konings JE et al: Diagnosis and treatment of malignant pheochromocytoma with ^{131}I-meta-iodobenzylguanidine: A case report. *Radiother Oncol* 1990;**17:**103.

Limone P et al: ^{131}I-meta-iodobenzylguanidine for the diagnosis and treatment of pheochromocytoma. *Panminerva Med* 1988;**30:**169.

Malone MJ et al: Preoperative and surgical management of pheochromocytoma. *Urol Clin North Am* 1989;**16:**567.

Nakagani Y et al: A case of malignant pheochromocytoma treated with ^{131}I-metaiodobenzylguanadine and alpha methyl-p-tyrosine. *Jpn J Med* 1990; **29:**329.

Samaan NA et al: Diagnosis, localization and management of pheochromocytoma: Pitfalls and follow-up in 41 patients. *Cancer* 1988;**62:**2451.

Shapiro B, Fig LM: Management of pheochromocytoma. *Endocrinol Metab Clin North Am* 1989;**18:**443.

Sheps SG et al: Recent developments in the diagnosis and treatment of pheochromocytoma. *Mayo Clin Proc* 1990;**65:**88.

Sisson JC et al: Radiopharmaceutical treatment of malignant pheochromocytoma. *J Nucl Med* 1984;**25:**197.

Stein PP, Black HR: A simplified diagnostic approach to pheochromocytoma: A review of the literature and report of one institution's experience. *Medicine* 1991;**70:**46.

Troncone L et al: The diagnostic and therapeutic utility of radioiodinated metaiodobenzylguanidine (MIBG): 5 years experience. *Eur J Nucl Med* 1990;**16:**325.

Velchik MG et al: Localization of pheochromocytoma: MIBG, CT and MRI correlation. *J Nucl Med* 1989;**30:**328.

Incidentally Discovered Adrenal Mass

Baker ME et al: MR evaluation of adrenal masses at 1.5 tesla. *Am J Roentgenol* 1989;**153:**307.

Bitter DA et al: Incidentally discovered adrenal masses. *Am J Surg* 1989;**158:**159.

Copeland PM: The incidentally discovered adrenal mass. *Ann Intern Med* 1983;**98:**940.

Hubbard MM et al: Nonfunctioning adrenal tumors: Dilemmas in management. *Ann Surg* 1989;**55:**516.

Ross NS, Aron DC: Hormonal evaluation of the patient with an incidentally discovered adrenal mass. *N Engl J Med* 1990;**323:**1401.

Virkkala A et al: Endocrine abnormalities in patients with adrenal tumours incidentally discovered on computed tomography. *Acta Endocrinol (Copenh)* 1989;**121:**67.

Calcium & Bone Metabolism | 7

Dolores Shoback, MD, & Michael W. Draper, MD, PhD

PHYSIOLOGY

Maintenance of mineral homeostasis is a complex process requiring the integrated function of several different organs. The mineral ions, namely, calcium, magnesium, and phosphorus, are important constituents of the skeleton and also participate in a variety of vital biochemical reactions involving muscle contraction, blood clotting, hormone action, and secretion. For these reasons, serum concentrations of these ions are precisely regulated.

Maintenance of Serum Calcium

The mineral metabolic system maintains a normal serum calcium concentration by balancing gastrointestinal calcium absorption with calcium loss. In the normal North American adult, daily calcium loss in the urine and feces is about 600 mg. The ordinary, daily North American diet contains 0.5–1 g elemental calcium. The gastrointestinal tract may vary the fractional calcium absorption between 0.1 and 0.7, and thus excreted calcium can be replaced by absorbed calcium. During periods in which positive calcium balance is required (growth, pregnancy, lactation), a combination of increased intake and maximal absorption will meet the need. In older persons, both calcium intake and fractional calcium absorption usually decline, and the potential for calcium deficiency develops.

Parathyroid hormone (PTH) regulates the serum calcium concentration through its effects on bone and kidney. Secretion of PTH from the parathyroid glands is regulated by serum calcium levels. A low serum calcium concentration stimulates PTH secretion, while a high calcium level suppresses it. Calcium metabolism exhibits the characteristics of a classical "negative feedback" physiologic system.

PTH acts on the kidney in 2 ways: the kidney regulates short-term calcium concentrations via selective tubular reabsorption of calcium. This process is stimulated by PTH. The kidney also generates one of the hormones vital to mineral homeostasis: 1,25-dihydroxyvitamin D [1,25(OH)$_2$-D]. 1,25(OH)$_2$-D is the most biologically potent

SOME ACRONYMS USED IN THIS CHAPTER

CRF	Chronic renal failure
DHT	Dihydrotachysterol
FHH	Familial hypocalciuric hypercalcemia
iPTH	Immunoreactive PTH
IRMA	Immunoradiometric assay
MEN	Multiple endocrine neoplasia
MTC	Medullary thyroid carcinoma
PHP	Pseudohypoparathyroidism
PTH	Parathyroid hormone
PTHRP	PTH–related peptide
RTA	Renal tubular acidosis

vitamin D metabolite known. The renal 1-hydroxylase enzyme responsible for production of $1,25(OH)_2$-D is stimulated by elevated PTH levels and by hypophosphatemia. In turn, $1,25(OH)_2$-D enhances mineral absorption from the gastrointestinal tract.

PTH regulates calcium turnover in the skeleton in a complex and poorly understood manner. Other bone-derived factors and vitamin D metabolites are also involved in the control of skeletal mineral metabolism.

Bone turnover involves both resorption of preformed bone and new bone formation in a carefully balanced, continuous process. When local skeletal metabolic activities are properly balanced, bone turnover rates can vary over a wide range, with no net effect on overall calcium homeostasis.

Under normal circumstances, any perturbation of serum calcium concentration will elicit an appropriate compensatory response, resulting in a return of serum calcium to normal levels. In a hypercalcemic state, PTH secretion will be suppressed. Renal reabsorption of calcium falls, and $1,25(OH)_2$-D production declines. Gastrointestinal calcium absorption is thereby decreased. These processes return the elevated serum calcium level toward normal. Hypocalcemia, on the other hand, elicits the opposite set of responses, also leading toward normal serum calcium concentration.

HYPERCALCEMIA

Determining the cause of hypercalcemia is one of the most important diagnostic challenges in clinical endocrinology (Table 7–1). The most significant disorders are treated individually in follow-

Table 7–1. Causes of hypercalcemia.

Artifact	Immobilization (especially with
Laboratory error	Paget's disease)
High serum protein concentration	Thyrotoxicosis
Dehydration	Adrenal insufficiency
Excess tourniquet time	Granulomatous disease (eg,
Primary hyperparathyroidism	sarcoidosis or histoplasmosis)
Sporadic cases	Acute renal failure (especially
Familial variants	diuretic phase)
Familial hypocalciuric	Infancy
hypercalcemia	Idiopathic (sensitivity to
Hypercalcemia of malignancy	vitamin D)
Solid tumors	Maternal gestational
Multiple myeloma	hypocalcemia
Adult T-cell leukemia/lymphoma	
Medications	
Thiazides	
Lithium carbonate	
Vitamin preparations (vitamins A	
and D)	
Calcium and antacids	
(milk-alkali syndrome)	

ing sections. Others will be mentioned in the discussion of related problems. In dealing with any case of hypercalcemia, establishing the correct diagnosis is of prime importance. Management, specific treatment, and prognosis all depend heavily on the cause of the elevated serum calcium.

Elevated serum calcium may be first encountered in a patient on a multichannel screen of serum chemistry values, or as one of a number of abnormal values in a seriously ill patient. When clinical conditions permit, repeat determination is warranted. If total serum calcium is indeed elevated, an estimate should be made of the active fraction of serum calcium, ie, ionized calcium. Under normal conditions of pH and protein concentration, plasma calcium will be about 50% free (ionized) and about 50% complexed or protein-bound. Albumin is the most important binding protein for calcium in the plasma, although under unusual conditions (such as in multiple myeloma), other plasma proteins may contribute significantly to calcium binding. A simple formula permits conversion of the total serum calcium to reflect an estimate of true ionized calcium in states of abnormal albumin concentration. If 4 g/dL is taken as normal reference level for serum albumin, then 0.8 mg/dL should be added to the observed serum calcium for every 1 g/dL of serum albumin above this reference level, and 0.8 mg/dL subtracted from serum calcium for every 1 g/dL serum albumin below this level. This correction is adequate for most clinical purposes. Acidemia will increase the fraction of free calcium in the serum, while alkalemia will reduce it, but this correction is significant only in severe cases of acid-base imbalance. In an occasional case, a difficult diagnostic problem may be resolved by direct determination of ionized calcium, a determination now available in many large reference laboratories. For most clinical purposes, however, total serum calcium is sufficiently precise and reproducible.

In dealing with a case of hypercalcemia, an assessment of plasma volume status should be made before a hypercalcemic workup is initiated. Total serum calcium is inversely related to plasma volume, and appropriate rehydration may fully correct a volume-contraction hypercalcemia and eliminate the need for further workup. The prudent course in a volume-depleted patient is to assume that hypercalcemia is real until volume status has been corrected, but then to proceed only if hypercalcemia persists.

Manifestations of Hypercalcemia

Symptoms may be "constitutional," with weakness, dizziness, anorexia, nausea, abdominal pain, constipation, and emotional irritability most commonly described in association with mild hypercalcemia. Polyuria and polydipsia may reflect nephrogenic diabetes insipidus induced by the hypercalcemic state. More severe hypercalcemia may be accelerated by dehydration from poor oral intake and may present with confusion, ataxia, frank psychosis, coma, cardiac arrhythmias, and even convulsions and death. In the patient on digitalis, hypercalcemia predisposes to digitalis toxicity. This may be either a direct effect or one due to iatrogenic hypokalemia induced by therapeutic diuresis for the hypercalcemic state. Hypertension, muscle weakness, or pancreatitis may occur with hypercalcemia of any origin. Deposits of calcium salts may occur in the sclera, resulting in band keratopathy.

PRIMARY HYPERPARATHYROIDISM

Primary hyperparathyroidism is one of the most common of all endocrine disorders (incidence in adults is about 1/1000). Since many patients with this disease are asymptomatic for many years, the disorder only became widely diagnosed with the advent of autoanalyzer screening of serum calcium. With increased detection, however, controversies have arisen concerning prudent management.

PARATHYROID ANATOMY & PHYSIOLOGY

Under normal circumstances, the parathyroid glands occur in 2 pairs, with the 4 glands weighing a total of 120–150 mg. The superior pair arises from the fourth branchial pouch and usually resides just dorsolateral to the thyroid, on either side, at the level of the thyroid isthmus. The inferior pair arises from the third branchial pouch and has a variable final location in the adult. Inferior parathyroid glands are usually found somewhere between the inferior pole of the thyroid and the superior mediastinum. In addition, nearly one in 20 individuals has 5 or more parathyroid glands. The supernumerary glands usually reside inferior to the thyroid or in the mediastinum. The variable location and number of parathyroid glands sometimes lead to problems for the parathyroid surgeon.

The parathyroid glands secrete PTH (an 84-amino acid peptide) in response to hypocalcemia. Secretion is inhibited by hypercalcemia, as well as by severe hypermagnesemia or hypomagnesemia. PTH raises serum calcium by directly stimulating bone resorption and by stimulating renal secretion of $1,25(OH)_2$-D, which causes increased calcium absorption from the gut. PTH also stimulates the renal tubular reabsorption of calcium; however, severe or extended hypercalcemia will overwhelm this effect and produce hypercalciuria. PTH also causes the renal tubule to excrete phosphate and bicarbonate.

The pathophysiology of primary hyperparathyroidism has not been clearly defined. The increase in functioning parathyroid mass that accompanies primary hyperparathyroidism clearly plays a role. An altered ''set-point'' for calcium (defined as the calcium concentration required for half-maximal suppression of PTH secretion) has been demonstrated in tissues from patients with this disease. This set-point abnormality may be responsible for the hypersecretion of PTH—despite the presence of hypercalcemia—which is the hallmark of primary hyperparathyroidism.

CLINICAL FEATURES

Primary hyperparathyroidism is a disease of adults, with significantly rising incidence after age 45 and a female predominance of about 2:1. A single parathyroid adenoma is found in over 80% of cases, while hyperplasia of multiple parathyroid glands accounts for about half of the remaining cases. Multiple adenomata and parathyroid carcinoma occur unusually in this disease. Primary hyperparathyroidism may present (about 5% of cases) in a familial form, including its association with various multiple endocrine neoplasia (MEN) syndromes. Diffuse parathyroid hyperplasia accounts for a disproportionately large number of cases when a positive family history is obtained. Clinical features do not distinguish between adenomatous and hyperplastic hyperparathyroidism. Previous neck irradiation is a significant risk factor for primary hyperparathyroidism, in addition to its established association with thyroid cancer.

Symptoms

Since most primary hyperparathyroidism is now discovered through routine serum calcium screening, many patients are asymptomatic at the time of diagnosis. When symptoms are present, they are usually those described in association with hypercalcemia of any cause.

Gastrointestinal complaints may suggest the presence of peptic ulcer disease or pancreatitis, both of which may appear more frequently than usual in patients with primary hyperparathyroidism. Typical renal or ureteral colic may lead to a diagnosis of kidney stones. Bone pain is not usually associated with mild primary hyperparathyroidism, although osteitis fibrosa cystica, the bone disease of severe hyperparathyroidism, may be manifested by bone pain and symptomatic fractures.

Signs

In mild to moderate cases of hyperparathyroidism, few clinical signs are apparent. Those present are probably related to the degree of elevation of the serum calcium. Hypertension and tachycardia may be associated with hyperparathyroidism, although cause-and-effect relationships are ill-defined. Altered mental status is commonly ascribed to another cause until hypercalcemia is suspected and confirmed, particularly in the hyperparathyroid patient who presents with little else to suggest this disease.

LABORATORY FEATURES

Laboratory Tests

Hypercalcemia, without appropriate suppression of PTH values, is the sine qua non for the diagnosis of primary hyperparathyroidism. Hypercalcemia may be mild and even intermittent, or it may be masked by complicating conditions, such as calcium malabsorption in Vitamin D–deficient patients. In normal individuals, hypercalcemia would be associated with suppressed serum immunoreactive parathyroid hormone (iPTH) levels. Hypercalcemia with elevated or high-normal iPTH values is, therefore, suggestive of hyperparathyroidism. An inverse relationship between serum calcium levels and iPTH is seen in most patients with primary hyperparathyroidism who are studied over time. This finding suggests that the parathyroids in this disorder are not totally autonomous but rather respond in a qualitatively normal, but quantitatively altered fashion, to serum calcium levels.

PTH is measured in the serum by RIA using one of a number of antisera raised against the intact PTH molecule or its fragments. The amino-terminal portion of the molecule is responsible for biological activity; however, antisera directed toward this region detect principally short-lived species of the hormone. In the past, mid- and carboxy-region antisera proved to be most useful in measuring clinically relevant levels of PTH, in spite of the fact that these antisera recognize a biologically inactive region of the molecule. The fact that clearance of carboxy-terminal fragments occurs in the kidney results in artifactually high iPTH values in renal failure. In primary hyperparathyroidism, mid- and carboxy-region PTH values are virtually always elevated or are inappropriate to the level of the hypercalcemia. In the best of these assays, at a given serum calcium level, there is minimal overlap between PTH levels in primary hyperparathyroidism (high) and those in other hypercalcemic disorders (normal or low), although no level of iPTH is absolutely diagnostic of any particular disease. Interpretation of iPTH levels must be made in the context of the serum calcium and with attention to situations that may lead to *secondary* hyperparathyroidism.

In recent years, mid- and carboxy-terminal PTH assays have been largely supplanted by intact assays in many laboratories. The immunoradiometric assay (IRMA) for PTH utilizes both N-terminal and mid-region or carboxy-terminal antisera to determine the level of biologically active PTH in serum (Fig 7–1). The N-terminal antiserum is radiolabeled, while the mid-region or carboxy-terminal antiserum is coated to a solid phase such as a bead. Species of PTH in the serum that contain the N-terminal sequence of the hormone are bound to the first antibody. PTH fragments that contain mid-region or carboxy-terminal determinants of the hormone will bind to the other antibody. The solid and liquid phases are then separated. Only intact, full-length PTH, containing both N- and mid-region or carboxy-terminal determinants, is bound to both the labeled N-terminal antiserum and to the antibody coated to the solid phase and will be counted in the assay.

Serum iPTH levels rise with age. This effect is probably due to decreased gastrointestinal absorption of calcium (vitamin D deficiency?), or decreased functional renal mass in this age group. If only "very healthy" elderly individuals are examined, the iPTH levels tend to be relatively normal.

In mild hyperparathyroidism, especially in its early stages, urinary calcium excretion may be suppressed owing to increased,

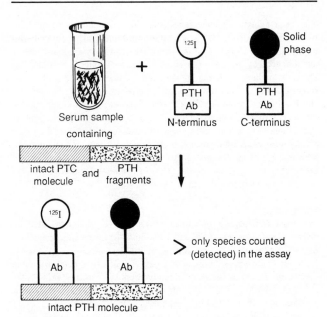

Figure 7–1. Two-site immunoradiometric assay for PTH. Serum sample containing intact PTH and its fragments is reacted with 2 region-specific antisera for PTH. One antibody for example, the C-terminal antibody, is bound to a solid-phase, and the other, which recognizes the N-terminal portion of the molecule, is ^{125}I-labeled. Only intact PTH containing the ^{125}I-label and bound to the solid phase shown by the uppermost drawing is counted in the assay.

PTH-mediated, calcium reabsorption in the kidney. In established hyperparathyroidism, however, the increased filtered calcium load ultimately leads to hypercalciuria. Serum phosphorus levels are usually decreased in hyperparathyroidism owing to PTH-mediated suppression of tubular phosphorus threshold (TmP/GFR). In severe or long-standing hyperparathyroidism, non-anion-gap metabolic acidosis may be seen. Serum alkaline phosphatase level is elevated in 10–20% of cases of hyperparathyroidism, reflecting the PTH-induced increase in metabolic turnover in skeletal tissue.

X-Rays

In mild hyperparathyroidism radiologic findings are seldom, if ever, significant. Nephrolithiasis or nephrocalcinosis may be revealed by routine x-rays or nephrotomograms, but these are not specific for hyperparathyroidism. Hand films done on high-grade industrial film may reveal subperiosteal resorption of the tufts or radial surfaces of distal phalanges, which is specific for hyperparathyroidism (Fig 7–2). Distal clavicular osteopenia, generalized osteoporosis, and evidence of fractures may be seen in cases of hyperparathyroidism, but are not specific for this disorder. Osteitis fibrosis cystica, the classic skeletal disorder of hyperparathyroidism, is no longer commonly seen, but an occasional case appears with severe bone disease. Cystic radiolucent areas and regions of increased bone density (osteosclerosis) may be seen (especially in the long bones). Skull demineralization may take on an irregular "ground glass" pattern. Chondrocalcinosis may also be seen, especially in the knee.

Special Tests

Bone densitometry may be helpful in some cases to determine the degree of osteopenia and treatment options. Nephrogenous production of cyclic AMP is a direct result of circulating bioactive PTH levels. Difficult diagnostic dilemmas can occasionally be solved with this measurement; however, increasingly popular intact PTH assays (IRMA) have largely replaced this test.

Because of the technical challenges that face the parathyroid surgeon, several techniques have been developed to preoperatively localize hyperfunctioning parathyroid tissue. The resolution using ultrasound or CT scan has now been refined to the point that most parathyroid adenomas larger than 1 cm can be localized. Another promising technique for noninvasive localization of parathyroid tissue is a thallium scan of the neck enhanced by subtraction of a technetium scan of the thyroid. Sensitive CT scanning is often helpful in detecting occult parathyroid adenomas, especially those in the mediastinum. Parathyroid angiography, selective venous catheterization, or magnetic resonance imaging may be useful in selected cases, particularly when reoperation has become necessary. The trend has been away from invasive tests.

TREATMENT

Acute Hypercalcemia (Hypercalcemic Crisis)

It has become unusual for a case of primary hyperparathyroidism to present with hypercalcemic crisis. Because the disease is slowly progressive, relatively high levels of serum calcium may be tolerated with few symptoms. In cases that are misdiagnosed, or in which denial or ignorance on the part of the patient or family delay diagnosis, genuine hypercalcemic crisis may still be seen in this disorder. Thera-

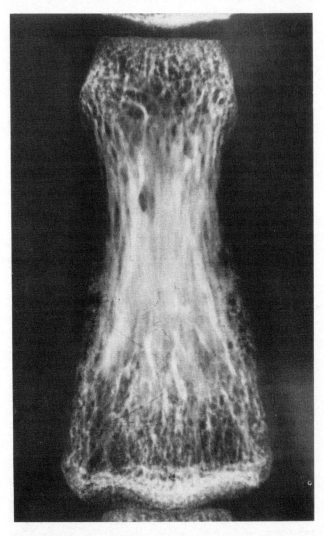

Figure 7–2. Finger showing subperiosteal resorption of bone found in hyperparathyroidism.

py of the hypercalcemic crisis is outlined below, in the section on hypercalcemia of malignancy.

Chronic Hypercalcemia

A. Medical: Medical management of primary hyperparathyroidism includes several options but often proves to be a difficult and frustrating endeavor. Mild degrees of hypercalcemia need only be treated in symptomatic cases or in situations in which the likelihood of development of complications is high. First-line treatment is to increase oral fluid intake with or without additional sodium chloride or furosemide (or both). This regimen is difficult for most patients to maintain, and potassium and magnesium deficiencies may develop if supplements are not given. Oral phosphate therapy may be very effective, but deposition of calcium phosphate salts in the soft tissues is a potential complication. Such therapy is contraindicated in the presence of renal failure, or if the patient is taking glucocorticoids. Phosphate therapy has a cathartic effect in many patients, and this limits long-term therapy.

B. Surgical: Surgery is required eventually for most patients with hyperparathyroidism, despite the generally indolent and asymptomatic progression of the disease. About half of asymptomatic patients will eventually develop a significant complication (renal stone, bone disease). With an experienced parathyroid surgeon, surgery is usually curative. When a single adenoma is clearly identified, simple removal of the gland containing the adenoma is usually sufficient. In hyperplastic disease, a subtotal ($\sim$3.5 of 4 glands) parathyroidectomy is commonly performed; such patients with hyperplasia have an increased risk for postoperative hypoparathyroidism or persistent hyperparathyroidism. Recurrent or persistent hyperparathyroidism may be due to supernumerary or ectopic glands. These glands may be deep in the mediastinum, in the thyroid, or in unusual locations. Most cases of persistent hyperparathyroidism, despite multiple operations, ultimately are shown to involve obscure, supernumerary glands. Increasing use is being made of preoperative localization techniques (see above) to guide the surgeon.

Surgical complications are rare with an experienced parathyroid surgeon. Recurrent laryngeal nerve damage is probably the most common. Postoperatively, hypocalcemia is a common occurrence. Early on, hypocalcemia may be due to suppression of residual normal parathyroid tissue by the hypercalcemic state, which may require a few days to adjust to normal function. Hypocalcemia may also reflect ''bone hunger,'' a process in which serum minerals are taken up by remineralizing osteopenic bone. In either case, if serum calcium falls below 8 mg/dL or if symptoms are reported, or signs can be elicited (see hypoparathyroid section), supplementation with calcium may be necessary. Oral supplements are usually sufficient (dairy products with high phosphorus content should be avoided), but occasionally intravenous calcium may be required. Persistent hypocalcemia may indicate that hypoparathyroidism has been induced. Recurrence of hypercalcemia will be seen if the hyperparathyroid state persists, and reoperation may be necessary. Uncomplicated cases are usually followed at least every 6 months to deal with the possibilities of hypoparathyroidism or recurrence of the hyperparathyroid state.

Parathyroid Carcinoma

This is a rare cause of parathyroid disorders ($< 2\%$ of primary hyperparathyroidism). It may be associated with rapid development of primary hyperparathyroidism, although some tumors are totally nonfunctional. It may remain relatively confined, spread locally, or even (rarely) metastasize. It may present as a mass in the neck, as the tumor invades and adheres to local tissues. Treatment is surgical, and multiple operations have often aided prolonged survival. Radiotherapy is ineffective.

MULTIPLE ENDOCRINE NEOPLASIA

In the evaluation of hypercalcemia a detailed family history is important, since hypercalcemia may be the presenting sign of one of a number of disorders of genetic origin known as multiple endocrine neoplasia (MEN). It is well recognized that certain kinds of tumors are seen with high prevalence within certain families. Furthermore, some of these tumors appear together in an individual patient in characteristic patterns. The MEN syndromes were once considered rare, but with heightened awareness and improved diagnostic techniques, MEN is now much more commonly and correctly diagnosed. The MEN syndromes may account for 5% of all hyperparathyroidism. Isolated familial hyperparathyroidism may merge into MEN syndromes; some consider it a simple variant of MEN and others the forme fruste of full-blown MEN.

Several theories have been advanced to explain the associations between the tumors of MEN, including those based on the neural-crest origin of tumor-producing tissues and others based on the presence of a circulating growth factor in MEN I patients that is mitogenic for parathyroid cells. None of the theories thus far presented adequately explains all the clinical observations. In addition, there are increasing reports of ''mixed'' or ''overlap'' cases in which the usual delineations within MEN syndromes break down. The gene for MEN IIA and

IIB has been recently mapped to chromosome 10, and intensive research efforts are under way to characterize the responsible gene or genes for these syndromes. The traditional classifications will be used in this brief discussion, but better pathophysiologic understanding of new MEN cases will eventually lead to revised categories within the MEN syndromes.

CLINICAL FEATURES

The traditional classification of MEN recognizes three distinct syndromes: MEN I, MEN IIa, and MEN IIb (Table 7–2). Patients with these syndromes are identified principally by one of 2 means. First, a patient may present with one of the individual tumors associated with MEN. The astute physician will consider the possibility that MEN may be involved, and appropriate investigation then defines the syndrome. Because of the autosomal dominant, high-penetrance nature of the MEN syndromes, family history must be vigorously pursued and family members given appropriate screening examinations. By this means, each time a new kindred is defined, a number of asymptomatic (preclinical) cases of MEN will be identified in the family of the presenting patient.

Table 7–2. Multiple endocrine neoplasia (MEN) syndromes.

	MEN I	MEN IIa	MEN IIb
Synonym	Wermer's syndrome	Sipple's syndrome	—
Genetics	Autosomal dominant	Autosomal dominant	Autosomal dominant(?)
Tumor types (% incidence)			
Parathyroid	>80%	50%	Rare
Pancreatic	75%	—	—
Pituitary	60%	—	—
Medullary thyroid carcinoma	—	>90%	80%
Pheochromocytoma	—	20%	60%
Mucosal and gastrointestinal ganglioneuromas	—	Rare	>90%
Lipoma	Occasional	—	—
Adrenocortical adenoma	Occasional	—	—
Carcinoid	Occasional	—	—
Thyroid adenoma	Occasional	—	—

MEN I is characterized by the presence of parathyroid, pancreatic, and pituitary tumors in the approximate incidence noted in Table 7–2. The hyperparathyroidism differs from that seen in sporadic primary hyperparathyroidism. Hyperparathyroidism in MEN is usually hyperplastic or involves multiple adenomas. Many patients with MEN I have recurrent hyperparathyroidism and supernumerary parathyroid glands. Pancreatic tumors involve endocrine cells of the pancreas (islet cells), and disease of this organ represents the most serious feature of MEN I. Gastrinoma (pancreatic delta cells) is the most common pancreatic tumor and may result in Zollinger-Ellison syndrome with peptic ulcer disease or secretory diarrhea. Insulinoma may be present in the MEN I patient presenting in hypoglycemic coma or complaining of ravenous appetite and weight gain. Pancreatic tumors producing glucagon or somatostatin have also been reported. Pancreatic tumors are the only tumors of MEN I complex that have frequent malignant potential. Pituitary tumors in MEN I may be functional or nonfunctional. Functional tumors are typically growth hormone– or prolactin–secreting. The majority of pituitary tumors in MEN I are nonfunctinal chromophobe adenomas, which may, by virtue of their size, produce pituitary insufficiency.

MEN II is discussed in Chapters 5 and 6.

MEN IIa is characterized by various combinations of thyroid, adrenal medullary, and parathyroid tumors (Table 7–2). Medullary thyroid carcinoma (MTC) is the characteristic thyroid tumor and is usually the first recognized of MEN IIa tumors. Pheochromocytoma is the second most common tumor. The pheochromocytoma of MEN II is more frequently multicentric, extraadrenal, and bilateral than that seen in isolated pheochromocytoma. Parathyroid tumors are seen in about half of MEN IIa cases, and as in MEN I, hyperplasia and multiple adenomata are much more commonly seen (more than 70%) than in isolated hyperparathyroidism (about 10%).

MEN IIb includes MTC and pheochromocytoma. Hyperparathyroidism is not commonly seen in MEN IIb.

LABORATORY FEATURES

No particular laboratory features are unique to the MEN syndromes. The laboratory presentation of each component tumor should be considered separately and these features used to characterize and manage that particular element of the patient's disease. Some laboratory features require complicated interpretation. Serum gastrin levels, for example, may be elevated secondary to the hypercalcemia of primary hyperparathyroidism, and diagnosis of a gastrinoma may thus be very difficult. Likewise, secretory diarrhea in MEN II may be associated with a gastrinoma, or even with hypokalemia or other electrolyte abnormalities, and yet be difficult to distinguish from manifestations of MTC, mucosal neuromas, or other, unrelated causes (eg, infection).

If a suspected kindred is being screened for MEN, there is disagreement about the extent of workup necessary in asymptomatic relatives. In the case of MEN I, serum calcium, prolactin, sella turcica evaluation on a lateral skull x-ray, and serum gastrin probably constitute the minimum workup, with more extensive investigation following clinical suspicions or initial findings. The initial workup for MTC in MEN II is described in Chapter 5.

TREATMENT

Treatment is essentially the treatment of each tumor present in the individual patient. Parathyroidectomy requires careful evaluation of the amount of tissue to be removed and the amount of tissue to be left behind. The practice of autotransplanting viable parathyroid tissue to the forearm has been used in cases of parathyroid hyperplasia, in an attempt to protect against hypoparathyroidism while avoiding multiple neck explorations. Pancreatic surgery can be very difficult in MEN I, as the multifocal nature of this tumor sometimes requires subtotal pancreatic resection (particularly with insulinomas) or gastric resection for uncontrollable peptic ulcer disease. Most pituitary tumors in MEN I can be successfully approached by the transsphenoidal route.

Treatment of MEN II involves the management of MTC (Chapter 5) and pheochromocytoma (Chapter 6).

FAMILIAL HYPOCALCIURIC HYPERCALCEMIA

Familial hypocalciuric hypercalcemia (FHH) is an unusual but important cause of hypercalcemia. FHH belongs in the differential diagnosis of hypercalcemia. This disorder has been described in a small number of kindreds, but considering the fact that virtually all affected individuals are asymptomatic, FHH may be grossly under-diagnosed. The disorder is characterized by mild to moderate hypercalcemia and hypocalciuria. The serum iPTH levels for a given serum calcium level are normal to slightly elevated but clearly lower than those seen with a comparable degree of hypercalcemia in primary hyperparathyroidism.

CLINICAL FEATURES

Most patients with FHH are asymptomatic and are discovered either on routine serum chemical screening or during investigations of FHH kindreds. Those with significant hypercalcemia will sometimes complain of the nonspecific constitutional symptoms noted in other forms of hypercalcemia. Physical signs of hypercalcemia can be elicited only in the most severely affected cases. Family history is of great interest, as the penetrance of this autosomal dominant disorder is high. In an affected kindred, about 50% of family members of all ages will be hypercalcemic. Several cases of severe neonatal hyperparathyroidism have been described in kindreds with FHH, and these children have been successfully treated with parathyroidectomy.

LABORATORY FEATURES

Hypercalcemia is, by definition, the universal finding in affected patients with FHH. In most cases, hypercalcemia is mild, although values up to 14 mg/dL have been reported in otherwise uncomplicated cases. Serum phosphorus may be low normal and serum magnesium borderline high (characteristic but not highly significant findings). The most important laboratory determinations in FHH are the serum iPTH and the urinary calcium. PTH levels in FHH are normal or slightly elevated. For a given serum calcium level, iPTH is significantly lower than in primary hyperparathyroidism but higher than that seen when, for example, calcium is infused into a normal individual. Urinary calcium excretion, expressed as the ratio of calcium clearance to creatinine clearance, is significantly lower in FHH than in comparable primary hyperparathyroidism.

TREATMENT

Distinguishing between FHH and primary hyperparathyroidism is often difficult and may depend on astute, chronic clinical observation and on extensive investigation of family members. Once a diagnosis of FHH has been made, patients can usually be followed without treatment. Patients in some FHH kindreds probably have lived with constant hypercalcemia for more than 50 years without any demonstrable ill effect. On the other hand, some patients with FHH have undergone parathyroidectomy because of the belief that FHH is merely part of the spectrum of primary hyperparathyroidism. The parathyroids in FHH may occasionally show diffuse hyperplasia, but partial parathyroidectomy does not result in restoration of eucalcemia. Current data on the long-term effects of hypercalcemia in FHH do not support a surgical approach.

HYPERCALCEMIA OF MALIGNANCY

Hypercalcemia of malignancy is the most frequent cause of hypercalcemia in hospitalized patients and the second most frequent cause (next to primary hyperparathyroidism) of hypercalcemia in all patients. Accelerated and uncontrolled resorption of bone appears to be the key pathologic process. This may be due to the local release of bone-resorbing substances such as interleukin-1 and transforming growth factor–α by tumor cells present in the bone, production of $1,25(OH)_2$-D by certain leukemia or lymphoma cells, or elaboration into the circulation of a parathyroid hormone–related peptide (PTHRP) and potentially other humoral factors.

Understanding of the pathophysiology of cancer-associated hypercalcemia has advanced substantially with the recent cloning of the gene for PTHRP. Based on predictions from the PTHRP gene, this hormone may exist as a 139-, 141-, or 173-amino acid peptide; however, the exact forms of PTHRP that circulate have not been firmly established. PTHRP shares significant sequence identity ($\sim$ 62%, 8 of 13 amino acid residues) with authentic PTH in the first 13 amino acids (Fig 7–3). The sequences for PTH and PTHRP, thereafter, diverge significantly. Despite this fact, PTHRP appears to bind with high affinity to PTH receptors in kidney and bone and to activate adenylate cyclase. Radioimmunoassays have been developed to detect PTHRP in the sera of cancer patients. Studies indicate that at least 70–80% of patients with hypercalcemia and solid tumors have elevated PTHRP levels. Other tumor-related hypercalcemic factors may yet be identified; however, PTHRP clearly plays an important role in the pathogenesis of hypercalcemia in a large group of cancer patients.

CLINICAL FEATURES

Hypercalcemia may be the presenting feature of a malignant condition, or it may develop only as a preterminal event. Generally, the underlying cancer is not occult. In most cases (> 90%) of cancer-associated hypercalcemia, the tumor is evident on the initial workup. In large clinical series, 25% of patients with malignancy-associated

```
                 1            10           20           30
Human PTH:   S V S E I Q L M H N L G K H L N S M E R V E W L R K K L Q D V H N
Human PTHRP: A V S E H Q L L H D K G K S I Q D L R R R F F L H H L I A E I H T
```

Figure 7–3. Comparison of the primary amino acid sequences of the first 34 residues of human PTH and PTHRP. Amino acids are represented by their single-letter codes. Boxed sequences represent sequence identity between the 2 different peptides.

hypercalcemia have lung cancer and 20% have breast cancer. Tumors of the head and neck, multiple myeloma, renal cell and urinary tract carcinomas, and various other solid tumors account for the remainder of hypercalcemic cancer patients. Fewer than half of patients with cancer-associated hypercalcemia survive 3 months from diagnosis. Signs and symptoms of mild hypercalcemia (confusion, ataxia, nausea, fatigue) may be indistinguishable from those of the cancer itself. Some patients become severely dehydrated owing to vomiting, anorexia, or hypercalcemia-induced nephrogenic diabetes insipidus. Such patients may become markedly hypercalcemic over the course of their disease.

LABORATORY FEATURES

Distinguishing between primary hyperparathyroidism and hypercalcemia of malignancy may be difficult. Since both disorders are quite common, they may coexist. Serum calcium levels in hypercalcemia of malignancy may range from slightly elevated to greater than 20 mg/dL. Serum phosphate levels may be normal or slightly depressed. With the availability of assays specific for intact PTH, the clinician should be able to exclude with certainty the diagnosis of primary hyperparathyroidism in the majority of patients with cancer-associated hypercalcemia. Circulating tumor-derived factors such as the PTHRP do not typically cross-react in these newer PTH assays. Intact N-terminal PTH levels as determined by these assays should be suppressed in hypercalcemia due to cancer. If only the more traditional mid-region or carboxy-terminal PTH assays are available for diagnostic purposes, normal to somewhat elevated iPTH levels may be observed in hypercalcemia of malignancy. It is clear, however, that iPTH levels in this disorder are usually not as high as would be seen with a comparable degree of hypercalcemia in primary hyperparathyroidism, but they are also not suppressed to the degree expected in hypercalcemia from exogenous sources. The availability of assays for PTHRP in the near future should simplify diagnosis.

TREATMENT

Therapy of the underlying cancer is the only definitive treatment. Most cases require temporizing measures, aimed at the hypercalcemia itself. The degree of hypercalcemia and the severity of accompanying symptoms will determine the specific hypocalcemic therapy. Fluid administration is the mainstay of therapy for hypercalcemia of malignancy. Many patients present in a hypovolemic state. Correction of this state may relieve symptoms and stabilize serum calcium at a lower level. In the fully alert patient, oral fluids may be given, although sodium chloride tablets may need to be included to maintain adequate calcium diuresis. If intravenous fluids are used, normal saline is preferred, and the patient must be carefully monitored to avoid fluid overload. As euvolemia is achieved, a diuretic that blocks tubular reabsorption of calcium (such as furosemide) may be administered to further increase calcium excretion. As vigorous diuresis is continued, hypokalemia and hypomagnesemia may develop, and such deficiencies must be anticipated and prevented with supplements.

If the condition is severe enough that fluid and diuretic therapy fail to relieve the acute state, or if chronic therapy is required, other approaches must be considered. Important therapeutic agents for hypercalcemia include plicamycin, calcitonin, and diphosphonates (Table 7–3).

Plicamycin, (mithramycin, Mithracin) a cytotoxic agent, has been used for more than 15 years in the management of life-threatening hypercalcemia. It may be administered initially in doses of 7–25 µg/kg body weight, intravenously over 30 minutes. This corrects hypercalcemia in most cases within 48 hours. The clinical response may last for 7 or more days before retreatment is necessary. Care must be taken to use the smallest effective dose to reduce calcium to an asymptomatic range, tolerating mild hypercalcemia. For less severe or recurrent hypercalcemia, lower doses of about 5–15 µg/kg body weight may be used as required to maintain calcium in an elevated but noncritical range. Plicamycin therapy may produce nausea, and repeated dosing is often limited by drug-induced thrombocytopenia or hepatic or renal insufficiency.

Calcitonin (salmon calcitonin, Calcimar) is a moderately successful agent for the acute therapy of hypercalcemia. Calcitonin directly inhibits osteoclast-mediated bone resorption and may be administered subcutaneously or intramuscularly in doses of 4 IU/kg every 6–12 hours (Table 7–3). A test dose of 1 IU intracutaneously should be given to patients before initiating therapy. The drug is usually well tolerated, but side effects may include nausea, flushing, and skin rash. Although calcitonin can lower serum calcium levels quickly (peak effects within 12 hours), chronic therapy is limited by the nearly universal development of drug tolerance. This result is believed to be

Table 7–3. Acute therapy of hypercalcemia.

Drug	Doses and Route of Administration	Onset of Action	Duration of Response	Side Effects
Etidronate disodium	7.5 mg/kg by intravenous infusion in D5W over 2 hours for 3–5 days	24–48 hours	7 days, or may be prolonged	Nausea, vomiting, abdominal pain
Calcitonin	4 IU/kg subcutaneously or intramuscularly every 6–12 hours after one intravenous test dose	2–4 hours	Tolerance may develop unless combined with glucocorticoid	Nausea, flushing, skin rash
Plicamycin	7–25 µg/kg intravenously over 30 minutes	24–48 hours	5–7 days	Thrombocytopenia, hepatic and renal toxicity

secondary to the production of neutralizing antibodies to the peptide and may be prevented or delayed by the concomitant administration of glucocorticoids (eg, prednisone, 30 to 60 mg/d). The development of drug tolerance, frequency of parenteral administration, and cost limit the overall usefulness of calcitonin in the chronic management of hypercalcemia of malignancy.

Etidronate disodium (Didronel), the only diphosphonate available in the USA, has been approved for intravenous use in cancer-associated hypercalcemia. Etidronate is thought to act by binding to bone matrix and directly blocking osteoclastic bone resorption. Etidronate is given as an intravenous infusion typically for 3–5 days (Table 7–3) and is highly effective ($\sim$ 50–75%) in acutely restoring normocalcemia in hypercalcemic cancer patients. Chronic oral therapy with etidronate may then be initiated; however, studies of patients on this form of therapy indicate a far lower succeses rate in maintaining normocalcemia (< 30%). Side effects are minimal and include nausea, vomiting, and gastrointestinal discomfort. There are rare reports of renal toxicity in cancer patients with underlying renal dysfunction. The tendency of etidronate to induce a mineralization defect in bone is rarely an important consideration in the therapeutic options for this group of patients because of their short life expectancy.

After acute stabilization of the hypercalcemia, a chronic regimen must be selected. Oral fluid therapy, with or without diuretics, may be successful in certain cases, but most patients have difficulty maintaining such a regimen for long periods. In addition, if at all possible, ambulation should be encouraged. Oral etidronate may be tried, but chronic therapy has had limited success (see above). Oral phosphate may be very effective over a period of time (begin therapy with the equivalent of 1–2 g elemental phosphorus/d; see Table 7–4), but diarrhea is a limiting side effect in most patients. Care must be taken to avoid hyperphosphatemia (more than 5 mg/dL), as soft tissue calcifications and renal impairment may develop when the serum calcium phosphate product rises too high (above 40). Glucocorticoid therapy appears to be effective in some cases of multiple myeloma but is probably not indicated in hypercalcemia associated with other malignancies. Research is in progress toward the development of more potent diphosphonates and PTHRP antagonists that should prove highly effective in controlling cancer-associated hypercalcemia.

HYPOPARATHYROIDISM

Hypocalcemia is the hallmark of hypoparathyroidism and can result from a variety of causes (Table 7–5). These possible etiologies should be vigorously pursued in the hypocalcemic patient. If such

Table 7–4. Oral phosphate preparations.

	Amount Equivalent to 1 g Elemental Phosphorus
K-Phos Neutral	4 tablets
Neutra-Phos or Neutra-Phos-K (sodium free)	4 capsules (contents)
pHos-pHaid	8 tablets (0.5 g each)
Phospho Soda	6.2 mL (1.5 tsp)
Phosphaljel	4 oz

causes have been ruled out, and if hypocalcemia is accompanied by hyperphosphatemia, the differential diagnosis is virtually restricted to the various forms of hypoparathyroidism. The kidney cannot maintain normal mineral levels in the blood unless calcium conservation and phosphate excretion are stimulated by circulating PTH. Renal insufficiency itself may result in hypocalcemia and hyperphosphatemia. The pathogenesis of hyperphosphatemia is thought to be reduced phosphate excretion by the failing kidney. Hypocalcemia may result from the binding of calcium to phosphate and from decreased renal 1,25 $(OH)_2$-D production. The latter leads to gastrointestinal malabsorption of calcium. In addition, skeletal resistance to PTH action in renal insufficiency may exacerbate the hypocalcemia.

Hypoparathyroidism may result from one of 2 general pathologic mechanisms. PTH secretion may be deficient, or the end organs may be insensitive to circulating PTH. PTH deficiency (primary hypoparathyroidism) commonly presents after surgical damage to the parathyroids. During thyroidectomy or radical neck dissection, the parathyroids may be inadvertently damaged. Resection of parathyroid

Table 7–5. Causes of hypocalcemia.

Artifact (low serum albumin; rapid volume expansion)	Acute pancreatitis
Hypoparathyroidism	Malabsorption (may or may not have diarrhea) (calcium; vitamin D; magnesium)
Pseudohypoparathyroidism	
Postoperative resection of parathyroid adenoma (transient)	Chelation (EDTA; large transfusions of citrated blood)
Hypomagnesemia	Plicamycin
Hypermagnesemia	Diphenylhydantoin
Chronic renal failure (hyperphosphatemia)	Neonatal (maternal hypercalcemia; diabetes mellitus; cow's milk or high phosphate formula; respiratory distress syndrome)
Postoperative thyroidectomy for Graves' disease (transient)	
Metastatic carcinoma (especially prostate and breast)	Hyperphosphatemia [IV, oral, or enema phosphate; chemotherapy of responsive tumors (especially leukemias, lymphomas)]
	Vitamin D resistance syndromes

tissue, particularly in parathyroid hyperplasia, always carries the risk of transient or permanent hypoparathyroidism.

Damage to the parathyroid glands occasionally results from infection, metastatic tumor, or infiltration by granulomata (eg, tuberculosis, sarcoidosis) or by heavy metals (eg, hemochromatosis, transfusion hemosiderosis, Wilson's disease). Parathyroid function may be transiently suppressed by radiation therapy to the neck. Occasional cases of hypoparathyroidism are due to dysembryogenesis (eg, DiGeorge's syndrome), while others fall into the idiopathic category. Idiopathic hypoparathyroidism often appears as a familial disorder, may have an autoimmune basis, and is frequently associated with mucocutaneous candidiasis due to underlying immunodeficiency. Hypoparathyroidism occasionally accompanies other endocrine deficiency states.

Hormone-resistant hypoparathyroidism is an unusual inherited disorder. This condition is known as **pseudohypoparathyroidism** (PHP). PHP results from an apparent end-organ resistance to the action of PTH, plasma levels of which are high in response to hypocalcemia. The pathogenetic defect in PHP is characterized by the inability of PTH to generate an increase in urinary cyclic AMP (PHP types Ia and Ib) or a phosphaturic response (PHP type II). PTH-sensitive tissues (kidney or bone) may be differentially involved in cases of PHP, and the manifestations of the disorder can thus be quite varied. Decreased activity of G_s, the stimulatory guanyl nucleotide binding protein coupled to adenylate cyclase, is postulated to be an etiologic factor in PHP type Ia. The molecular defects responsible for PHP types Ib and II are unknown. (Figs 7–4 and 7–5.)

CLINICAL FEATURES

Hypocalcemia may result from inadequate gastrointestinal absorption owing to calcium or vitamin D deficiency, may accompany acute pancreatitis or osteoblastic malignancy, may be related to complexing by excessive circulating levels of certain anions (albumin, citrate, phosphate), may be due to coexistent hypomagnesemia, or may be seen in renal insufficiency. If these causes have been ruled out, however, and especially if hyperphosphatemia is present, hypoparathyroidism should be considered the likely explanation for hypocalcemia, particularly with a history of thyroid surgery.

Symptoms

Symptoms, if present, result from hypocalcemia (and possibly hyperphosphatemia). Carpopedal spasm, paresthesias, and muscle cramps are most commonly reported, but tetany and convulsions may occur. Symptoms of L-dopa–resistant parkinsonism and visual prob-

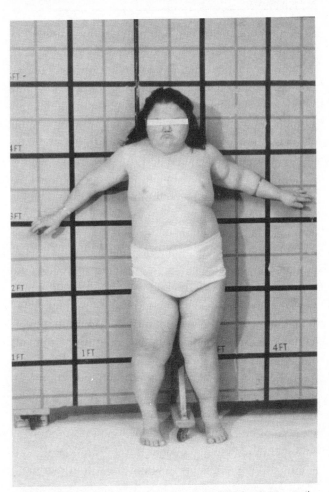

Figure 7–4. Patient with pseudohypoparathyroidism demonstrating commonly associated features: short stature, round face, stocky habitus, and mental retardation. Patients frequently also have manifestations of hypocalcemia such as seizures or tetany, cataracts, dental abnormalities, and calcification of the basal ganglia. Ectopic calcification also occurs. Manifestations vary considerably.

lems from pseudotumor cerebri have been reported in hypoparathyroidism, but they usually resolve with normalization of serum mineral levels. Alopecia and mucocutaneous candidiasis are also occasionally reported.

Signs

Most signs are directly attributable to hypocalcemia. Chvostek's sign (contraction of facial muscles when the facial nerve is gently tapped) and Trousseau's sign (carpopedal spasm within 3 minutes of impeding blood return from the forearm with a blood pressure cuff) are signs of latent tetany, but they may be positive in about 20% of normal persons. Hyperreflexia may be seen. Papilledema may reflect the increased intracranial pressure occasionally associated with this condition. Dermatologic findings may include dry skin, brittle hair, alopecia, and transverse ridging of nails. Dental examination will often reveal enamel hypoplasia and caries. Pseudohypoparathyroidism sometimes presents with a characteristic physiognomy, including short stature, round facies, short neck, short metacarpals and metatarsals, and mild mental retardation. This is known as Albright's hereditary osteodystrophy. The pattern of inheritance is controversial. Symptomatic hypocalcemia usually appears in childhood in patients with PHP. A variant disorder, called pseudopseudohypoparathyroidism, presents with the characteristic somatic features often seen in PHP family members but without hypocalcemia or increased iPTH.

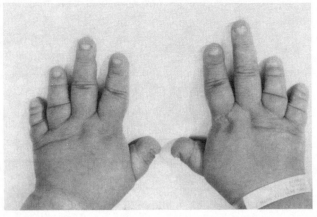

A

Figure 7–5. A. Hands of a patient with pseudohypoparathyroidism. (*continued*)

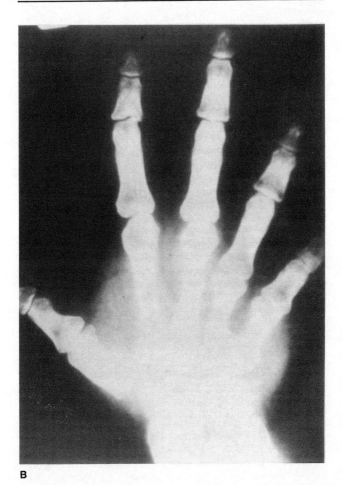

B

Figure 7–5. (*cont'd*) **B.** X-ray of patient's hand with pseudohypoparathyroidism demonstrating short metacarpals. Metatarsals are frequently short as well.

LABORATORY FEATURES

Laboratory Tests

The hallmark of hypoparathyroidism is hypocalcemia, which may range from very mild to severe, with roughly corresponding degrees of symptomatology. Serum phosphate may be elevated owing to the lack of PTH suppression of phosphate reabsorption in the kidney, but this is not a universal finding in hypoparathyroidism. Measurement of serum immunoreactive PTH is key in this workup: iPTH will be low to undetectable in primary hypoparathyroidism but elevated in pseudohypoparathyroidism. Serum magnesium should always be measured. Very high (> 3.5 mg/dL) or very low (< 1 mg/dL) levels of serum magnesium may be associated with suppressed PTH secretion. Renal function should be evaluated in all hypoparathyroid patients, since a hypocalcemic hyperphosphatemic picture is often seen in azotemia. Immunoreactive PTH levels (measured by mid-region or carboxy-terminal PTH assays) are usually markedly elevated in chronic renal failure but may be only slightly elevated in newer assays for intact PTH.

X-Rays

Ectopic ossification may be seen on x-rays, particularly in young patients with PHP. The short metacarpals and metatarsals of PHP are also best evaluated on x-rays. Patients with PHP and intact skeletal responsiveness to PTH may present with hyperparathyroid bone changes including osteitis fibrosa cystica. Patients with advanced vitamin D deficiency may present with radiologic findings of osteomalacia. Typically, radiologic investigations are not helpful in the evaluation of hypoparathyroidism.

TREATMENT

Some hypoparathyroid patients become severely hypocalcemic. Such patients may display surprisingly few signs and symptoms because the hypocalcemia has developed very gradually. In the symptomatic hypocalcemic patient, blood should be drawn for renal function tests and iPTH and treatment begun immediately. In severely hypocalcemic patients with life-threatening complications such as seizures or laryngospasm, intravenous calcium must be given. Calcium chloride and calcium gluconate are available as concentrated intravenous solutions, but they should be diluted in order not to irritate infusion sites and administered at rates of up to 200 mg of elemental calcium over 10 minutes. Intravenous calcium therapy must be monitored by serum calcium measurement. Oral calcium remains the foundation of therapy for chronic hypocalcemia. Calcium carbonate preparations are preferred, since other calcium salts (see Table 7–9) contain less calcium. Up to 2 g of elemental calcium may be required daily; dosage should be divided and titrated against serum calcium and urinary calcium. As long as the patient is asymptomatic, serum calcium is best maintained near 8 mg/dL. If calcium absorption appears to be the limiting factor (urinary calcium remaining low with increased oral calcium), vitamin D usually needs to be added to the regimen. Commonly used vitamin D preparations are listed in Table 7–6. The most practical preparation is ergocalciferol. Patients with hypoparathyroidism require 25,000–150,000 U/d, depending on the severity of the disorder. Dihydrotachysterol (DHT) and $1,25(OH)_2$-D are potent and short-acting. Their expense and propensity to cause fluctuations in serum calcium levels makes them less suitable alternatives in most cases, but occasionally they may be useful. Care must be taken to avoid vitamin D toxicity and hypercalcemia. Hypercalcemia due to vitamin D toxicity is treated with hydration and glucocorticoids. If calcium excretion is limiting (unacceptably high urinary calcium levels despite symptomatically subnormal serum calcium levels), a low-sodium diet plus a diuretic such as chlorthalidone may be indicated. Oral phosphate binders (eg, Amphojel) may be helpful adjuncts in the therapeutic regimen. Treatment principles are similar for primary hypoparathyroidism and pseudohypoparathyroidism. Calcium absorption, however, is usually more nearly normal in psuedohypoparathyroidism, especially in forms in which renal PTH resistance is incomplete. The combination of low PTH levels and elevated serum phosphate in primary hypoparathyroidism is particularly potent in suppressing the production of $1,25(OH)_2$-D.

Complications

The most significant complications result from undertreatment or overtreatment. If hypoparathyroidism remains unrecognized or undertreated, hypocalcemic tetany and seizures may result. Patients on

Table 7–6. Vitamin D preparations.*

	Forms	Usual Starting Dose in Hypoparathyroidism	Persistence of Effect, Days
Ergocalciferol	25,000 U (0.625 mg) 50,000 U (1.25 mg)	25,000 U/d	20–60
Dihydrotachysterol (DHT)	0.125 mg 0.2 mg 0.4 mg	0.125 mg/d	3–14
25-OH-D₃ (calcifediol)	20 µg 50 µg	20 µg/d	7–30
1,25 (OH)₂-D (calcitriol)	0.25 µg 0.5 µg	0.25 µg/d	2–7

therapy, or the other hand, are at risk for developing hypercalcemia or hypercalciuria and nephrolithiasis, especially if urine calcium is not measured periodically (at least every 6 months). Patients should drink extra fluids, especially at bedtime, to dilute their urine. Screeening for excessive urine calcium concentration may be done with a 24-hour urine or a fasting morning "spot" urine for calcium concentration; greater than 30 mg/dL is considered excessive.

OSTEOPOROSIS

Osteoporosis is a public health problem of major proportions. Fractures attributable to this disorder cause considerable morbidity and mortality. The annual cost related to osteoporosis in the USA has reached nearly 20 billion dollars. Yet this disorder is generally underdiagnosed, underevaluated, and undertreated.

Osteoporosis is the most common form of osteopenia (Table 7–7), the latter describing any condition in which bone mass per unit volume of bony tissue is abnormally low. The distinguishing feature of osteoporosis is that while bone mass is decreased, the remaining bone collagen matrix is normally mineralized. Osteoporosis usually involves all parts of the skeleton, but the most striking effects are seen in trabecular (cancellous) bone. Cortical bone is the predominant component (80%) of the skeleton. Trabecular bone is, however, concentrated in certain areas of the skeleton (axial structures, eg, the vertebral bodies) that are most prominently affected by the osteoporotic process because the rate of bone turnover is greater in trabecular than in cortical bone.

Several pathophysiologic processes may be involved in osteopenia: (1) decreased rate of bone formation (appositional rate), (2) increased rate of bone resorption, (3) decreased gastrointestinal absorption of calcium, and (4) increased urinary excretion of calcium. Some less common forms of osteopenia can be clearly defined in terms of one or more of these pathophysiologic mechanisms. Osteoporosis, on the other hand, probably describes a group of disorders, any one of which may be due to one or a combination of the possible pathophysiologic mechanisms.

Table 7–7. Major classifications of osteopenia.

Osteoporosis (see Table 7–8)	Osteogenesis imperfecta
Osteomalacia	Malignancy
Osteitis fibrosa	

Clinically, there are 4 main types of osteoporosis (Table 7–8).

Senile osteoporosis is an extremely common, if not universal, condition associated with the aging process. Loss of both cortical and trabecular bone is involved, and an underlying etiologic factor may be the decrease in gastrointestinal calcium absorptive capacity that occurs with age. The ultimate severity of senile osteoporosis is a function of both the skeletal mass at maturity and the rate of loss of bony mineral. The morbid event in senile osteoporosis is usually the hip fracture.

Estrogen-deficiency osteoporosis, commonly known as postmenopausal osteoporosis, is responsible for the marked preponderance of elderly women among osteoporotic patients. Although postmenopausal osteoporosis affects both trabecular and cortical bone, trabecular involvement predominates and may lead to vertebral crush fractures. Postmenopausal loss of bone mineral in the axial skeleton occurs at a rate of about 1–2% per year. Presentation of symptomatic disease in any particular patient, however, may be a function of several factors, possibly triggered by sufficient trauma to cause the first vertebral fracture. Key issues remain unresolved in postmenopausal osteoporosis, including the role played by PTH and the mechanism by which estrogen protects against bone loss. Other estrogen-deficiency states, such as hyperprolactinemia, may also be associated with abnormally low bone density. It is uncertain whether osteoporosis in males, which has been attributed to relative androgen deficiency, is directly comparable with postmenopausal osteoporosis.

Osteoporosis of glucocorticoid excess affects trabecular bone almost exclusively, and its severity may represent the summation of multiple adverse effects on the bone-mineral system. Exogenous glu-

Table 7–8. Classification of osteoporosis.

Senile	**Genetic disorders**
Hormone deficiency	Osteogenesis imperfecta
Estrogen (women)	Ehlers-Danlos syndrome
Androgen (men)	Marfan's syndrome
Hormone excess	Menke's syndrome
Cushing's syndrome or glucocorticoid administration	Homocystinuria
	Miscellaneous
Thyrotoxicosis	Diabetes mellitus
Hyperparathyroidism	Protein-calorie malnutrition
Excessive vitamin D administration	Liver disease
	Rheumatoid arthritis
Immobilization	Heparin therapy
Hematologic malignancy, especially multiple myeloma	Vitamin C deficiency
	Juvenile osteoporosis
	Systemic mastocytosis
	Alcoholism-induced

cocorticoids inhibit ACTH secretion, resulting in decreased production of adrenal androgens and estrogens. Glucocorticoids inhibit bone formation and stimulate bone resorption. Finally, renal calcium excretion is increased while gastrointestinal calcium absorption is decreased by glucocorticoids. It is estimated that about 50% of patients receiving chronic glucocorticoid therapy will eventually suffer from symptomatic osteoporosis.

Immobilization osteoporosis is characterized by markedly increased urinary and fecal excretion of calcium, thus fitting a resorptive hypercalciuria model. It becomes a major problem in cases of long-term immobilization, such as quadriplegia, and may be a devastating complication of the recovery period from an immobilizing osteoporotic hip fracture.

Neither the features nor types of osteoporosis are clearly distinguishable from one another. Osteoporosis in a particular patient may be multifactoral, characterized by features unique to that patient. Furthermore, it does not appear that preferred treatment strategies will distribute according to rigid classifications of osteoporosis, but rather will best be specifically tailored to each individual case. The implications are discussed below.

CLINICAL FEATURES

The initial task in evaluating any potential case of osteoporosis is to distinguish it from other causes of osteopenia (Table 7–7). Although other osteopenic disorders are less common than osteoporosis, some are curable, and all have therapeutic and prognostic features different from those of osteoporosis.

A careful medical history is of great value both in differential diagnosis and baseline evaluation. Skeletal mass at maturity is greater in black than in light-skinned races, and greater in men than in women. There is a low-grade, baseline mineral loss from the axial skeleton of all humans, the rate of which is linear with age. Menopause triggers an acceleration of loss from both the axial and the appendicular skeleton in women, and decline in androgen levels may be accompanied by a similar process in men. Multiparity and a history of breast feeding may be protective factors in some women against subsequent skeletal mineral loss.

Sunlight exposure (activation of endogenous vitamin D) and physical activity appears to be positive factors in skeletal mineral retention. Diet plays a complex role. Dietary levels of calcium and vitamin D are important factors in overall calcium absorption. Older patients generally decrease calcium intake at the time the gastrointestinal tract decreases fractional absorption of calcium. In fact, malabsorption in any patient may first be suggested by the finding of osteopenia on x-ray. Severe protein deficiency interferes with bone formation, in that bone matrix production is limited. On the other hand, diets very high in protein result in increased production of inorganic acids, and the acidosis may adversely affect bone turnover. Excessive alcohol use and smoking also impair skeletal calcium retention, although mechanisms have not been elucidated.

A positive family history for osteoporosis is often obtained but may be trivial in light of the common nature of the disease and due to the clustering of many of the above-mentioned factors within families. Drugs must be identified in the history. Most important are the sex steroids (postitive factors) and the glucocorticoids (negative factors), whether exogenous or endogenous. Excessive thyroid hormone from any source is believed to adversely affect skeletal mineralization. Isoniazid and the tetracycline antibiotics have been found to inhibit normal bone turnover.

Symptoms & Fractures

In patients who will eventually become osteoporotic, there is generally a long symptomatically silent period during early stages of bone demineralization. Symptoms in clinically evident osteoporosis may also be minimal and nonspecific unless a fracture has already occurred. Back pain, often of sudden onset, is the cardinal symptom of vertebral crush fractures, but many osteoporotic patients may complain of back pain in the absence of x-ray–detectable fractures.

Osteoporosis results in fractures that can be painful, debilitating, deforming, and even fatal. It is estimated that in the USA about 40,000 individuals die yearly of complications (eg, pulmonary emboli) of osteoporotic hip fractures. Fractures may occur spontaneously or with minimal trauma.

Signs

Weight and body habitus should be documented in all osteopenic patients, since osteoporosis is more common and often more severe in slender individuals. On the other hand, excessive weight may lead to dangerous mechanical stresses on the skeleton of an osteoporotic patient. Careful and frequent documentation of height and comparison with arm span, and previously recorded measurements of height are helpful in following patients with osteoporosis. Unless fractures of the extremities occur, deformities and changes in length of the extremities are not seen in osteoporosis. A single vertebral crush fracture results in about 1 cm loss in height in the average patient, and multiple vertebral fractures will often lead to severe kyphosis and the so-called dowager's hump sometimes seen in elderly women.

LABORATORY FEATURES

Laboratory Tests

A. Total Serum Calcium: Total serum calcium is the cornerstone of the laboratory workup of osteopenia. High serum calcium suggests primary hyperparathyroidism or hypercalcemia of malignancy, although serum calcium may also be elevated in the osteoporosis of immobilization. If normal mineral homeostatic processes are operative, a high serum calcium suggests either accelerated bone resorption or increased intestinal calcium absorption. Most cases of osteoporosis present with normal to low-normal serum calcium. Low serum calcium raises the question of a calcium absorptive defect. Serum phosphorus may be abnormally low in nutritionally inadequate or malabsorptive states, and is often elevated in renal failure. Primary hyperparathyroidism often presents with low serum phosphorus.

B. Quantitative Urinary Calcium: Quantitative urinary calcium is a simple, inexpensive determination of great utility in the evaluation and the management of osteopenia. Baseline calcium excretion on the patient's usual diet should be determined in every osteoporotic patient. High urinary calcium excretion is frequently seen in osteoporosis associated with cancer, immobilization, and glucocorticoid excess, reflecting a net skeletal resorptive state. On the other hand, senile osteoporosis may be associated with calcium malabsorption and significant hypocalciuria.

C. Serum PTH: A serum PTH level should be obtained in the course of the evaluation of the osteopenic patient. Mild elevation in iPTH, coupled with low-normal serum calcium, is characteristic of the hypoabsorptive state of "normal" aging; this pattern is even more pronounced in osteomalacia. Estrogen-deficiency osteoporosis is usually characterized by normal serum calcium and iPTH levels. The osteopenic patient with high serum calcium and high iPTH should receive a thorough evaluation for primary hyperparathyroidism.

D. Serum Alkaline Phosphatase: Serum alkaline phosphatase is usually normal in osteoporosis unless there has been a recent fracture. Elevated serum alkaline phosphatase level in the osteopenic patient should also raise suspicion of osteomalacia, primary hyperparathyroidism, or cancer. Serum alkaline phosphatase may also originate from the hepatobiliary system. Measurement of gamma glutaryl transferase, an enzyme exclusively of hepatobiliary origin (which appears in the circulation in parallel with alkaline phosphatase), will help identify the source of an elevated serum alkaline phosphatase.

X-Rays

Generalized osteopenia, if severe enough, will be apparent on virtually any plain radiograph of bone. Mild to moderate osteopenia, on the other hand, is undetectable on plain x-ray. In the clinical diagnosis and management of osteoporosis, it is important to recognize osteopenia as early as possible. Certain radiologic features, although not absolutely specific for osteoporosis, are useful in this effort. In osteoporosis, the vertebral bodies, as viewed on spine films or a lateral chest x-ray, will show gradual loss of transverse trabeculations, sometimes resulting in an accentuaton of vertical trabeculations and a thinning and sharpening of the cortical margins. Wedging and collapse of vertebral bodies are signs in the development of vertebral crush fractures. Evidence of old fractures, often clinically silent, may be seen in other bones as well. Severe osteoporosis is sometimes recognized by cortical thinning in the distal clavicles. The only method for precisely quantifying the severity of osteoporosis is by measuring bone mineral content as described below. Whenever x-rays of an osteopenic patient are examined, careful search should be made for signs specific for other disorders, such as Looser's zones (osteomalacia) or subperiosteal resorption in the distal phalanges (primary hyperparathyroidism).

Special Tests

The following special tests are not indicated for every osteoporotic patient. However, when a patient is identified at risk for severe osteoporosis, when osteoporosis appears to be rapidly advancing, when osteomalacia cannot be definitely eliminated, or when intensive or experimental therapies are to be undertaken, such procedures are available and should be used for careful, objective, ongoing patient management.

A. Bone Densitometry: A number of techniques have been developed to measure bone mineral content. Single-photon absorptiometry of the forearm can be conveniently performed and serves as an index of cortical bone mineral content. The precision of this method is generally excellent. Only recently have methods emerged that are suitable for its precise measurement in the vertebral bodies, which are the sites of most rapid bone loss in most forms of osteoporosis. Dual photon absorptiometry is the most commonly used method. Its advantages are excellent precision and low radiation exposure. This method cannot be focused exclusively on trabecular bone, however, and cost remains fairly high. Quantitation of vertebral bone density using CT scan is available at some centers. This method is more specific for trabecular bone and is comparable in cost to other techniques, but higher radiation dosage and limited availability still hamper its use. Most recently, techniques have been introduced for measuring bone mineral content in the spine and hip by quantitative digital radiography (QDR) and dual energy x-ray absorptiometry (DEXA). These techniques are precise, use readily available x-ray sources, and have lower radiation exposures than densitometry by CT. These methods are becoming increasingly popular and will enable reproducible measurements of bone mineral content to be made at most centers.

B. Bone Scan: Differential diagnosis of osteopenia may be aided by bone scanning after administration of technetium-labeled diphosphonates. In this procedure, Paget's disease and various neoplastic processes show localized increased uptake. The bone scan in osteoporosis will identify recent fractures but is otherwise negative.

C. Percutaneous Bone Biopsy: In unusual cases of osteopenia, histologic examination of bone is necessary. Percutaneous bone biopsy after double tetracycline labeling is now an established and reliable method to this end. This is an invasive procedure; however, in the proper hands, the risks are low, and if both nondecalcified and fixed sections of the biopsy are read by an experienced bone pathologist, the yield of useful diagnostic information is high.

TREATMENT

Since the reversibility of adult osteoporosis is limited, most attention is justifiably focused on prophylaxis. Initiation of estrogen replacement in postmenopausal or hypogonadal women will markedly reduce subsequent vertebral bone loss. Calcium supplements also reduce bone loss due to aging, particularly in patients with daily calcium intakes below the recommended daily allowance (RDA). High-risk patients, such as those with premature gonadal failure, those receiving chronic corticosteroids, or those with multiple risk factors for bone loss, should receive either gonadal steroids, the conservative therapy outlined below, or both. There is a growing opinion that all aging female patients should receive such prophylactic therapy.

Elimination of Avoidable Risk Factors

Excessive bed rest should be avoided in chronic illness in the elderly, and prudent early ambulation after surgery is encouraged. Bone mineral may also be preserved by elimination of alcohol, tobacco, and unnecessary analgesics. Dosage of necessary drugs (eg, corticosteroids) should be minimized or administered in a (presumably) less harmful manner (ie, alternate day regimen, or direct delivery of drug to the affected organ).

The elderly, disabled, or known osteoporotic patient must have a well-lighted obstacle-free "fall safe" home. Walking aids, handrails, padded stairs, and other measures can decrease fracture risk.

Calcium Balance

Maintenance of calcium balance requires increased calcium intake in older individuals, mainly because of decreased gastrointestinal capacity for absorption of calcium. The actual calcium content in the North American diet decreases with age, to the point that nearly 1 g/d of elemental calcium deficit is present in the average senior citizen. Dietary changes and supplemental calcium can be provided to bring most elderly patients back into calcium balance, but vigilance is required. Increasing dietary dairy product intake has practical limits. Cow's milk products have high phosphate content, leading to lower fractional calcium absorption. Many elderly patients have a degree of lactose intolerance, such that high dairy product intake may lead to gastrointestinal disturbance and flatulence. A wide variety of commonly available calcium salts differ considerably in their content of elemental calcium (Table 7–9). Because of low cost, high calcium content, and availability in flavored, chewable form, calcium carbonate is a practical supplement in many patients. Each 500-mg tablet contains 200 mg of elemental calcium. Thus, 6 tablets per day provide 1200 mg of supplemental calcium. For patients who do not tolerate calcium carbonate, other forms of oral calcium are available (Table 7–9). Lower proportionate calcium content and greater expense may be drawbacks to some of these supplements. Calcium supplements do not appear to prevent trabecular bone loss and have only a modest effect on cortical bone. Therefore, *calcium supplements cannot substitute for estrogen* in preventing osteoporosis.

Diet

Excessive fat in the diet may interfere with calcium absorption. Calcium may also be complexed in the gastrointestinal lumen by oxalate (tea, coffee, spinach, rhubarb), and phosphate (dairy products). Excessive phosphate also inhibits production of active forms of vitamin D, with resultant decreases in calcium absorption. Protein intake must be sufficient to support skeletal anabolic processes. Excessive protein intake may, however, lead to increased production of inorganic acids and metabolic acidosis. Acidosis decreases calcium reabsorption in the kidney and may increase bone resorption.

Table 7–9. Elemental calcium content (% weight) of some commonly used oral calcium supplements.*

	% Elemental Calcium
Calcium carbonate	40%
Calcium glycerophosphate	19%
Calcium gluconate	9%
Calcium lactate	13%
Dicalcium phosphate	23%
Calcium citrate	21%

*Commonly used preparations of calcium carbonate include oyster shell calcium (250 mg/tablet); Titralac (400 mg/5 mL); Tums (200 mg/tablet); dolomite (140 mg/tablet); Titralac (168 mg/tablet); Citracal (200 mg/tablet).

Exercise

Moderate, regular, weight-bearing exercise appears to be beneficial in the prevention and treatment of osteoporosis. Accompanying sunlight exposure will increase endogenous vitamin D levels. The osteoporotic patient has to be wary of trauma or strain to weakened areas of the skeleton, however, and the form of exercise should be chosen accordingly.

Drugs

A. Thiazides: In patients with relative hypercalciuria (with or without calcium supplementation), addition of thiazides may stimulate retention of calcium in the circulation and may have positive effects on bone mineral density. Thiazides must be used with great care, especially in eldery patients, as they commonly induce dehydration or hyponatremia in this population. Thiazides may lead to hypercalcemia in the calcium-supplemented patient, and periodic serum calcium determinations are essential in this group. Vitamin D has not been shown to be beneficial in preventing osteoporosis in the post-menopausal patient, and this therapy should be reserved for the osteoporotic patient in whom malabsorption is a probable component of the problem.

B. Estrogen: The most significant therapeutic modality in prevention and treatment of osteoporosis is hormone replacement in estrogen-deficient women. The role of estrogen deficiency in osteoporosis has been directly demonstrated in a number of studies in which oophorectomized women demonstrate rapid and consistent decreases in vertebral bone density and increases in fracture rates, unless they are protected with appropriate doses of supplemental estrogens. Significant benefit is also apparent in women begun on such supplements at the time of natural menopause.

Estrogen should be given within 20 years after menopause to be effective in retarding bone loss. Doses of at least 0.625 mg/d of conjugated estrogens in a cycled regimen seem to be necessary to achieve a protective effect. Because the 1.25-mg dose of conjugated estrogens may be effective in reversing established osteoporosis, this dose may be preferable in treating older osteoporotic patients. In the patient with an intact uterus, estrogen should be cycled (periodically with a progestin) in order to reduce the risk of endometrial cancer. Other contraindications to estrogen therapy, such as gallbladder disease or thrombophlebitis, must also be considered. Some patients will object to the use of estrogens because of continued cyclic bleeding after the menopause, or to the relatively benign but troublesome estrogen-associated weight changes and fluid shifts.

Estrogens decrease skeletal resorption. This effect may be an estrogen-mediated decrease in skeletal sensitivity to PTH or to

1,25(OH)$_2$-D. Estrogens have also been shown to increase gastrointestinal absorption of calcium. There is considerable variation in skeletal response to estrogen replacement. Estrogen deficiency may not fully explain the disease pattern encountered in postmenopausal osteoporosis; ovarian inactivity may lead to other crucial deficits.

C. Testosterone: There is good evidence that androgen deficiency in males leads to osteoporosis. Therefore, any hypogonadal male should be treated with testosterone to preserve skeletal integrity as well as libido and sexual function.

D. Calcitonin: Calcitonin has been approved by the FDA for the therapy of osteoporosis. This drug has been used extensively in Europe for this indication. Calcitonin is given in doses of 50 or 100 IU/d subcutaneously. Beneficial effects include mild analgesia, which may be helpful in patients with pain due to acute vertebral compression fractures and (over the long term) an increase in bone mineral content. Calcitonin has been particularly efficacious in high-turnover osteoporosis. When administered chronically for 2 years, calcitonin increases spinal bone density by approximately 7%. Side effects are minimal, but the main disadvantages are cost and the required parenteral route of administration.

E. Diphosphonates: Since these agents block bone resorption, trials investigating their efficacy in the treatment of osteoporosis have been undertaken. The only diphosphonate currently available in the USA is etidronate disodium. Reports from the USA and Europe indicate that etidronate given cyclically in doses of 400 mg/d for 2 weeks repeated every 3 months over 2–3 years is effective in halting bone loss and increasing bone density in postmenopausal osteoporotic patients. This regimen increases vertebral mineral content by 4–5% in this time period as assessed by dual-photon absorptiometry. Most importantly, vertebral fracture rates were significantly reduced compared with osteoporotic controls. Since therapy is oral and has minimal side effects, these studies have stimulated much interest in this class of agents in osteoporosis treatment programs. Etidronate has not been approved by the FDA for this indication.

Monitoring Long-term Therapy

When a therapeutic regimen is started in the osteoporotic patient, it is essential to decide how frequently and by what means to monitor disease progression and response to therapy. Bone densitometry, because of its simplicity, precision, and noninvasiveness, is the best means available.

Another useful test for monitoring the osteoporotic patient is quantitative urinary calcium. The traditional method for quantifying urinary calcium has been the measurement of calcium in a 24-hour urine collection. Nearly as accurate and much more convenient, however, is the measurement of calcium-to-creatinine ratio in a spot morning urine. Quantitative urine calcium is helpful to assure the adequacy of calcium supplementation while avoiding hypercalciuria (> 4 mg Ca/kg body weight/24 h or > 230 mg Ca/g creatinine).

Investigational Drugs

Diphosphonates and fluoride remain investigational drugs for the treatment of severe osteoporosis. Etidronate has been shown to be effective in reducing bone mineral loss and decreasing spinal fracture rate (see above). Clinical trials indicate that while sodium fluoride may increase spinal bone mineral density, the incidence of fractures is not decreased in fluoride-treated osteoporotic patients. Human PTH has anabolic effects on bone in low doses and is undergoing research testing alone and in combination with different antiresorptive drugs.

OSTEOMALACIA

Osteomalacia is a disorder of skeletal mineralization. It is due to skeletal deficiency of calcium or phosphorus; in the past the most common cause was calcium malabsorption due to a nutritional deficiency of vitamin D. In the USA nutritional causes of osteomalacia have become less common due to dietary supplementation with vitamin D, and genetic defects now account for most of the cases of osteomalacia seen in the usual adult practice. Despite a myriad of potential causes (Table 7–10), a general approach can be taken in evaluation, and most osteomalacic cases respond to standard treatment.

CLINICAL FEATURES

In children, inadequate mineralization of growing bone leads to a characteristic clinical picture known as rickets. In adults, this condition is known as osteomalacia, which is usually asymptomatic in its early stages. Generalized muscle weakness and skeletal pain (which may or may not be associated with a fracture) are the hallmarks of symptomatic osteomalacia. Fractures frequently occur in untreated cases, and signs and symptoms related to fractures (including loss of height) may eventually become the dominant clinical features.

As can be seen from Table 7–10, clinical history is vital in the evaluation of suspected osteomalacia. Dietary habits, physical activity, and sunlight exposure should be carefully documented. Associated diseases must be characterized. Drugs that affect mineral absorption, bone mineralization, or vitamin D metabolism should be noted.

Table 7–10. Causes of osteomalacia.

Vitamin disorders
  Decreased availability of vitamin D
    Insufficient sunlight exposure
    Nutritional deficiency of vitamin D
    Malabsorption
    Nephrotic syndrome
  Abnormal response to vitamin D
    Vitamin D dependent rickets–type II
    Gastrointestinal disorders
  Abnormal vitamin D metabolism
  Vitamin D dependent rickets—type I
  X-linked hypophosphatemic rickets
  Tumoral hypophosphatemic osteomalacia
  Liver disease
  Chronic renal failure
  Diphenylhydantoin or barbiturate therapy

Calcium deficiency

Phosphate deficiency
  Decreased intestinal absorption
    Nutritional deficiency of phosphorus
    Malabsorption
    Phosphate-binding antacid therapy
  Increased renal loss
    Vitamin D resistant rickets
    Tumoral hypophosphatemic osteomalacia
    Association with other disorders, including paraproteinemias, glycogen storage diseases, galactosemia, tyrosinemia, cystinosis, neurofibromatosis, Wilson's disease, Fanconi's syndrome

Disorders of bone matrix
  Hypophosphatasia
  Fibrogenesis imperfecta
  Axial osteomalacia

Inhibitors of mineralization
  Aluminum
  Diphosphonates

LABORATORY FEATURES

Calcium and phosphorus determinations in the serum and urine form the basis for laboratory evaluation of osteomalacia. Serum calcium may be low but often is normal owing to a compensatory increase in PTH. Serum phosphorus is often subnormal, reflecting decreased mineral absorption. Low urinary excretion of calcium (often < 40 mg/24 h) or phosphorus supports a hypoabsorptive state, while renal defects leading to osteomalacia may present with inappropriately high excretion of mineral. Secondary hyperparathyroidism may also induce a relative hyperphosphaturia. Serum $1,25(OH)_2$-D levels will detect most vitamin D deficiency states but may not identify vitamin D metabolic abnormalities. Because of calcium deficiency, a state of secondary hyperparathyroidism usually exists, with elevated PTH; alkaline phosphatase is usually high-normal or elevated. In most cases of osteomalacia, urinary excretion or serum mineral levels can be used to monitor the progress of the disease and response to therapy. Exceptions occur in situations in which PTH secretion is inhibited (eg, aluminum intoxication), or in intrinsic skeletal defects (eg, fibrogenesis imperfecta), where overall mineral homeostasis remains balanced.

X-Rays

The osteopenia of mild osteomalacia is radiologically indistinguishable from that of other causes. In more advanced disease, Looser's fractures may be seen, which are quite characteristic of osteomalacia. These radiolucent lines are found in the long bones of the extremities, the ribs, the clavicles, and the scapulae. Looser's fractures may begin as pseudofractures but can progress to more classical features, eventually resulting in deformity. Bone mineral content measurement is not very helpful in cases of osteomalacia. Although osteopenia is the rule, some instances of osteomalacia (eg, in renal failure) actually present with increased bone density.

Bone Biopsy

Bone biopsy is the standard for diagnosing the presence of osteomalacia. In most clinical cases, however, the diagnosis is available by other means, or it can be confirmed by a clinical therapeutic trial. For these reasons, bone biopsy is not necessary in most patients with osteomalacia. Double-labeling of the bone with tetracyclines should precede the biopsy itself. In osteomalacic bone, osteoid seams are wide and unmineralized. These findings, along with a low appositional rate and an increased mineralization lag time, form a histologic picture pathognomonic for osteomalacia.

TREATMENT

In adults, most cases of osteomalacia can be successfully treated, leading to normalization of clinical, biochemical, and radiologic abnormalities. To achieve this goal without inducing hypercalcemia, ectopic calcification, hyperphosphatemia, hypercalciuria, or nephrolithiasis, however, requires vigilance by both patient and physician. Most patients with osteomalacia do not display clearly diagnostic laboratory critiera for osteomalacia. However, if the clinical and radiological features fit a diagnosis of osteomalacia, a therapeutic trial of treatment may be justified as a route to confirming the diagnosis.

Correction of complicating medical conditions and repletion of necessary minerals is the first treatment priority. If vitamin D therapy (Table 7–6) is necessary, requirements may range from 2000 IU/d in simple nutritional deficiency up to 100,000 IU/d in severe malabsorption. Equivalent doses of more potent vitamin D metabolites (eg, 1-hydroxylated derivatives in renal failure) are reasonable alternatives in some specific forms of osteomalacia. In X-linked hypophosphatemia, 1–3 g of oral phosphorus (Table 7–4) must be given daily in divided doses. Because of gastrointestinal intolerance (eg, diarrhea), this therapy is associated with poor compliance. Vitamin D (25,000–100,000 U/d) and calcium (1–3 g/d) must usually be given as well, to prevent hypocalcemia. If calcium is given, it must be administered temporally remote from phosphate administration, to minimize calcium phosphate salt formation in the gut. In addition, such therapy must be handled carefully to avoid ectopic deposition of calcium salts.

Ironically, serum calcium may decrease and alkaline phosphatase increase early in the course of therapy with vitamin D; this should not be regarded as a treatment failure. The bone disease of osteomalacia usually takes several months of appropriate therapy to heal, at which point therapeutic doses must be cut back to maintenance levels. Patients being treated for osteomalacia should be carefully monitored with determinations of serum calcium, phosphorus, alkaline phosphatase, and immunoreactive iPTH as well as urinary calcium. Adequacy of therapy can thus be assessed while avoiding hypercalcemia and hypercalciuria.

RENAL OSTEODYSTROPHY

Some disturbance in skeletal metabolism is present in every patient with chronic renal failure (CRF). The complexity and the extent of this disease, or group of diseases, known as renal osteodystrophy, has become apparent as dialysis and transplantation for CRF have become more widespread. As improved techniques are developed for directly combating renal failure, the relative importance of renal osteodystrophy in the overall health of the CRF patient continues to increase. Means for dealing with this progressive bone disease are far from adequate.

PATHOPHYSIOLOGY

As kidney disease progresses, phosphate is retained and production of $1,25(OH)_2$-D declines, leading to decreased absorption of calcium. The parathyroid glands are stimulated by this combination of hypocalcemia and hyperphosphatemia, and PTH production increases. In addition, the uremia and acidosis associated with CRF have adverse effects on normal bone turnover. To complicate matters further, therapy for CRF may contribute to the development of renal osteodystrophy. Aluminum retained from antacid therapy or rarely from the dialysate leads to suppression of bone formation and perhaps to inhibition of both calcium absorption and PTH secretion. Dialysis may deplete the body of vital mineral stores if careful attention is not given to dialysate composition and mineral replacement. Physiologic compensatory mechanisms are rapidly overwhelmed in CRF, and the skeleton and other vital organs suffer as the body attempts to maintain mineral balances.

The bone disease associated with CRF is, therefore, a combination of disorders, including osteomalacia, osteosclerosis, and osteitis fibrosa cystica. Each case of renal osteodystrophy is unique, and evaluation and therapy should be tailored to findings in the individual patient.

CLINICAL FEATURES

The most common signs and symptoms of renal osteodystrophy are bone pain and muscle weakness. These nonspecific findings are difficult to characterize in the setting of chronic renal failure. Soft tissue calcifications or fractures may be seen in some cases. Calcium-salt deposition sometimes leads to pruritus or conjunctivitis. Most cases of renal osteodystrophy have no specific clinical features. In an individual patient, a feature may be identifiable that can be helpful in following the progress of the disease.

LABORATORY FEATURES

Laboratory Tests

Renal osteodystrophy develops in 3 fairly well characterized stages: (1) In early renal failure (serum creatinine < 3 mg/dL), serum PTH slowly rises to maintain serum mineral concentrations close to the normal values. (2) As renal failure progresses, the capacity for increased PTH secretion to correct the electrolyte abnormalities is overwhelmed, and serum phosphate rises and serum calcium concentration may fall. (3) At some point in the untreated case, the continuing stimulus to PTH hypersecretion leads to relative autonomy of the parathyroid glands. PTH-mediated bone resorption results in a rise in serum calcium, often into the frankly hypercalcemic range. This state, sometimes referred to as "tertiary" hyperparathyroidism, eventually leads to severe bone disease and impairment of vital organ function and is a strong indication for surgical resection of parathyroid tissue.

Very high iPTH levels may be seen in CRF. This may be due to increased secretion of bioactive, intact PTH or the type of PTH radioimmunoassay used. Many mid-region or carboxy-terminal radio-immunoassays for PTH detect intact hormone as well as bioinactive fragments, which are slowly cleared in the uremic patient. In spite of the fact that the iPTH value may not correspond directly to the true bioactive PTH level, the serial determination of iPTH by mid-region or carboxy-terminal PTH assays in the CRF patient is helpful in evaluating the effects of various therapeutic maneuvers and in charting the overall progress of the disease. Elevated PTH levels may be inappropriately low in some patients with the osteomalacic form of renal osteodystrophy, contributing to a low-turnover state. PTH levels, as assessed by 2-site IRMA assays or other intact PTH assays, may be normal or elevated. These assays should detect the earliest stages of secondary hyperparathyroidism and may provide better diagnostic discrimination of the type and severity of renal osteodystrophy.

Alkaline phosphatase is frequently elevated in renal osteodystrophy, but it is a reliable indicator of neither osteitis fibrosa cystica nor osteomalacia in this setting. Levels of $1,25(OH)_2$-D may be normal if diet and sunlight exposure are adequate in the CRF patient. Nevertheless, $1,25(OH)_2$-D levels are usually very low, and the resultant decreased calcium absorption may be manifest as decreased renal calcium clearance, even in the face of active skeletal resorption.

Serum and bone aluminum assays have been applied to investigation of the role of aluminum in renal osteodystrophy. Total body aluminum burden appears to be best estimated by measuring the serum aluminum level after an infusion of deferoxamine, an aluminum chelator.

X-Rays

X-ray changes in renal osteodystrophy may reflect osteoporosis, osteomalacia, osteitis fibrosa, osteosclerosis, or a combination of disorders, depending on the nature of the disease in the particular patient and in the area examined. Osteosclerosis in the vertebral bodies, or "rugger jersey spine," is probably the most characteristic x-ray change. Patients with CRF may be followed radiologically with industrial-grade hand films.

Bone Biopsy

Percutaneous bone biopsy in a patient with renal osteodystrophy will always contribute definitive information on the specific pathologic processes involved. In most cases, however, such information is either available through less invasive means or is not crucial in making therapeutic decisions. Bone biopsy specimens can be routinely stained for aluminum, and the percent of bone surface covered by aluminum can be estimated. This diagnostic step may prove particularly useful, along with assessment of iPTH and other clinical parameters, in determining the cause of low-turnover bone disease in patients with CRF. Such a determination may have important ramifications for treatment.

TREATMENT & PREVENTION

Calcium & Vitamin D

Since every patient with renal failure is at high risk for renal osteodystrophy, measures designed to prevent or retard the development of this disorder are of prime importance. Daily intake of at least 1500 mg of calcium is required to compensate for decreased calcium absorption in CRF. Since minimization of dietary phosphorus is also important, calcium availability from the usual "renal" diet is limited, and calcium supplements must be given (Table 7–9). Vitamin D preparations may improve calcium (and phosphorus) absorption, and they may be helpful in treating the bone disease of renal osteodystrophy as well. The 1-hydroxylated derivatives [1,25(OH)$_2$-D and DHT] are particularly effective in renal osteodystrophy (Table 7–6), but extreme care must be taken to anticipate and avoid hypercalcemia in an oliguric patient.

Diet & Phosphate Binders

Another goal is the prevention of metabolic acidosis by limiting animal protein intake. This measure may also be helpful in limiting dietary phosphorus, but it severely restricts the dietary supply of calcium. Perhaps the most difficult goal to achieve in prevention of renal osteodystrophy is the maintenance of near-normal serum phosphate levels. Dietary restrictions are seldom adequate, and the common approach is to add phosphate binders (aluminum hydroxide–containing antacids; calcium carbonate also is a weak phosphate binder). Over an extended time period, however, the constipating and anorexic effects of these substances become limiting in many patients. Unfortunately, various dietary measures, each of which may be helpful in preventing renal osteodystrophy, combine to make a diet that is unpalatable to many patients. Patients with aluminum overload have been successfully managed with high doses of calcium carbonate, which serves as a phosphate binder.

Estrogen or Androgen

In the patient with CRF who has developed hypogonadism, supplemental estrogens may be given to women and androgens to men. These steroids may play a role in protecting the skeleton as well as in contributing to the patient's sense of well-being. Vaginal bleeding may limit estrogen use in women who are already anemic owing to CRF.

Dialysis

Treatment for renal osteodystrophy must be, to a large extent, treatment for CRF itself. Frequent dialysis helps maintain mineral balance and thus slows the progression of renal osteodystrophy. A high calcium dialysate (usually 6 mg/dL or higher) should be used in nonhypercalcemic cases. In addition, the dialysate may be a major source of aluminum retained in the system of the patient with CRF. Since aluminum-containing phosphate binders contribute additionally to this load, dialysate aluminum content should be kept as low as possible. Deferoxamine may be useful in minimizing aluminum accumulation and in treating aluminum overload in patients with CRF.

Renal Transplantation

Renal transplantation is the definitive therapy for CRF, and provided that improved renal function is maintained in the transplanted state, it usually has a beneficial effect on renal osteodystrophy as well. With respect to the bone disease, early transplantation is desirable. Mild hyperparathyroidism may persist for a time after transplantation, as the glomerular filtration rate does not immediately return to normal. Since glucocorticoid therapy is a usual component of peritransplant management, glucocorticoid-induced osteoporosis might be induced as an adverse component of this otherwise beneficial therapy. Newer approaches deal with transplant rejection by employing shorter courses and lower doses of glucocorticoids in combination with other immunosuppressive agents. Such approaches may aid in establishing transplantation therapy as the definitive treatment for renal osteodystrophy.

Surgery

Parathyroid surgery plays an important role in the management of renal osteodystrophy. Considerations in the timing of surgery and extent of parathyroid resection are complex. Removal of parathyroid tissue decreases the stimulus to bone turnover and suppresses hypercalcemia. On the other hand, phosphate excretion and 1-hydroxylation of vitamin D may be further compromised (if any renal function remains) by parathyroid resection. Removal of parathyroid tissue also introduces the risk of hypoparathyroidism. Parathyroid resection may convert the bone disease of CRF from a high-turnover osteitis-like picture to a low-turnover osteomalacia–like state. This conversion may be a net loss to skeletal health, since the PTH-induced skeletal turnover may be vital to remodeling and repair processes in the patient with CRF. The prudent approach is to minimize the stimulus to hyperparathyroidism by maintaining serum phosphorus in the high-normal range for as long as possible. When hypercalcemia becomes a problem, when high-turnover bone disease must be suppressed, or when marked, sudden rises in serum immunoreactive PTH herald "tertiary" hyperparathyroidism, resection of parathyroid tissue is probably the only alternative. Since parathyroid resection accelerates aluminum deposition in bone, patients should be evaluated for aluminum toxicity, preferably by bone biopsy, before surgery. Chelation could be done preoperatively. Postoperatively, aluminum intake must be restricted. Removal of at least 3.5 glands is usual practice, and parathyroid tissue can be transplanted to the forearm as an extra hedge against hypoparathyroidism. This general approach must be carefully modified to meet the specific needs of the individual patient.

PAGET'S DISEASE OF BONE

Paget's disease is one of the most common metabolic bone diseases. This and a variety of uncommon genetic disorders are generally classified as the osteoscleroses: disorders with localized or generalized increases in bone density. Paget's disease occurs in 3–5% of adults over age 50 in the United Kingdom, Central Europe, Australia, New Zealand, and the USA. On the other hand, it is rare in Asia, Africa, the Middle East, and Scandinavia. The disease is occasionally familial. Paget's disease is chronic and slowly progressive. It begins with an osteolytic phase, involving giant osteoclasts and leading to osteoporosis circumscripta cranii. An osteoblastic response follows, with eventual formation of patchy areas of sclerosis. Paget's disease is a high-turnover disorder, with mixed osteolytic and osteoblastic processes. Pagetic bone is structurally unsound due to the highly disordered architecture. Current theories ascribe a viral cause.

CLINICAL FEATURES

Symptoms

Most patients with Paget's disease have no symptoms, and the disease is often detected when plain x-rays or bone scans of affected areas have been obtained for other reasons. In some patients, the disease is discovered when an unexplained elevation of alkaline phosphatase appears on a screening blood test. Pain is the most common symptom and is usually localized to affected areas. Pain is often described as a deep, bony ache; it is usually due to the disease itself but may also be caused by a pathologic fracture. Bony overgrowth occurs in severe cases and may lead to a variety of important symptoms. Skeletal deformity may be merely unsightly or may actually impair function. Neurologic involvement ranges from focal deficits to myelopathy or radiculopathy due to disease in the vertebrae. Some degree of deafness will eventually appear in half of all patients with pagetic skull involvement. Deafness may result from both nerve and conduction defects.

Signs

Clinical findings in the asymptomatic patient are seldom significant. In more severely affected cases, bony overgrowth may be apparent in the skull and long bones. Skull circumference may be a useful way to follow this process. Blood flow increases significantly to skeletal areas affected by Paget's disease owing to increases in vascularity that accompany progression of the disease. Skin temperature sometimes increases over affected areas. Localized increased blood flow occasionally leads to vascular steal syndromes. In severe long-standing Paget's disease (not frequently seen today), increased vascularity may even become manifest as high-output congestive heart failure. Extramedullary hematopoiesis may occasionally be seen with attendant organomegaly or masses adjacent to affected bone.

LABORATORY FEATURES

Laboratory Tests

Osteoclastic overactivity during the osteolytic phase of Paget's disease results in collagen breakdown, which can be detected as increased urinary hydroxyproline. Osteoblastic activity is reflected in an elevation of serum alkaline phosphatase. The alkaline phosphatase level usually correlates fairly well with disease activity, and this test is also used to monitor the effectiveness of therapy. Increased erythrocyte sedimentation rate and elevated uric acid may be seen, probably reflecting the markedly increased metabolic activity and high cellular turnover that characterize this disease. Because Paget's disease (as well as other osteosclerotic disorders) results from a defect within bony tissues, mineral homeostasis will not be affected unless normal control mechanisms are overwhelmed. Serum calcium and phosphorus are usually normal. Extensive disease may deliver a calcium load to the kidney that is large enough to result in hypercalciuria. This process may result in mild secondary hyperparathyroidism, with elevated iPTH.

X-Rays

Radiologic studies are key to diagnosis and follow-up. Paget's disease probably begins as, and may remain, an anatomically localized disease. Patches of activity are most commonly seen in bones of the pelvic girdle and in the skull. Bones may be expanded or deformed. Affected areas are usually rather sharply demarcated from normal bone (the "osteoporosis circumscripta" phenomenon). V-shaped resorption fronts are often identifiable in areas of pagetic activity. The bony trabecular pattern is disrupted with mixed areas of porosis and sclerosis in an active patch. As the disease becomes more generalized, the asymmetry that is the rule in localized involvement may tend to disappear. Technetium bone scan should be obtained in every patient with Paget's disease. Areas of active disease show markedly increased uptake. Sites of active disease should be confirmed by plain x-ray. Bone scan may be used, along with serum alkaline phosphatase, to monitor disease activity periodically.

Special Tests

Many cases of atypical Paget's disease, when investigated, turn out to be examples of other osteosclerotic disorders. When osteo-sclerosis is seen in a young person, if family history is particularly striking, if the x-ray pattern is symmetrical or generalized, or if there are unusual deviations from the laboratory findings described above, suspicion should be high for one of the numerous, but uncommon, genetic osteosclerotic disorders. Because therapeutic issues seldom arise in the differential diagnosis of osteosclerosis, there is not always strong incentive to investigate a case thoroughly. Conclusive diagnosis in many osteosclerotic disorders depends on careful histologic analysis of a bone biopsy, and this procedure cannot always be justified in this patient population.

TREATMENT

Most patients are asymptomatic and require no specific treatment. This group includes those in whom the disease is discovered incidentally and those with inactive disease (no symptoms and normal alkaline phosphatase values, in spite of often extensive x-ray changes). These patients should be followed clinically, keeping in mind that fluctuating cycles of disease activity are common in Paget's disease. Patients who are symptomatic and those who have biochemical or radiologic evidence of extensive or progressive disease (including *any* skull involvement) should receive treatment.

Drugs

A. Calcium: Calcium supplements may help to reduce the risk of osteomalacia and secondary hyperparathyroidism in Paget's disease. Bone pain may also be reduced in the calcium-supplemented patient. In the nonambulatory patient, calcium supplements should be given with care, if at all, because of the tendency of immobilized patients with active Paget's disease to develop hypercalciuria and hypercalcemia.

B. Calcitonin: Calcitonin has been the mainstay of treatment in Paget's disease. Therapy is confined to the parenteral route of administration at present and is usually begun with 50 IU/d subcutaneously. Effects on clinical and biochemical parameters are usually seen in 2–4 weeks, and side effects are usually minimal (see above). Occasionally, 100–150 IU/d will be necessary. Maintenance dosage is usually 50 IU, 3 times a week. Therapy may be given in 6- to 12–month courses with observation periods between. Effectiveness of prolonged or repeated therapy is occasionally limited by antibody formation. An increase in bone pain is an indication to discontinue or change therapy or look for complications (see below).

C. Diphosphonates: In the USA, only one diphosphonate (etidronate) is available for clinical use, but it has become important in the treatment of Paget's disease. In contrast to calcitonin, etidronate can be given orally. Gastrointestinal side effects are fairly common but usually not severe. Therapy is begun with doses of 5–10 mg/kg/d. Limited absorption may affect drug potency in a given patient. The dose should be used that just maintains clinical and biochemical parameters at the desired (not necessarily normal) level. Treatment courses should not exceed 6 months, with a rest period prior to a new course of therapy. Prolonged remissions have been reported after 6 months. Paradoxical increases in bone pain may occur during diphosphonate therapy, and a serious osteomalacia-like picture is a rare side effect. Osteomalacia secondary to etidronate therapy is usually observed when doses of 20 mg/kg have been used. Such complications may be related to the state of secondary hyperparathyroidism, which may accompany severe Paget's disease, and may be treated with oral calcium supplements. Development of such a picture (usually heralded by increased bone pain) requires a termination of or change in therapy.

D. Plicamycin: In severely progressive, refractory cases of Paget's disease, plicamycin has proved to be effective alternative therapy. Initially, infusions are given every 2–3 days, but some patients have maintained for several weeks on a once-a-week infusion. Potential toxicity makes this therapy a last resort in Paget's disease.

Complications

Several major complications of Paget's disease must be recognized. The high-turnover state may lead to negative calcium balance and secondary hyperparathyroidism. For this reason, calcium supplements are given routinely by some, or in response to rising iPTH levels by others. Diphosphonate therapy may accentuate secondary hyperparathyroidism, which in turn may be involved in the development of the osteomalacia-like complication. For this reason, calcium supplements are especially recommended for Paget's disease patients on diphosphonates. Prolonged bedrest should be avoided, since it may add a resorptive component to Paget's disease. Pagetic bone may be osteoporotic, be osteosclerotic, or (most often) display mixed defects, but it is always mechanically deficient. For this reason, the patient with Paget's disease is prone to fractures in areas of disease. This may be a consideration in therapeutic decisions in a borderline-symptomatic patient. Precautions against trauma are indicated in all patients with Paget's disease. About 1% of patients eventually develop bone tumors in regions of active disease. These tumors may range from benign giant cell reparative granulomas to malignant sarcomas. Sudden symptomatic deteriorations (including fractures), a rapid and marked increase in alkaline phosphatase activity compared with baseline levels, and suggestive x-ray changes should alert the clinician to possible tumor development.

NEPHROLITHIASIS

Nephrolithiasis is a common medical problem which, although it seldom progresses to fatality, is most debilitating and disruptive. At least 3% of North Americans have the disease, but its prevalence varies greatly from area to area within the USA and even more throughout the world (Table 7–11). The incidence by stone composi-

Table 7–11. Classification of renal stones by composition.

		% Incidence in USA
Calcium salts		90%
Oxalate	75%	
Phosphate and mixed	12%	
Triple phosphate (struvite)	3%	
Uric acid		6%
Cystine		2%
Miscellaneous		<1%

tion also varies greatly worldwide—over half of all renal stones in some parts of Israel are uric acid stones. Both the prevalence and the distribution of renal stone disease are functions of a myriad of factors—genetic, dietary, environmental, and cultural. The interplay of these factors is not well understood.

EVALUATION

Renal stones are made up of an organic matrix onto which a sparingly soluble salt has crystallized. The formation of the matrix, the sources and interactions of the salt components, the concentrations and solubility products of minerals in the urine, and local factors affecting solubility and crystallization all play a role in stone formation. Paradoxes are common; many patients with very high urinary calcium excretion never form renal stones, while some formers of calcium stones can never be shown to be hypercalciuric.

Hypercalciuria is nevertheless a strong predisposing factor to nephrolithiasis, and most stones in the USA contain calcium (Table 7–11). There are 3 possible mechanisms for hypercalciuria. (1) Primary absorptive hypercalciuria involves abnormally high gastrointestinal absorption of calcium, which suppresses PTH. (2) Renal phosphate leak leads to a secondary increase in $1,25(OH)_2$-D levels, and resultant calcium hyperabsorption suppresses PTH. (3) Renal calcium leak leads to negative calcium balance and elevated PTH levels. Primary hyperparathyroidism or hypersensitivity to PTH causes a secondary form of the renal phosphate leak or a gastrointestinal hyperabsorption mechanism for nephrolithiasis.

CLINICAL FEATURES

Nephrolithiasis is frequently a manifestation of another disorder. A renal stone is frequently the presentation of hyperparathyroidism and is occasionally the first sign of gout. There is a high incidence of nephrolithiasis in patients with renal malformations, especially medullary sponge kidney. Malabsorption disorders, such as inflammatory bowel disease, or intestinal bypass surgery may lead to enteric hyperoxaluria. The mechanism is probably increased absorption of oxalate. Oxalate absorption is normally limited by intraluminal complexation with calcium; in gastrointestinal disease a significant portion of that calcium may be competitively complexed with nonabsorbed fatty acids.

Urate stone disease is also more common in patients with gastrointestinal disorders. In patients who have severe renal stone disease, the incidence of struvite stones may be as high as 20%. This patient group should be vigorously investigated for possibly primary or secondary infection in the urinary tract. Family history may be revealing, since both genetic and environmental factors may cluster within families. For example, type I (distal) renal tubular acidosis (RTA) is usually transmitted as an autosomal dominant trait although some cases are sporadic. Cystinuria is transmitted as an autosomal recessive trait. Hyperparathyroidism may also be familial.

Patients with type I RTA are prone to calcium phosphate stones and nephrocalcinosis. In hereditary type I RTA, chronic hyperchloremic acidosis causes hypercalciuria, secondary hyperparathyroidism, and deficient urine citrate (which usually binds to 40% of urine calcium). Untreated children have short stature and rickets; adults have osteomalacia. In hereditary type I RTA, hypokalemia and polyuria are common. Patients with acquired RTA are less likely to have hypokalemia and hypercalciuria unless the RTA was caused by nephrocalcinosis induced by hereditary idiopathic hypercalciuria. Other diseases that cause acquired RTA may be present, eg, Ehlers-Danlos syndrome, medullary sponge kidney, galactosemia, hereditary elliptocytosis, or Fabry's disease.

Some patients with nephrolithiasis are identified when asymptomatic microscopic hematuria is detected, or when examination of an abdominal x-ray reveals an abnormal renal density. Most patients, however, present with gross hematuria or pain. Renal colic may localize to any area of the abdomen, but is characteristically in the flank on the side of involvement. The pain is sharp, usually intermittent, and often severe. Pain episodes may be associated with nausea, vomiting, and occasionally fever. Patients describe this pain to be unlike any other and often as the most severe ever experienced.

LABORATORY FEATURES

The laboratory evaluation of nephrolithiasis should be guided by the severity and frequency of the disease in the particular patient. A limited workup is recommended for every nephrolithiasis patient, with aggressiveness in both diagnosis and treatment increasing with frequency or severity of attacks. Even the patient who has experienced only a single stone episode may benefit from knowledge of the possible pathophysiology involved.

Laboratory Tests

The initial workup includes routine urinalysis, blood tests, and evaluation of 24-hour urine samples (Table 7–12). Urinalysis permits identification of blood in the urine, evaluation of urinary tract infec-

Table 7–12. Evaluation for Nephrolithiasis.

1. History: Any preceding dehydration, bone fracture, gout, urine infection; any ingestion of calcium, vitamin D, glucocorticoids, triamterene, or large dose of ascorbic acid (vitamin C). Any personal or family history of nephrolithiasis, hyperparathyroidism, pituitary adenomas, pancreatic neoplasms, or peptic ulcer disease.
2. Send any stone that is passed or recovered at operation for analysis. Stones may be sent to Louis C. Merring and Co., PO Box 2191, Orlando, FL 32802.
3. Urinalysis to include analysis for pH, crystals, pyuria.
4. Urine culture.
5. Urine excretion of calcium and uric acid, creatinine clearance, and phosphate.
6. Serum calcium, uric acid, bicarbonate. If serum calcium is high, a serum PTH is obtained.
7. Intravenous pyelogram to look for renal anomalies and other stones.
8. Chest x-ray to look for sarcoidosis.

tions that may be either the cause or the result of renal stones, and determination of urine pH and specific gravity. A urine pH repeatedly alkaline suggests renal tubular acidosis or urine infection. Serum electrolytes, calcium, phosphorus, uric acid, creatinine, and iPTH should be determined. The 24-hour urine sample is analyzed for calcium, oxalate, urate, sodium, and creatinine. In the hypercalcemic patient or in the patient with known calcium-containing stones, the urine evaluation should be repeated after a 14-hour fast (with care not to precipitate a stone episode by excessive urine concentration) or on a low (or occasionally high) calcium diet. In this way, inexpensive and noninvasive determinations of the characteristics of calcium absorption can be made.

A morning urine specimen may be acidified and centrifuged and the sediment examined under low microscopic power for the translucent, hexagonal crystals that are pathognomonic of cystinuria. The presence of calcium crystals is less helpful.

Hypercalciuria is defined as calcium excretion of greater than 4 mg calcium/kg body weight/24 h. Urinary concentration is a more crucial determinant of stone formation than urinary excretion, but the patient with hypercalciuria is at risk for stones and should be identified. If the patient is hypercalciuric owing to excessive calcium absorption, serum calcium will be normal to high-normal, and serum iPTH will be suppressed. A secondary hyperabsorptive state may result from a renal phosphate leak, with resulting low normal serum phosphate and elevated $1,25(OH)_2$-D levels. If abnormally high renal excretion of calcium is involved, serum calcium levels will be low-normal with resultant secondary hyperparathyroidism. Hypercalcemia with high iPTH levels, of course, suggests primary hyperparathyroidism. The hypercalciuric patient seldom fits exclusively into one of the categories outlined, but consideration of operative mechanisms allows choice of rational, goal-directed therapy.

Stone Analysis

The patient should be impressed with the importance of collecting and delivering any renal stone to the physician. Thorough crystallographic stone analysis should be performed, including analysis of the core or nidus of the stone. Some stones appear to form around a nidus of a distinct material (eg, calcium oxalate stones on a urate nidus). Another common scenario is a patient with small stones of metabolic origin who develops a urinary tract infection involving urease-producing bacteria (eg, *Proteus* sp). The small metabolic stones may then provide a nidus for development of large "infection stones" (struvite). Patients with calcium phosphate stones must be evaluated for RTA. Urate or cystine stones similarly direct further evaluation and treatment.

X-Rays

All calcium-containing stones are radiopaque (uric acid stones are radiolucent). Since many cases of calcium nephrolithiasis are first detected incidentally after examination of an abdominal x-ray, sequential radiographs can be helpful in monitoring the progress of a stone during therapy. If more precise information on the size or location of the stone is necessary, ultrasound analysis or CT scans may be necessary. Patients with nephrocalcinosis should be evaluated for RTA. Patients with staghorn calculi must be evaluated for cystinuria and chronic urinary tract infections, especially *Proteus* sp.

TREATMENT

If the stone composition is known, or if laboratory workup has identified a urinary solute that may be involved, attempts to decrease the concentration of that solute in the urine are worthwhile.

Fluids

The cornerstone of nonsurgical treatment is increased fluid intake. Although this may be simple in principle, it is difficult for most patients to comply with an intake of 2 L/d of fluid, and considerable time is required in patient education and persuasion. In addition, some drinking water sources are high in calcium content, and a few cases of hypercalciuria *due* to excessive ingestion of drinking water have been reported.

Diet

If stones are composed of calcium salts, especially if high calcium excretion appears to be based on excessive gastrointestinal absorption, moderate dietary restriction of calcium may be warranted. Severe calcium restriction may, however, lead to osteopenia or to increased absorption of oxalate and paradoxical increases in stone formation. In the patient with calcium oxalate stone disease, prudence dictates restriction of oxalate-rich foods and of dietary calcium. Oxalate-rich foods include dark-green leafy vegetables (eg, spinach), black pepper, rhubarb, tea, coffee, cola, chocolate, and some fruit juices (grapefruit, cranberry); ascorbic acid (vitamin C) administration also increases urine oxalate concentrations. Low sodium diets and thiazide diuretics promote calcium reabsorption and may be particularly helpful in patients who display a renal calcium leak. Mild protein restriction may limit acid load (particularly in urate lithiasis). Low carbohydrate and high fiber diets may be helpful in calcium stone disease; however, such diets are not very palatable.

Drugs

A. Thiazide Diuretics: Hydrochlorothiazide and similar thiazides inhibit urine excretion of calcium if dietary salt is restricted. The dose begins with 50 mg/d and is titrated upward if needed, while urine calcium concentration is monitored. Combined diuretics containing triamterene should not be used, since this drug itself may cause nephrolithiasis.

B. Phosphate: Elemental phosphorus, 1–2 g/d, is sometimes administered to limit calcium absorption from the gastrointestinal tract. This therapy is not always well tolerated.

C. Allopurinol: In uric acid stones, dietary measures (avoidance of sweetbreads, some cheeses, wines) and alkalinization of urine often need to be supplemented with allopurinol (200–400 mg/d), although the potential marrow and liver toxicity of this drug must be recognized. Some cases of calcium-containing stone disease have been shown to benefit from allopurinol therapy, presumably owing to the influence of urinary urate on deposition of calcium salts. Allopurinol is given prophylactically before chemotherapy of responsive cancers (such as lymphomas or leukemias) to prevent renal uric acid sludge.

D. Potassium Citrate: In 1985, the FDA approved potassium citrate for use in patients with nephrolithiasis associated with distal RTA, hypocitraturia and calcium oxalate stones, and gouty diathesis. Administration of this agent lowers tubular reabsorption of citrate and increases citrate excretion. The resulting hypercitraturia enhances urinary inhibitor activity against calcium oxalate crystallization and may also reduce urate-induced crystallization of calcium oxalate. In addition, potassium citrate provides an alkali load that increases urinary pH and further reduces the likelihood of uric acid crystal formation.

Urine pH

Alteration of urinary pH to favor soluble, ionic forms of stone salts can be a useful adjunct to therapy. Alkalinization (sodium bicarbonate, 1–3 mg/kg/d) favors soluble salts for patients with documented urate, cystine, or calcium phosphate stones due to RTA.

Other Therapy

In some cases, treatment of infection (overt or subliminal) in the urinary tract may be the key to therapy. A urease inhibitor, acetohydroxamic acid, may prove helpful in some struvite-stone cases. Additional approaches have been applied specifically to calcium oxalate stones. Cholestyramine (along with pyridoxine supplement) can be used to inhibit oxalate absorption, and sodium cellulose phosphate has been used to decrease gastrointestinal calcium absorption. Magnesium oxide (MgO, 200–300 mg/d) may be effective as an inhibitor of stone formation. With cystine stones that are refractory to increased fluid and alkali therapy, D-penicillamine has proved useful, but side effects are common.

Surgery

In cases unresponsive to medical therapy, or when stones are large enough to cause mechanical obstruction or recurrent infections, removal of the stone becomes the only alternative. Occasionally, renal colic from a stone is so severe that intervention is required before more conservative measures take their course. Many stones can be fragmented by **lithotripsy**, a procedure that localizes the stone and concentrates sound waves on it, resulting in fragmentation of the stone. The gravel and small fragments of the stone are subsequently passed by the patient generally without complications. This technique has largely replaced surgical procedures for the removal of stones in centers where the instrumentation and expertise are available. When surgery is necessary in the patient with nephrolithiasis, retrograde procedures are used for smaller stones, particularly those lodged in the lower urinary tract. Larger stones in the renal pelvis require nephrolithotomy.

Complications

Continuing debilitating pain and narcotic dependence are serious complications of untreated or unresponsive nephrolithiasis. Such cases lead to significant blood loss through hematuria. Partial obstruction from renal stones predisposes to urinary tract infections. The complications of long-standing nephrolithiasis may eventually lead to renal failure.

PHOSPHATE METABOLISM

HYPERPHOSPHATEMIA

Hyperphosphatemia creates no definitive symptoms. However, chronic hyperphosphatemia may produce extraskeletal calcium-phosphate deposits. By binding to calcium, excess phosphate produces a stimulus for PTH secretion. Causes of hyperphosphatemia are listed in Table 7–13. This is one factor involved in renal osteodystrophy, and treatment is discussed in that section.

HYPOPHOSPHATEMIA

Hypophosphatemia may be asymptomatic when it is of acute onset. Persistent hypophosphatemia, however, may produce symptoms of muscular weakness, anorexia, dizziness, bone pain, rickets in children, and osteomalacia in adults. Some patients develop congestive heart failure. Severe hypophosphatemia may cause rhabdomyolysis with increased serum creatine phosphokinase levels. Children with hypophosphatemia have impaired growth. Causes of hypophosphatemia are listed in Table 7–14. Available phosphate preparations are found in Table 7–4.

FIBROUS DYSPLASIA

Fibrous dysplasia is a rare disorder of bone that is frequently associated with other seemingly unrelated endocrine disorders. It is also known as Albright's syndrome and as McCune-Albright syndrome. It is usually recognized in childhood, and 3 abnormalities are

Table 7–13. Causes of hyperphosphatemia.

Renal failure
Hyperparathyroidism with renal failure
Hypoparathyroidism and pseudohypoparathyroidism
Youth
Phosphate preparations: intravenous or oral
Severe hyperglycemia
Growth hormone excess: acromegaly and gigantism

Table 7–14. Causes of hypophosphatemia.

Poor nutrition	Acute insulin therapy for
Malabsorption	hyperglycemia (especially
Hyperparathyroidism	ketoacidosis)
Total parenteral nutrition or	Renal phosphate loss: genetic,
administration of large amounts	tumor, or other disease
of carbohydrates (eg, glucose,	Volume expansion (acute)
fructose, glycerol)	Alcoholism: chronic and withdrawal
Calcium infusion	Alkalosis: hyperventilation or
Phosphate-binding antacids	bicarbonate administration
(aluminum hydroxide)	Refeeding patients with protein-
	calorie malnutrition

often present: bone lesions, precocious puberty (especially girls), and cafe-au-lait skin pigmentation with irregular (coast-of-Maine) borders. The pigmentation occurs most frequently over the low back and cervical spine. Patients are afflicted by bone pain, deformities, fractures, and altered gait. On x-ray, the bone lesions have a ground-glass appearance with multiple lesions thinning the cortex and deforming the bone. Serum alkaline phosphatase and urine hydroxyproline excretion are usually increased. Bone lesions may become sarcomatous.

The syndrome is frequently associated with hyperplasia or adenomas of endocrine glands that can produce acromegaly or gigantism, hyperprolactinemia, hyperparathyroidism, hyperthyroidism, Cushing's syndrome, hypophosphatemic (vitamin D–resistant) rickets, and hypothalamic hypogonadism.

Attempts at treatment have been disappointing. Calcitonin has not proved beneficial in limited trials. Radiation therapy may increase the risk of sarcomatous degeneration. Symptomatic treatment and corrective surgery are often required. Associated endocrine problems are watched for and treated individually as described elsewhere.

REFERENCES

Reviews
Berner YN et al: Consequences of phosphate imbalance. *Annu Rev Nutr* 1988;**8**:121.
Strewler GJ, Nissenson RA: Nonparathyroid hypercalcemia. *Adv Intern Med* 1987;**32**:235.

Hypercalcemia
Adams JS et al: Vitamin D metabolite–mediated hypercalcemia and hypercalciuria in patients with AIDS- and non-AIDS-associated lymphoma. *Blood* 1989;**73**:235.

Bilezikian JP: Surgery or no surgery for primary hyperparathyroidism. *Ann Intern Med* 1985;**102:**402

Blind E et al: Two-site assay of intact parathyroid hormone in the investigation of primary hyperparathyroidism and other disorders of calcium metabolism compared with midregion assay. *J Clin Endocrinol Metab* 1988;**67:**353.

Budayr AA et al: Increased serum levels of a parathyroid hormone–like protein in malignancy-associated hypercalcemia. *Ann Intern Med* 1989;**111:**807.

Fitzpatrick LA, Bilezikian JP: Acute primary hyperparathyroidism. *Am J Med* 1987;**82:**275.

Fukumoto S et al: Clinical evaluation of calcium metabolism in adult T-cell leukemia/lymphoma. *Arch Intern Med* 1988;**148:**921.

Harinck HIJ et al: Role of bone and kidney in tumor-induced hypercalcemia and its treatment with bisphosphonate and sodium chloride. *Am J Med* 1987;**82:**1133.

Jacobs TP et al: Neoplastic hypercalcemia: Physiologic response to intravenous etidronate disodium. *Am J Med* 1987;**82(Suppl 2A):**42.

Kristiansen JH et al: Familial hypocalciuric hypercalcemia. II. Intestinal calcium absorption and vitamin D metabolism. *Clin Endocrinol* 1985;**23:**511.

Law WM Jr, et al: Parathyroid glands in familial benign hypercalcemia (familial hypocalciuric hypercalcemia). *Am J Med* 1984;**76:**1021.

Law WM Jr, Heath H, III: Familial benign hypercalcemia (hypocalciuric hypercalcemia): Clinical and pathogenetic studies in 21 families. *Ann Intern Med* 1985;**102:**511.

Motokura T et al: Parathyroid hormone–related protein in adult T-cell leukemia-lymphoma. *Ann Intern Med* 1989;**111:**484.

Nussbaum SR et al: Highly sensitive two-site immunoradiometric assay of parathyrin, and its clinical utility in evaluating patients with hypercalcemia. *Clin Chem* 1987;**33:**1364.

Parisien M et al: The histomorphometry of bone in primary hyperparathyroidism: Preservation of cancellous bone structure. *J Clin Endocrinol Metab* 1990;**70:**930.

Potts JT Jr: Management of asymptomatic hyperparathyroidism. *J Clin Endocrinol Metab* 1990;**70:**1489.

Strewler GJ et al: Parathyroid hormone–like protein from human renal carcinoma cells: Structural and functional homology with parathyroid hormone. *J Clin Invest* 1987;**80:**1803.

Strewler GJ et al: Peptide mediators of hypercalcemia in malignancy. *Annu Rev Med* 1990;**41:**35.

Suva LJ et al: A parathyroid hormone-related protein implicated in malignant hypercalcemia: Cloning and expression. *Science* 1987;**237:**893.

Winzelberg GG: Parathyroid imaging. *Ann Intern Med* 1989;**107:**64.

Hypoparathyroidism

Ahn TG et al: Familial isolated hypoparathyroidism: A molecular genetic analysis of 8 families with 23 affected persons. *Medicine* 1986;**65:**73.

Carter A et al: Reduced expression of multiple forms of the alpha subunit of the stimulatory GTP-binding protein in pseudohypoparathyroidism type 1a. *Proc Natl Acad Sci USA* 1987;**84:**7266.

Deasi TK et al: Prevalence and clinical implications of hypocalcemia in acutely ill patients in a medical intensive care setting. *Am J Med* 1988;**84:**209.

Levine MA et al: Activity of the stimulatory guanine nucleotide–binding protein is reduced in erythrocytes from patients with pseudohypoparathyroidism and pseudopseudohypoparathyroidism: Biochemical, endocrine, and genetic analysis of Albright's hereditary osteodystrophy in 6 kindreds. *J Clin Endocrinol Metab* 1986;**62**:497.

Levine MA et al: Genetic deficiency of the α subunit of G$_s$ as the molecular basis for Albright hereditary osteodystrophy. *Proc Natl Acad Sci USA* 1988; **85**:617.

Mallette LE: Synthetic human parathyroid hormone 1-34 fragment for diagnostic testing. *Ann Intern Med* 1988;**109**:800.

Okano O et al: Comparative efficacy of various vitamin D metabolites in the treatment of various types of hypoparathyroidism. *J Clin Endocrinol Metab* 1982;**55**:238.

Osteoporosis

Avioli LV: *The Osteoporotic Syndrome: Detection Prevention and Treatment*, 2nd ed. Grune & Stratton, 1987.

Civitelli R et al: Bone turnover in postmenopausal osteoporosis: Effect of calcitonin treatment. *J Clin Invest* 1988;**82**:1268.

Cummings SR: Are patients with hip fractures more osteoporotic? Review of evidence. *Am J Med* 1985;**78**:487.

Dawson-Hughes B et al: A controlled trial of the effect of calcium supplementation on bone density in postmenopausal women. *N Engl J Med* 1990; **323**:878.

Eastell R et al: Unequal decrease in bone density of lumbar spine and ultradistal radius in Colles' and vertebral fracture syndromes. *J Clin Invest* 1989; **83**:164.

Ettinger B et al: Long-term estrogen replacement therapy prevents bone loss and fractures. *Ann Intern Med* 1985;**102**:319.

Gallagher JC et al: The effect of calcitriol on patients with postmenopausal osteoporosis with special reference to fracture frequency. *Proc Soc Exp Biol Med* 1989;**191**:287.

Greenspan SL et al: Importance of gonadal steroids to bone mass in men with hyperprolactinemic hypogonadism. *Ann Intern Med* 1989;**110**:526.

Gruber HE et al: Long-term calcitonin therapy in postmenopausal osteoporosis. *Metabolism* 1984;**33**:295.

Heaney RP et al: Calcium absorption in women: relationships to calcium intake, estrogen status, and age. *J Bone Min Res* 1989;**4**:469.

Hui SL et al: Age and bone mass as predictors of fracture in prospective study. *J Clin Invest* 1988;**81**:1804.

Jackson JA et al: Bone histomorphometry in hypogonadal and eugonadal men with spinal osteoporosis. *J Clin Endocrinol Metab* 1987;**65**:53.

Jackson JA, Kleerekoper M: Osteoporosis in men: Diagnosis, pathophysiology and prevention. *Medicine* 1990;**69**:139.

Johnston Jr CC et al: Clinical indications for bone mass measurements. *J Bone Miner Res* 1989;**4**:1.

Lufkin EG et al: Estrogen replacement therapy: Current recommendations. *Mayo Clin Proc* 1988;**63**:453.

Mazzuoli GF: Effects of salmon calcitonin in postmenopausal osteoporosis: A controlled double-blind clinical study. *Calcif Tissue Int* 1986;**38**:3.

Melton LJ et al: Lifetime fracture risk: An approach to hip fracture risk assessment based on bone mineral density and age. *J Clin Epidemiol* 1988; **41**:985.

Nordin BEC et al: Relative contributions of age and years since menopause to postmenopausal bone loss. *J Clin Endocrinol Metab* 1990;**70**:83.

Ott SM et al: Ability of four different techniques of measuring bone mass to diagnose vertebral fractures in postmenopausal women. *J Bone Miner Res* 1987;**2**:201.

Ott SM et al: Calcitriol treatment is not effective in postmenopausal osteoporosis. *Ann Intern Med* 1989;**110**:267.

Pacifici R et al: Dual energy radiography versus quantitative computed tomography for the diagnosis of osteoporosis. *J Clin Endocrinol Metab* 1990; **70**:705.

Riggs BL et al: Clinical heterogeneity of involutional osteoporosis: Implications for preventive therapy. *J Clin Endocrinol Metab* 1990;**70**:1229.

Riggs BL et al: Effect of fluoride treatment on the fracture rate in postmenopausal women with osteoporosis. *N Engl J Med* 1990;**332**:802.

Slovik DM et al: Restoration of spinal bone in osteoporotic men by treatment with human parathyroid hormone (1-34) and 1,25-dihydroxyvitamin D. *J Bone Miner Res* 1986;**1**:377.

Storm T et al: Effects of intermittent cyclical etidronate therapy on bone mass and fracture rate in women with postmenopausal osteoporosis. *N Engl J Med* 1990;**322**:1265.

Watts NB et al: Intermittent cyclical etidronate treatment of postmenopausal osteoporosis. *N Engl J Med* 1990;**323**:73.

Multiple Endocrine Neoplasia (MEN)

Brandi ML et al: Familial multiple endocrine neoplasia type I: A new look at pathophysiology. *Endocr Rev* 1988;**8**:341.

Cance WG et al: Multiple endocrine neoplasia. Type IIa *Curr Probl Surg* 1985;**22**:1.

Gagel RF et al: The clinical outcome of prospective screening for multiple endocrine neoplasia type 2a: An 18-year experience. *N Engl J Med* 1988; **314**:478.

Marx SJ et al: Multiple endocrine neoplasia type I: Assessment of laboratory tests to screen for the gene in a large kindred. *Medicine* 1986;**65**:226.

Mathew CG et al: A linked genetic marker for multiple endocrine neoplasia type: 2A on chromosome 10. *Nature* 1987;**328**:527.

Rizzoli R et al: Primary hyperparathyroidism in familial multiple endocrine neoplasia type I: Long-term follow-up of serum calcium levels after parathyroidectomy. *Am J Med* 1985;**78**:467.

Simpson NE et al: Assignment of multiple endocrine neoplasia type 2a to chromosome 10 by linkage. *Nature* 1987;**328**:528.

Osteomalacia

Bell NH: Vitamin D endocrine system. *J Clin Invest* 1985;**76**:1.

Bikle DD: Osteomalacia and rickets. In: *Cecil Textbook of Medicine*, 18th ed. Wyngaarden JB, Smith LH (editors). Saunders, 1988.

Harrell RM et al: Healing of bone disease in X-linked hypophosphatemic rickets/osteomalacia: Induction and maintenance with phosphorus and calcitriol. *J Clin Invest* 1985;**75**:1858.

Henry HL, Norman AW: Vitamin D: Metabolism and biological actions. *Annu Rev Nutr* 1984;**4**:493.

Parfitt AM: Osteomalacia and related disorders. In: *Metabolic Bone Disease*, 2nd ed. Avioli LV, Krane SM (editors). Grune & Stratton, 1990.

Weidner N et al: Phosphaturic mesenchymal tumors: A polymorphous group causing osteomalacia or rickets. *Cancer* 1987;**8**:1442.

Osteonecrosis/Osteosclerosis

Mitchell DG et al: Femoral head avascular necrosis: Correlation of MR imaging, and clinical findings. *Radiology* 1988;**162**:709.

Strewler GJ: Osteonecrosis, osteosclerosis, and other disorders of bone. In: *Cecil Textbook of Medicine*, 18th ed. Wyngaarden JB, Smith LH (editors). Saunders, 1988.

Renal Osteodystrophy

Andress DL et al: Aluminum associated bone disease in chronic renal failure: High prevalence in a long-term dialysis population. *J Bone Miner Res* 1986;**1**:391.

Andress DL et al: Comparison of parathyroid hormone assays with bone histomorphometry in renal osteodystrophy. *J Clin Endocrinol Metab* 1986;**63**:1163.

Andress DL et al: Early deposition of aluminum in bone in diabetic patients on hemodialysis. *N Engl J Med* 1987;**316**:292.

Hercz G et al: Reversal of aluminum-related bone disease after substituting calcium carbonate for aluminum hydroxide. *Am J Kidney Dis* 1988;**11**:70.

Hodsman AB et al: Do serum aluminum levels reflect underlying skeletal aluminum accumulation and bone histology before or after chelation by deferoxamine? *J Lab Clin Med* 1985;**106**:674.

Milliner DS et al: Clearance of aluminum by hemodialysis: Effect of deferoxamine. *Kidney Int* 1986;**29(Suppl 18)**:100.

Norris KC et al: The iliac crest bone biopsy for the diagnosis of aluminum toxicity and a guide to the use of deferoxamine. *Semin Nephrol* 1986;**6(Suppl 1)**:27.

Slatopolsky E et al: Calcium carbonate as a phosphate binder in patients with chronic renal failure undergoing dialysis. *N Engl J Med* 1986;**315**:157.

Slatopolsky E et al: Marked suppression of secondary hyperparathyroidism by intravenous administration of 1,25-dihydroxycholecalciferol in uremic patients. *J Clin Invest 1984*;**74**:2136.

Slatopolsky E et al: The interaction of parathyroid hormone and aluminum in renal osteodystrophy. *Kidney Int* 1987;**31**:842.

de Vernejoul MC et al: Increased bone aluminum deposition after subtotal parathyroidectomy in dialyzed patients. *Kidney Int* 1985;**27**:785.

Paget's Disease of Bone

Altman RD: Long-term follow-up of therapy with intermittent etidronate disodium in Paget's disease of bone. *Am J Med* 1985;**79**:583.

Altman RD et al: Proceedings of the Kroc Foundation Conference on Paget's Disease of Bone. *Arthritis Rheum* 1988;**23**:1073.

Boyce BF et al: Focal osteomalacia due to low-dose diphosphonate therapy in Paget's disease. *Lancet* 1984;**1**:821.

El-Sammaa M et al: Calcitonin as treatment for hearing loss in Paget's disease. *AM J Otol* 1986;**7**:241.

Johnston CC et al: Review of fracture experience during treatment of Paget's disease of bone with etidronate disodium (EHDP). *Clin Orthop* 1983;**79**:186.

Nephrolithiasis

Broadus AE et al: Evidence for disordered control of 1,25-dihydroxyvitamin D production in absorptive hypercalciuria. *N Engl J Med* 1984;**311**:73.

Ettinger B et al: Randomized trial of allopurinol in the prevention of calcium oxalate calculi. *N Engl J Med* 1986;**315**:1386.

Finlayson B et al: Overview of surgical treatment of urolithiasis with special reference to lithotripsy. *J Urol* 1988;**141**:778.

Pak CYC et al: Correction of hypocitraturia and prevention of stone formation by combined thiazide and potassium citrate therapy in thiazide-unresponsive hypercalciuric nephrolithiasis. *Am J Med* 1985;**79**:284.

Pak CYC: Citrate and renal calculi. *Miner Electrolyte Metab* 1987;**13**:257.

Parks JH et al: A urinary calcium-citrate index for the evaluation of nephrolithiasis. *Kidney Int* 1987;**32**:749.

Uribarri J et al: The first kidney stone. *Ann Intern Med* 1989;**111**:1006.

Phosphate Metabolism

Knochel JP: The clinical status of hypophosphatemia. *N Engl J Med* 1985;**313**:447.

Fibrous Dysplasia

Cuttler L et al: Hypersecretion of growth hormone and prolactin in McCune-Albright Syndrome. *J Clin Endocrinol Metab* 1989;**68**:1148.

Feuillan PP et al: Treatment of precocious puberty in the McCune-Albright syndrome with the aromatose inhibitor testolactone. *N Engl J Med* 1986;**315**:1115.

Harris RI: Polyostotic fibrous dysplasia with acromegaly. *Am J Med* 1985;**78**:538.

Lever EG, Pettingale KW: Albright's syndrome associated with a soft-tissue myxoma and hypophosphatemic osteomalacia: Report of a case and review of the literature. *J Bone Joint Surg* 1983;**65[Br]**:621.

Membership and support are encouraged for:

The Paget's Disease Foundation, PO Box 2772, Brooklyn, NY 11202.

The American Brittle Bone Society, c/o Roberta DeVito, 1256 Merrill Drive, Marshalton, Westchester, PA 19380

The National Osteoporosis Foundation, 1625 Eye Street, N.W., Suite 822, Washington, DC 20006.

Male Reproductive Disorders | 8

Ira D. Sharlip, MD

ANATOMY OF THE TESTICLE

Each testicle is an ovoid shaped mass with a mean volume in the adult of 18.6 mL (range 13.8–23.4 mL). The average length is 4.6 cm (range 3.6–5.5 cm), and the average width is 2.6 cm (range 2.1–3.2 cm). Abnormally small testicles may be seen with any cause of hypogonadism. Abnormally large testicles are seen in hyperthyroidism, acromegaly, and mental retardation due to the fragile X chromosome, or they may be familial. Each testicle is divided into approximately 250 lobules by fibrous tissue septae. Each lobule contains 1–4 seminiferous tubules. Each tubule is approximately 60 cm in length and 165 μm in diameter. The seminiferous tubules account for approximately 90% of the testicular mass. The interstitial tissue accounts for the other 10%.

The interstitium of the testicle between the seminiferous tubules contains Leydig (interstitial) cells, blood vessels, lymphatic channels, macrophages, and mast cells. The function of the Leydig cells is production of androgenic steroids, predominantly testosterone, which is the most potent circulating androgen in the male.

Spermatogenesis

Spermatogenesis occurs in the seminiferous tubules. Within the tubule itself are located 2 cell types: germ cells and Sertoli cells. The most primitive of the germ cell line, the spermatogonia, are located in the periphery of each tubule. As these cells differentiate into primary spermatocytes, secondary spermatocytes, spermatids, and finally spermatozoa, they move progressively toward the inner lumen of the tubule. The Sertoli cells line the inside of the tubule wall. Within the tubule the Sertoli cells connect to one another in a system of tight junctions. The spermatogonia and primary spermatocytes are located peripheral to these tight junctions; this is known as the basal compartment. Secondary spermatocytes, spermatids, and spermatozoa are on the luminal side of the tight junctions; this is known as the adluminal compartment. The germ cells in the basal compartment are those

---

SOME ACRONYMS USED IN THIS CHAPTER

ABP	Androgen–binding protein
DHEA	Dehydroepiandrosterone
DHT	Dihydrotestosterone
FSH	Follicle–stimulating hormone
GnRH	Gonadotropin–releasing hormone
hCG	Human chorionic gonadotropin
hMG	Human menopausal gonadotropin
LH	Luteinizing hormone
TeBG	Testosterone–binding globulin

---

which reproduce by mitosis, whereas the germ cells in the adluminal compartment undergo meiosis. The tight junctions form the blood-testis barrier. Interstitial fluid has access through the tubular wall to the basal compartment, but the adluminal compartment is separated from the interstitial fluid and therefore becomes an immunologically privileged site. The Sertoli cells "unzip" their tight junctions to allow passage of developing spermatocytes from the basal to the adluminal compartment. Cytoplasmic extensions of the Sertoli cells completely surround the developing germ cells, nurturing and supporting them during germ cell development. In addition to these functions, the Sertoli cells phagocytose injured germ cells and residual bodies, secrete androgen-binding protein (ABP), and secrete inhibin, the substance responsible for negative feedback on the FSH arm of the hypothalamic-pituitary-gonadal axis (Fig 8–1). The Sertoli cells are also the testicular source of estrogen. In addition, in utero, they form the müllerian inhibiting factor that causes recession of the müllerian duct structures.

Approximately 45–205 million sperm are produced by both testes each day. The entire process of spermatogenesis takes 74 ± 4 days in the human male. Passage through the epididymis requires another 3–12 days so that an event or agent acting to improve spermatogenic function will not produce an observable change in ejaculated sperm until approximately 3 months later.

PHYSIOLOGY OF THE TESTICLE

The testicle is capable of synthesizing a variety of steroids. Fig 2–4 depicts the pathways for formation of the major sex steroids from cholesterol. The most important of these is testosterone. In males,

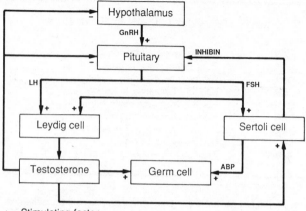

+ = Stimulating factor
− = Inhibiting factor

Figure 8–1. The hypothalamic-pituitary-testicle axis.

95% of circulating blood testosterone is produced by the testicle, while approximately 5% is produced by peripheral conversion of steroid precursors to testosterone in peripheral tissues of the body. Two other important sex steroids are dihydrotestosterone and estradiol. Only 20% of circulating blood levels of these hormones comes from testicular secretion, while 80% comes from peripheral conversion of testosterone.

Gonadotropin-Releasing Hormone

Under the influence of norepinephrine, dopamine, histamine, endorphins, and other neurotransmitters, neurons in the arcuate nucleus of the medial basal hypothalamus produce a decapeptide, gonadotropin-releasing hormone (GnRH). GnRH is produced in pulsatile fashion, the pulses occurring approximately every 60–90 minutes. It enters the hypothalamic-hypophyseal portal blood and reaches the anterior pituitary gland, where it binds to specific receptor sites on gonadotrope cell membranes. This in turn stimulates the gonadotropes to secrete the gonadotropins, luteinizing hormone (LH), and follicle-stimulating hormone (FSH). There is only one GnRH for stimulation of both LH and FSH. The gonadotropes secrete more LH than FSH following stimulation by GnRH. LH and FSH then enter the general circulation and reach the testis. Here, LH binds to receptors on the interstitial (Leydig) cells, while FSH binds to receptors on both Leydig cells and Sertoli cells.

Testosterone

In the Leydig cells, this process activates adenylate cyclase and generates cyclic AMP, initiating steroidogenesis. Increased levels of androgens, predominantly testosterone, then enter the testicular venous blood and become diffused throughout the body. In addition, some testosterone diffuses locally in the interstitial tissue and into the adjacent seminiferous tubules. Very high concentrations of testosterone are found within testicular tissue compared with circulating blood levels. Testosterone, which is admitted through the blood-testis barrier, then combines with androgen-binding protein produced by the Sertoli cells and travels within the seminiferous tubules and seminal duct system. Circulating testosterone exerts a negative feedback effect on the pituitary gland. Testosterone may also exert an inhibitory effect on secretion of GnRH from the hypothalamus, although it is currently thought that the proximate cause of this inhibition is estradiol, formed locally from conversion of testosterone to estradiol in the hypothalamus. Thus, the day-to-day control of the hypothalamic-pituitary-Leydig cell axis depends on this negative feedback system. There is in addition a positive feedback control for LH secretion, which is estrogen induced. The positive feedback mechanism is not important in normal men but is active in patients with Klinefelter's syndrome, with Sertoli-cell-only syndrome, and possibly in male patients being treated with estrogen.

Testosterone circulates as either free testosterone (2%), albumin-bound testosterone (38%), or globulin-bound testosterone (60%). The testosterone-binding globulin (TeBG) has a molecular weight of 80,000–94,000 and is synthesized in the liver. TeBG is distinct from androgen-binding protein secreted by the Sertoli cells, but they appear to have similar structure. Serum concentration of TeBG is increased by estrogen administration, hyperthyroidism, and cirrhosis and is decreased by androgen administration, growth hormone, hypothyroidism, acromegaly, and obesity. The degree of androgenicity produced by free, albumin-bound, and TeBG-bound testosterone in the human is not clear. Testosterone bound to TeBG is not available for intracellular action. The availability of circulating testosterone to target tissues is a complex function. It is related not to the availability of circulating testosterone for target tissues but to the affinity of tissue receptor sites and metabolic rates of testosterone as well. Clinically, the circulating testosterone can be measured as free, weakly bound, and tightly bound testosterone as well as total testosterone levels. The clinical significance of each level is not clear, since the contribution of each to production of androgenicity has not yet been elucidated.

Dihydrotestosterone

Once testosterone traverses the cell membrane of target tissues, it is converted to the more potent androgen dihydrotestosterone (DHT) by the microsomal enzyme 5α-reductase. DHT then binds to specific intracytoplasmic receptor proteins (R_c). The DHT-receptor complex then moves to the cell nucleus, where it is transformed to DHT-R_n and binds to nuclear chromatin. This in turn causes messenger RNA synthesis. The latter affects androgenicity by instructing new protein synthesis.

Metabolism of Testosterone

Circulating testosterone is broken down by the liver into various metabolites, including androsterone and etiocholanolone, which are conjugated with glucuronic or sulfuric acid and secreted in the urine as 17-ketosteroid. Only 20–30% of urinary 17-ketosteroids, however, are composed of testosterone metabolites. The other 70–80% are derived from weak androgens secreted by the adrenal gland. Therefore, urinary 17-ketosteroid levels cannot be used as an accurate reflection of testicular steroidogenesis.

Effects of Testosterone

The biologic effects of androgens include embryologic male genital differentiation, maturation of the internal and external male genitalia during puberty, skeletal muscle growth, deepening of the voice due to laryngeal growth, epiphyseal cartilage growth during puberty, male hair growth and distribution, erythropoiesis, stimulation of sebaceous glands, and male social behavior. These actions may be divided into androgenic and anabolic effect of testosterone.

Measurement of Testosterone

While LH is secreted in a pulsatile manner, there is no corresponding testosterone pulse in men. There are, however, oscillations in testosterone on a minute-to-minute basis, and there is evidence of a circadian rhythm of testosterone secretion in young men with an amplitude of 10–25%. The higher levels of testosterone are found on awakening in the morning, and the nadir is in the evening. Illness and certain drugs (Tables 1–4 and 8–1) may cause temporary decreases in serum testosterone. Because of the minute-to-minute variations of both LH and testosterone, a single serum measurement may be inaccurate. If serum levels are abnormal, several measurements should be obtained.

FSH Secretion & Effects

In response to GnRH stimulation, pituitary gonadotropes also secrete FSH, which enters the general circulation. Peripheral receptor

Table 8–1. Nonpituitary causes of male hypogonadism.

Idiopathic and male climacteric	Decreased androgen production
Testicular trauma	Congenital adrenal hypoplasia
Orchitis	Drugs: aminoglutethamide,
Mumps	spironolactone, ketoconazole,
Leprosy	alcohol, marijuana
Radiation	Leydig cell hypoplasia
Infiltrative disease	Chronic renal failure
(eg, lymphoma)	Decreased androgen sensitivity
Developmental	states
Klinefelter's syndrome	Myotonic dystrophy
XYY syndrome and variants	Adult seminiferous tubular failure
Sertoli-cell-only syndrome	Leydig cell tumor with
Noonan's syndrome	hyperestrogenism
Cryptorchidism	Wolfram syndrome
Anorchia	

sites for FSH are found on both Leydig and Sertoli cells. In the Leydig cell, FSH action results in an increase in LH receptor sites. In the Sertoli cells, FSH action stimulates AMP formation and this results in the formation of androgen-binding protein and inhibin. Production of ABP by the Sertoli cell is synergized by FSH and testosterone, the latter acting through specific androgen receptors on the Sertoli cell. It is probably ABP that maintains the androgen milieu of the seminiferous tubule.

Spermatogenesis

The initiation of spermatogenesis requires the presence of both testosterone and FSH. Once spermatogenesis is initiated, maintenance of sperm production no longer requires FSH. Once spermatogenesis has been established, a negative feedback mechanism exerted on the hypothalamic-pituitary axis reduces the secretion of FSH so that the seminiferous tubules are not overdriven. The exact agent producing this negative feedback is not clear. While it is known that testosterone, DHT, and estradiol are capable of inhibiting FSH secretion, the major inhibitory role is ascribed to inhibin, a nonsteroidal substance produced by the Sertoli cells. This substance suppresses pituitary secretion of FSH. It is not known whether it has an effect on the hypothalamus as well.

Prolactin

Prolactin is present in males as well as females (see Chapter 1). Prolactin has an ill-defined role in male reproduction. In the presence of increased prolactin secretion, lower plasma LH levels are found, and vice versa. Prolactin receptors have been identified on Leydig cells. In concert with testosterone, prolactin has been shown to act as an anabolic hormone. Finally, clinical hyperprolactinemia is associated with erectile dysfunction and infertility in a small number of cases. A role for prolactin in the physiology of the male reproductive tract likely will be more clearly defined in the future.

PRIMARY HYPOGONADISM*

EVALUATION

In establishing a diagnosis of hypogonadism, a careful examination of the genitalia is of great importance. This examination should be done in a warm room so that the scrotum is in a relaxed position that facilitates palpation of the scrotal contents. In the case of an infant, it is advisable to perform the examination of the scrotum in a warm bath. For either an adult or an infant, placing the patient in a cross-legged position facilitates the examination. First the testicles should be palpated. They normally have an ovoid shape and a rubbery consistency. Testicular size can be measured with a caliper or testicular volume can be closely estimated by comparison with an orchidometer, a group of varying sized ovoid masses of standard volumes. Standard sizes and volumes are given in Fig 8–2. (A Prader orchidometer may be purchased from Professor Andrea Prader, Kinderspital, Steinwiesstrasse 75, CH 8032, Zurich, Switzerland.)

Following examination of the testicle, the epididymides should be palpated. These will be indistinct, tubular masses of soft consistency forming an arc on the posterior or posterolateral aspect of the testicle. Occasionally, they can be nonpalpable though normal. Above the epididymis, the scrotal part of the spermadic cord with the vas deferens running through it may then be palpated. The vas deferens has a unique feeling on palpation that is best described as a firm, rubbery piece of spaghetti. The spermatic cord about the vas deferens is a soft, usually indistinct tubular mass leading up to the inguinal region. The penis should then be examined and its unstretched and stretched length noted. Normal values for penile length are listed in Fig 8–3. Abnormalities of the penis such as hypospadias, epispadias, and chordee should be noted. Finally, a rectal examination checking for perianal sensation, rectal sphincter tone, and prostate size should be completed. In hypogonadism, one finds small penis and testicular size if androgen

*The hypothalamic-pituitary causes of hypogonadism are covered in Chapter 1. This section is limited to testicular causes of hypogonadism, ie, hypergonadotropic hypogonadism.

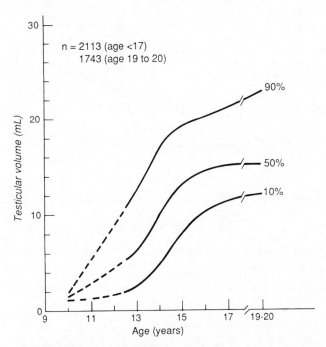

Figure 8–2. Normal testicular volume in boys and young men. (Reproduced, with permission, from Zachmann M et al: Testicular volume during adolescence: Cross-sectional and longitudinal studies. *Helv Pediatr Acta* 1974;**29**:61.)

deficiency occurs in utero or in infancy or childhood. In adult-onset hypogonadism, penile size does not change significantly, but the testicles become soft and mushy and may decrease in size slightly. The testicular findings in Klinefelter's syndrome are unique in that the testicles are characteristically small and firm due to peritubular sclerosis.

The clinical features of hypogonadism depend on the age of onset. When androgen deficiency occurs in the second to third month of fetal life, the result is ambiguous genitalia. Androgen deficiency developing before puberty results in failure of secondary sexual development and consequent skeletal eunuchoidism. The arm span will be 5 cm greater than the body height and the crown-pubis/pubis-floor ratio less than 1. These features occur because the epiphyseal plate of the long bones continues to grow under the influence of stimulated so-

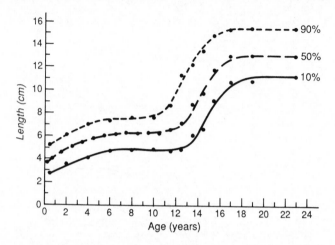

Figure 8–3. Length of the penis (stretched) from birth to maturity.

matomedin while the tissues of the body fail to undergo the normal pubertal growth spurt. In Klinefelter's syndrome, however, arm span may be less than body height. Further observations include a decrease in muscle mass associated with diminished muscle strength and endurance. The voice is high pitched because of the failure of thickening and maturation of the vocal cords. The failure of secondary sexual development leads to sparse facial, body, pubic, and axillary hair and persistence of the female scalp hairline. The genitalia have an infantile appearance, and sexual drive and erections are inadequate.

If androgen deficiency develops following puberty, it is more difficult to diagnose and may take many years before clinical features are apparent. Men first note a decrease in their rate of beard growth and consequently need to shave less often. Over many years, there may be a decrease in facial hair. These features are seen because high levels of testosterone are necessary to induce male sexual hair growth but lower levels are necessary to simply maintain it. There may be a decrease in sexual drive and erections. Fine wrinkles about the mouth and eyes and sparse beard are referred to as hypogonadal facies. In addition, the testicles may become smaller and softer than normal.

LABORATORY FEATURES

Semen Analysis

Semen is an easily accessible fluid for assessment of gonadal function. With rare exceptions, hypogonadism is ruled out if the semen analysis is normal. However, an abnormal semen analysis is usually not associated with endocrine causes of hypogonadism.

Testicular Biopsy

Testicular biopsy is rarely useful in the evaluation of hypogonadism. Its indications are limited to patients with azoospermia or severe oligospermia associated with normal testicular size, serum testosterone, and serum FSH. These patients may have obstruction of the duct system with completely normal spermatogenesis.

Laboratory Tests

The most important tests to obtain in the assessment of hypogonadism are the serum testosterone, FSH, and LH. In selected cases, it may be helpful to test for free and weakly bound testosterone, in addition to total testosterone, to get an estimate of TeBG level. In addition, serum prolactin and estradiol levels may be useful. The normal values for these steroids and gonadotropins in men are listed in the Appendix.

Most patterns of gonadotropin and sex steroid levels are easy to understand. The classic pattern seen with pituitary insufficiency is that of low gonadotropins and low testosterone. The classic pattern seen with gonadal dysfunction is that of high gonadotropins and low testosterone. In hyperprolactinemia, normal or low testosterone may be seen. Administration of testosterone will not be effective in these patients if the prolactin level remains elevated. With the androgen-insensitivity states, there are elevations of both testosterone and gonadotropin. The differential diagnosis of **elevated serum testosterone** includes exogenous testosterone administration, androgen-insensitivity state, and elevation of TeBG, which is seen in hypothyroidism, obesity, acromegaly, and cirrhosis. In these conditions, the absolute level of serum free testosterone remains normal and the percentage of free testosterone is low. Occasionally, a compensated form of hypergonadotropic hypogonadism is encountered. This is marked by elevation of LH with normal levels of testosterone. These patients may be clinically hypogonadal and may respond to exogenous testosterone administration. Most other patterns are due to sampling or laboratory error, and tests should be repeated. Occasionally, borderline normal testosterone values are associated with normal gonadotropins. In these cases, a double-blind trial of intramuscular testosterone and placebo may be used as a clinical test for hypogonadism. In this test, there is a good response to testosterone but no response to placebo.

Measurements of urinary 17-ketosteroids are rarely used, since 70% of this urinary steroid is metabolized from weak adrenal androgens such as androstenedione and DHEA-sulfate and the study is not reflective of gonadal function.

hCG Test

hCG has predominantly LH activity although it has some FSH activity as well. The hCG test is a test for Leydig cell function. It is indicated when the adequacy of Leydig cell function is in question, eg, in unpalpable, undescended testicles prior to puberty. hCG is administered to men or boys at 4000 IU intramuscularly daily for 4 days. This will produce at least a doubling of serum testosterone in 3–4 days. Failure to obtain this doubling indicates Leydig cell dysfunction. If there is no rise in testosterone, the test indicates Leydig cell absence as in anorchia.

GnRH Test

GnRH stimulates secretion of LH and FSH from the anterior pituitary gland. Following intravenous administration of 100 μg of GnRH, blood levels of LH and FSH are measured at 15, 30, 45, and 60 minutes. Some investigators carry the study out to 180 minutes. In adult men, a normal response is a maximum serum LH of 2.5 times the basal level and a maximum serum FSH of 2 times the basal level. GnRH is expensive and seldom helpful in establishing the diagnosis of hypopituitarism (Chapter 1) because of a significant incidence of false-negative and false-positive results.

Clomiphene Stimulation Test

This test may be used to identify secondary hypogonadism due to inadequate hypothalamic or pituitary secretion of gonadotropins. Clomiphene citrate is a nonsteroidal weak estrogen that acts as an estrogen receptor blocker in the hypothalamus. As noted previously, most of the feedback control at the level of the hypothalamus is mediated by peripherally or locally formed estradiol. Consequently, clomiphene leads to an increase in GnRH release and subsequently to LH and FSH release. To perform this test, 50–100 mg of clomiphene is administered twice daily for 10 days. Pooled samples of blood are obtained, and plasma LH and FSH are measured prior to clomiphene administration and on days 9 and 10. A 50–250% increase in LH, a 30–200% increase in FSH, and a 30–220% increase in testosterone on day 10 of the test is a normal response. Clomiphene produces little change in prepubertal boys whose testosterone levels are less than 100 ng/dL and therefore does not distinguish delayed puberty from hypogonadotropism. It is therefore useful predominantly in postpubertal hypogonadotropism with mild hypogonadism when the serum testosterone and gonadotropins are nearly normal. Because of its limited applicability, it is a rarely used test.

TREATMENT

Drugs

The most reliable form of therapy for hypogonadism is intramuscular **testosterone enanthate** or **testosterone cypionate** (Table 8–2), of which 100–200 mg every 10–14 days provides adequate levels of serum testosterone in most patients, though many are sustained by 200–400 mg every 3–4 weeks. Even higher doses may be needed for the induction of puberty. A 3.8-cm, 20-gauge needle should be used for injection in adults to ensure the intramuscular deposition of testosterone. After initiation of therapy, the interval between doses should be prolonged or the dose minimized in order to reduce the replacement therapy to the lowest dose that is compatible with maintenance of eugonadism. The effect should be judged by the patients' symptomatology. Decreased hair growth may persist if hypogonadism has been chronically untreated since childhood.

Several **oral preparations** are available as well. However, gastrointestinal uptake is variable and there is a 1–2% incidence of cholestatic jaundice or peliosis hepatis, which is reversible upon termi-

Table 8–2. Androgen Preparations.

Preparation	Size	Dosage
Oral		
Fluoxymesterone	2–, 5–, and 10–mg tablets	5–10 mg daily
Methyltestosterone	5–, 10–, and 25–mg tablets	10–50 mg daily
Mesterolone	25 mg (not available in USA)	30–60 mg daily
Sublingual		
Methyltestosterone	5– and 10–mg buccal tablets	5–25 mg daily
Intramuscular		
Testosterone cypionate	50–, 100–, and 200–mg/ mL in 1– or 10–mL vials	100–400 mg every 2–4 weeks
Testosterone enanthate	100– and 200–mg/mL in 5– or 10– mL vials	100–400 mg every 2–4 weeks
Testosterone propionate	25–, 50–, and 100–mg/mL in 10– or 30–mL vials	50 mg 2–3 times/ week
Subcutaneous		
Testosterone pellets	75 mg	450 mg every 4–6 months

nation of the drug. Hepatomas have been rarely reported with oral testosterone preparations. In general, the oral forms of testosterone therapy, even in larger doses, do not have the maximal androgenic effect that can be obtained by intramuscular therapy. The oral agents include fluoxymesterone, 5–10 mg/d; methyltestosterone, 10–15 mg/d orally or 5–25 mg/d sublingually; and mesterolone, which is not available in the USA. Mesterolone has not been reported to cause cholestatic jaundice.

A short-acting intramuscular preparation, **testosterone propionate,** is also available but it must be administered 2 or 3 times weekly by intramuscular injection. The usual dose is 50 mg. Its usage is limited to trial doses for men with prostatic hypertrophy whose obstructive voiding symptoms may be exacerbated by testosterone therapy. Since the duration of the effect is short, the risk of obstructive uropathy is less than during a trial with this preparation. Subcutaneous administration of testosterone pellets is rarely used. The usual dose is 450 mg every 4–6 months.

Side Effects

Side effects of androgen therapy may occur in a small number of patients. Androgens may cause premature epiphyseal fusion in a prepubertal male and therefore should not be given before the age of 13. Cholestatic jaundice and very rarely hepatoma and peliosis hepatis have been reported with the oral preparations. Because of feedback on the hypothalamus and pituitary gland, reduction of pituitary gonadotropins with suppression of sperm counts may occur. Several pounds of weight gain due to fluid retention, erythrocytosis, gynecomastia, acne, aggressive behavior, and reductions in globulins that bind thyroxin and cortisol have all been reported. Androgen therapy is contraindicated in the presence of prostatic cancer. However, there is no evidence that replacement of androgen in the hypogonadal male induces the development of prostatic cancer.

The use of gonadotropin to treat nonpituitary causes of hypogonadism is very limited. Replacement of gonadotropin should be limited to patients with hypothalamic-pituitary disease of dysfunction (Chapter 1).

Hot Flashes

When hypogonadism develops slowly, hot flashes do not occur. However, with acute hypogonadism, eg, following bilateral orchiectomy, hot flashes may result. Hot flashes may be eliminated by intramuscular administration of testosterone if it is not contraindicated by the patient's clinical condition. Other useful treatments include administration of oral estrogens; oral use of clonidine; and oral administration of a combination of phenobarbital, ergotamine, and belladonna. Oral administration of cyproterone has also been reported to be useful for treatment of hot flashes in men.

SYNDROMES OF PRIMARY HYPOGONADISM

KLINEFELTER'S SYNDROME

Klinefelter's syndrome (XXY seminiferous tubule dysgenesis) occurs in approximately 1 of every 400 males. It may become manifest at the time of expected puberty or thereafter. The syndrome consists of hypogonadism with small, firm testicles, gynecomastia, elevated gonadotropins, and reduction of the serum testosterone due to sclerosis of the seminiferous tubules. The chromosome karyotype in classical Klinefelter's syndrome is XXY. Other genotypes, including XXXY, XXXXY, XXYY, and XY/XXY mosaicism occur less frequently. The classical XXY genotype is due to nondisjunction of the sex chromosomes during meiosis. Less frequently the XXY constitution may arise from zygotic nondisjunction during mitosis. Advanced maternal age predisposes to meiotic disjunction, but paternal age is not a factor. Histologic characteristics of the testicle are fibrosis and hyalinization of the seminiferous tubules. This gives the appearance of Leydig cell hyperplasia, although the total number of Leydig cells is not increased. No increased incidence of testicular carcinoma occurs. The abnormalities in the seminiferous tubules are usually expressed as azoospermia although patients may have oligospermia and occasionally a normal sperm count as well. At puberty, despite the presence of normal appearing numbers of Leydig cells, Leydig cell dysfunction becomes apparent with reduced testosterone production and compensatory increase in serum LH. The increased LH concentrations stimulate Leydig cell secretion of estradiol, producing variable degrees of feminization and gynecomastia. Estradiol also causes the liver to increase TeBG so that the total testosterone is frequently in the low-normal range, although classically it is below normal.

Clinical Features

The diagnosis is suggested by clinical signs and symptoms and substantiated by the finding of low serum testosterone and elevated serum LH levels. Clinical and laboratory findings that occur in over 50% of men with Klinefelter's syndrome include azoospermia (95%), gynecomastia (80–90%), decreased sexual interest, impotence, and other manifestations of androgen insufficiency. Findings that occur in less than 50% of patients include clinodactyly, tall stature, eunuchoid proportions, and cubitus valgus. The skeletal proportions are not truly eunuchoid. Long-bone growth occurs in the lower extremities but not in the upper extremities. Consequently the pubis-floor/crown-pubis ratio is higher than 1, but the arm span is not greater than body height. This finding is unique to Klinefelter's syndrome. Children with this karyotype are generally not diagnosed until during or after expected puberty. In retrospect, however, they have a higher chance of congenital anomalies such as clinodactyly, immature emotional and social skills, and poor coordination. In addition, intellectual impairment and dissocial behavior are common. Associated diseases include chronic pulmonary disease, breast cancer, and varicosities of the lower extremities. Diabetes mellitus occurs in about 8% of patients and impaired glucose tolerance in another 19%.

Laboratory Features

A. Buccal Smear: Diagnosis may be aided by examination of a buccal smear for Barr (sex chromatin) bodies. A sterile metal spatula is used to scrape the buccal surface of the cheek and the cells are spread on a clean glass slide. It is good practice to make two slides from the same area. The slide is immediately fixed without air drying in 70% alcohol for 10 minutes to 24 hours. Barr bodies are present in 20–30% of cells examined in a normal XX female and in none of the cells from a normal XY male.

XXY Klinefelter's patients are positive for one Barr body. A drumstick configuration in polymorphonuclear leukocytes has the same significance as the Barr body in the buccal smear. One to 15% of polymorphonuclear leukocytes have the drumstick appearance in normal XX females.

B. Karyotyping: Chromosomal karyotyping is a further aid to diagnosis of Klinefelter's syndrome. Karyotyping may be done on bone marrow, amniotic fluid, fetal cells, skin solid tumors, and testicular tissue, but the most common tissue for this use is blood lymphocytes. Peripheral blood, 1 mL at room temperature in a sterile tube containing 20 U of preservative-free heparin, is needed. The laboratory should be notified in advance to prepare for lymphocyte culture. While more accurate than buccal smear, karyotyping is much more expensive and time consuming.

Treatment

Therapy consists of androgen replacement. Treatment of gynecomastia may be necessary if cosmetically displeasing. Life expectancy is not shortened.

XYY SYNDROME

In men possessing more than one Y chromosome, antisocial behavior is common. Some men with XYY syndrome have hypogonadism or infertility, but most have no abnormality of testicular function. XYY syndrome is associated with tall stature and severe acne.

SERTOLI-CELL-ONLY SYNDROME

This is an uncommon syndrome characterized by azoospermia, elevated or normal FSH levels, and small testicles. These patients do not have chromosome abnormalities or gynecomastia. Testicular biopsy shows absence of germ cells; only Sertoli cells are seen in the tubules, suggesting the syndrome's name. However, Leydig cells are present in the interstitium, and therefore serum testosterone levels are normal. The pathogenesis of Sertoli-cell-only syndrome is uncertain. It may be congenital in some cases and acquired in others. Diagnosis is made with certainty only with testicular biopsy. No treatment is available for this cause of infertility.

NOONAN'S SYNDROME (MALE TURNER'S SYNDROME)

Males with some of the classic stigmata of Turner's syndrome fall into this category. They are genotypically and phenotypically male. The syndrome has autosomal dominant inheritance with variable penetrance. Clinical characteristics include short stature, webbed neck, cubitus valgus, congenital heart disease, cryptorchidism, and hypogonadism. The serum testosterone level is low or low normal, while FSH and LH are elevated. The only therapy is testosterone replacement.

CONGENITAL ANORCHIA

Approximately 40% of unpalpable testicles are due to testicular absence. Bilateral anorchia occurs in approximately 1 of 20,000 males. The pathogenesis is probably due to an in utero testicular catastrophe such as torsion. That some functional testicular tissue must have been present is proved by the constant finding of regressed müllerian duct structures and normal development of the external genitalia at birth. The testicles, however, are not palpable, and at puberty eunuchoidism develops. It is sometimes called the vanishing testes syndrome. Diagnosis is established by an abnormal hCG stimulation test. Treatment is with testosterone replacement and testicular prostheses if desired for cosmetic purposes.

DRUGS THAT INHIBIT TESTOSTERONE SYNTHESIS

Several drugs are known to interfere with steroidogenesis. These include aminoglutethimide, spironolactone, marijuana, and mitotane. Ketoconazole interferes with cholesterol conversion to lanosterol and with the 17,20-desmolase conversion of 17α-hydroxypregnenolone to DHEA and of 17α-hydroxyprogesterone to androstenedione. Alcohol inhibits testosterone production by several mechanisms, including direct inhibition of Leydig cells and feedback inhibition of hypothalamic-pituitary axis due to increased levels of circulating estradiol in patients with liver disease.

Glucocorticoids (eg, prednisone) cause hypogonadism by suppressing gonadotropin secretion.

LEYDIG CELL HYPOPLASIA & APLASIA

Congenital Leydig cell aplasia has been identified as a cause of male pseudohermaphroditism with ambiguous genitalia. An adult form consisting of hypogonadism with Leydig cell agenesis has also been described. Its incidence is uncertain.

ORCHITIS

Orchitis occurs in about 20–25% of males with mumps. Of those men affected, 70% of cases are unilateral and 30% are bilateral; 85% have involvement of the epididymis as well as the testicle. Prepubertal mumps orchitis is associated with complete recovery. However, postpubertal mumps orchitis results in some degree of seminiferous tubule damage and testicular atrophy in 50% of affected testes. Even when orchitis is unilateral, functional abnormalities are often noted on the opposite side. While the incidence of sterility after mumps orchitis is about 5–10%, the true incidence of subfertility has not been clearly identified. Leydig cells are hardier than germ cells and usually appear to be normal following mumps orchitis. No effective therapy exists for acute mumps orchitis. Treatment with estrogens or corticosteroids during the acute phase has been advocated; their value is unproved. Orchitis may also be caused by leprosy, irradiation, and infiltrative diseases such as lymphoma.

CHRONIC RENAL FAILURE

Specific suppression of Leydig cell function has been found in some uremic patients. This is characterized by low testosterone and high LH levels. Treatment consists of testosterone replacement or renal transplantation. Prednisone administration to prevent rejection may then suppress LH and testosterone. In addition, some patients with chronic renal failure are hypogonadal owing to low LH levels associated with hyperprolactinemia.

MYOTONIC DYSTROPHY

Approximately 80% of men with myotonic dystrophy have testicular atrophy and hypogonadism, which is usually primary. Some men may have hypogonadotropic hypogonadism as well. The disease is characterized by myotonia, progressive weakness and atrophy of the facial, neck, hand, and lower extremity muscles, ptosis, frontal baldness, and cataracts. Initially, Leydig cell function is usually preserved while seminiferous tubular atrophy occurs. More advanced cases demonstrate Leydig cell dysfunction as well. No therapy is indicated unless the serum testosterone level is below normal.

ANDROGEN-INSENSITIVITY STATES

Several syndromes are characterized by insensitivity to androgen or absence of androgen receptor sites in peripheral tissues. The most full-blown of these is the testicular feminization syndrome, in which genotypic males are phenotypically female (Chapter 4). Several familial syndromes of male pseudohermaphroditism are due to varying degrees of partial androgen receptor deficiency (Chapter 2). These syndromes consist of partial androgen insensitivity that results variably in gynecomastia, hypospadias, and decreased male sexual hair development. The patients may be distinguished (eg, from Klinefelter's syndrome patients) by hypospadias and more common occurrence of cryptorchidism, bifid scrotum, and prostatic hypoplasia. Testosterone therapy is required, often in doses exceeding normal replacement. Correction of the gynecomastia and hypospadias is surgical. Variations on this familial syndrome are the syndromes described as Reifenstein's, Lubs, Dreyfuss, and Rosewater's.

Partial androgen insensitivity has been described as a cause of male infertility without other clinical evidence of androgen insensitivity. The characteristic features of the insensitivity states are increases in the levels of both LH and testosterone. The incidence of infertility due to occult partial androgen insensitivity is currently unknown.

OTHER CAUSES

Other causes of primary hypogonadism include hemochromatosis, cirrhosis, and feminizing adrenal carcinoma. Testicular and hypothalamic-pituitary function may both be suppressed.

Male Infertility

Infertility is defined as the inability of a couple to conceive after 12 months of trying for a pregnancy. Only 10–15% of couples are unable to have children, and another 10–15% have fewer children than desired. Approximately 50% of infertility problems are due to an abnormality in the female partner, approximately 40% to an abnormality in the male partner, and the remaining 10% to abnormalities in both partners.

Of men with infertility problems, over 50% have idiopathic adult seminiferous tubular failure. Approximately 20% have a varicocele with oligospermia. About 10% have ejaculatory abnormalities, 10% have obstructive causes of infertility, and 10% have endocrine abnormalities. Other conditions described below exist as well but are uncommon. The causes of male infertility may be classified as testicular, posttesticular, and pretesticular (Table 8–3).

Table 8–3. Causes of male infertility.

Testicular	**Posttesticular**
Seminiferous tubular failure	Abnormalities of ejaculation
Primary (idiopathic)	Increased volume
Secondary (cryptorchidism,	Decreased volume
drugs, testes cancer,	Retrograde ejaculation
endocrinopathy, chemotherapy	Absent ejaculation
[especially cyclophosphamide,	Obstruction of seminal ducts
chlorambucil, cisplatin,	(idiopathic, infection, trauma,
busulfan, mechlorethamine,	congenital, vasectomy)
thiotepa, ifosfamide])	Genitourinary infection
Varicocele	Immunologic infertility
Defective androgen production	
Pretesticular	
Endocrinopathy (hypothalamic-	
pituitary dysfunction, androgen	
insensitivity states)	
Sexual dysfunction	

TESTICULAR CAUSES

Adult Seminiferous Tubular Failure

Most infertile men have an idiopathic decrease in sperm count or sperm motility. These men have normal sexual function, normal testicular size, normal serum gonadotropins, and no history of cryptorchidism, infection, inflammation, or varicocele.

In some cases, a specific cause of seminiferous tubular failure can be identified. **Cryptorchidism** is one such cause and is discussed separately, below.

Certain **medications** may suppress spermatogenesis. These include estrogens, antiandrogens, intramuscular testosterone, high-dose nitrofurantoin, many antineoplastic agents, marijuana, phenytoin, MAO inhibitors, and sulfasalazine. Some chemotherapeutic agents, notably cyclophosphamide and ifosfamide, may produce temporary and reversible reductions in spermatogenesis. Cimetidine acts as an antiandrogen and reduces sperm production. A higher than normal incidence of oligospermia and developmental defects of the genitalia occurs in the sons of mothers treated with diethylstilbestrol during pregnancy. There has been much speculation that environmental agents and workplace toxins may cause infertility. The only specific agents known to produce male infertility are the pesticide dibromochloropropane (DBCP), toluene diamine, ethylene dibromide, and lead. Exposure to significant amounts of these agents is limited to workers in industries that produce or use high concentrations of these agents.

There is no evidence that specific nutritional factors cause or cure infertility in the male, nor that the routine emotional stress found in Western culture is responsible for subfertility, although the physical stress of illness may suppress spermatogenesis. The various non-pituitary causes of **hypogonadism** (see above) may present with seminiferous tubular failure in their early or mild form prior to the development of endocrine hypogonadism. Three-fourths of patients with **testicular cancer** have infertility, even after removal of the cancerous testicle and before chemotherapy or radiation therapy. The **immotile cilia syndrome** is caused by the absence of dynein arms in the ultrastructure of the sperm tail; this causes absence of sperm motility. This same abnormality may occur in the cilia of the respiratory tract, causing bronchitis, bronchiectasis, and sinusitis.

Varicocele

An association between varicocele and infertility has long been recognized. Varicocele is found in 15% of normal men and up to 40% of infertile men. Abnormalities of semen analysis have been demonstrated in 50–66% of men with varicoceles. About 80–90% of varicoceles are on the left side, about 5% are on the right side, and the rest are bilateral. The reasons for the left-sided predominance of varicoceles is probably related to the difference between the venous anatomy of the left internal spermatic vein, which inserts into the left renal vein, compared to that of the right internal spermatic vein, which inserts directly into the inferior vena cava. However, the exact mechanism by which this anatomic difference produces left-sided varicoceles has not been clearly identified. The pathogenesis of oligospermia due to varicocele is uncertain, but the most commonly accepted explanation is disturbance of intratesticular thermoregulation. The size of the varicocele has no relationship to the degree of its effect in reducing sperm production. A nonspecific stress pattern of sperm morphology is often produced by a varicocele. This consists of greater than 10% tapered or 4% immature sperm.

Defective Androgen Production

Inadequate androgen production may cause oligospermia. It is found in certain forms of congenital adrenal hyperplasia (Chapters 2 and 4). Inadequate androgen production may also occur as a side effect of certain drugs including aminoglutethimide, spironolactone, ketoconazole, alcohol, and marijuana. It may also occur as a side effect in some cases of uremia.

POSTTESTICULAR CAUSES

Ejaculatory Abnormalities

Abnormalities of ejaculation account for approximately 10% of cases of male infertility. These abnormalities include small volume of ejaculate and retrograde, absent, and partial ejaculation. The most common causes of retrograde or absent ejaculation are diabetic or other autonomic neuropathy, sympatholytic drugs (most commonly phenoxybenzamine), retroperitoneal lymph node dissection for testicular tumor, trauma, transurethral surgery (such as transurethral prostatectomy), or YV-plasty of the bladder neck.

Obstruction of Seminal Ducts

It has long been recognized that one cause of azoospermia is obstruction of the seminal duct system. Obstruction may also be associated with oligospermia. In these cases, the obstruction is not complete; high-grade but not total obstruction allows for a few sperm to come through the diseased area and mix with the products of the seminal vesicle and prostate gland, resulting in a low sperm count. Approximately 10–20% of those men with oligospermia have obstructive causes. The most common naturally occurring site of obstruction is the epididymis. Causes are trauma, infection, and idiopathic. Congenital absence of the vasa differentia occurs in 1–2% of men with infertility. Vasal aplasia is the cause of sterility in cystic fibrosis. Ejaculatory duct obstruction occurs in other men due to trauma, retroprostatic surgery, transurethral surgery, and congenital cysts of the prostate, seminal vesicle, ejaculatory duct, or müllerian duct remnants. The most common cause of obstructive azoospermia is vasectomy.

Genitourinary Infection

The relationship between genitourinary infection and infertility is inconclusive. T mycoplasma, chlamydia, *Escherichia coli,* and other gram-negative rods have been implicated by some authors. Most infections of the seminal duct system are either uncommon or easily recognized. Infection is not thought to be a common cause of male infertility.

Immunologic Infertility

There is disagreement about the importance of immunologic infertility. The generally accepted concept is that sperm antibodies do cause infertility in some individuals, particularly when antibody levels are high in the serum or semen. The diagnosis is established by testing the semen for the presence of sperm antibodies using an immunobead binding test. This test uses polyacrylamide gel to identify IgA, IgM, and IgG antibodies on sperm heads or tails.

PRETESTICULAR CAUSES

Endocrinopathy

Hypothalamic-pituitary dysfunction is discussed in Chapter 1. Androgen insensitivity states are discussed in a previous section.

In the past, thyroid dysfunction, adrenal dysfunction, and diabetes mellitus were thought to be endocrine causes of infertility, but there is little convincing evidence that this is the case. At present, it is proper to consider that these conditions are not direct causes of infertility in the male, aside from ejaculatory disturbances that may occur in a small percentage of diabetic men.

Sexual Dysfunction

Sexual dysfunction occurs in less than 5% of men with infertility. Included in this category are men with erectile impotence, premature ejaculation, inadequate coital technique, and ejaculation of excessive frequency. The optimal frequency of sexual intercourse in the peri-ovulatory period of the female partner is every 24–48 hours.

EVALUATION

Fig 8–4 shows an algorithm for the diagnostic evaluation of a potentially infertile male.

History & Physical Examination

These should be keyed to the various causes of male infertility discussed in the previous section. Body measurements for eunuchoid proportions should be taken. Visual field examination, testing for anosmia, and breast examination for gynecomastia should be done. Particular attention to the examination of external genitalia is important. Testicular size should be estimated.

Laboratory Tests

The basic endocrine studies include measurement of serum testosterone, FSH, LH, and prolactin levels. Serum estradiol may be helpful in cases of suspected alcoholism. Measurement of serum 17α-hydroxyprogesterone or DHEA-sulfate is seldom indicated for assessment of adrenal function except in men with suspected congenital adrenal hyperplasia. Urinalysis and examination of expressed prostatic secretions for prostatitis, urine or semen culture for infection, and serum creatinine for occult renal failure are indicated when appropriate.

Semen Analysis

The basic study for evaluation of infertility is the semen analysis. Semen is obtained by masturbation in a wide-mouthed glass jar after a period of abstinence of at least 2 days. It must be examined within 2 hours of collection. In temperate climates, preservation at room temperature is acceptable. Normal values following a period of sexual abstinence of 2–5 days include volume 2–5 mL; viscosity 0; liquefaction complete in 30 minutes; color opalescent. The pH should be 7.5–8. The currently accepted normal value for sperm concentration is greater than 20 million/mL and greater than 60/mL/ejaculate. Over '60% of the sperm should be motile if examined within 2 hours of ejaculation. Using a grading system of motility from 0–4, the grade of motility should be $2+$ or more. Approximately 60% of the sperm heads should have normal oval morphology. When the ejaculatory ducts are blocked or the seminal vesicle is absent, the semen contains no fructose. The normal range of fructose concentration in semen is

120–450 mg/dL. However, measurement of semen fructose is rarely helpful, since semen of pH 7 or less and volume less than 1 mL are usually diagnostic of ejaculatory duct obstruction regardless of the fructose measurement.

A new way to assess sperm function is to measure the ability of human sperm to penetrate zona-free hamster eggs. Sperm are incubated overnight with 10–20 zona-free hamster eggs. More than 10% of the hamster eggs should be penetrated by the sperm. There is moderately good correlation between sperm penetration of zona-free hamster eggs and of human eggs. The cause of abnormal sperm penetration is unknown, and no treatment exists with the possible exception of surgical correction of varicocele.

Testicular Biopsy

Testicular biopsy is indicated for selected cases. These include patients with azoospermia, if the serum FSH is normal or less than 2 times normal. Biopsy may also be useful in selected cases of severe oligospermia. The aim is to identify those patients with azoospermia or oligospermia in whom spermatogenesis continues to be completely normal. In these patients, obstructive infertility is present and surgical treatment is possible.

Vasography

In most cases with azoospermia or oligospermia and completely normal spermatogenesis, scrotal exploration and radiologic opacification of the vas deferens are indicated to identify the obstruction. If found, surgical bypass can be performed.

Miscellaneous Studies

Serum testing for sperm antibodies is indicated by sperm clumping or agglutination, poor motility with a normal sperm count, and abnormal postcoital tests along with otherwise unexplained infertility. Buccal smear and chromosome karyotype are useful in suspected genetic abnormalities.

TREATMENT

Primary Seminiferous Tubular Failure of the Testicle

If gross testicular atrophy has occurred and the FSH level is greater than 2 times normal, no treatment is possible. Most cases are not associated with elevated FSH or testicular atrophy. Spermatogenic depressants such as drugs or excessive heat should be eliminated. Marijuana smoking should be stopped. There is meager evidence that cigarette smoking is deleterious to spermatogenesis.

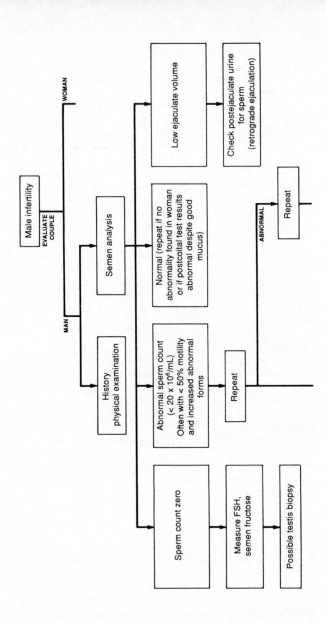

376

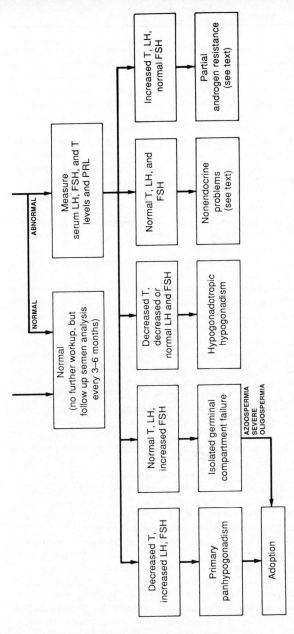

Figure 8-4. Evaluation of male infertility. (Adapted from Swerdloff RS, Boyers SM: Evaluation of the male partner of an infertile couple: An algorithmic approach. *JAMA* 1982;**247**:2418.)

377

Pharmacologic attempts to stimulate spermatogenesis are generally unsuccessful. The most common treatment involves intramuscular injection of hCG, oral clomiphene citrate, or testosterone rebound treatment. In assessing the results for treatment of male infertility, it must be remembered that some pregnancies will occur without any therapy at all. The spontaneous pregnancy rate in untreated, idiopathic seminiferous tubular failure with oligospermia is 20–25%.

If empirical administration of **hCG,** 4000 U intramuscularly, twice weekly for 10 weeks, is used, the results of gonadotropin therapy for eugonadotropic oligospermia have produced pregnancy rates of 7–30%. In some cases, hCG may even temporarily suppress spermatogenesis for several months after completion of therapy. The addition of human menopausal gonadotropin, which has a stronger FSH action, adds nothing to the results of therapy. While gonadotropin therapy has been unimpressive statistically, it is a reasonably safe method. Side effects include transient nipple tenderness, gynecomastia, weight gain, and increased libido in a small percentage of patients.

Clomiphene citrate has been used to increase endogenous LH and FSH production but is not approved by the FDA for use in the male. The optimal dosage is unknown. Currently used regimens include 100 mg 3 times weekly and 25 mg/d for the first 25 days of each month. Pregnancy rates of approximately 30% have been reported.

Exogenous intramuscular **testosterone** has been used to promote spermatogenesis by initially inhibiting sperm production. Following termination of testosterone treatment, there may be a rebound effect with improvement of sperm count. The dosage schedule is testosterone enanthate or testosterone cypionate, 200 mg intramuscularly weekly for 10 weeks and then every other week for 10 weeks. Again, pregnancy rates of approximately 30% are reported. However, 4% of men fail to return to pretreatment sperm counts after termination of testosterone injections.

Pharmacologic stimulation of spermatogenesis by tamoxifen, hCG, clomiphene, or intramuscular testosterone is not efficacious and is not frequently used. Empirical therapy with thyroid hormone, prednisone, vitamin E, or arginine is not effective for the treatment of male infertility of any cause and should not be considered.

Because excessive heat interrupts spermatogenesis, prolonged hot baths and tight clothing such as jockey shorts and jeans should be avoided. Application of artificial ice to the scrotum has been advocated but is unproved.

Because of the inefficacy of drugs in improving sperm counts, specialists in reproductive medicine have turned increasingly to techniques of ''assisted reproduction'' to achieve pregnancy in couples with oligoasthenospermia. Intrauterine insemination of processed or washed sperm has not been effective, but more complex techniques such as in vitro fertilization, gamete intrafallopian transfer, and micromanipulation of human ova do offer some experimental hope. Micromanipulation involves the manipulation of individual sperm into a single ovum, by microsurgical techniques.

Varicocele

Approximately 10–15% of men have a varicocele. In one-third of these, the varicocele interferes with spermatogenesis by altering the temperature-cooling mechanism of the scrotal wall. Surprisingly, size of a varicocele is not related to severity of effect. Surgical correction of varicocele is accomplished through a groin rather than scrotal incision. Seventy percent of men who undergo such an operation will have a significant improvement in semen analysis, and the average pregnancy rate is 40% compared with 15% in untreated cases. If the preoperative sperm count is greater than 10 million, better results are obtained.

Ejaculatory Abnormalities

For **excessive ejaculate volume,** a split ejaculate technique may be successful in producing pregnancy. The ejaculate is collected in 2 separate containers, each containing approximately one-half. The sperm-rich first portion of the ejaculate may be used for artificial insemination. Alternatively, a coital technique of early withdrawal may be used. The first several spurts of the ejaculate containing most of the sperm are deposited intravaginally and the remainder discarded.

Low ejaculate volume requires artificial insemination timed to the female partner's ovulation.

Retrograde ejaculation is diagnosed by finding large numbers of sperm in the urine sediment obtained after ejaculation. Retrograde ejaculation may be treated by ephedrine, 25–50 mg, 30 minutes before intercourse, or 25–50 mg 3 times daily. Imipramine, 25 mg 3 times daily, has also been used with success. In addition, antihistamines such as pseudoephedrine hydrochloride, 60 mg every 8 hours; phenylpropanolamine, 25–50 mg every 8 hours; or chlorpheniramine plus phenylpropanolamine every 12 hours, have been used to convert retrograde to antegrade ejaculation in approximately 60% of cases.

If pharmacologic treatment of retrograde ejaculation is unsuccessful, sperm may be recovered from the urine or bladder following ejaculation and used for artificial insemination. The urine is alkalinized with baking soda or sodium bicarbonate tablets for 24 hours. The patient urinates and then ejaculates. The postejaculatory urine is obtained either by repeat urination or catheterization. The urine is centrifuged for 5 minutes at 2000 rpm, and the sperm-rich pellet at the bottom of the centrifuge tube is used for artificial insemination. Because this form of therapy is rarely used, success rates are uncertain.

Recently, a technique of electro-ejaculation has been developed, primarily for use in spinal cord injury patients but also for other conditions if combined with general anesthesia. An electric stimulator is placed transrectally against the anterior rectal wall, seminal vesicles, and prostate. Electro-ejaculation is fairly reliable in producing an ejaculate with motile sperm. Pregnancy chances are not yet known but seem to be less than 50%.

Obstructive Oligospermia or Azoospermia

The treatment of obstructive infertility is surgical. When the obstruction is in the epididymis, pregnancy rates of 20–35% may be achieved by current methods of microsurgical vasoepididymostomy.

Vasectomy reversal has become more successful in recent years. Microsurgical techniques produce a normal sperm count in 75–90% of cases and pregnancy in 50–65% of cases.

Endocrinologic Infertility

Infertility due to hypergonadotropic hypogonadism is not treatable. In the hypogonadotropic forms of infertility, hCG, 2000–5000 U intramuscularly, 3 times weekly, should be tried for 3–6 months. If normal serum testosterone levels and masculinization are achieved without improvement in the sperm count, addition of hMG, 1–2 ampules (75 IU of FSH and 75 IU of LH per ampule) 3 times weekly, should be added. Once spermatogenesis is initiated, hMG is discontinued while hCG therapy is maintained. With congenital forms of hypogonadotropic hypogonadism, the sperm counts with such therapy are usually not over 10 million/mL, but pregnancy may occur nonetheless. Intranasal, subcutaneous, or intravenous GnRH may supplant these forms of therapy in the future as clinical experience with this agent increases. If hyperprolactinemia is present, it should be treated with either bromocriptine or surgical ablation of the pituitary tumor. Further discussion of the treatment of hypogonadotropic hypogonadism is found in Chapter 1.

Sexual Dysfunction

See Erectile Dysfunction, below

Infection

Obvious infection of the genitourinary system should be treated with appropriate antibiotics. The value of antibiotic therapy for infertility associated with asymptomatic genitourinary infection remains to be proved.

Immunotherapy

In the presence of sperm antibodies in the male, glucocorticoid therapy for suppression of antibody formation effects pregnancy in approximately one-third of couples. Methylprednisolone, 96 mg daily for 7 days, or prednisone, 20 mg every other day for 3 months, has been used to treat immunologic infertility, as has in vitro fertilization.

Evaluation of the Female Partner

Regardless of the cause of male infertility, gynecologic evaluation is appropriate for the female partner after attempting for pregnancy for 1 year without success.

CRYPTORCHIDISM

Cryptorchidism is the unilateral or bilateral absence of the testicles from the scrotum due to the lack of full descent of the testicles through the inguinal canal or due to absence of the testicle. Undescended testes may be located in intra-abdominal, inguinal, prescrotal, or ectopic positions. About 20% of cryptorchid testes are due to a mechanical or developmental abnormality such as ectopic insertion of the gubernaculum or inguinal hernia. In 80% of cases, subtle endocrine abnormalities, such as inadequate LH production in utero, or occasionally frank endocrinopathy cause the failure of normal testicular descent. The physiology and pathophysiology of testicular descent have not been fully elucidated.

The incidence of cryptorchidism is 9–30% in premature males, 3–6% in full-term births, and 1–2% at 1 year of age. Following 1 year there is no significant change in the incidence, showing that spontaneous descent after the first year of life is unlikely to occur. The location of the undescended testicle is as follows: intra-abdominal (8%), inguinal (63%), prescrotal (24%), ectopic (11%). Anorchia occurs in 3–4% of unpalpable testicles. Cryptorchidism is bilateral in 30% and unilateral in 70%. It occurs on the left side in 30% and on the right side in 70%.

CLINICAL FEATURES

Absence of the testicle on one or both sides is the presenting complaint. There is an increased incidence of torsion of the testicle, which produces acute pain at the site of the undescended testicle. An associated indirect inguinal hernia is present in 50–95% of cases but is usually asymptomatic.

LABORATORY FEATURES

Basal gonadotropin and testosterone levels are normal except in bilateral anorchia or severe testicular atrophy, which result in low testosterone levels and elevated gonadotropins in adults. Basal and stimulated gonadotropin and testosterone levels are not useful in diagnosing cryptorchidism. However, failure of serum testosterone to rise following hCG stimulation is diagnostic of bilateral anorchia. Ultrasound of the inguinal region, pelvic CT scan, and laparoscopy may be used in that order to identify the position of the unpalpable testicle.

Because of cost ineffectiveness, assessment of cryptorchid males with intravenous pyelography is not indicated.

INCREASED INCIDENCE OF TESTICULAR CANCER

The incidence of malignant neoplasm of the testicle is approximately 2/100,000 males. The incidence of testicular cancer in cryptorchid males is approximately 4–40 times greater. The higher the position of the testicle, the higher is the chance for development of testicular cancer. The chance for development of cancer in an intra-abdominal testicle may be as high as 5%. Surgical or endocrine transposition of the undescended testicle to the scrotum after age 10 does not increase the chance for development of neoplasia. Statistical study of transposition before age 10 is not yet available. Some preliminary data suggest that transposition before age 10 may reduce the chance for testicular cancer.

Scrotal transposition of the undescended testicle places the testicle in a palpable position so that it may be carefully followed. Theoretically, this would make it possible to diagnose cancer at an earlier stage and improve the chances for cure. However, the stage of cancer at the time of diagnosis and the 5-year survival rate were almost identical for testicular cancer developing in surgically corrected undescended testicles compared with testicular cancer in still cryptorchid testicles. The increased incidence of testicular cancer in cryptorchid testes includes all cell types, and the distribution of seminoma and nonseminoma is the same as is found in normally descended testicles.

REDUCED FERTILITY

Reduced fertility is often seen in men with cryptorchidism. Even when the cryptorchidism is unilateral, bilateral histologic and functional abnormalities are often present. Fertility is present in 50% of adult men with unilateral cryptorchidism and 25% of men with bilateral cryptorchidism. Research suggests that endocrine or surgical treatment of cryptorchidism before age 2 will preserve fertility potential because testicular damage begins at this age. However, data will not be clearly documented for another 15 years because of a widespread policy of correction of cryptorchidism before age 2. If the cryptorchidism is corrected surgically in late childhood, fertility rates of about 65% for unilateral and about 40% for bilateral cryptorchidism are later found. Postpubertal correction of cryptorchidism does not improve fertility, because of permanent damage to the seminiferous tubules.

TREATMENT

In any patient the possibility of a retractile testicle due to an active cremasteric reflex must be ruled out. These testicles have normal histologic characteristics and fertility. The patient should be examined in the cross-legged position in a warm room or bath. In this position, it may be possible to milk the testicle from the inguinal region into the scrotum. About 50% of patients referred for possible cryptorchidism actually have retractile testicles and require no therapy.

Correction of true cryptorchidism should be accomplished at age 12 months because it is at this age when irreversible testicular damage begins. Therapeutic options include surgical orchiopexy, orchiectomy, and endocrine therapy with GnRH or hCG (or both).

GnRH

GnRH has been used in Europe with good success, and it appears to be the endocrine therapy of choice. The dose is 400 μg 3–4 times a day by nasal insufflation for 4 weeks. In European studies, scrotal descent has occurred in 50–60% of cases. For patients who fail on GnRH therapy, administration of hCG produces scrotal descent in another 25% of cases.

hCG

Prior to the use of GnRH, hCG injections were the traditional method of endocrine treatment. No standard dose or duration of treatment was agreed upon, and results were extremely variable. In the past, commonly used regimens of hCG included a short course of 10,000–15,000 U in divided doses intramuscularly over 3–5 days or a long course of 10,000–50,000 U in divided doses over 6–8 weeks. The current recommendation consists of a 5-week course of intramuscular hCG given twice weekly. For patients below 2 years of age, 250 IU is given with each injection; for ages 2–6, 500 IU is given with each injection; and beyond age 6, 1000 IU is given with each injection.

Approximately 20% of cryptorchid testes treated with hCG descend to the scrotum whether the hCG therapy is used de novo or following failure of GnRH.

Surgery

Should endocrine therapy be unsuccessful, surgical therapy is indicated. If the contralateral testicle is adequate, **orchiectomy** is an alternative for a poorly developed testicle or very high testicle for which orchiopexy would be difficult. Surgical **orchiopexy**, however, has been the traditional method of treatment. If there is concurrent indirect inguinal hernia or true ectopy of the testicle, hormonal therapy should be omitted and surgery should be the treatment of choice. Patients with severe mental retardation or independent causes of infertility such as ejaculatory failure (eg, prune-belly syndrome or exstrophy of the bladder) should not undergo orchiopexy because fertility is either not desirable or not possible. Treatment does not alter the chances of testicular neoplasia.

Selection of Treatment

Bilateral cryptorchidism before puberty warrants a trial of hCG or GnRH analog. If this is unsuccessful, the more palpable testicle should have an orchiopexy first. The other side may then be considered for either orchiopexy or orchiectomy.

Unilateral cryptorchidism in a palpable position also warrants a trial of endocrine therapy. Atrophic or dystrophic nonpalpable testicles should be removed as should unilateral cryptorchid and abdominal testicles.

Bilateral intra-abdominal testicles are difficult to manage. A good option is to place the better testicle in the scrotum so that it can be followed by palpation and allowed to maintain its hormonal function. The other testicle can be brought down but also can be removed without compromising the patient.

Contraindications to surgical orchiopexy include severe mental retardation, ejaculatory failure, and finding testes with abnormal adnexae. Such testes are unable to contribute sperm to the ejaculate because of obstruction of the seminal duct. In cases of genetic abnormality such as Klinefelter's syndrome or Sertoli-cell-only syndrome, fertility is usually not possible and orchiopexy should not be considered. The choices in these situations are no treatment or orchiectomy. In patients with severe endocrine hypogonadism due to cryptorchidism, particularly when the cryptorchidism is intra-abdominal, bilateral orchiectomy is probably advisable. These testicles have failed in spermatogenesis and endocrine function and have a significant risk of malignancy. The risk of operation is less than the risk of cancer.

Patients being treated after age 13 have little chance that fertility will be improved by scrotal transposition, so orchiectomy or no treatment becomes more viable alternatives, particularly if the contralateral testicle appears to be normal. Before the advent of current therapeutic regimens for disseminated testicular cancer, the risk of death from cancer exceeded the risk of anesthesia and orchiectomy up to age 32. For that reason orchiectomy was considered preferable to no treatment. However, the efficacy of current chemotherapy for testicular cancer may prove that it is equally acceptable to advocate no treatment for the unilateral undescended testicle. This hypothesis awaits confirmation.

TESTICULAR CANCER

Testicular tumors are rare. They account for approximately 1% of all male malignancies and 5–10% of all genitourinary malignancies. However, they are one of the most common types of cancer in men aged 20–35. The overall incidence of testicular tumors is 2/100,000 men in the USA.

GERM CELL TUMORS

Germ cell tumors account for 95% of testicular tumors, and most are malignant. Of germ cell tumors, 40% are seminomas and 60% are nonseminomas. The nonseminomatous germ cell tumors are made up of embryonal cell carcinoma, teratocarcinoma, choriocarcinoma, mixed patterns, endodermal sinus tumor (yolk sac tumor, the most common germ cell neoplasm in infants), and occasionally benign teratomas.

Germ cell tumors may be hormonally active. They may produce 2 serum markers: hCG and alpha-fetoprotein. Alpha-fetoprotein has no clinical endocrine effect, but hCG may produce gynecomastia. About 10% of tumors present with gynecomastia. In the seminoma type of testicular cancer, alpha-fetoprotein is not elevated and 5–10% of seminomas have measurable serum levels of hCG. However, in the nonseminomatous type, 90% of tumors produce one or the other of these serum markers. Seventy-five percent of tumors produce hCG alone, 60% produce alpha-fetoprotein alone, and 50% produce both hCG and alpha-fetoprotein. hCG must be measured in the serum by the beta subunit radioimmunoassay method. It does not appear in urinary assays in 50% of men who have elevated serum levels of β-hCG.

LEYDIG & SERTOLI CELL TUMORS

About 5% of testicular tumors are Leydig and Sertoli cell tumors, most of which are malignant. Other tumors of the testicular stroma are very rare.

Some Leydig and Sertoli cell tumors are hormonally active. About 75% of Leydig cell tumors produce estrogens and are feminizing. They produce not only gynecomastia but impotence, decreased hair growth, and increased urinary estrogen levels. Leydig cell tumors, both benign and malignant, occasionally produce androgens also. In children, the result of androgen production is sexual precocity. In adults, there is no change in secondary sexual characteristics but gynecomastia may develop. Of Sertoli cell tumors, about 30% produce feminization owing to estrogen secretion and about 25% are associated with gynecomastia probably because of hCG secretion.

CLINICAL FEATURES

Classically, testicular tumors are described as painless lumps in the testicle. In fact, about 30% of testicular tumors are painful. In 10% a coexisting, acute, reactive hydrocele may obscure the underlying mass. For that reason, any acute-onset hydrocele in a young man should be cause for suspicion of testicular cancer.

The differential diagnosis includes any other scrotal mass (eg, hydrocele, epididymitis, spermatocele), but the main difficulty is distinguishing epididymitis from testicular tumor. With epididymitis the inflammation initially is confined to the epididymis; its causes include gram-negative rods, tuberculosis, gonococcus, and chlamydia. In more advanced cases, the usual landmarks in the scrotum are obliterated and it is not possible to tell whether the mass is in the epididymis or in the testicle. With epididymitis there is often a history of dysuria, prostatitis, or gonorrhea. Pyuria is usually present. The urine should then be cultured and appropriate antibiotics given. Initial therapy is with tetracycline, the antibiotic of choice, while the cultures are incubating. The mass in epididymitis resolves over a period of weeks, whereas the mass in testicular tumor increases in size. Any case in which there is a reasonable suspicion of testicular cancer should be explored surgically.

LABORATORY FEATURES

The most important laboratory studies are the serum markers β-hCG, and alpha-fetoprotein. With functioning Leydig cell tumors, urinary 17-ketosteroids and serum DHEA sulfate are increased. In addition, urinary and serum estrogen levels are increased in about 25%. Serum androgen levels may also be elevated. Sites of metastasis in the bones, liver, retroperitoneal lymph nodes, mediastinum, lungs, and supraclavicular lymph nodes may be reflected in abnormalities of studies directed at these tissues. Of particular importance are CT scans of the chest, abdomen, and pelvis, and bone scans.

TREATMENT

The initial treatment is inguinal orchiectomy. For testicular cancer, a scrotal approach should not be used because this may change the pattern of lymph node metastases, inducing involvement of the inguinal nodes in addition to the retroperitoneal nodes. Once the pathologic diagnosis is established, staging of the tumor by CT scan of chest, abdomen, and pelvis, bone scan, and liver function tests should be accomplished.

Seminoma is a very radiosensitive tumor. When seminoma is limited to the testicle, options for clinical management following orchiectomy are (1) careful clinical surveillance or (2) radiation therapy of 2500–3000 rads to the retroperitoneal lymph nodes. If there is spread of seminoma to the retroperitoneum, radiation therapy to the retroperitoneum and mediastinum is appropriate. If the tumor has spread above the diaphragm or to other metastatic sites, chemotherapy is the next mode of treatment. Extremely effective cisplatin-based multiple drug chemotherapy captures nearly 100% of metastatic seminomas, but toxic side effects include myelosuppression, pulmonary fibrosis, and renal damage.

For nonseminomatous germ cell tumors confined to the testicle, the options for clinical management following orchiectomy are (1) careful clinical surveillance or (2) retroperitoneal lymph node dissection. If there is tumor involvement of the retroperitoneal lymph nodes, orchiectomy and retroperitoneal lymph node dissection are appropriate. For those tumors which have spread above the diaphragm or to other metastatic sites, chemotherapy should be initiated. Surgical removal of residual masses may be advisable following chemotherapy. Remission rates with cisplatin-based multiple drug chemotherapy are over 90%.

Most Leydig and Sertoli cell tumors are benign and are adequately treated by orchiectomy. Those which are malignant have a poor prognosis, regardless of additional surgical or chemotherapeutic treatment. Men with Leydig cell tumors producing estrogen usually have hypogonadism and infertility owing to pituitary and direct testicular suppression by estrogen. Following gonadectomy, gonadotropin levels rise but testicular function usually remains abnormal.

PROGNOSIS

For seminoma, the cure rate for stage I tumor (limited to the testicle) is 98%. For stage II (retroperitoneal metastasis), it is approximately 90%. For nonseminomatous germ-cell tumors, chances for survival are approximately 90–100% for stage I and 80–90% for stage II. When either seminoma or nonseminomatous tumor is disseminated (stage III), remission rates over 90% are now being achieved and long-term survival chances are significantly better than in the past.

Benign Leydig cell tumors have an excellent prognosis, whereas malignant Leydig cell tumors have a very poor prognosis.

GYNECOMASTIA

Gynecomastia is benign glandular enlargement of the male breast. Bilateral gynecomastia is more common than unilateral and must be distinguished from fatty enlargement (pseudogynecomastia). Unilateral gynecomastia must be distinguished from tumors such as carcinoma, neurofibroma, and lipoma. Mammography may help this distinction.

CAUSES

Gynecomastia is associated with a wide variety of conditions and drugs (Table 8–4). In many cases the pathogenesis is unknown, conjectural, or a combination of 2 or more factors. Gynecomastia appears to be caused by a high estradiol:testosterone ratio in most cases. Since most estradiol, as well as testosterone, is produced by the testes, castration does not cause gynecomastia, whereas testicular injury may. An imbalance of the estradiol:testosterone ratio may be produced in a variety of ways. There may be a decrease in free testosterone (primary hypogonadism) or an increase in TeBG, reducing the percentage of free testosterone (hyperthyroidism and cirrhosis). Overstimulation of testicular interstitial cells by LH changes the patterns of steroidogenesis, resulting in a relative imbalance favoring estradiol over testosterone. This is probably the mechanism of gynecomastia in primary hypogonadism and perhaps puberty, when the incidence of gynecomastia may be as high as 70%.

Patients who are malnourished or who have severe systemic disease sometimes develop gynecomastia with nutritional replacement or recovery from chronic disease. It is thought that pituitary suppres-

Table 8–4. Causes of gynecomastia.

Drugs

Increasing estrogen activity: Estrogen, diethylstilbestrol, androgen, hCG, digitalis, opiates, marijuana, creams containing estrogen.

Inhibitors of testosterone production: Cancer chemotherapeutic agents (especially busulfan, carmustine, estamustine, phosphate sodium, flutamide), alcohol.

Competitive inhibitors of androgen receptors: Spironolactone, cimetidine, cyproterone acetate, progestine, flutamide.

Prolactin stimulators: Phenothiazines, butyrophenones, metoclopramide, reserpine, methyldopa, opiates, methadone, cimetidine, hydroxyzine.

Unknown mechanisms: Isoniazid, tricyclic antidepressants, ethionamide, thyroid hormone excess, amphetamines, ?meprobamate, amiodarone.

Physiologic

Neonates; puberty; old age; familial.

Conditions increasing estrogen production

Testicular tumors, hCG-secreting carcinoma (usually lung or liver), liver disease, ?thyrotoxicosis, adrenal adenoma or carcinoma, obesity, true hermaphroditism.

Conditions decreasing testosterone production

Klinefelter's syndrome, chronic illness (eg, tuberculosis, Hodgkin's disease), orchiectomy, orchitis, injury, enzyme defects (17β–hydroxy-steroid oxidoreductase deficiency).

Conditions with testosterone insensitivity

Androgen-insensitivity syndrome: Complete (testicular feminization syndrome) to partial.

Conditions with selective insensitivity of breast tissue to testosterone

Idiopathic or familial gynecomastia (usually bilateral but often unequal or unilateral).

Conditions with increased prolactin

Drugs, pituitary tumors, hypothyroidism, renal failure.

Conditions with recovery of LH secretion

Refeeding after malnourishment, hemodialysis, recovery from liver failure.

Conditions with increased TeBG

Hyperthyroidism, cirrhosis.

sion occurs during malnutrition and with recovery rising gonadotropin secretion overstimulates interstitial cells. This is referred to as refeeding gynecomastia and is seen in chronic malnutrition, hemodialysis for renal failure, and recovery from liver dysfunction. Overstimulation of Leydig cells may also occur from hCG-producing testicular tumors such as testicular cancer and some primary liver cancers. Hyperprolactinemia directly stimulates breast tissue and may also interfere with the peripheral action of testosterone. Consequently, any of the causes of hyperprolactinemia (Chapter 1) may be associated with gynecomastia. Breast enlargement may be familial.

Clinically, gynecomastia may be associated with the following conditions: increased estrogen secretion (relative to testosterone secretion; found in Leydig cell tumors); tumors of the adrenal cortex; and some forms of hypergonadotropism. Decreased androgen secretion is seen in Klinefelter's syndrome and any cause of testicular atrophy. End-organ insensitivity to testosterone will also produce gynecomastia; this abnormality is seen in the various forms of testicular feminization. Increased gonadotropin secretion is found in some pituitary tumors. hCG secretion is found with testicular cancer and bronchogenic and other carcinomas.

Drugs that have estrogen action of antiandrogens may also produce gynecomastia. Cimetidine given clinically in high doses causes gynecomastia, impotence, or both in 50% of men. Ranitidine, another effective inhibitor of gastric acid secretion, does not have antiandrogen effects and is therefore preferred for chronic treatment in men.

Chronic diseases associated with gynecomastia either during recovery or at other times include malnutrition, tuberculosis, diabetes, cirrhosis, renal failure, and Hodgkin's disease.

Chemotherapy for malignancy may also produce gynecomastia, perhaps by blocking the final steps in Leydig cell synthesis of testosterone, thereby producing an increased estradiol:testosterone ratio.

CLINICAL FEATURES

The presenting complaint is breast enlargement. In about 25% of patients this is painful. In 4% there is galactorrhea. Symptoms and signs of associated diseases may be present as well. Since gynecomastia is occasionally a presenting sign of testicular cancer, a careful gonadal examination must be performed.

LABORATORY FEATURES

Laboratory findings depend on the cause. For mild physiologic gynecomastia, no laboratory evaluation is necessary. Otherwise appropriate laboratory tests include measurement of serum β-hCG, serum estradiol and estrone, and serum prolactin, and assessment of the hypothalamic-pituitary-testicular axis with measurement of serum LH, FSH, free testosterone, and total testosterone. If there is any suspicion of testicular tumor, a serum alpha-fetoprotein should be obtained. CT scan of the pituitary and chest x-ray should be done as well. Buccal smear, chromosome karyotyping, mammography, and assessment for other organ function should be tailored to the individual case. If no other explanation is present, assessment of thyroid function is appropriate. Finally, excisional biopsy should be considered if it is not possible to rule out other causes of breast enlargement by physical examination.

TREATMENT

The most common cause of gynecomastia is puberty. Over 50% of pubertal boys experience transient, mild gynecomastia. The condition is usually self-limited, and no treatment is indicated. However, if gynecomastia becomes chronic and psychologically disturbing, excision of the subcutaneous breast tissue may be done through a transaxillary or periareolar approach, thus preserving the nipple and avoiding obvious scars. Correction of any underlying disorder causing gynecomastia should be accomplished. Regardless of the cause, in severe cases, tamoxifen (a nonsteroidal antiestrogen), 10 mg, orally twice daily, may induce a remission. In addition, clomiphene citrate can reverse gynecomastia or relieve breast pain. Radiation therapy is not indicated for gynecomastia. However, it is useful in preventing the development of painful gynecomastia in patients with metastatic prostate cancer who will be receiving estrogen treatment. In such cases, each breast is radiated with 400 rads for 3 days.

Gynecomastia of puberty resolves spontaneously in 1–2 years in almost all patients. Regardless of the cause of gynecomastia, resolution will not occur if it is allowed to persist until the breast tissue becomes fibrotic.

ERECTILE DYSFUNCTION

The term erectile dysfunction refers to the entire range of erection problems often referred to as impotence. The pathophysiology of erectile dysfunction includes psychogenic, vasculogenic, pharmacogenic, neurogenic, and endocrinologic disorders.

Each of the 4 parts of the male sexual response—erection, emission, ejaculation, and orgasm—has a separate neurologic mechanism. Though these mechanisms are usually integrated, it is possible to drop out any one or more while the others remain intact. Erection is a complex autonomic nervous system function with both sympathetic and parasympathetic components. Emission is a purely sympathetic activity, while ejaculation is mediated by the somatic nervous system via the pudendal nerves. Orgasm is a psychic integration of these various events.

CAUSES

Psychogenic Causes

Psychogenic causes of erectile dysfunction are more common in men under age 40. Recent advances in diagnostic techniques have identified organic disease especially of vasculogenic origin in many patients formerly thought to have psychogenic impotence. It is now estimated that erectile dysfunction is of psychogenic origin in less than 50% of patients. In men over 50 years of age, psychogenic causes are even less common. In these patients, underlying depression or marital problems may be causal.

Certain symptoms are pathognomonic of psychogenic erectile dysfunction. These include normal and sustained erections in foreplay lost at the moment of intromission; normal erection with some sexual partners but failure with others; normal erection with masturbation but failure with partners; sudden onset of total impotence in a man under the age of 40; and alternating periods of normal function and total impotence. Organic disease, especially vasculogenic disorders, may be present even though morning, nocturnal, or partial erections occur. Many organic causes of erectile dysfunction have waxing and waning periods of function; it is rare for a man to have totally absent erections.

Vasculogenic Causes

A. Arteriogenic Disease: Vasculogenic impotence accounts for many cases of impotence that fail to respond to psychotherapy or are of unknown cause. Arterial insufficiency of the penis is a common cause of impotence, especially in men over the age of 40. It may occur from lesions in one or more areas. Aortic or iliac atherosclerosis may compromise arterial supply to the penis, as in the Leriche syndrome. Obstruction may also occur in the hypogastric artery although it is rarely limited to this site. Blockage of the internal pudendal and penile arteries is probably the most common cause of penile arterial insufficiency.

B. Venogenic Disease: Primary and secondary impotence may be caused by abnormal venous drainage of the corpus cavernosum in an unknown percentage of cases. While primary venogenic impotence is unusual, secondary venogenic impotence is much more common, especially with increasing age. The mechanism by which corporo-venous leakage develops is not understood, but its presence may be identified by cavernosometry and cavernosography.

Pharmacologic Causes

Many commonly used drugs have undesirable effects on erectile function (Table 8–5). The most common of these are the antihypertensive agents. The incidence of erectile dysfunction has been reported to be as much as 50% with the use of methyldopa, beta-blockers, clonidine, spironolactone, and guanethidine. On the other hand, antihypertensives that are less likely to cause erectile dysfunction include thiazides, angiotensin-converting enzyme inhibitors, calcium channel blockers, prazocin, phenoxybenzamine, hydralazine, minoxidil, and metoprolol.

Anticholinergic agents, phenothiazines, antihistamines, and antidepressants may all be associated with erectile dysfunction due to central or peripheral neurogenic effects. Estrogens and the various antiandrogens produce impotence by alteration of hormone status. Cimetidine may be associated with impotence in a small percentage of cases because it acts as an antiandrogen. Ranitidine, another inhibitor of gastric acid secretion, does not have antiandrogen effects and does not cause impotence. The antifungal agent ketoconazole interferes with androgen synthesis in the testicle and may also produce endocrine impotence. Drugs that cause hyperprolactinemia (Chapter 1) may also cause endocrine impotence, as may alcohol and marijuana. Alcohol elevates plasma estrogen by causing hepatic dysfunction and decreases testosterone by direct effect on the Leydig cells. Marijuana also causes a reversible depression of serum testosterone. Most barbiturates, sedatives, tranquilizers, and street drugs have been reported to be associated with erectile dysfunction, although the exact mechanism of action is unknown.

Table 8–5. Some drugs that may be associated with impotence.

Alcohol	Cimetidine, ranitidine
Amphetamines	Cocaine
Antihypertensives, eg, prazocin, diuretics, guanethedine, hydralazine, guanabenz, indapamide, clonidine, methyldopa, reserpine.	Estrogens
	Ketoconazole
	Marijuana
	Metoclopramide
	Narcotics, eg, heroin, morphine, methadone.
Anticholinergics	Phenothiazines
Antihistamines	Phenytoin
Antidepressants, eg, tricyclics, lithium, MAO inhibitors.	Sedatives, eg, butyrophenones, barbiturates, benzodiazepines
Beta-blockers	Spironolactone
Carbamazepine	
Cardiovascular drugs, eg, digitalis, clofibrate, verapamil, beta-blockers	

Diabetes

Impotence ultimately occurs in over 50% of diabetic men. In juvenile diabetics, the age of presentation is commonly the 30s while in adult-onset diabetes the common age of presentation is the 50s and 60s. Rarely, impotence is the presenting manifestation of diabetes. The pathogenesis is neuropathic (especially in patients with concomitant neuropathy), vasculogenic, or psychogenic, and may frequently be of mixed etiology, especially when the patient is taking antihypertensive agents, is under poor blood glucose control, or is azotemic.

Surgery

Men with aortoiliac atherosclerosis frequently have organic erectile dysfunction caused by inadequate blood flow. Aortoiliac reconstruction can reverse this impotence especially if a surgical technique that preserves the sensitive autonomic nerves is used. Otherwise, neurogenic impotence will frequently result. In addition, about 30% of patients become impotent after aortoiliac surgery because of further compromise of the blood flow to the hypogastric system in aorto-femoral bypass surgery. Radical pelvic surgery for cancer of the prostate, bladder, or rectum may also be associated with erectile dysfunction because of neurologic injury. Prostatectomy for benign prostatic hypertrophy is infrequently complicated by impotence. The incidence of impotence following transurethral or suprapubic prostatectomy is less than 5%. Certain neurosurgical procedures such as pudendal neurectomy of complicated spinal cord operations may also interfere with erections.

Neurogenic Causes

Intact neurologic innervation to the penis is necessary for erection. Thus, any form of encephalopathy, myelopathy, or peripheral neuropathy that interferes with the cerebral cord or peripheral structures necessary for erection may cause dysfunction. Prominent among these are spinal cord injury, tabes dorsalis, multiple sclerosis, myelodysplasia, and various peripheral neuropathies including diabetes.

Renal Failure

Impotence occurs frequently with renal failure. Approximately 50% of patients stabilized on hemodialysis and 25% of patients with functioning renal transplants have erectile dysfunction. The pathogenesis in these cases is multifactorial including accelerated arteriosclerosis, use of antihypertensive agents, uremic neuropathy, Leydig cell dysfunction specific to renal failure, and psychologic factors.

Trauma

Penile injuries may result in damage to the erectile tissue. Pelvic fractures due to severe pelvic trauma are associated with neurologic and vascular injury to the cavernous nerves and pudendal arteries. About 30% of men with such injury have erectile dysfunction.

Local Penile Diseases

Peyronie's disease is the deposition of fibrous tissue on the tunica albuginea. It causes a penile curvature with erection that is sometimes painful. Previous priapism and primary or metastatic penile tumors may so damage the erectile tissue as to make erection impossible.

Chronic Disease States

Sexual dysfunction often complicates chronic systemic illness. The pathogenesis in these cases is not clear. Psychogenic factors, especially decreased sexual interest, are the most obvious, but organic factors may also be present. Chronic prostatitis and benign prostatic hypertrophy have been unfairly blamed for impotence. There is currently no documented causal relationship between chronic prostate disease and erectile impotence.

Endocrinopathy

Less than 5% of men with organic impotence have significant endocrine disease. Most of these men have hypogonadotropic hypogonadism due to age, alcohol, and unknown factors. Some have primary gonadal dysfunction. Hyperprolactinemia can directly cause impotence by interfering with testosterone action, even when the serum testosterone level is normal. Hyper- or hypothyroidism may cause impotence; hypothyroidism may cause hyperprolactinemia, and hyperthyroidism may increase TeBG and so reduce the percentage of free testosterone. It has been claimed in the past that erectile dysfunction may be due to either hyper- or hypoadrenal dysfunction but currently there is no known pathophysiologic relationship between the two.

Any of the conditions discussed in the section on hypogonadism that significantly reduce serum testosterone or increase serum prolactin may produce impotence.

EVALUATION

Sexual History

Detailed information should be obtained concerning the patient's sexual background, previous sexual experience, sexual expectations, marriage, and methods of adjusting to the state of dysfunction. The review of systems and past medical history should focus on the causes of erectile dysfunction discussed above.

Physical Examination

A thorough physical examination with emphasis on the vascular, neurologic, endocrine, and genitourinary systems is important.

LABORATORY TESTS

Basic laboratory data should include serum free and total testosterone, serum LH, and serum prolactin levels. In addition, measurements of serum creatinine, blood glucose, and liver function should be done. Examination of prostatic secretions, urinalysis, and a VDRL are also important.

Several recently developed diagnostic techniques are being widely used to help determine the causes of impotence.

A. Nocturnal Penile Tumescence and Rigidity (NPTR) Monitoring: Nocturnal erections occur in healthy males of all ages. Most occur during REM phases of sleep. A typical nocturnal pattern consists of erectile periods each lasting 10–30 minutes, or approximately 100 minutes per night. A monitoring device for nocturnal tumescence and rigidity consists of gauges placed about the penile shaft and connected to a recorder. This may be done in a formal sleep laboratory with concomitant EEG and EOG or it may be done using a portable monitor in the patient's home. Sources for portable monitors include the Lifetech Company in Houston, Texas, and the Dacomed Company in Minneapolis (Rigiscan). These monitors cost many thousands of dollars, the total amount depending on the readout equipment that is selected for them. A simpler but less informative technique is the snap gauge device (Dacomed). This consists of a ring connected by 3 small plastic bands that will withstand pressures of approximately 80, 120, and 160 mm Hg. The ring is placed about the base of the penis just prior to falling asleep. The intracavernous pressure developed during nocturnal erection will then break plastic bands of different strengths, thus giving the physician an estimate of the maximum intracavernous pressure during one night of sleep. The simplest test of all is the "stamp test," in which a ring of postage stamps can be used as a screening test for the presence or absence of erections. Nocturnal erection monitoring is used to assist in distinguishing psychogenic from organic impotence. Patients with psychogenic impotence have nocturnal erections and will therefore show normal nocturnal patterns. Organic impotence is revealed by abnormal patterns of nocturnal erections. Recently, however, the sensitivity and specificity of nocturnal erection testing has been questioned. Visual sexual stimulation using videotapes may produce a more natural stimulation test.

B. Penile Circulation: A screening test for vasculogenic impotence is the intracavernous injection of a vasoactive drug such as papaverine, phentolamine, or prostaglandin E_1. Typical doses are 30–60 mg of papaverine, 0.5–1 mg of phentolamine, and 5–20 mg of prostaglandin E_1. A normal response is a full or nearly full erection lasting for more than 30 minutes. Failure to achieve this response shows that the patient has a vasculogenic problem, but this test does not distinguish arteriogenic from venogenic abnormalities.

Arterial insufficiency of the corpus cavernosum may be diagnosed by duplex sonography of the corpus cavernosum before and after injection of a stimulating vasoactive agent. If this study is abnormal, anatomic abnormalities of the penile arteries may be identified by penile arteriography. Performance and interpretation of these x-rays require skill and experience.

The diagnosis of venogenic impotence requires dynamic infusion cavernosometry. Following cavernosometry, cavernosography using fluoroscopy or permanent x-rays is used to identify the location of the venous leak.

C. Neurogenic Impotence: The bulbocavernous reflex is a somatic reflex that passes through the sacral spinal cord. Electrical stimulation of the penile skin results in contraction of the bulbocavernous muscle, which can be monitored using a needle electrode. The normal range of latency time is 27–42 msec. Prolongation of the reflex time shows the presence of pudendal neuropathy and provides a means of identifying obscure evidence of peripheral neuropathy of genitalia. In addition, biothesiometry, dorsal penile nerve conduction times, and evoked sacral potentials may produce data concerning the afferent arm of erection neurophysiology. However, no clinical means of directly testing the neurologic function of the corpus cavernosum currently exists.

TREATMENT

In patients with psychogenic erectile dysfunction, counseling or antidepressants may help when indicated. Testosterone injections have a placebo effect only. In general, medical therapy for erectile dysfunction is limited to those patients with endocrine disease. Androgen replacement therapy as discussed in the section on hypogonadism is highly effective for these patients. In the presence of hyperprolactinemia, the prolactin level must be normalized with bromocriptine or surgical removal of a pituitary tumor before testosterone replacement therapy is effective.

Yohimbine is an alpha-adrenergic blocking agent that is helpful to occasional patients when taken by mouth in divided doses of 15–40 mg/d. Double-blind studies show a true response rate in only 20% of patients.

Semi-rigid Penile Prosthesis

Semi-rigid penile prostheses are a reliable form of surgical treatment for erectile dysfunction when psychological and endocrine therapy are unsuccessful. These consist of a pair of silicone cylinders surgically implanted within the corpora cavernosa. They create a permanent semi-erection of sufficient internal rigidity to allow for normal sexual function. Several different companies manufacture semi-rigid prostheses; there is little difference among these, and the selection should be based on the surgeon's experience and preference. All are surgically successful in approximately 97% of cases; 3% require removal for persistent pain, infection, or inadequate size. Of those who have had a semi-rigid prosthesis operation, 80–90% experience good or excellent sexual function.

Inflatable Penile Prosthesis

The inflatable penile prosthesis (Fig 8–5) consists of a pair of expandable cylinders connected to a reservoir of radioopaque fluid with a pump between the 2 to transfer the fluid from reservoir to

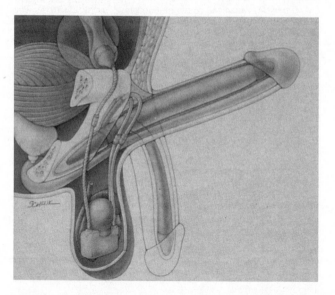

Figure 8–5. 700 Ultrex device, a surgically insertable, inflatable penile prosthesis for male erectile dysfunction. Inflation and deflation controlled with intrascrotal pump and valve. (Reproduced, with permission, from American Medical Systems, Minnetonka, MN.)

cylinder and back. The cylinder is placed within the corpora cavernosa, the pump is placed within the scrotum, and the reservoir is placed behind the abdominal wall. To achieve erection, the pump is digitally compressed 10–15 times, and detumescence is achieved by pressing a release valve on the pump, allowing the fluid to flow back into the reservoir. Inflatable prostheses consisting of one or 2 rather than 3 components are also available. Biologic complications such as infection occur in 2–3% of patients. Mechanical malfunctions occur in approximately 10–25% and are surgically correctible by replacing the faulty part. The advantages of the inflatable prosthesis are its more natural and physiologic function and ease of concealment. Disadvantages include problems with mechanical function and higher cost.

Intracavernous Pharmacotherapy

Intracavernous injection of vasoactive drugs may be used for therapy as well as for diagnosis. Patients who have a good response to the intracavernous injection of vasoactive drugs may be taught to self-administer injections, as often as 2 times per week. Risks include an approximately 1% chance of prolonged erection, the possibility of subclinical hepatic dysfunction in patients who use papaverine, and an approximately 25% incidence of corporal fibrosis occurring at the site of repeated injections.

External Vacuum Device

An external vacuum device to induce erections (Fig 8–6) consists of a plastic cylinder closed at one end and connected to a hand-operated suction pump. When the cylinder is placed over the penis and the suction pump activated, subatmospheric pressure is created about the penis, drawing blood into the corpora cavernosa and creating a reasonably good erection. A rubber constricting ring must then be placed about the base of the penis to trap the blood in the corpora when the cylinder is removed. Such devices (eg, Erec-Aid, PO Box 1478, Augusta, GA) produce satisfactory erections in 80% of men who use them, regardless of the cause of impotence.

Penile Vascular Surgery

For patients with purely arteriogenic dysfunction, anastomosis of the inferior epigastric artery to the penile arteries provides a method of revascularization. For patients with pure venogenic impotence, ligation or resection of penile veins, including the crural veins, may reduce or eliminate the corporo-venous leak. For patients with combined arteriogenic and venogenic impotence, the inferior epigastric artery may be anastomosed to the deep dorsal vein. Surgical success has been variable.

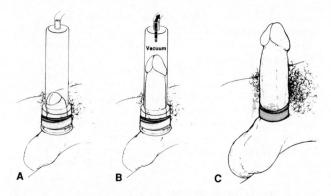

Figure 8–6. External vacuum therapy for male erectile dysfunction. **A.** Tube is placed over penis and air seal is made with gel. **B.** Partial vacuum is produced by hand-held pump (not pictured), thereby inducing penile engorgement. **C.** Elastic constriction ring is slipped off tube onto base of penis, thereby maintaining erection. (Reproduced with permission from Osbon Medical Systems, LTD, Augusta, GA.)

REFERENCES

Carlson HE: Gynecomastia. *N Engl J Med* 1980;**303:**795.

Gabrilove JL et al: Feminizing and nonfeminizing. Sertoli cell tumors. *J Urol* 1980;**124:**757.

Gasser TC et al: Intracavernous self-injection with phentolamine and papaverine for the treatment of impotence. *J Urol* 1987;**137:**678.

Giwereman et al: Testicular cancer risk in boys with undescended testis: A cohort study. *J Urol* 1987;**138:**1214.

Hadziselimovic F: *Cryptorchidism.* Springer-Verlag, 1983.

Howards, SS, Lipschultz LI (eds): Male infertility. *Urol Clin North Am* 1987;**14:**441.

Johnson DE, Swanson DA, von Eschenbach AC: Tumors of the testis, Chapter 19 in Smith's *General Urology,* Tanagho EA, McAninch JW (editors). Appleton & Lange, 1988.

Krane, RJ (editor): Impotence. *Urol Clin North Am* 1988;**15:**1.

Lange PH, Chang WY, Fraley EE: Fertility issues in therapy for nonseminomatous testicular tumors. *Urol Clin North Am* 1987;**13:**731.

Li SP, Connelly RR, Myers M: Improved survival rates among testicular cancer patients in U.S. *JAMA* 1986;**247:**825.

Loehrer PJ, Williams SD, Einhorn LH: Status of chemotherapy for testis cancer. *Urol Clin North Am* 1987;**14:**713.

Lue TF, Tanagho EA: Physiology of erection and pharmacologic management of impotence. *J Urol* 1987;**137:**829.

Mineur P et al: Feminizing testicular Leydig cell tumor: Hormonal profile before and after unilateral orchidectomy. *J Clin Endocrinol Metab* 1987;**64**:686.

Murray FT et al: Gonadal dysfunction in diabetic men with organic impotence. *J Clin Endocrinol Metab* 1987;**65**:127.

Norcross WA, Schmidt JD: Hot flashes in men with testicular insufficiency. *West J Med* 1986;**145**:515.

Parker LN et al: Treatment of gynecomastia with tamoxifen: A double-blind crossover study. *Metabolism* 1986;**35**:705.

Paulsen CA et al: Klinefelter's syndrome and its variants: A hormonal and chromosomal study. *Recent Prog Horm Res* 1968;**24**:321.

Schonfeld WA: Primary and secondary sexual characteristics: Study of their development in males from birth through maturity, with biometric study of penis and testes. *Am J Dis Child* 1943;**63**:535.

Swerdloff RS, Boyers SM: Evaluation of the male partner of an infertile couple: An algorithmic approach. *JAMA* 1982;**247**:2418.

Wilson JD, Aiman J, McDonald PC: The pathogenesis of gynecomastia. *Adv Intern Med* 1980;**25**:1.

Zachman M et al: Testicular volume during adolescence: Cross-sectional and longitudinal studies. *Helv Paediatr Acta* 1974;**29**:61.

Female Reproductive Disorders | 9

Robert D. Nachtigall, MD

MENSTRUAL CYCLE

During reproductive life, the brain, pituitary, ovaries, and genital tract of a woman are in a complex harmony that has pregnancy as its goal. Every month of this 30-year span is hormonally dedicated to the development, maturation, release, and fertilization of an egg. Reproductive endocrinology is the study of the normal menstrual cycle and its pathologic forms—when it begins (menarche, puberty) and ends (climacteric, menopause); when it is interrupted (amenorrhea, contraception); when it is painful or abnormal (dysmenorrhea, premenstrual syndrome, dysfunctional uterine bleeding); and when it fails in its basic function (infertility).

The menstrual cycle is directed by the pituitary gonadotropins follicle-stimulating hormone (FSH) and luteinizing hormone (LH). FSH and LH release are stimulated by hypothalamic gonadotropin-releasing hormone (GnRH; see Chapter 1). Their release is modulated by estradiol, which tends to inhibit FSH release while stimulating LH.

It is conventional to consider a normal menstrual cycle as one of 28 days, with the first day of bleeding referred to as "day 1."

FOLLICULAR (PROLIFERATIVE) PHASE

Initial ovarian follicle growth is initiated in the waning days of the preceding menstrual cycle and can take place independently of outside hormonal stimulation. However, this initial growth phase will be limited and followed by regression of the follicle (atresia) unless stimulated by FSH.

Early follicle growth is maintained by FSH; at day 7–8, estradiol

---

SOME ACRONYMS USED IN THIS CHAPTER

DHEAS	Dehydroepiandrosterone sulfate
DHT	Dihydrotestosterone
FSH	Follicle–stimulating hormone
GnRH	Gonadotropin–releasing hormone
HDL	High–density lipoprotein
hCG	Human chorionic gonadotropin
hMG	Human menopausal gonadotropin
IUD	Intrauterine device
LDL	Low–density lipoprotein
LH	Luteinizing hormone
PID	Pelvic inflammatory disease
PMS	Premenstrual syndrome
SHBG	Sex hormone–binding globulin
T_3	Triiodothyronine
T_4	Thyroxine
TSH	Thyroid–stimulating hormone

---

begins to increase. Local estradiol increases the follicle's FSH receptors, thereby ensuring the follicle's continued response to FSH; but by days 7–12, rising systemic estradiol concentrations suppress the actual FSH levels. An early-developing follicle becomes dominant, producing more estradiol than do the other follicles; the local estradiol concentration surrounding this dominant follicle is high enough to protect it from falling FSH levels by promoting enough FSH receptors to utilize whatever FSH is available. This dominant follicle eventually ovulates. The smaller follicles undergo atresia (atrophy), since they do not produce enough local estradiol (and therefore FSH receptors) to augment the action of declining FSH levels.

OVULATION

The positive feedback effect of estradiol upon LH secretion occurs when the circulating estradiol concentration exceeds 200 pg/mL for approximately 48 hours. This causes an increased pulsatile release of GnRH, which results in a pulsatile surge of LH (accompanied by a smaller surge of FSH). Ovulation (expulsion of the oocyte) occurs approximately 36 hours following initiation of the LH surge.

LUTEAL (SECRETORY) PHASE

Following ovulation, ovarian granulosa cells become vascularized, enlarge, and accumulate the yellow pigment (lutein) that characterizes the corpus luteum. LH levels return to a basal state and support the synthesis of estrogen and, for the first time, progesterone. Progesterone changes the histology of the endometrium from its proliferative state during the follicular phase to a secretory state during the luteal phase. These histologic changes are so characteristic that a sample of endometrium may be accurately dated with respect to time of ovulation. The hormone secretion from the corpus luteum spontaneously declines 9–11 days after ovulation, with menstruation (shedding of the endometrium) occurring 12–14 days following ovulation. What controls the biologic clock of the corpus luteum is unknown; however, falling estrogen and progesterone levels (1) release the negative feedback on gonadotropins, allowing for increasing FSH secretion and recruitment of a new crop of follicles for the following cycle, and (2) cause the synthesis and release of prostaglandins in the endometrium, resulting in the focal arteriolar vasospasm and uterine contractions associated with menstruation.

PREGNANCY

If pregnancy does occur, the implanting trophoblast produces human chorionic gonadotropin (hCG), which acts just like LH; this rescues the corpus luteum, which produces the increasing amounts of progesterone and estradiol necessary for the maintenance of pregnancy for the first trimester. By 12 weeks the placenta has formed and produces enough estradiol (from fetal adrenal DHAS) and progesterone to make continued corpus luteum function unnecessary.

SECONDARY AMENORRHEA*

Secondary amenorrhea is defined as the absence of visible menstruation for 3 consecutive months in a woman who has passed the menarche (first menstrual period), and it is found in 2–3% of women aged 15–40. With the exception of uterine disorders, all forms of amenorrhea are caused by anovulation. Whether a patient with anovulation presents with amenorrhea or dysfunctional uterine bleeding

---

* Primary amenorrhea, the absence of spontaneous menarche, is discussed in Chapter 4.

is most significantly dependent on the amount and fluctuation of estrogen secretion. Look for signs and symptoms of pregnancy, hypo- or hyperthydroidism, galactorrhea, hot flashes, hirsutism, virilization, weight loss, recent uterine surgery, chronic renal or liver disease, or psychologic stress. Initial laboratory evaluation should include serum measurement of the β-subunit of hCG (if pregnancy is even *remotely* possible), prolactin, TSH, LH, and FSH. Estrogen assays are misleading and are not clinically useful.

If pregnancy has been excluded, the patient may then be given medroxyprogesterone, 10 mg orally, every day for 7–10 days as a bioassay of the endogenous estrogen level. Estrogen levels sufficient to cause proliferation of the endometrium will be revealed by conversion of the endometrium to a secretory state by the progestin and will result in shedding of the endometrium within a week after the progestin is discontinued (progestin withdrawal bleeding). The amount of bleeding response may range from a brownish spotting or staining to flow consistent with a heavy menstrual period. A scanty or absent bleeding response to progestin withdrawal implies low estrogen levels. This may result from (1) lack of appropriate GnRH or gonadotropin stimulation from the hypothalamus and pituitary, (2) ovarian failure, or (3) interference by overproduction of other hormones. Progestin-induced withdrawal bleeding demonstrates the presence of endogenous estrogen and functional integrity of the uterus, ovaries, and higher centers, and it implies a state of chronic anovulation.

CENTRAL NERVOUS SYSTEM DISORDERS CAUSING AMENORRHEA

Hypothalamic Amenorrhea

Secondary amenorrhea is most commonly hypothalamic in origin; such patients usually have normal laboratory values and progestin withdrawal bleeding. The term hypothalamic amenorrhea is used because no disease of the pituitary gland, ovaries, or uterus is found. Frequent associations include young age, normal pubertal development, relatively low body weight, a history of irregular menses dating from menarche, and acute psychologic stress (especially involving acute separation from home and family). The pathophysiologic mechanism is decreased hypothalamic GnRH secretion resulting in chronic anovulation with normal but noncyclic gonadotropin release.

Spontaneous resolution is common, and treatment should include reassurance, psychologic referral if needed, and medroxyprogesterone administration, 10 mg orally, every day for 10 days, every 3 months, to prevent unopposed estrogen stimulation of the endometrium and to detect any decline in estrogen secretion.

When GnRH release is insufficient, hypogonadotropic hypogonadism results; patients have low, nonpulsatile basal LH levels and hypoestrogenemia. These patients do not menstruate following a progestin challenge because gonadotropin secretion is insufficient to stimulate enough ovarian estrogen release for endometrial proliferation. Spontaneous remission is unlikely, and patients are candidates for estrogen replacement therapy to prevent premature development of osteoporosis and genital tract atrophy. If fertility is desired, a small number of patients will respond to high doses of clomiphene but most will require treatment with hMG (Pergonal) and hCG.

Lesions of the Pituitary or Hypothalamus

Pituitary dysfunction may cause amenorrhea through hyposecretion of gonadotropins, hypersecretion of other hormones (usually prolactin), or both. Secreting tumors may produce gigantism, acromegaly, or Cushing's disease (Chapter 1).

Weight Loss & Exercise

Amenorrhea may follow weight loss of any cause: crash dieting, strenuous physical exercise, and anorexia nervosa. In postmenarchal women, loss in body fat below 17% has been associated with the development of secondary amenorrhea. A 10–15% reduction in body weight represents a 33% decrease in body fat and may lower body fat percentage from an average of 28% in sedentary women to below 22%, the level at which menstrual disturbances may begin to appear.

Vigorous physical exercise (especially running, gymnastics, ballet, and rowing) appears to be synergistic with loss of body fat in predisposing to amenorrhea. Menstrual dysfunction occurs in about 24% of runners and in about 58% of ballet dancers. Women athletes who are 6% below ideal body weight are 10 times more likely to be amenorrheic than nonathletes. In addition, athletes may decrease body fat without loss of body weight by replacing fat with dense, heavier muscle. Risk factors for the development of weight-loss amenorrhea include premenarchal physical training, late menarche, light weight prior to weight loss, overachieving personality, and a high level of athletic performance. Weight-loss amenorrhea is a form of hypogonadotropic hypogonadal amenorrhea. If menstruation does not occur after progestin challenge, hypoestrogenemia is present, and estrogen replacement therapy will be necessary for cyclic withdrawal bleeding (which may be psychologically important for the adolescent). Osteoporosis is a risk in the young athlete. Regular exercise usually helps to maintain bone mass; however, women athletes are at higher risk for stress fractures than male athletes. Estrogen replacement therapy using conjugated estrogens 0.9–1.25 mg/d for days 1–25 of the calendar month with medroxyprogesterone, 5 mg, added for

Table 9–1. Causes of secondary amenorrhea.

Pregnancy or trophoblastic disease	**Ovarian disorders**
	  Polycystic ovary syndrome
	  Premature failure (menopause)
	  Chromosomal anomalies

Central nervous system disorders
  Idiopathic (hypothalamic)
    Mild—anovulation
    Severe—hypogonadism
      (isolated; hypopituitarism)
  Lesions of the pituitary or
    hypothalamus
    Trauma; surgery; radiation
    Tumor (destructive or
      secreting prolactin or
      ACTH)
    Infection
  Weight loss and exercise
    Mild—dieting
    Severe—anorexia nervosa,
      systemic illness
  Stress—psychological or due to
    illness
  Flying
  Pseudocyesis
  Drug use
	Autoimmune disorders
	  Virilizing ovarian tumor
	  Insensitive ovary syndrome
	  Destruction
	    Irradiation
	    Chemotherapy (eg,
	      cyclophosphamide)
	    Infection (eg, mumps)
	
	Uterine disorders
	  Endometrial scarring
	    (Asherman's syndrome)
	  Infection
	    Tuberculosis
	    Schistosomiasis
	    Other
	
	Endocrine disorders
	  Cushing's syndrome
	  Addison's disease
	  Hyperthyroidism

Renal failure	
Chronic active hepatitis	

days 12–25, is recommended. (See Recommended Estrogen Regimen, below.)

Anorexia nervosa is the most extreme form of weight-loss amenorrhea and is associated with a variety of endocrine and psychologic disturbances. Anorexia nervosa may be distinguished from simple weight-loss amenorrhea by the patient's abnormal food ideation, altered and inappropriate body image, and self-induced vomiting or laxative abuse. Patients are 10–25 years of age, often intellectually bright and overachieving, manipulative, and evasive, and they deny any problems associated with their cachectic appearance. The incidence of anorexia nervosa is 0.5% and is associated with a mortality rate of 5–10%. Amenorrhea results from the loss of pulsatile LH secretion associated with decreased GnRH release. Basal gonadotropins are extremely low with LH usually less than FSH, a pattern seen in premenarchal girls. With weight gain, sleep-associated pulsatile LH activity returns (an initial event in normal girls entering puberty).

Signs and symptoms include weight 15% below ideal body weight for height and age, or a weight loss of more than 25% of ideal body weight, constipation, hypotension, bradycardia, hypothermia, dry skin, lanugo hair on the back and malar eminences, and yellow-orange discoloration of the palms.

Many laboratory tests are abnormal and may include leukopenia, hypoplastic bone marrow, electrolyte imbalance with hypokalemic alkalosis (resulting from emetic and laxative abuse), hyper-carotenemia, azotemia, decreased T_3 and elevated reverse T_3, hypoglycemia, elevated levels of cortisol (with reversed circadian rhythm), elevated growth hormone, and hypercholesterolemia. Most laboratory abnormalities are not specific for anorexia nervosa but reflect the state of chronic starvation.

Hypopituitarism may be ruled out by finding an elevated serum cortisol or finding a normal ACTH stimulation test and elevated GH level. Abnormalities return to normal with return to normal body weight, although amenorrhea persists in 30% of patients.

Treatment requires experienced psychiatric care and may require hospitalization with hyperalimentation to avoid death.

Stress

Moderate to severe acute psychologic stress may result in amenorrhea, especially in adolescents leaving home for the first time, or in older women undergoing prolonged hospitalization or incarceration. Previous irregular menses with anovulation is a predisposing factor. Menstrual dysfunction occurs in 14–21% of college students and has been attributed largely to stress. The amenorrhea is usually self-limited, and reassurance is appropriate.

Flying

Menstrual dysfunction occurs in 18–28% of airline stewardesses. The disorders are worse with jet flying and intercontinental flights. They tend to resolve with time. Normal menstruation and fertility ordinarily resumes after flying is discontinued.

Pseudocyesis

Pseudocyesis (false pregnancy) is a psychiatric problem that can cause hypothalamic dysfunction severe enough to cause amenorrhea. Patients have a strong desire for pregnancy and are often infertile, poorly educated, and depressed. Patients mimic the signs of pregnancy and distend their abdomens through air swallowing. Pelvic examination reveals a normal sized uterus and negative β-hCG. Psychiatric consultation is mandatory.

Substance Abuse

Menstrual abnormalities (amenorrhea or oligomenorrhea) occur in 64–70% of women using heroin. They persist with methadone use but usually resolve after the drug use is stopped.

OVARIAN DISORDERS CAUSING AMENORRHEA

Premature Ovarian Failure

This accounts for 10% of secondary amenorrhea and presents with serum FSH levels > 40 mIU/mL in a woman under 40 years of age. It is caused by accelerated atresia (oocyte degeneration), the process by which the 6 million fetal oogonia decline to 2 million oocytes at birth and 400,000 at menarche. Only about 400 oocytes are ever ovulated; the rest are lost by atresia. Premature ovarian failure might therefore be caused by a decreased number of original oogonia, acceleration of atresia, or destruction. Menopausal amenorrhea occurs when there are no follicles left capable of maturation even under maximal gonadotropin stimulation.

A. Chromosomal Abnormalities: Chromosomal abnormalities can cause amenorrhea that is usually primary. However, sex chromosome abnormalities such as mosaicism, deletions, rings, translocations, and isochromosomes may cause premature ovarian failure and secondary amenorrhea. Patients under 30 years of age with an elevated serum FSH should have a karyotype to detect a cell line carrying a Y chromosome, which confers a 25% risk of formation of a malignant ovarian neoplasm (dysgerminoma, gonadoblastoma) and necessitates bilateral oophorectomy. These tumors are not found in patients over 30 years of age. Even without detectable chromosomal abnormality, an inherited pattern of premature ovarian failure has been noted to occur in certain families, including some with known genetic enzyme defects, such as galactosemia.

Postnatal destruction of germ cells has been described following pelvic irradiation (400–500 rads over 4–6 weeks will induce ovarian failure in 50% of women), chemotherapy (especially cyclophosphamide and other alkylating agents), and rarely infection (mumps oophoritis).

B. Autoimmunity: Autoimmunity is responsible for at least 20% of premature ovarian failure. The diagnosis is based on the presence of circulating antiovarian antibodies, lymphocytic infiltration of ovarian biopsy specimens, or association with other autoimmune diseases; eg, Hashimoto's thyroiditis, Grave's disease, Addison's disease, hypoparathyroidism, type I diabetes mellitus, pernicious anemia, alopecia vitiligo, autoimmune hemolytic anemia, idiopathic thrombocytopenic purpura, myasthenia gravis, and mucocutaneous candidiasis. Among the collagen-vascular diseases, only juvenile rheumatoid arthritis has been associated with ovarian failure.

C. Insensitive Ovary Syndrome: Insensitive ovary syndrome refers to finding primordial follicles on ovarian biopsy in a patient with elevated gonadotropins. There is absence or functional failure of the ovarian FSH receptor, or immunologically active but biologically inactive gonadotropins are being released. Ovarian biopsy requires laparotomy (laparoscopic biopsies are inadequate) and is not routinely recommended because of the questionable clinical significance of finding ovarian follicles in terms of patient management or fertility prognosis. Pregnancy may occur in 5% of women following the diagnosis of premature ovarian failure, most commonly in patients given estrogen replacement therapy, and isolated occurrences follow treatment with hMG (Pergonal), gluocorticoids, and thymectomy. Patients should be told that the condition is irreversible and be started on cyclic estrogen and progestin replacement.

The evaluation of premature ovarian failure includes a karyotype for patients under 30 years of age and a history, physical examination, and laboratory examination directed toward detection of associated autoimmune diseases (antiovarian antibodies, thyroid function tests with TSH, antithyroid antibodies, antinculear antibodies, erythrocyte sedimentation rate, complete blood count, platelet count, calcium, phosphorus, glucose, electrolytes, and rheumatoid factor). If the patient has signs of Addison's disease, she should be tested with cosyntropin.

Polycystic Ovary Syndrome

Polycystic ovary syndrome classically presents with chronic anovulation in association with elevated androgen levels. Half of patients have amenorrhea and 70% have hirsutism. Irregular menses usually begin in adolescence. Patients are in a self-perpetuating steady-state in which estrogen, unopposed by postovulatory progesterone, acts on the anterior pituitary to depress FSH secretion (negative feedback) while sensitizing the pituitary to GnRH so that an augmented LH release results (positive feedback). The combination of inadequate follicle stimulation (due to decreased FSH) and increased intraovarian androgen formation (due to increased stromal stimulation by increased LH) causes premature atresia of ovarian follicles, which gives the characteristic polycystic appearance to the ovaries. Obesity is found in 40% of patients. Adipose tissue is a site for aromatization of androgens to estrogens, supporting the estrogen-mediated chronic anovulatory state. Infertility will also be found as a result of anovulation.

A. Diagnosis: Physical examination may demonstrate the presence of excessive hair growth on face, chest, breasts, and abdomen.

The cervix has abundant mucus with a characteristic ferning pattern when viewed under low power on an air-dried microscope slide. Palpably enlarged ovaries are not necessary for the diagnosis, since they will be of normal size in 40% of cases. Testosterone, androstenedione, and DHAS may be mildly elevated (testosterone < 200 ng/dL; DHAS < 700 ng/dL) or normal, and the LH:FSH ratio is >2 in 80% of cases. Serum progesterone levels are low. As estrogen secretion is not decreased, administration of medroxyprogesterone will so predictably result in withdrawal bleeding that failure to observe this response casts doubt on the diagnosis of polycystic ovary syndrome.

B. Treatment: Treatment consists of ovulation induction in cases of infertility, or cyclic progestin treatment with either a combination oral contraceptive or medroxyprogesterone, 10 mg/d for 10 days a month, to prevent constant unopposed estrogen stimulation of the breast and endometrium.

Ovarian Neoplasms

Ovarian neoplasms may produce amenorrhea associated with virilization evidenced by temporal pattern balding, deepening of the voice, clitorimegaly, breast atrophy, or hypermuscularity and prompts a search for an adrenal or ovarian androgen-secreting tumor. Ovarian androgen-secreting tumors (hilus cell, arrhenoblastoma, Sertoli-Leydig cell) are extremely rare and are especially suggested by the *rapid* development of masculinization (months rather than years), a serum testosterone level above 200 ng/dL, and a palpable adnexal mass.

UTERINE DISORDERS CAUSING AMENORRHEA

Secondary amenorrhea may result from endometrial scarring following intrauterine infection (Asherman's syndrome). Such patients have regular menses until an episode of endometritis is followed by decreasing menstrual flow, culminating in hypomenorrhea or amenorrhea. Subjective premenstrual symptoms (breast tenderness, bloating, mood changes) will still be present and cyclic. The usual cause is endometritis following delivery, D&C, or uterine surgery. Diagnosis is suggested by finding a biphasic basal body temperature graph in an amenorrheic patient and is confirmed by finding irregular filling defects on hysterosalpingogram.

Optimally, confirmation of diagnosis and treatment is by lysis of adhesions under direct hysteroscopic vision; however, a blind D&C may suffice if hysteroscopy is not available. At the completion of the procedure, a pediatric Foley catheter is used as a stent to separate the anterior and posterior uterine walls while broad spectrum antibiotics are given orally for 14 days. The catheter is removed in 7 days; an IUD may remain for 1–2 months. Conjugated estrogens, 2.5 mg 2–4 times daily, are administered for 1–2 months to stimulate endometrial proliferation and regeneration. Medroxyprogesterone, 10 mg, is given daily for 10 days at the completion of the estrogen therapy. Treatment will be successful in 75% of patients, but subsequent pregnancies have an increased risk of spontaneous abortion and placenta previa, placenta accreta, and abruptio placentae.

Tuberculous endometritis is rare in the USA and is diagnosed by culture of an endometrial biopsy specimen. Uterine schistosomiasis is also rare and is diagnosed by identification of eggs in endometrial biopsy, urine, or feces.

ENDOCRINE DISORDERS CAUSING AMENORRHEA

Cushing's Syndrome

Cushing's syndrome is associated with amenorrhea in 75% of cases. The mechanism most likely involves disturbance of cyclic gonadotropin release (basal FSH is normal, and LH may be slightly low) by increased conversion of adrenal androgens to estrogens, especially in adipose tissue, resulting in a cyclic estrogen feedback and the development of polycystic ovaries.

Addison's Disease

Addison's disease is associated with amenorrhea in 25% of cases. Ten to 25% of patients with idiopathic Addison's disease will also have premature ovarian failure on an autoimmune basis. Antibodies may not be organ-specific and may cross-react with steroid-producing cells of the adrenal and ovaries with a cytotoxic effect.

Hyperthyroidism

Hyperthyroidism usually leads to hypomenorrhea but may also be associated with secondary amenorrhea. Increased thyroid hormone induces an increase in plasma sex hormone–binding globulin, which reduces the metabolic clearance rate of androgens and estrogens. Testosterone levels are elevated, and there is an increase in the conversion of testosterone to androstenedione. The net effect is an increase in circulating estrogen from increased peripheral conversion of testosterone to androstenedione. The elevated acyclic estrogen may result in chronic anovulation as in the polycystic ovary syndrome and may be associated with an increased LH:FSH ratio.

Hypothyroidism

Hypothyroidism is not a common cause of secondary amenorrhea, but primary hypothyroidism may present with hyperprolactinemia causing amenorrhea and galactorrhea. Amenorrhea can also result from the peripheral effects of hypothyroidism. These include an increased metabolic clearance rate of testosterone to estradiol. Estradiol metabolism is also shifted from estradiol toward estriol, a weaker estrogen, with the subsequent disruption in estrogen-gonadotropin feedback causing anovulation.

RENAL FAILURE CAUSING AMENORRHEA

Amenorrhea is found in most women with severe renal disease. Hyperprolactinemia may also be found owing to insensitivity of the lactotropes to dopamine, although galactorrhea is uncommon. The metabolic clearance rate for LH is reduced, resulting in an elevated LH:FSH ratio and polycystic ovaries, although without elevated serum androgens. Uremic toxins may prevent the ovaries and breasts from responding to the elevated LH and prolactin levels with hyperandrogenemia and galactorrhea as might be expected.

CONDITIONS TREATED WITH ESTROGEN REPLACEMENT THERAPY

HYPOGONADISM

Hypogonadism in women is the loss of synthesis and systemic release of ovarian steroid hormones (estrogen and progesterone) and may be classified as primary or secondary. Secondary hypogonadism refers to the loss of ovarian stimulation by pituitary FSH and LH or inappropriate over-production of other hormones. These disorders are discussed in Chapter 1 and in this chapter under Secondary Amenorrhea. Primary hypogonadism refers to the failure of the ovaries themselves as an estrogen-secreting organ and may be caused by genetic errors (gonadal dysgenesis), surgical removal (for conditions such as chronic salpingo-oophoritis and endometriosis), radiation therapy for pelvic cancer, chemotherapy, autoimmunity, and physiologic circumstances (menopause).

MENOPAUSE

The transition from full reproductive potential to final ovarian failure is referred to as the *climacteric* and begins at approximately age

40. At birth the ovaries contain approximately 2 million primordial follicles. Beginning at menarche these follicles are cyclically stimulated by pituitary LH and FSH to develop and secrete estradiol, which during reproductive life, triggers a surge of LH release (positive feedback) that results in ovulation and corpus luteum formation. Beginning at age 40, the follicles remaining in the ovary are those which were least sensitive to gonadotropin stimulation and require increasing levels of FSH to develop and secrete estradiol. A lowered estradiol level may result in menstrual irregularities by either shortening the follicular phase of the cycle or, in failing to induce ovulation, by creating anovulatory menometrorrhagia (dysfunctional uterine bleeding). In the final event no follicles are capable of responding to even maximal pituitary stimulation (as measured by a serum FSH over 40 IU/mL), estradiol levels fall below those necessary to induce endometrial proliferation, and menses cease.

The menopause is the last episode of physiologic uterine bleeding. The diagnosis is therefore retrospective and is usually made after 6–12 months of amenorrhea. The median age of menopause in the USA is 51.4 years, with the normal range being from 48 to 55. Cessation of menses before age 40 is referred to as premature ovarian failure. The diagnosis is made clinically on the basis of characteristic symptoms, which can be classified as early or late. Early symptoms include disturbances in menstrual function, psychologic symptoms (anxiety, mood depression, irritability), and vasomotor instability (the hot flush or flash). Late symptoms include those resulting from urogenital atrophy and pathologic fractures secondary to osteoporosis.

Women in the USA lead one-third of their total life span after the age of menopause, and successful treatment of their symptoms requires an individualized assessment of the patient's hormonal, genetic-cultural, and psychological status as well as the advantages and disadvantages (risks) of estrogen replacement therapy.

Hormonal Factors

Symptoms may depend on the amount of estrogen depletion and the rate at which it is withdrawn. Postmenopausal estrogen is not estradiol of follicular origin but estrone, which results from the extragonadal conversion of ovarian (15%) and adrenal (85%) androstenedione. Since the endogenous estrogen level (now estrone) will not be influenced by pituitary-ovarian negative feedback, exogenous estrogen replacement will be additive to whatever endogenous level exists. Obesity, liver disease, and hyperthyroidism enhance peripheral aromatization of androstenedione to estrone. Functioning ovarian tumors (eg, granulosatheca cell) may secrete estrogen or androgen directly.

Genetic-Cultural Factors

The aging process is the result of inherited and acquired propensities including overall health, stress, diet, activity and race. For example, thin, sedentary, cigarette-smoking Caucasian women are at the highest risk for menopausal symptoms while active, obese, black women are at the lowest. These factors will be alluded to more specifically below.

Psychological Factors

The "change of life" has differing psychological impact on women—for some, the final loss of reproductive capacity may signal the end of womanliness; for others, it is the start of a new life free from the burdens of contraception and child-rearing. Fatigue, irritability, headache, insomnia, depression, and nervousness are common subjective complaints that are difficult to ascribe to hormonal changes alone. Many women, however, describe increased psychological well-being from estrogen replacement therapy, an effect possibly related to reduced hot flushing.

ADVANTAGES OF ESTROGEN REPLACEMENT THERAPY

Some advantages of estrogen replacement therapy are (1) control of vasomotor instability; (2) prevention of urogenital atrophy; (3) prevention of osteoporosis; (4) probable decreased heart disease; (5) possible increased psychologic well-being; (6) possible prolongation of life.

Vasomotor Symptoms

Vasomotor symptoms (hot flash, hot flush) are experienced by 75–85% of postmenopausal women as an episodic disturbance consisting of the sudden onset of a feeling of intense heat rising through the chest, neck, and head, often followed by profuse perspiration. The flush usually lasts from seconds to minutes and may recur infrequently or every 10–30 minutes. Flushes may be more frequent and severe at night (resulting in loss of REM sleep) or be triggered by emotional stress. Of those having flushes, 80% will experience them for more than 1 year, and 25–50% may complain of the symptoms for more than 5 years. A close temporal association between the occurrence of flushes and the pulsatile release of LH has been demonstrated, but as flushes may occur after hypophysectomy, the likelihood is that the flush originates in the hypothalamic or central nervous system pathways leading to hypothalamic GnRH release. A low-estrogen state alone is not sufficient for the development of flushes, but the presence of estrogen followed by its withdrawal is. Treatment is most effective with estrogen replacement, but medroxyprogesterone may be effective in patients who do not want to take estrogen, and clonidine may be beneficial for patients in whom estrogen is contraindicated.

Urogenital Atrophy

Urogenital atrophy is the result of estrogen deprivation on the vaginal epithelium, endocervical glands, endometrium, and myometrium. The bladder and urethral epithelium may undergo partial atrophy also. The appearance of the vagina changes as the rugae progressively flatten, allowing the capillary bed to shine through as diffuse or patchy reddening. Further atrophy of the capillary bed results in a final smooth, shiny, whitened epithelial surface. Local bacterial invasion may initiate vaginal pruritus and leukorrhea. The vagina is easily traumatized and may bleed after douching or coitus. Dyspareunia may result from vaginal thinning, dryness (due to diminished vaginal and cervical mucus secretion), and stenosis. Urethritis with dysuria, urgency incontinence, and urinary frequency are the results of mucosal thinning of the urethra. Estrogen is the only effective treatment for atrophy.

Osteoporosis

Osteoporosis caused by estrogen deficiency is discussed in Chapter 7.

RISKS OF ESTROGEN REPLACEMENT THERAPY

A major source of prescribing difficulty is the confusion of the risks associated with combination oral contraceptive pill use and those associated with estrogen replacement therapy. Contrary to the experience with oral contraceptives, no increased risk of hepatoma, hypertension (in nonobese individuals), arterial thromboembolic events (myocardial infarction and cerebrovascular accident) or venous thromboembolic events (thrombophlebitis, pulmonary emboli) is associated with estrogen replacement. As with oral contraceptives, however, estrogen slightly increases the risk of gallbladder disease.

Absolute contraindications to estrogen therapy are (1) cholestatic hepatic dysfunction; (2) acute or active vascular thrombotic disorder; (3) neuroophthalmologic vascular disease; (4) undiagnosed vaginal bleeding; (5) known or suspected estrogen-dependent neoplasia (breast, ovary, uterus, cervix, vagina); (6) past history of thromboembolic disorders associated with previous estrogen use.

Risk of Endometrial Cancer

Several retrospective case-control studies performed in the 1970s suggested a 4- to 8-fold increased risk of adenocarcinoma of the endometrium in women receiving estrogen. The risk appears to increase with the duration of exposure and dose and is greater if estrogens are given continuously. Almost all cancers were stage I, and no excess mortality has been reported. Accumulated evidence suggests that *the monthly addition of a progestational agent to estrogen will reduce the incidence of endometrial cancer to below that of patients receiving no estrogen.* The hypothesis is that extended periods of relative estrogen excess and progesterone deficiency can result in progressive endomentrial proliferation leading to adenocarcinoma. Progestins "oppose" the mitogenic potential of estrogen by preventing the recycling and replenishment of estrogen receptors through suppressed DNA synthesis. In addition, progestins convert proliferative and hyperplastic endometrium to a secretory state in which (1) there is an altered pattern of intracellular protein production with induction of dehydrogenase and sulfotransferase enzymes that convert the more potent estradiol to the weaker estrone; and (2) the endometrium is more completely shed when the estrogen-progestin combination is withdrawn. To avoid giving estrogen to a patient with a hyperplastic endometrium, it is recommended that either an endometrial biopsy or a progestin challenge test be performed before treatment is begun.

Risk of Breast Cancer

No direct cause-and-effect relationship between exogenous estrogen and breast cancer has been demonstrated; however, given that breast cancer may be associated with estrogen receptors and is essentially a condition of postpubertal women, a permissive role of estrogen in breast neoplasia is a possibility. The weight of clinical evidence continues to indicate no increased risk of breast cancer in women using estrogen. All postmenopausal patients with preexisting benign breast disease should be carefully monitored with routine palpation, mammography, fine-needle aspiration, and surgical biopsy when indicated.

Risk of Heart Disease

Data from cohort studies suggest a cardioprotective effect for estrogen replacement therapy, with most studies showing at least a 50% reduction in coronary heart disease and related mortality. The protective effect is believed to be mediated by a decrease in LDL cholesterol through the induction of LDL receptors, an increase in HDL cholesterol through the destruction of HDL-degrading hepatic lipase, and a direct effect on blood vessel walls through an increase in local prostacyclin production.

RECOMMENDED ESTROGEN REGIMEN

The decision to use estrogen must be individualized and based on the likelihood of benefit to the patient. Obese patients may make sufficient endogenous estrone from adrenal androstenedione to remain asymptomatic. Thin Caucasian women with a family history of osteoporosis are at greatest risk for postmenopausal fractures, while black women may be at reduced risk. Patients with early or surgically induced menopause will be without estrogen for a longer time and have a greater risk of hypoestrogenemic sequelae. The cardioprotective effect of estrogen suggests that estrogen therapy be offered to all postmenopausal women who do not have an absolute contraindication. If prescribed, estrogen therapy should be continued indefinitely, since its advantages disappear rapidly following discontinuation of therapy. No oral estrogen formulation has been shown to be superior to any other, but some generic estrogen preparations may have reduced potency and should be prescribed with caution. An estradiol-containing transdermal patch (Estraderm) is available and is effective in preventing flushes, atrophy, and osteoporosis. The nonoral absorption reduces the estrogen impact on hepatic coagulation factors but also may blunt the beneficial estrogen mediated increase in HDL cholesterol. Clinical data are insufficient to discern whether estrogen administered transdermally has less cardioprotective effect than when taken orally. Approximate bioequivalents for estrogen supplements are 0.625 mg conjugated estrogens = 0.75 mg estrone = 1 mg estradiol = 0.05 mg transdermal estrogen.

Addition of a progestin to estrogen decreases the risk of endometrial and possibly breast cancer and is recommended in postmenopausal women with an intact uterus, but there is no clear consensus on the optimal type, dosage, and duration of progestin supplementation. Progestins derived from the progesterone molecule, eg, medroxyprogesterone, are recommended because they are less likely to lower HDL levels than 19-nortestosterone derivatives (eg, norethindrone). Although current progestins have not been shown to have an adverse effect on the cardioprotective effect of estrogen, newer progestins with less effect on HDL levels are being tested. To minimize the risk of starting hormone replacement in a woman with an existing endometrial hyperplasia or cancer, it is recommended that new patients be given a "progestin challenge test" with medroxyprogesterone, 10 mg/d for 14 days. Patients who do not have withdrawal bleeding may be started on estrogen immediately, while patients who do withdraw should have a second 14-day course of medroxyprogesterone. Patients who do not withdraw to the second course may then start estrogen, while patients who bleed in response to the second challenge should undergo endometrial biopsy before starting estrogen replacement. Two regimes of hormone replacement therapy are currently recommended. **Sequential therapy** mimics the hormone sequence of the menstrual cycle and results in predictable bleeding following progestin withdrawal in 70% of patients and in amenorrhea in 30%. This bleeding pattern may lead to patient apprehension and compliance difficulty unless the basis for this endometrial shedding (and its protective effect against endometrial cancer) are clearly explained. **Combination therapy** mimics the hormone pattern of oral contraceptives and has the induction of amenorrhea as its goal for patients who are uncomfortable with regular withdrawal bleeding.

Sequential Therapy

1. For days 1–25 of the month, administer conjugated estrogens (or equivalent), 0.625 mg/d. For patients under age 40, administer 0.9–1.25 mg/d. Older patients, especially if thin or with established osteoporosis, may have less endogenous estrogen and may require 0.9–1.25 mg/d.

2. For days 12–25 of the month, medroxyprogesterone, 5 mg/d. (Medroxyprogesterone is sometimes given at other doses or for shorter intervals, eg, days 16–25.)

3. For days 25–31 of the month, no medication is taken and withdrawal bleeding is expected. Bleeding during the first 12 days of estrogen-only administration requires endometrial biopsy for evaluation. In general, bleeding that begins before the completion of the progestin may indicate the need for a lower estrogen or higher progestin dose.

4. Women who have had a hysterectomy do not require supplemental progestin and may take estrogen every day.

Combination Therapy

Conjugated estrogens, 0.625 or 0.9 mg, and medroxyprogesterone, 2.5 mg, are taken daily. Most patients will become amenorrheic within 3 months but should be counseled to expect some irregular spotting until that time.

DYSMENORRHEA & ENDOMETRIOSIS

DYSMENORRHEA

Dysmenorrhea is painful menstruation that interferes with normal function in women and requires medication. Estimates of incidence for primary dysmenorrhea run as high as 50%, with approximately 10% of patients suffering incapacity for 1–3 days a month. The disorder is of considerable importance because it is incapacitating.

Primary Dysmenorrhea

Primary dysmenorrhea presents without any macroscopically identifiable pelvic disease. It is caused by myometrial contractions induced by prostaglandin $F_{2\alpha}$ originating in the endometrium. Other symptoms such as headache, nausea, and diarrhea represent effects of prostaglandins entering into the systemic circulation.

The history usually dates back to the onset of menarche or shortly thereafter (when ovulatory menses are established). Anovulatory cycles are generally painless because there is no prostaglandin synthesis induced by falling progesterone levels. Pain usually starts with the menstrual flow and rarely lasts more than 72 hours. Symptoms are less common in older patients regardless of parity.

Laboratory values in primary dysmenorrhea are those of normal ovulatory women. The diagnosis is based on the characteristic history, lack of abnormal findings on pelvic and rectovaginal examinations, and clinical response to either antiprostaglandin medication or ovulation suppression with combination oral contraceptives.

About 80% of dysmenorrheic women experience clinical relief with the use of an oral nonsteriodal prostaglandin synthetase inhibitor. These medications should be started immediately with the onset of menses and continued for 3 days. All antiprostaglandins may cause central nervous system side effects (headaches, visual disturbances, dizziness) and gastrointestinal discomfort (which may be reduced by taking the medication with milk or food).

Arylpropionic acid derivatives have been extensively tested and have the highest efficacy with the fewest side effects. These include ibuprofen, 400–600 mg 4 times daily; naproxen, 250–375 mg twice daily; and naproxen sodium, 275 mg 3–4 times daily.

Fenamates including mefenamic acid, 250 mg, 4 times daily, are about equal in effectiveness to the arylpropionic derivatives.

Indolacetic acid derivatives (indomethacin) 25 mg 4 times daily, may have more gastrointestinal side effects than other nonsteroidal antiinflammatory agents. Aspirin is ineffective for primary dysmenorrhea in that the uterus is relatively insensitive to the benzoic acid derivatives. Butyrophenones (phenylbutazone, oxyphenbutazone) should be avoided because of the potential for blood dyscrasias and the availability of safer, more effective alternatives.

If the patient desires birth control and has no contraindication, a combination oral contraceptive will relieve primary dysmenorrhea in 90–100% of cases. Menstrual fluid prostaglandins are reduced by converting the endometrium to an atrophic decidualized state.

If the above measures fail after a 3–4 month trial, it is appropriate to reconsider the possibility of a pelvic disorder and perform laparoscopy and D&C. If no pathologic process is found, a trial of a betamimetic agent such as isoxsuprine hydrochloride, terbutaline sulfate, or ritodrine hydrochloride may be considered.

Analgesics combined with psychotherapy are reserved for the very few patients who are resistant to the above treatment options.

Secondary Dysmenorrhea

Secondary dysmenorrhea presents as a result of some pathologic pelvic condition. It can be distinguished from primary dysmenorrhea by a history of several prior years of pain-free menses and abnormal findings on pelvic or rectovaginal examination. Additionally, any dysmenorrheic patient who fails to respond to treatment with antiprostaglandin medication or combination oral contraceptives should be evaluated for other pain-producing conditions.

The most common causes of secondary dysmenorrhea include endometriosis (see below); recurrent or chronic pelvic inflammatory disease (PID); the presence of an intrauterine device; uterine myomas, polyps, and adhesions; cervical strictures or stenosis; congenital malformation of the müllerian system (bicornuate and septate uterus, transverse vaginal septum); and ovarian cysts.

Evaluation may include complete blood count, erythrocyte sedimentation rate (often elevated in recurrent or chronic PID), pelvic ultrasound, hysterosalpingography, and genital cultures for gonorrhea, chlamydia, and if an IUD is present, actinomycosis. Laparoscopy, hysteroscopy, and D&C may be necessary to complete the workup or confirm the diagnosis. Treatment of the underlying condition will ordinarily relieve the dysmenorrhea.

ENDOMETRIOSIS

Endometriosis is the ectopic location of endometrium (glands, stroma, hemosiderin). Endometriosis is usually confined to the abdominal cavity but rarely may be found in distant sites (eg, lung). It is most likely caused by retrograde menstruation through the uterine tubes. Both genetic and immunologic factors may influence the susceptibility of a woman to endometriosis. Endometriosis does not occur before menarche and is most common in nulliparous women in their 30s, although it is not rare in adolescence or as a cause of secondary infertility.

Endometriosis should be suspected in any patient complaining of secondary dysmenorrhea or other cyclic abdominal or pelvic pain. Other symptoms include dyspareunia, infertility, and rectal or low back pain. Premenstrual spotting or menorrhagia are less common historical events. The extent of endometriosis does not always correlate well with the degree of the patient's symptoms. Extensive endometriosis may be asymptomatic. Cyclic hematuria, dysuria, hematochezia, or painful defecation are uncommon but may point to bladder or rectal/sigmoid involvement.

Examination findings may include nodularity of the uterosacral ligaments, a tender uterus fixed in retroversion, pelvic or adnexal mass, and pelvic tenderness.

Pelvic ultrasound may be useful in the evaluation of a pelvic or adnexal mass, but direct visualization by laparoscopy is necessary for definitive diagnosis prior to institution of therapy. Only the young, asymptomatic patient with minimal findings may be treated by observation or cyclic use of oral contraceptives.

Endometriosis has a strong association with infertility; 30–40% of patients with endometriosis are infertile (twice the rate of the general population); and among infertile patients, 6–15% have endometriosis. The pregnancy rate after treatment correlates inversely with the severity of the disease.

Staging & Treatment

A uniform system of classification that takes into account the presence, location, and quality of adhesions, endometriomas, and tubal distortion has been formulated by the American Fertility Society (available by writing the Society at 1608 13th Avenue South, Suite 101, Birmingham, AL 35256) and classifies the disease into 4 stages—mild (I), moderate (II), severe (III), and extensive (IV). Staging is derived from a numerical score in which the presence, location, size, and severity of adhesions, tubal occlusion, or endometriomas are evaluated. Treatment may be surgical or hormonal and is based upon a confirmed diagnosis, the patient's age and fertility status, and the stage of the disease.

Hormonal Treatment

Implants of endometriosis have estrogen, progesterone, and androgen receptors. Implants retain hormonal responsiveness similar to that of normal endometrial cells. Hormone therapy interrupts the stimulation and bleeding of the implants that follows the fluctuations of estrogen and progesterone during the menstrual cycle; it is suppressive rather than curative. Hormonal treatment is indicated for symptomatic relief and prevention of progression of disease in patients with endometriosis who are delaying conception. It is also indicated for treatment of infertility in patients under 30 with mild disease or moderate disease without adhesions (infertility patients over 30 are generally best treated by surgery).

A. Combination Oral Contraceptives: Given in a daily continuous fashion for 6–9 months (pseudopregnancy), any estrogen-progestin pill will convert endometrial implants into decidualized cells associated with inactive endometrial glands. The contraindications and side effects of treatment are those associated with birth-control pills, although weight gain, abdominal swelling, mastalgia, and breakthrough bleeding may be more common with continuous versus cyclic use. Lo/Ovral is recommended because of its relatively potent progestin component. Oral contraceptives are more commonly used for milder cases, when conception is being delayed, and when the expense or side effects of danazol are factors.

B. Danazol: Danazol (Danocrine) produces a relatively hypoestrogenic state by direct inhibition of ovarian steroidogenesis and by androgen-mediated inhibition of follicular development. Danazol produces a hypoprogestational environment by inhibiting ovulation, binding to progesterone receptors without translocating to the nucleus, and increasing the metabolic clearance rate of progesterone. Danazol has a direct androgenic effect leading to atropy of implants. Finally, the amenorrhea that is produced prevents new seeding from the uterus into the peritoneal cavity.

Side effects of danazol are related both to its androgenic properties and to the hypoestrogenic environment it creates and include weight gain, fluid retention, fatigue, decreased breast size, acne, oily skin, deepening of the voice, hirsutism, atrophic vaginitis, hot flashes, muscle cramps, emotional lability, and breakthrough bleeding. Danazol also increases LDL and decreases HDL cholesterol. Even though 80% of treated patients have some of these effects, they are usually mild and only 10% will discontinue treatment because of them. Danazol is contraindicated in patients with liver disease, severe hypertension, congestive heart failure, or impaired renal function.

Danazol should be started with the onset of a menstrual period and should not be given if there is a possibility of pregnancy, because of the risk of masculinization of a female fetus. The standard dose is 800 mg/d (400 mg twice daily or 200 mg 4 times daily), but because of high cost and high incidence of side effects, lower doses have been utilized. For treatment of infertility, doses of 400–800 mg/d are indicated, while lower doses may give symptomatic relief in patients delaying conception. Suppression of ovulation and amenorrhea are not consistent in doses lower than 400 mg/d, and the risk of pregnancy must be acknowledged. Pregnancy rates after danazol treatment are approximately 45% and may possibly be superior to treatment with oral contraceptives.

C. GnRH Analogs: GnRH analogs (leuprolide, nafarelin) of the hypothalamic decapeptide GnRH, when given by injection or nasal spray, suppress pituitary gonadotropin release, which in turn prevents follicle development, ovulation, and menstruation and results in profound hypoestrogenemia. Endometriosis deprived of estrogen undergoes atrophy within 3–6 months. Leuprolide (Lupron) is available in a short-acting form for daily subcutaneous injection and in long-acting depot form for intramuscular injection once a month. Nafarelin (Synarel) is available as a short-acting nasal spray used twice daily. Both forms are equally effective, and pregnancy rates after treatment are equivalent to those seen after danazol therapy. Treatment with GnRH analogs should begin approximately a week after ovulation so that the initial stimulation phase will be suppressed by the progesterone secreted by the corpus luteum. Side effects related to hypoestrogenemia include hot flashes, vaginal dryness, decreased libido, dyspareunia, and irregular spotting. Headaches, depression, and weight loss or gain have been reported less frequently. It is thought that GnRH analogs do not cause significant bone loss if used for 6 months or less. Protection against osteoporosis may be afforded by norethindrone, 1–2 mg/d.

D. Medroxyprogesterone: Medroxyprogesterone is a progestational agent that induces a decidual reaction in endometrial implants and inhibits ovulation by suppression of cyclic gonadotropin release. It may be given orally (30 mg/d) or by injection (Depo-Provera, 100 mg every 2 weeks for 4 doses and then 200 mg every month for an additional 4–6 months). Breakthrough bleeding is common and may be treated by the administration of ethinyl estradiol (20 μg) or conjugated estrogens (2.5 mg) daily for 7 days. A significant drawback to the use of Depo-Provera for the treatment of infertility is the occasionally prolonged interval to resumption of ovulatory menses after discontinuation.

Surgical Treatment

Total abdominal hysterectomy and bilateral oophorectomy is the definitive treatment for patients over 35 who are symptomatic.

Surgical therapy is necessary for all patients with a pelvic mass (endometrioma), which usually is adnexal in location but may involve the bowel and urinary tract. Intra-abdominal rupture of an endometrioma presents as an acute abdomen and requires immediate laparotomy, lavage, and resection of involved tissues.

Conservative surgery has the objective of restoring normal anatomic relationships, with excision or fulguration of as much of the endometriosis as possible. In the hands of an experienced surgeon, laparoscopy with laser ablation of implants and adhesions is an alternative to laparotomy where microsurgical technique (atraumatic tissue handling, use of magnification, reperitonealization of raw areas, and use of fine suture material) should be used. Suspension of a retroverted uterus and plication of the uterosacral ligaments may aid in preventing the ovaries from adhering to raw areas in the cul de sac. Presacral neurectomy does not enhance fertility, although many surgeons advocate it to alleviate dysmenorrhea, albeit with the risk of intraoperative bleeding and postoperative bowel dysfunction. The success of surgery in relieving infertility is directly related to the severity of endometriosis with 60% pregnancy rates following surgery for moderate disease and 35% for severe disease. The highest pregnancy rates following conservative surgery occur in the first year after surgery.

Conservative surgery is indicated for patients with (1) mild to moderate disease (stage I–II) who remain symptomatic or infertile after hormonal treatment and laparoscopic fulguration have failed and (2) severe disease (stage III–IV) who are infertile or desire future fertility.

INFERTILITY

Infertility is defined as the inability of a couple to conceive after 1 year of unprotected intercourse. If no pregnancy has ever occurred, the condition is referred to as primary infertility, whereas secondary infertility means that a previous pregnancy has taken place, even if it resulted in fetal loss. Infertility is common, affecting 15% of reproductive age couples. *Participation of both partners is recommended.* Approximately 30% of couples will be diagnosed as having a male factor, 40% a female factor, 20% a combination of factors, and 10% no satisfactory explanation of their infertility. Because of the psychologic stress caused by infertility, referral to specialists should not be unnecessarily delayed. Infertility studies are notorious for their lack of control groups, making objective analysis of different therapies difficult. Empirical treatments should be avoided whenever possible. Factors causing amenorrhea or hypopituitarism also cause infertility.

COITAL FACTOR

A sexual history must note the frequency of intercourse, use of lubricants, anorgasmia, impotence, and dyspareunia. Coital frequency less than once a week is associated with a prolonged conception interval and may suggest ambivalence or psychosexual difficulty; if such is the case the couple is referred to a qualified sex therapist or counselor. Lubricants can be spermicidal and, if needed, natural vegetable oils may be used. Severe hypospadias, neurologic impotence, and retrograde ejaculation refractory to medical therapy may be indications for Artificial Insemination with Husband's sperm (AIH). However, AIH has not proved to be a satisfactory treatment for oligospermia except in certain cases of intrauterine insemination using sperm-enhancement techniques. Optimal coital frequency is approximately every 48 hours for the middle 2 weeks of the menstrual cycle, but couples should be discouraged from allowing intercourse to become mechanical or scheduled by the basal body temperature chart. The loss of feelings or privacy, control, and spontaneity will damage the couple's relationship and in the long run hamper the evaluation more than it will enhance fertility.

MALE FACTOR

A complete discussion of the male factor appears in Chapter 8. *A semen analysis should be the first step in the infertility evaluation.* If the analysis is abnormal in terms of volume, count, motility, or morphology, it should be repeated 1 week later after an abstinence period of 48 hours. If it is still abnormal, the man should be referred to a specialist in male infertility for further evaluation.

OVULATION FACTOR

Endocrinologic problems account for 30–40% of female infertility and may be manifested as secondary amenorrhea, irregular menses (representing chronic anovulation or oligo-ovulation), or luteal phase defect. Irregular cycle lengths (under 25 days or over 36 days, or variation in consecutive cycle lengths of over 7 days) are suggestive of ovulation defects, especially if premenstrual symptoms (molimina), dysmenorrhea, and amount and duration of menstrual flow is variable from one cycle to the next.

Basal Body Temperature (BBT) Graph

The BBT graph is a daily record of oral or rectal temperature taken upon arising and is a useful adjunct when interpreting postcoital tests, response to ovulation induction, serum progesterone measurements, or endometrial biopsy. Prolonged chart graphing or using the graphs in an effort to pinpoint ovulation for coital timing should be discouraged, since it often leads to patient frustration and anxiety. The graphs should be started with the first day of a menstrual period (referred to as day 1) and, if ovulatory, should show a transition from a consistently lower temperature (usually < 36.7°C) to a consistently higher temperature (usually > 36.7°C) occurring 11–16 days prior to the following menstrual period. A temperature dip before the rise may indicate the day of ovulation, but not all women show a dip nor should a slowly rising temperature be interpreted as necessarily indicating a hormonal abnormality. The temperature rise results from the early periovulatory release of progesterone on thermoregulatory centers in the central nervous system. If the temperature rise is not sustained for 11 days or more, suspect a luteal phase defect.

Serum Progesterone Level

Serum progesterone is measured to document ovulation and, in conjunction with endometrial biopsy, to diagnose a luteal phase defect. Progesterone is undetectable before ovulation, reaches a peak 7 days later, and declines before menses unless conception has occurred (in which case, hCG of trophoblastic origin rescues the corpus luteum and progesterone secretion continues). It should be measured 7 days before expected menses and if > 15 ng/mL is usually indicative of not only ovulation but overall hormonal normality of the cycle. Values < 3 ng/mL are suspicious for anovulation, and intermediate values are suggestive of a luteal phase defect if menses occurs within 6–8 days of the progesterone measurement.

Endometrial Biopsy

Endometrial biopsy is used to diagnose a luteal phase defect. It is performed 2–3 days before expected menses by means of a Pipette. The risk of interrupting an early gestation is small. The biopsy should be interpreted by an observer familiar with the histologic dating criteria of Noyes and Rock. The histologic report will assign a date from 14 to 28 to the specimen. The patient's menstrual period following the biopsy is arbitrarily designated day 28 (regardless of actual cycle day) and the date of the biopsy determined by counting days backward from the following period to the day when the biopsy was performed. This biopsy date and the histologic date should be within 2 days of agreement. Discrepancy of more than 2 days is suggestive of a luteal phase defect. Waiting until day 1 of the following cycle to perform the biopsy (theoretically avoiding the possible interruption of an early pregnancy) gives inaccurate results because of the tissue disruption associated with the onset of menstrual flow.

Induction of Ovulation

Once it is determined that a patient has an ovulation disorder, characterization of the disturbance will indicate the choice of treatment (Table 9–1). History and physical examination should be directed toward the elicitation of symptoms and signs suggestive of hyper- or hypothyroidism, hirsutism, obesity, galactorrhea, hot flashes, weight loss, and severe psychologic stress. Laboratory measurements should include measurements of thyroid function with TSH, prolactin, LH, and FSH (if amenorrhea exists). Abnormal thyroid function should be corrected (Chapter 5) although routine empiric use of thyroid supplements is not justified. Menstrual irregularities associated with hirsutism or obesity usually represent polycystic ovary syndrome with chronic anovulation, especially if associated with an LH:FSH ratio greater than 2:1. Weight loss and severe psychologic stress may also induce anovulation. Hyperprolactinemia may be associated with a clinical spectrum ranging from amenorrhea with galactorrhea and hypoestrogenemia to subtle luteal phase defects. Ovulation disturbances may then be classified as those with normal but acyclic estrogen production (eg, polycystic ovary syndrome), for which the treatment is clomiphene; subnormal estrogen production (eg, weight loss), for which the initial treatment may be with clomiphene but more likely by hMG/hCG; and hyperprolactinemic states, for which the treatment is with bromocriptine.

A. Bromocriptine (Parlodel): Approximately 15% of ovulation disturbances are due to hyperprolactinemia. Primary hypothyroidism with elevated TSH must be excluded, since it is more directly treatment with thyroid replacement. Hyperprolactinemia, bromocriptine, and pituitary tumors are discussed in Chapter 1. For infertility, only enough bromocriptine is given to bring the prolactin level into the normal range. Persistent nausea may be ameliorated by using the tablets as vaginal suppositories.

B. Clomiphene (Clomid, Serophene): Clomiphene is an orally active nonsteroidal chemical with a structure resembling the synthetic estrogen diethylstilbestrol. It binds but does not activate the estradiol receptors in the hypothalamus and pituitary such that a lower estradiol level is perceived. This effect enhances FSH secretion, which stimulates follicular development and results in increased estradiol secretion and activation of an estradiol-mediated LH surge (positive feedback) followed by ovulation. For clomiphene to be successful, (1) there must be some endogenous estrogen and (2) the patient must have an intact positive feedback mechanism. The clinical criterion for patient selection is the demonstration of endogenous estrogen without ovulation. Amenorrheic patients who do not have withdrawal bleeding are poor candidates for clomiphene, although even in this group clomiphene should be tried before the more expensive and complex hMG/hCG regimen.

Clomiphene is administered for 5 days beginning on the fifth day of a spontaneous cycle, or 5 days after progestin-induced withdrawal bleeding. The initial dose is 50 mg/d (10 mg/d if *cis*-clomiphene is used), and the cycle is evaluated with a BBT graph. Ovulation usually takes place 7–14 days after the initiation of drug taking. If ovulation does not occur at the 50-mg level, the dose is increased by 50 mg each cycle until ovulation or a maximal dose of 250 mg/d is reached. Once the ovulation dosage has been established, the patient remains at that level for 3–6 months. If no conception ensues, the patient continues clomiphene for a total of 12 months while the remainder of the infertility evaluation is completed. Ovulation can be induced in 80% of patients; however, the term pregnancy rate is only half of those ovulating, or 40%. Spontaneous abortion rate may be slightly increased at 20% and the twinning rate is 8–10%. Multiple births greater than twins are rare. There is no increase in congenital anomalies in offspring delivered after clomiphene therapy, but the drug should not be administered to women who may be pregnant.

1. Side effects–Side effects of clomiphene are usually mild but can be disturbing and include mood alterations, headache, abdominal bloating, visual disturbances, hot flushes, painful ovulation, nausea, and hair loss. If side effects are sufficiently severe to cause discontinuation of the drug, clomiphene may be reinstituted at 25 mg/d after a 1–2 month hiatus. Ovarian enlargement may result from multiple follicle stimulation. Functional cysts (follicular or luteal) usually regress within 1 week after menses, and monthly ovarian palpation rarely changes patient management. If pain develops, evaluation for cyst rupture or torsion or ectopic pregnancy may be facilitated by pelvic ultrasound. True hyperstimulation syndrome is rare with clomiphene and is discussed below under hMG/hCG treatment.

2. Failure–Clomiphene failure is the inability to ovulate at the 250-mg daily dose level or to conceive after 12 months of therapy.

The following adjunctive therapies are empirical but may be tried before proceeding to hMG/hCG therapy.

(a) Addition of hCG, 10,000 IU intramuscularly, 7 days after the last clomiphene dose.

(b) Extension of clomiphene at the 250-mg daily dose level for 8 days with or without the addition of hCG.

(c) Addition of dexamethasone, 0.5 mg, orally at bedtime (reserved for patients with elevated androgen levels or hirsutism) while restarting the clomiphene cycle at the 50-mg level.

(d) Addition of bromocriptine (despite normal serum prolactin).

C. hMG/hCG (Pergonal): Human menopausal gonadotropin (hMG) is the combination of 75 IU of FSH and 75 IU of LH extracted from the urine of postmenopausal women and supplied in dessicated form in ampules that are rehydrated with sterile saline (1 mL/ampule) just before use. Injected intramuscularly, it has ovarian effects very similar to pituitary gonadotropins.

hCG is needed to trigger ovulation by mimicking the LH surge. Because of its expense and risks (multiple gestation, hyperstimulation syndrome), only physicians trained or experienced in its use should undertake Pergonal therapy. Patients must have completed a complete infertility evaluation to exclude other treatable forms of reproductive failure.

The optimal patient is one with secondary amenorrhea associated with low (< 50 pg/mL) estrogen levels (and who therefore would not be expected to respond to clomiphene) without hyperprolactinemia (which is better treated by bromocriptine). Optimal monitoring utilizes rapid (same-day) serum estradiol measurements in conjunction with ultrasonic monitoring of ovarian follicular diameter. Pergonal is given as a daily intramuscular injection with monitoring beginning at the first sign of cervical mucus production. Serum estrogen and ultrasound follicular diameter measurements are then begun and repeated every 1–3 days. Pergonal dosage is adjusted in an attempt to have 1–4 dominant follicles reach a diameter of 17–24 mm while the estrogen is in the range of 750–1500 pg/mL. hCG, 10,000 IU, is then given intramuscularly and ovulation is anticipated in 36 hours. Pregnancy rates of 60–80% may be achieved in patients having normoprolactinemic hypogonadotropic hypogonadism, but success in patients with estrogen production but chronic anovulation (eg, polycystic ovary syndrome) or clomiphene failure is lower (20–30%). The risks of Pergonal are multiple gestation rate and hyperstimulation syndrome. Twins are conceived in 20% of pregnancy cycles, triplets in 5%, and quadruplets or greater in 1%. Pregnancy reduction in the early second trimester is safe and effective but must be discussed with the couple before treatment with Pergonal is begun.

Hyperstimulation syndrome is a risk in patients who develop high preovulatory estradiol levels (> 2,000 pg/mL) in association with multiple intermediate (8–12 mm) follicles. Hyperstimulation will not occur if the ovulatory hCG injection is withheld and usually can be prevented if the patient has overshot the anticipated estradiol level or has unfavorable ultrasonic findings. Nonetheless, hyperstimulation may complicate 3–5% of Pergonal cycles and may vary from mild (ovarian enlargement with small cysts, abdominal distention, and weight gain of 2–3 kg) to severe (massive ovarian enlargement, ascites, hypovolemia, azotemia, and hyperkalemia). Symptomatic patients should be hospitalized for maintenance of fluid and electrolyte balance, prevention of thrombosis, and observation for ovarian rupture. Severe hyperstimulation syndrome may be life-threatening, and experienced consultation is mandatory. Hyperstimulation syndrome resolves spontaneously in 1 week in a nonpregnant patient but may last for 2–3 weeks in the patient who has conceived during that cycle.

Luteal Phase Defect

Luteal phase defect is a term applied to a poorly understood group of subtle hormonal alterations in which ovulation appears to take place but progesterone secretion is inadequate to allow or support a pregnancy. Clinically, it has been linked to infertility (5% of infertile women) and habitual abortion. The presumed defect is inadequate progesterone output by the corpus luteum. The diagnosis may be suggested by a temperature rise of less than 11 days on BBT graph (the short luteal phase); midluteal phase progesterone values of less than 15 ng/mL; or most reliably, an endometrial biopsy more than 2 days out of phase. Because luteal phase defect is known to occur sporadically in many women, it should be documented in 2 successive cycles for maximum diagnostic validity. Once hyperprolactinemia has been excluded, treatment options include administration of clomiphene, progesterone, or both.

A. Clomiphene: See above.

B. Progesterone: Progesterone is used to replace a postulated hormone deficiency. Progesterone is not orally absorbable; it must be administered in vaginal/rectal suppository form. These suppositories are neither FDA-approved nor commercially available in the USA. The dose is 25 mg inserted twice daily, starting 2–3 days after ovulation and continuing until the onset of menses. Progesterone may be less conveniently administered as an intramuscular injection of 12.5 mg/d. Synthetic progestins are contraindicated owing to the possible risk of congenital limb-reduction defects and a luteolytic effect.

CERVICAL FACTOR

The endocervix contains glands that respond to estradiol with the formation of mucus, a hydrogel containing 98% water with traces of salts, soluble proteins, enzymes, and immunoglobulins. The mucus increases in quantity by 30-fold as ovulation approaches and changes in quality by increasing its stretchability (spinnbarkeit) and clarity (acellularity) and is generally associated with slight dilatation of the cervical os. The function of cervical mucus is to (1) act as a reservoir for sperm for continued release into the upper genital tract; (2) filter the semen to exclude bacteria, particulate debris, seminal plasma, and nonmotile sperm; (3) buffer and protect the sperm from the acid environment of the vagina (mucus should have a pH above 7); and (4) guide the sperm into the uterus by forming linear fibrinous filaments (micelles) that are arranged to form parallel rods that direct the sperm into columns (phallanx formation). An inadequate cervical factor may account for 5–10% of infertility in women.

Postcoital (Sims-Huhner) Test

This test is an in vivo evaluation of sperm-mucus interaction. After 48 hours of sexual abstinence, the couple has intercourse and the mucus is examined within 2–8 hours. The test is timed 15 or 16 days before the following menses, ie, 24–48 hours before presumed ovulation. Mucus is most easily removed from the endocervical canal with nasal polyp forceps after its quantity, clarity and spinnbarkeit are assessed (should be more than 8 cm). A small amount of mucus is air-dried on a slide and examined under low power for ferning, a crystalline pattern reflecting salt concentration. If ferning is not present, inflammation, infection, or poor timing of the test relative to ovulation should be suspected. The remainder of the mucus is placed on a slide under a coverslip and examined at a magnification of 400× for the number and progressive motility of sperm and cellularity (epithelial cells, red and white blood cells). The finding of more than 5 progressively motile sperm/hpf in clear mucus is considered normal.

The following represent the most common causes and treatments of an abnormal postcoital test:

A. Absent or Low Quantity of Mucus: This may result from congenital cervical stenosis, previous cervical trauma (cone biopsy, electric cautery, obstetrical trauma), or prenatal exposure to DES. Be sure timing is correct relative to ovulation. Treatment is intrauterine insemination with "washed sperm." Sperm can be washed by being passed through fine glass wool or a silica bead gradient or centrifuged mixed with a doubling volume of tissue culture media with added protein (albumin, follicular fluid, or fetal cord serum) at 300 rpm for 10 minutes. The supernatant is discarded and the pellet resuspended with 1 mL of media and recentrifuged. The 0.5 mL of media is layered over the sperm pellet and the tube incubated at 37° C for 1 hour, after which the most motile sperm will "swim up" into the media. The medium is removed and used for insemination with a 5F pediatric feeding tube or 16-gauge Teflon angiocath, which is gently threaded into the uterus without mechanically dilating the cervix. Timing of insemination is either by urinary LH kit or by hCG-induced ovulation in clomiphene-treated patients scanned with vaginal ultrasound for follicular maturity. The risk of endometritis-salpingitis is approximately 0.2%.

B. Poor Quality Mucus: This is usually thick, tenacious, and cellular and may show poor spinnbarkeit and the presence of red and white blood cells. If cervicitis is present, cultures for bacteria, T mycoplasma, and chlamydia should be taken and appropriately treated (doxycycline, 100 mg twice daily for 14 days for both partners starting on day 1 of the following cycle). Blood-tinged mucus usually represents a fragile and friable epithelium and is treated with estrogen or cryosurgery as is resistant cervical inflammation.

C. Few or Absent Sperm: Good quality mucus but few or absent sperm requires a reevaluation of the male factor. If the earlier semen analysis was normal, faulty coital technique (including the use of spermicidal lubricants), low volume (less than 1 mL), or unexpected variations in sperm count may be discovered.

D. Antisperm Antibodies: Male or female antisperm antibodies may cause a poor postcoital test owing to sperm agglutination, poor motility, or a vibrating or "shaking" pattern. There are numerous techniques for detecting antibodies, but the immunobead method is currently preferred. Antibodies directed at the sperm head are most ominous, while tail-directed antibodies may not be clinically significant. Antisperm antibodies are commonly found in men who have undergone vasectomy reversal but can also be found in fertile couples and even virgins. Treatment is by intrauterine insemination with washed sperm or by in vitro fertilization. Treatment with corticosteroids has been associated with serious side effects including aseptic necrosis of the femur.

PELVIC FACTOR

The pelvic factor includes disorders of the uterus, uterine tubes, ovaries, and adjacent pelvic structures and is responsible for 30–50% of infertility in women. It is suggested by a history of pelvic infection, IUD use, dysmenorrhea, DES exposure in utero, pelvic tuberculosis, ectopic pregnancy, septic abortion, or ruptured appendix. Physical examination may reveal pelvic tenderness, mass, decreased mobility, or irregular uterine contour; however, 50% of patients with a pelvic factor are asymptomatic. A cervical culture for gonococcus and chlamydia should be performed.

The initial evaluation is by **hysterosalpingography** under fluoroscopic imaging. Contraindications include allergy to iodine or radiocontrast dye as well as infection, which may present as a pelvic mass or tenderness or an elevated sedimentation rate. Risks include dye embolization (extremely rare) and salpingitis (1–3%). Hysterosalpingography should be performed in the proliferative phase of the cycle after cessation of menstrual flow. Both oil- and water-soluble contrast media are available. Oil-soluble may have the therapeutic advantage of enhancing the posthysterosalpingography pregnancy rate for up to 1 year and is less painful. Water-soluble dye gives a better image of the tubal epithelial folds. Dye injection should be under fluoroscopic control under minimal pressure at a rate of 1–2 mL/min. The procedure should be terminated if pain or signs of venous dye extravasation occur. A delayed flat plate (20 minutes when using water dye, 24 hours when using oil) is taken for the diagnosis of persistent dye collections (eg, pelvic adhesions or hydrosalpinx). Abnormal findings on hysterosalpingography include congenital malformations of the uterus, submucous leiomyomata, intrauterine synechiae (Asherman's syndrome), intrauterine polyps, salpingitis isthmica nodosa, tubal tuberculosis, and tubal block (proximal or distal).

If the semen analysis, ovulation indicators, postcoital test, and hysterosalpingogram are normal, it is appropriate to wait 6 months; then if no conception has taken place, **laparoscopy** with chromotubation is performed using dilute indigo carmine or methylene blue.

Laparoscopy should be performed sooner if hysterosalpingography was contraindicated or is abnormal, or if the history or physical findings strongly suggest a pelvic factor. Simultaneous hysteroscopy may be useful for defining intrauterine disorders at the time of laparoscopy. Laparoscopy/hysteroscopy should be performed by the surgeon who will be performing the definitive surgical procedure (eg, tuboplasty) if appropriate.

Treatment

A. Uterine Disorders:

1. Diethylstilbestrol (DES) syndrome–Characteristic changes in the vagina (adenosis), cervix (ectropion, hood), and uterus (small and T-shaped on hysterosalpingography) are markers of in utero exposure to DES, which was given to pregnant women in the 1950s and 1960s. An increased incidence of infertility, spontaneous abortion, and premature labor has been associated with the DES syndrome. There is no specific treatment.

2. Intrauterine synechiae (Asherman's syndrome)–These are adhesions that form in the uterus, resulting in amenorrhea, hypomenorrhea, infertility, or habitual abortion. They are seen following pregnancy, uterine surgery, abortion, or D&C complicated by endometritis. It certain endemic areas of the world synechiae may result from endometritis caused by schistosomiasis or tuberculosis. Diagnosis is by hysterosalpingography. Treatment is done under direct vision with hysteroscopically guided lysis of adhesions. A pediatric Foley catheter may be used as a stent postoperatively (the catheter is removed in 7 days). Broad-spectrum antibiotics are given orally for 14 days, and high-dose estrogen (conjugated estrogens 2.5 mg, 2–4 times daily) is administered for 1–2 months to stimulate endometrial proliferation. Patients will usually be anovulatory at this estrogen dose, and medroxyprogesterone, 10 mg/d, should be given for 7–10 days at the end of estrogen treatment. Treated patients have an increased risk of spontaneous abortion and placenta previa, placenta accreta, and abruptio placentae.

3. Congential abnormalities and leiomyomata–These are rarely a cause of primary infertility and should be surgically treated only after the remainder of the evaluation is negative. Both conditions are more likely associated with habitual abortion.

B. Tubal Disorders:
The physiologic roles of the uterine tubes in fertilization include sperm transport and capacitation, ovum pickup and transport, and embryo nourishment and transport. Inflammation resulting in tubal damage is the most common infertility factor in women (30–50%). Tubal disorders may result from pelvic inflammatory disease, endometriosis, peritubal adhesions from previous pelvic surgery, complications of IUDs, previous ectopic pregnancy, and tuberculous salpingitis. Treatment is surgical correction (tuboplasty)

or in vitro fertilization with embryo transfer. Prognosis is primarily dependent on the degree of original inflammatory damage to the tube (the integrity of the fimbria and ciliated and secretory cells); the site of tubal block (distal occlusion with hydrosalpinx usually having a poorer outcome than more proximal blocks); the causative pathogen, if known (tuberculous salpingitis with tubal block is a contraindication to tuboplasty); the postoperative length of viable tube; and the skill and experience of the surgeon. Most tubal surgery should be performed by specialists using microsurgical techniques. Pregnancy rates following tuboplasty may range from 15% or less for large hydrosalpinges to 70% or more for reversal of sterilization where tissue trauma has been minimal. All tuboplasty patients have an increased risk of ectopic gestation.

1. Endometriosis–Endometriosis is commonly associated with infertility and is discussed above.

2. In Vitro Fertilization–In vitro fertilization and embryo transfer has been successful in achieving human pregnancies since 1978. Details of the procedure are continually evolving and involve the following general steps:

(a) Development and stimulation of multiple follicles with GnRH agonists, clomiphene, and/or Pergonal (superovulation).

(b) Precise monitoring of follicular maturity by transvaginal ultrasound and rapid assays for estradiol, progesterone, and LH.

(c) Transvaginal recovery of mature oocytes by follicular aspiration under ultrasonic guidance.

(d) Fertilization of oocytes with washed, capacitated, diluted sperm.

(e) Embryo culture for 1–2 days, usually until the 4-cell stage.

(f) Transcervical transfer of 4–6 normally developing embryos into the uterus via a thin catheter.

Pregnancy rates are currently 10–25% per embryo transfer. In vitro fertilization is expensive and psychologically stressful to patients. Indications include inoperable tubal disease, unexplained infertility, and oligospermia.

Variations on in vitro fertilization include GIFT (gamete intrafallopian transfer), which is performed by placing washed sperm and aspirated oocytes directly into the uterine tubes under laparoscopic guidance, and ZIFT (zygote intrafallopian transfer), in which aspirated, fertilized, and incubated embryos are transferred to the uterine tubes via laparoscopy.

HABITUAL ABORTION

Habitual abortion is defined as 3 consecutive pregnancy losses before 20 weeks' gestation or 500-g fetal weight. It is an extremely difficult physical and psychological burden for couples. The frequency of spontaneous clinical abortion is 15–20%, but if clinically undetected (but hCG assay positive) pregnancies are included, the true spontaneous abortion rate may be closer to 50% of all fertilized ova. The risk of a subsequent abortion after each abortion is approximately 25–35%. A previous or intervening full-term pregnancy improves the prognosis, while a history of stillbirth of fetal malformation worsens it. Approximately 70% of patients who have spontaneous abortions will eventually carry to term.

The cause of habitual abortion can be detected in up to 60% of patients studied. The major etiologic factors are genetic, anatomic, hormonal, immunologic, infectious, and environmental.

Genetic Factors

Some 50–60% of spontaneous abortions are chromosomally abnormal with trisomy, polyploidy, and monosomy X being most frequently found. When karyotypes of couples experiencing habitual abortion are studied, 5–10% will have an abnormality, usually a balanced translocation (where the total amount of genetic material is normal, but a nonlethal chromosomal rearrangement exists). If the history also reveals a fetal malformation, the chance of an abnormal karyotype in a couple increases to 25%. Thus, most fetal chromosomal aberrations arise spontaneously in either the sperm or egg and may be randomly affected by parental age, delayed fertilization, or environmental factors. If a paternal balanced translocation is found, donor insemination may be considered. If maternal, there is no treatment, but a 50% chance of normal pregnancy still exists.

Anatomic Factors

A. Congenital Uterine Anomalies: Congenital uterine anomalies are found in 10–15% of women with habitual abortion. These defects may be detected by hysterosalpingography (but septate and bicornuate uteri may not be distinguished by hysterosalpingography alone). Inadequacy of septal blood supply may be the cause of recurrent abortion. Term pregnancy rates of up to 80% may be achieved following corrective surgery (Tompkins, Jones, Strassman, or hysteroscopic metroplasty). Urinary tract anomalies including renal agenesis will be found in 10% of these patients, and preoperative intravenous pyelogram should be performed.

B. Incompetent Cervix: Incompetent cervix may be diagnosed by a history of painless cervical dilation resulting in repeated second trimester abortions. The ability to painlessly pass a number 9 dilator in the nonpregnant state confirms the diagnosis. A cerclage procedure should be curative.

C. DES Syndrome: DES syndrome is often associated with a small, T-shaped uterus and an increased risk of premature labor. It is unclear whether there is an increased risk of habitual abortion.

D. Uterine Synechiae (Asherman's Syndrome): Uterine synechiae can cause of infertility or secondary amenorrhea, but 15% of these patients may present with habitual abortion. Treatment is as for infertility.

E. Uterine Leiomyomata: These are associated more with recurrent pregnancy loss than with primary infertility. Submucous myomas will appear as crescent-shaped filling defects on the hysterosalpingogram, while an enlarged, irregular uterus is characteristic on pelvic examination. Myomectomy is followed by a successful pregnancy in 50% of cases. The prognosis is poorer for patients with fibroids larger than 12-week size or who are over age 35.

Endocrine Factors

A. Hypothyroidism: Hypothyroidism is rarely responsible for abortion but should be excluded even in the clinical euthyroid patient.

B. Diabetes Mellitus: Diabetes mellitus is responsible only in the poorly controlled patient.

C. Luteal Phase Defects: These may occur in habitual aborters. If an endometrial biopsy is more than 48 hours out of phase or the luteal phase is less than 11 days by BBT, luteal phase defects should be treated. *There is no place for any hormonal therapy that begins after a missed menstrual period or in the face of a threatened abortion.*

D. Hyperprolactinemia: Mild hyperprolactinemia may be a cause of luteal phase defects and should be treated with bromocriptine (Parlodel).

Immunologic Factors

A normal embryo is protected from immunologic rejection by the formation of trophoblast-stimulated maternal blocking antibody, which is also required as a stimulus for further fetal cell division and growth. Habitual abortion may occur if the female partner's HLA antigens are insufficiently different from the male partner's to stimulate the production of blocking antibody. Immunizing the woman with the man's lymphocytes, has been reported to result in a living child in 60–80% of treated couples. A second immunologic mechanism is suggested by the presence of anticardiolipin antibody (indicating an autoimmune reaction to fetal phospholipids) and a clotting abnormality detected as circulating lupus anticoagulant. Even unaborted pregnancies are at increased risk for intrauterine growth retardation, preeclampsia/eclampsia, and fetal death. Treatment protocols that include aspirin (80 mg/d), heparin, and prednisone are undergoing clinical evaluation and should be administered only by physicians experienced with immunotherapy.

Infectious Factors

Any acute infectious illness may possibly cause a single abortion, but only a chronic endometrial infection should be associated with recurrent loss. Although a causal relationship has not been proved, the most likely suspects in humans are herpesvirus, toxoplasmosis, chlamydia, and T mycoplasma. Positive cervical cultures should be appropriately treated.

Environmental Factors

With the exception of chronic exposure to ethylene oxide by female operating room personnel, no specific toxic substance has been definitively linked to abortion. Possibilities include cigarette smoking, alcohol abuse, lead, mercury, polychlorinate biphenyl (PCB), radiation, chemical, chemical wastes, and pesticides.

DYSFUNCTIONAL UTERINE BLEEDING

Dysfunctional uterine bleeding refers to irregular bleeding patterns that result from anovulation. This is a diagnosis of exclusion and must be distinguished from other conditions such as those listed in Table 9–2. It should not be confused with dysmenorrhea.

The bleeding has no characteristic pattern and may range from an interval of several months of amenorrhea followed by profuse hemorrhage to continuous daily bleeding or spotting that may persist for months. The common feature of dysfunctional uterine bleeding is estrogen production without postovulatory progesterone secretion. Because there is no progesterone-induced prostaglandin secretion to cause menstrual cramps, the bleeding is usually painless. The amount and rapidity of bleeding roughly correlates with the amount of proliferative endometrium present (which is a function of the estrogen level and the duration of anovulation). The presence of estrogen alone causes endometrial proliferation, which continues unabated until the uterine lining reaches a stage of vascularity, hyperplasia, and fragility unaccompanied by the compact structure and stromal support induced by progesterone; finally, spontaneous superficial bleeding begins. Without the coiling of blood vessels, rhythmic vasoconstriction, and full-thickness collapse of the endometrium to induce hemostasis, bleeding will continue unabated.

Dysfunctional uterine bleeding is most common during puberty and the climacteric because anovulation is most common at the beginning and end of reproductive life. Cyclic ovulatory menses may not become well established for 1–3 years after menarche because of

Table 9–2. Causes of abnormal vaginal bleeding.

Dysfunctional uterine bleeding (anovulation) Menarche Menopause Polycystic ovaries Hyperandrogenism Hyperprolactinemia	**Uterine lesions** Carcinoma or sarcoma Polyps Adenomyosis Leiomyomata IUDs
Abnormal gestation Threatened or incomplete abortion Ectopic pregnancy Gestational trophoblastic disease	**Ovarian lesions** Granulosa–theca cell tumor **Coagulopathy** Hemophilia Von Willebrand's disease Leukemia Thrombocytopenia
Vaginal lesions Lacerations due to trauma or foreign body insertion Sarcoma botryoides Clear cell carcinoma	**Thyroid dysfunction**
Cervical lesions Polyps Sarcoma or carcinoma Chronic cervicitis	

immaturity of the central nervous system–hypothalamic centers. Before menopause, the remaining ovarian follicles are relatively gonadotropin resistant and may not produce adequate estradiol to induce an LH surge, yet still produce enough estradiol to produce dysfunctional uterine bleeding or hyperplasia after accumulation over months or years.

Dysfunctional uterine bleeding is commonly associated with obesity, hirsutism, and infertility (polycystic ovary syndrome). Regular menses with excessive blood loss is suggestive of coagulopathy or uterine leiomyomata. Physical examination should include thyroid palpation, notation of hirsutism or obesity, spleen palpation, and a vaginal speculum and bimanual pelvic examination. Laboratory evaluation should include a complete blood count with a platelet count, Papanicolaou smear, and if indicated, serum β-hCG (early pregnancy test), thyroid function tests, prothrombin and partial thromboplastin time, and serum progesterone 1 week before expected menses (if the diagnosis of anovulation remains uncertain). For patients over age 40, an office endometrial biopsy should be performed to exclude an endometrial malignancy or precursor before initiation of therapy.

TREATMENT

Treatment is based on the degree of abnormal bleeding. Profuse hemorrhage may require conjugated estrogens given as 20 mg, intravenously every 3 hours until bleeding stops or until 4 doses have been given. Meanwhile, hypotension is treated with intravenous normal saline; severe anemia may require blood transfusion and later iron supplements. If bleeding does not abate, D&C is indicated. If intravenous conjugated estrogens are used, medroxyprogesterone should be given concomitantly at 10 mg orally every day for 10 days with the patient told to expect a withdrawal bleeding episode within a week following discontinuation. For milder bleeding, any combination oral contraceptive may be given as one pill 4 times daily for 5 days. The expected response is cessation of bleeding within 5 days followed by withdrawal bleeding within a week after the last pill. If not contraindicated, oral contraceptives should then be continued in the usual cyclic manner for 3 months to prevent recurrent dysfunctional uterine bleeding and ensure complete endometrial sloughing. For patients in whom estrogens are contraindicated, medroxyprogesterone, 10 mg/d for 10 d/mo for 3 months, may be substituted for oral contraceptives. A failure of hormonal therapy to control irregular bleeding mandates a D&C to exclude an intrauterine lesion.

MEDICAL ABORTION

RU 486 (mifepristone), 600 mg orally followed in 36–48 hours by a prostaglandin analog by vaginal suppository or intramuscular injection, is 90% successful in inducing medical abortion. Bleeding continues on average for 9 days.

PREMENSTRUAL SYNDROME

Premenstrual syndrome (PMS) is a poorly understood, loosely organized group of symptoms that appear in reproductive-age women in a cyclical fashion. Most commonly, symptoms appear up to 2 weeks before menses, become progressively worse in the premenstrual phase, and diminish markedly within 24–72 hours after the onset of menstruation.

The incidence of PMS varies widely with an average reported incidence of 30%, with 5% of women suffering severe functional impairment.

More than 150 symptoms have been attributed to PMS, but the following are most commonly reported: nervous tension, anxiety, irritability, mood swings, weight gain, lower abdominal bloating, increased appetite, craving for sweets, headache, depression, forget-fulness, confusion, and insomnia.

Risk and severity factors for PMS include multiparity (especially with a history of preeclampsia), marriage, increased age (third and fourth decades of life most commonly), exposure to stress, poor nutrition, and sedentary lifestyle. Dysmenorrhea is not a common symptom, and if it is associated with other PMS symptoms, the patient should be evaluated for endometriosis.

Hypotheses concerning the cause of PMS include the following: vitamin B_6 deficiency, hypoglycemia, progesterone allergy, prolactin excess, aldosterone excess, altered estrogen/progesterone ratio, prostaglandin excess, decreased endorphins, and psychosomatic factors.

TREATMENT

Remedies for PMS are commonly applied, although few if any stand up to scrutiny when studied in a controlled manner. The placebo effect of these therapies may be substantial, especially if offered in a sympathetic and supportive manner. Pharmacologic treatment may be directed at a specific symptom complex or globally through ovulation suppression.

Lifestyle Alteration
Reduction of stress through relaxation techniques and decreased caffeine, nicotine, and alcohol use. Regular exercise.

Nutritional Alteration
Reduction in intake of salt, refined sugar, animal fats, dairy products, and animal protein. Increased intake of whole grains, legumes, complex carbohydrates.

Mastalgia
Bromocriptine is effective especially if symptoms are associated with hyperprolactinemia or galactorrhea. Use the lowest effective dose, starting at 1.25 mg at bedtime and increasing to as high as 2.5 mg twice a day. Side effects include nasal stuffiness, headache, malaise, nausea, and orthostatic symptoms. Primrose oil (1.5–2 g/d) is a linoleic acid nutritional supplement taken during the luteal phase. Side effects are gastrointestinal symptoms and skin rash.

Fluid Retention
Primrose oil and thiazide diuretics or spironolactone may be taken during the luteal phase beginning 24–48 hours before anticipated weight gain.

Anxiety/Depression

Mefenamic acid (Ponstel) 250 mg three times a day is especially effective if dysmenorrhea accompanies mood dysphoria. Because of potential hematologic, renal, and neurologic toxicity, it should not be taken for more than 7 consecutive days. Alprazolam (Xanax), 0.25 mg at bedtime up to 0.25 mg three times a day, may be taken during the luteal phase, with tapering of dosage during menstruation. Side effects are anticholinergic and sedative, with abuse and tolerance potential.

Ovulation Suppression

Danazol (Danocrine), 200 mg twice a day, effectively suppresses ovulation in most women, although barrier contraception is recommended until amenorrhea is established. Side effects include weight gain, acne, increased skin oiliness, and breakthrough bleeding. Side effects are fewer at the 200 mg/d dose, but ovulation is not suppressed, and barrier or IUD contraception is required to avoid the potential for virilization of a female fetus in early pregnancy. GnRH agonists (leuprolide, nafarelin) cause profound suppression of pituitary gonadotropins with resultant hypoestrogenemia and amenorrhea. Since all cyclic ovarian function is abolished, GnRH agonists may be used as a diagnostic as well as a therapeutic trial when the diagnosis of PMS is in doubt. Long-term therapy is limited by development of clinically detectable osteoporosis after 6 months. Estrogen replacement therapy may be added at that time, although the effectiveness of this combination has not been evaluated. Depot leuprolide may be given once a month as an intramuscular injection, while nafarelin is used as a nasal spray twice daily. Side effects related to hypoestrogenemia include hot flashes, vaginal dryness, decreased libido, dyspareunia, and irregular spotting.

Unsuccessful Treatments

Progesterone suppositories, pyridoxine (vitamin B_6), and lithium were no more effective than placebo in controlled trials. Oral contraceptives are usually poorly tolerated.

HIRSUTISM*

Hirsutism is the presence of excessive or coarse body or facial hair in women. It results when factors (usually androgens) stimulate hair in the resting phase (telogen) to enter the growth phase (anagen)

* By Robert D. Nachtigall and Paul A. Fitzgerald

or when androgens act upon the hair follicle to increase its diameter and pigmentation, progressing from fine vellus hair to coarse terminal hair. Hair density is normally highest in Caucasian women, especially those of southern Mediterranean ancestry; it is lowest in blacks, Asians, and those of northern European ancestry. Many women note an increase in facial hair following the menopause.

Female hyperandrogenism may cause hirsutism or acne. It may cause or result from anovulation and may be associated with menstrual irregularity and infertility. Severe hyperandrogenism may cause hirsutism associated with virilization, ie, male pattern baldness, muscular development, clitoromegaly, breast atrophy, and deepening of the voice.

PHYSIOLOGY

The clinically significant androgens are testosterone, androstenedione, and dehydroepiandrosterone sulfate (DHEAS). In hyperandrogenic women, testosterone is secreted by the ovary (60%) and derived from the peripheral conversion of androstenedione (40%), while androstenedione is secreted about equally by the ovary and the adrenal. DHEAS is secreted exclusively by the zona reticularis of the adrenal cortex.

Testosterone is by far the most potent androgen. Androstenedione is a much weaker androgen, and DHAS has minimal androgen activity. Androstenedione and DHAS circulate in an unbound state. Testosterone is 98% bound—65% strongly bound to sex hormone–binding globulin (SHBG) and 33% weakly bound to albumin. Such binding decreases the availability of testosterone, since only the unbound (free) testosterone and a small portion of the weakly bound testosterone can enter target cells and exert androgen action. Elevated levels of androgens cause a reduction in SHBG production, which results in a greater percentage (3–4%) of total testosterone circulating in the free state. As a result, total circulating testosterone may be normal or only mildly elevated, while free testosterone may be increased 2- to 3-fold.

Androgens actually exert their effects upon hair follicles and sweat glands through conversion to dihydrotestosterone (DHT) via 5α-reductase. DHT is metabolized to androstanediol glucuronide, which is an inactive marker for hyperandrogenism.

CAUSES

Increased androgen secretion in women most commonly results from functional disorders of the ovaries (polycystic ovary syndrome, hyperthecosis). Many of these women have concomitant functional adrenal androgen hypersecretion. Ovarian tumors are uncommon. ACTH-dependent Cushing's syndrome and adrenal carcinoma are relatively rare causes of hirsutism. Five percent of hyperandrogenic women will have the associated syndrome of insulin resistance, compensatory hyperinsulinemia, and acanthosis nigricans.

Adrenal enzyme defects need not present at birth with ambiguous genitalia. Some patients (1–6%) have late-onset congenital adrenal hyperplasia in which the expression of their enzyme defect is not detected until adolescence or adulthood. The most common enzyme disorder is 21-hydroxylase deficiency. Patients with 11-hydroxylase deficiency often have hypertension. Patients (46,XY) with the rare 17,20 desmolase deficiency may appear to be phenotypic females, who undergo virilization at puberty.

Other rare causes of hirsutism include acromegaly (10–15% incidence of hirsutism), central nervous system lesions (encephalitis, head trauma, multiple sclerosis), and pregnancy associated with an ovarian luteoma. Drugs that may cause hirsutism include phenytoin, anabolic steroids, diazoxide, progestins, cyclosporine, minoxidil, hexachlorobenzene, and aminoglutethimide.

CLINICAL EVALUATION

A history is recorded of the onset and rapidity of development of hirsutism as well as the menstrual and fertility history and family history. Hypertension should be noted, since it may be seen with 11-hydroxylase deficiency and Cushing's syndrome. The pelvic examination must be performed for evaluation of ovarian enlargement or clitorimegaly. The patient must be examined closely for any signs of Cushing's syndrome. Any acne present should be noted. Hirsutism must be distinguished from virilization, which is masculinization of the female body habitus consisting of hirsutism, temporal or occipital pattern balding, hypermuscularity, and clitorimegaly. Virilization suggests the presence of an androgen-secreting neoplasm.

LABORATORY EVALUATION

The diagnosis of hirsutism is really a clinical one; the very presence of spontaneous hirsutism indicates an increased androgen effect. When increased hair growth is obvious, the diagnosis should not be thought to be dependent upon a laboratory test. Practically speaking, the main usefulness for laboratory hormone testing in hirsutism is to help detect the presence of an occult ovarian or adrenal neoplasm or Cushing's syndrome. Fig. 9–1 portrays one approach to the evaluation of hirsutism. Typical androgen profiles measure serum testosterone and DHEAS. After these serum androgen levels are drawn, if the patient has any manifestations of Cushing's syndrome, a 1-mg dexamethasone suppression test is performed as a screening test.

Elevated Testosterone

Critically high serum testosterone levels indicate the likelihood of an ovarian neoplasm. Critical serum levels are generally considered to be total testosterone > 200 ng/dL or free testosterone > 40 ng/dL. Such high levels or rapid virilization indicate the need for pelvic examination and ultrasound. If the pelvic ultrasound does not disclose an ovarian mass, magnetic resonance imaging or CT scan of the ovaries and CT scan of the adrenals are indicated. Half of women with a total testosterone > 100 ng/dL will have insulin resistance and a compensatory hyperinsulinemia that stimulates ovarian androgen production in the presence of adequate LH.

Elevated DHEAS

If the initial serum DHAS is elevated above 700 μg/dL, an adrenal neoplasm must be excluded. Adrenal suppression is carried out with dexamethasone, 0.5 mg orally every 6 hours for 5 days, with a repeat DHAS measurement performed on the fifth day. If the DHAS is suppressed to less than 170 μg/dL, an adrenal tumor is virtually excluded and the diagnosis of adrenal hyperplasia is made. If dexamethasone does not suppress DHAS levels, a CT scan of the adrenals should be performed to search for an autonomous adrenal neoplasm. The most common form of adrenal hyperplasia is 21-hydroxylase deficiency (complete or partial). Evaluation requires an ACTH stimulation test. A baseline 17-hydroxyprogesterone blood sample is followed by an intramuscular injection of ACTH, 0.25 mg, and by a second blood sample 30–60 minutes later. The normal response is a baseline < 1 ng/mL and < 5 ng/mL after ACTH. Patients with congenital adrenal hyperplasia will have a baseline > 1 ng/mL or > 10 ng/mL after ACTH.

Cushing's Syndrome Evaluation

A screening test for hypercortisolism should be undertaken. Dexamethasone, 1 mg at 11 PM, is given and a plasma cortisol obtained at 8 AM the following morning. In adults, a value < 5 μg/dL virtually excludes Cushing's syndrome; a higher value can indicate Cushing's syndrome or cortisol resistance and requires further investigation (Chapter 6).

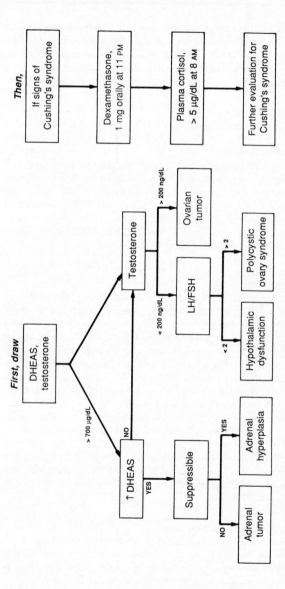

Figure 9–1. Diagnostic algorithm for hirsutism. (Exceptions occur that do not fit this algorithm. The evaluation of hirsutism requires clinical judgment.)

Polycystic Ovary Syndrome Evaluation

Most women presenting with hirsutism have polycystic ovary syndrome. Four-fifths of these patients are anovulatory and half have amenorrhea or dysfunctional uterine bleeding. In some, excessive adrenal androgen secretion appears to cause increased peripheral production of estrone; hyperestrogenemia may induce polycystic ovary syndrome, thus causing excessive androgen secretion by both adrenals and ovaries. Hyperandrogenism is ordinarily suppressible with an oral contraceptive. It may also sometimes be suppressed with a low dose of dexamethasone (eg, 0.5 mg at bedtime). Baseline LH:FSH ratios are frequently greater than 2:1. The pathophysiology, diagnosis, and treatment of this syndrome are discussed above, under Secondary Amenorrhea.

Other Laboratory Tests

As noted above, the diagnosis of hirsutism is a clinical one, not a laboratory one. However, if laboratory confirmation of the diagnosis is desired, certain hormone levels are more sensitive to the presence of an increased androgen effect. The most sensitive test is serum $3\alpha17\beta$-androstanediol glucuronide, which is elevated in a high percentage of cases of clinical hirsutism. The next most sensitive test is measurement of serum free testosterone, which is elevated in 75% of cases. Serum dihydrotestosterone is elevated in about 50% of cases.

TREATMENT

The underlying cause of hirsutism must be treated when possible. Any adrenal or ovarian neoplasm must be resected. Cushing's syndrome, if present, must be diagnosed and treated (Chapter 1). Drugs known to be the cause of hirsutism may be discontinued. For patients with polycystic ovaries and infertility, ovulation can be induced with clomiphene. For other patients, the goals are correction of menstrual irregularities, prevention of endometrial neoplasia, and cosmetic improvement. Patients with late-onset adrenal hyperplasia ordinarily do not require hydrocortisone; glucocorticoids are not as efficient as estrogen or antiandrogens in the treatment of their hirsutism. For severe hirsutism, an oral contraceptive is usually combined with an antiandrogen such as spironolactone or cyproterone.

Oral Combination Contraceptives

Oral combination contraceptives lower free testosterone levels by suppressing LH-dependent ovarian androgen synthesis and by increasing SHBG. Endometrial hyperplasia secondary to unopposed estrogen will be prevented and effective contraception provided. There is no universal agreement about the best combination oral contraceptive to use.

Progestins with Low Androgen Effect

In patients for whom oral contraceptives are contraindicated or unwanted, medroxyprogesterone will suppress LH, prevent endometrial hyperplasia, and increase testosterone clearance from the circulation by inducing hepatic enzyme activity. Dosage must be individualized. In some patients, medroxyprogesterone, 10 mg/d for 10 days each month, will result in regular withdrawal bleeding while minimizing breakthrough bleeding and provide adequate improvement in hirsutism. Other patients may require up to 30 mg/d, which may be associated with weight gain.

Spironolactone

Spironolactone, 50–100 mg twice daily on days 5–25 of the menstrual cycle or daily if combined with oral contraceptives, inhibits ovarian biosynthesis of androgens and also competes for the androgen receptors in the hair follicle. Patients receiving such treatment may have an initial diuresis and may rarely develop hyperkalemia or hyponatremia.

Glucocorticoids

Dexamethasone, 0.25–0.5 mg orally at bedtime, may be used in patients having elevated, suppressible androgen levels. It is also effective in many cases of hirsutism and acne without demonstrably increased serum androgens. Some patients may best be managed with 0.25 mg of dexamethasone orally at bedtime. Side effects of even a 0.5 mg/d dose are unusual but include weight gain, fluid retention, and psychiatric disturbances. Patients treated with glucocorticoids chronically may develop osteoporosis, so periodic bone densitometry is recommended.

Cyproterone Acetate

This is an effective antiandrogen with progestational activity that is not approved for use in the USA. Women using this drug should therefore be vigorously counseled regarding contraception. The usual dose is 50–100 mg on days 5–14 of the menstrual cycle. Ethinyl estradiol, 40 μg/d or a low-dose oral contraceptive is also given on days 5–15 of the menstrual cycle. Side effects include decreased libido, mental depression, nausea, and fatigue.

Estrogen

Conjugated estrogens may be used in postmenopausal women and cycled with a progestin. This treatment increases SHBG and reduces free testosterone levels.

Ketoconazole

Ketoconazole, 400 mg orally every 12 hours (maximum dose 1000 mg/d in 3 divided doses), may be given and the dose lowered depending on clinical response. Doses must be decreased in patients who drink alcohol. Absorption is decreased by H_2-blocking drugs. Other drugs that interact with ketoconazole include rifampin, isoniazid, cyclosporine, phenytoin, oral hypoglycemics, and warfarin. This antifungal agent inhibits 17,20-desmolase and later 17α-hydroxylase and 11β-hydroxylase. Menses frequently resume without signs of adrenal insufficiency. Because liver enzymes are frequently increased and must be monitored, it is used only rarely.

Local Treatment

Hormonal treatment of hirsutism does not yield rapid, dramatic results. Decrease in the rapidity and coarseness of new hair growth may require 6–12 months to be appreciated. During hormonal treatment, hirsutism can be treated with depilatories, waxing, bleaching, or shaving. After maximal benefit has been achieved from the treatment selected, electrolysis may be employed to permanently remove hair but is painful, expensive, and time consuming. Some women refuse to appropriately treat their hirsutism locally owing to cultural bias against facial shaving or to the ungrounded fear that removing hair stimulates its growth. Other patients are inappropriately self-conscious over a small amount of hair. Such women benefit from counseling and a frank discussion of their psychological reaction to the problem.

CONTRACEPTION

Contraceptive methods are chosen for efficacy, safety, and ease of use. Failure rates per year in Table 9–3 are approximate and reflect actual use.

ORAL CONTRACEPTIVES

Oral contraceptives (Table 9–4) are either a combination estrogen-progestin given cyclically or a progestin-only pill given continuously. The combination oral contraceptive is by far the most widely prescribed.

The estrogen component of oral contraceptives is either ethinyl estradiol or its 3-methyl ether, mestranol. Mestranol is converted to ethinyl estradiol in the liver, and there is little difference in potency between the 2 forms. The progestin component of oral contraceptives

Table 9–3. Failure rates for contraceptive devices.

Tubal ligation, vasectomy	1%
Combination oral contraceptive	2%
Progestin-only contraceptive	3%
Intrauterine device	4%
Condoms	10%
Diaphragm	13%
No method	80%

may be one of 5 synthetic forms of norethindrone, which is a synthetic 19-nortestosterone derivative. The potency of progestins varies (Table 9–4).

The combination pill exerts its contraceptive action by multiple mechanisms, primarily prevention of ovulation by suppression of the hypothalamic-pituitary axis. Gonadotropin release is inhibited by both the estrogenic suppression of FSH and the progestational suppression of LH. Additionally, the progestin induces endometrial gland atrophy and transforms cervical mucus to a form that is impenetrable by sperm. The estrogen component stabilizes the endometrium to prevent irregular shedding (breakthrough bleeding) and potentiates the effects of the progestin component.

The safe use of oral contraceptives depends upon adherence to the following procedures:

1. Carefully evaluate patient for the presence of contraindications (see below).

(a) Initial history and physical examination including blood pressure measurement, urinalysis, glucose, CBC, and pelvic examination with Pap smear.

(b) Interval history and blood pressure check at 3 months.

(c) Annual blood pressure, breast, abdominal, and pelvic examination with Pap smear.

2. For a woman over 35 years of age or at any age with a family history of vascular disease, obtain fasting cholesterol and triglyceride measurements. With a previous history of hepatic disease, perform a liver panel.

3. Exclusively use a pill with 35 μg of estrogen or less unless unacceptable breakthrough bleeding or amenorrhea develops (see Adverse Reactions, below).

Absolute Contraindications to Oral Contraceptive Use

1. History of predisposition to thromboembolic phenomena (thrombophlebitis, pulmonary embolism, stroke, myocardial infarction or angina, polycythemia, leukemia).

2. Known or suspected pregnancy (oral contraceptives may induce congenital cardiac and limb anomalies).

Table 9–4. Oral contraceptives available in the USA.

Drug	Estrogen*	(μg)	Progestin	(mg)	Progestin potency
Fixed combinations					
Ortho-Novum 2 mg	M	100	Norethindrone	2	Medium
Ortho-Novum 1/80	M	80	Norethindrone	1	Low
Demulen 1/50	EE	50	Ethynodiol diacetate	1	High
Norinyl 1 + 50	M	50	Norethindrone	1	Low
Norlestrin 2.5/50	EE	50	Norethindrone acetate	2.5	Medium
Norlestrin 1/50	EE	50	Norethindrone acetate	1	Medium
Ortho-Novum 1/50	M	50	Norethindrone	1	Low
Ovcon-50	EE	50	Norethindrone	1	Low
Ovral	EE	50	Norgestrel	0.5	High
Brevicon	EE	35	Norethindrone	0.5	Low
Demulen 1/35	EE	35	Ethynodiol diacetate	1	High
Modicon	EE	35	Norethindrone	0.5	Low
Norinyl 1 + 35	EE	35	Norethindrone	1	Low
Ortho-Novum 1/35	EE	35	Norethindrone	1	Low
Ovcon-35	EE	35	Norethindrone	0.4	Low
Norcept-E 1/35	EE	35	Norethindrone	1	Low
Levlen	EE	30	Levonorgestrel	0.15	Medium
Loestrin 1.5/30	EE	30	Norethindrone acetate	1.5	Medium
Lo/Ovral	EE	30	Norgestrel	0.3	High
Nordette	EE	30	Levonorgestrel	0.15	Medium
Loestrin 1/20	EE	20	Norethindrone acetate	1	Medium
Biphasic combination					
Ortho-Novum 10/11	EE	35	Norethindrone	0.5	Low
Followed by	EE	35	Norethindrone	1	Low
Triphasic combinations					
Ortho-Novum 7/7/7	EE	35	Norethindrone	0.5	Low
Followed by	EE	35	Norethindrone	0.75	Low
Followed by	EE	35	Norethindrone	1	Low
Trilevlen	EE	30	Levonorgestrel	0.005	Medium
Followed by	EE	40	Levonorgestrel	0.075	Medium
Followed by	EE	30	Levonorgestrel	0.125	Medium
TriNorinyl	EE	35	Norethindrone	0.5	Low
Followed by	EE	35	Norethindrone	1	Low
Followed by	EE	35	Norethindrone	0.5	Low
Triphasil	EE	30	Levonorgestrel	0.005	Medium
Followed by	EE	40	Levonorgestrel	0.075	Medium
Followed by	EE	30	Levonorgestrel	0.125	Medium
Progestin-only (minipill)					
Micronor			Norethindrone	0.35	Low
Nor-Q.D.			Norethindrone	0.35	Low
Ovrette			Norgestrel	0.075	Low

*EE = ethinyl estradiol; M = mestranol.

3. Known or suspected estrogen-dependent neoplasia (carcinoma of breast, endometrium, and cervix; melanoma).

4. Undiagnosed abnormal genital bleeding (requires diagnostic evaluation).

5. History of hepatic adenoma.

6. Cigarette smoking in women over 35 years of age (associated with excessive mortality due to cardiovascular complications).

Relative Contraindications to Oral Contraceptive Use

The following require clinical judgment to assess an individual's risk-benefit ratio. The patient should give informed consent.

1. Markedly impaired liver function (acute hepatitis or a history of cholestatic jaundice).

2. Sickle cell disease (predisposes to thromboembolic phenomena).

3. Diabetes mellitus. Oral contraceptives, especially the progestin component, induce insulin resistance and increase insulin requirements or latent diabetes.

4. History of cholecystitis/cholelithiasis (increased cholesterol saturation of bile).

5. Hypertension (lowest risk if under 30 years of age, otherwise healthy, with good control over medication. Patients with a history of renal disease, pregnancy-induced hypertension, family history of hypertension).

6. Migraine headaches (increased risk of thrombotic stroke).

7. Epilepsy (increased risk of seizures).

8. Elective surgery (increased risk of postoperative thrombosis).

9. History of moderate-to-severe depression.

Risks (Morbidity & Mortality) of Oral Contraceptives

There is no increased risk of death for women under age 35 with 35-µg estrogen (or less) pills unless they have additional risk factors.

Oral contraceptives cause metabolic changes that may explain their effects on vascular disease. They increase blood levels of procoagulant and fibrinolytic system components, alter the renin-angiotensin-aldosterone system, and increase blood levels of triacylglycerols, lipoproteins, cholesterol, and glucose. These effects may increase the risk of atherogenic and other vascular diseases, but the associations have not been proved.

A. Myocardial Infarction and Stroke: The frequently cited risks of stroke and myocardial infarction in oral contraceptive users are based on epidemiologic evidence gathered in Great Britain in the early 1970s when the steroid content of oral contraceptives was up to 5 times greater than current pill formulations. Although it is postulated that the progestin content of oral contraceptives may have an adverse effect on

HDL and LDL measurements, these changes are of questionable clinical significance in that no evidence to date indicates that these biochemical changes lead to atherosclerotic changes in blood vessels. Although oral contraceptives may act synergistically with other risk factors (cigarette smoking, hypertension, obesity, diabetes mellitus, hypercholesterolemia), myocardial infarction and stroke are rare in nonsmoking, low-dose pill users.

B. Thrombosis: The description of an elevated thrombotic risk was based on experience with pills containing 3–5 times the estrogen content of current low-dose formulations. Since the risk of deep vein thrombosis is directly related to estrogen content, current oral contraceptives should have minimal thrombotic risk.

C. Hypertension: Early British studies demonstrated the development of hypertension in 5% of women who used oral contraceptives for more than 5 years. Recent studies have found no association. The pill has been shown to increase plasma angiotensinogen; most women have a compensatory decrease in plasma renin to prevent excessive vasoconstriction. There is no clear-cut predictive association with variables such as pregnancy-induced hypertension or previous renal disease. If hypertension does develop, it usually will revert to normal within 3–6 months once the oral contraceptive is discontinued.

D. Hepatic Tumors: Hepatocellular adenomas are very rare (less than 1 in 30,000 users), and the risk appears to be related to duration of pill use. The adenomas are not related to any particular estrogen and may regress when the pill is discontinued. The risk lies in rupture and potentially fatal hemorrhage. Tumors may be asymptomatic or present with acute right upper quadrant or epigastric pain. CT scanning is recommended for diagnosis and follow up. Definitive treatment is surgical excision.

E. Gallbladder Disease: A 2-fold increased risk of gallbladder disease has been reported and may be due to an estrogen-induced increased cholesterol saturation in bile.

F. Oncogenic Potential: Evidence currently does not support a causative role for oral contraceptives in the development of cancer.

Adverse Reactions to Oral Contraceptives

Adverse reactions may be related to estrogenic, progestational, or combined effects. They are usually mild and may subside after 2–3 pill cycles. If persistent, these reactions may necessitate changing pill brands or using an alternative form of contraception.

1. Nausea, breast tenderness, and fluid retention with up to 2–3 kg of weight gain are common estrogenic side effects. Greater weight gains may represent an additional anabolic response to progestins and, if not responsive to dietary restriction, may require pill discontinuation for weight loss.

2. Depression and mood changes may result from altered tryptophan metabolism with decreased brain serotonin levels. Increased vitamin B_6 intake (pyridoxine; 100–200 mg/d orally) may have a beneficial effect.

3. Urinary tract infections and cervicitis with vaginal discharge may be increased.

4. Chloasma is uncommon but may require skin-blanching medication for treatment.

5. Breakthrough bleeding increases in incidence with a reduction in the estrogen content of the pill and is common in the first few months of pill use. Persistent breakthrough bleeding results from the progestin-induced conversion of the endometrium to a shallow decidualized state with a tendency toward breakdown and asynchronous bleeding. Bleeding in the first 3 months may be managed by encouragement and reassurance. Persistent bleeding is treated by prescribing conjugated estrogens, 2.5 mg/d for 7 days, while continuing the usual pill schedule. Doubling up of oral contraceptive pills is not effective.

6. Amenorrhea that develops while taking the pill is more common with low-dose pills because the estrogen content is not sufficient to promote endometrial proliferation. The progestin effect leads to endometrial atrophy, which is neither permanent nor dangerous. Physician and patient anxiety over possible pregnancy may require changing the brand of pill to one with a higher estrogen dosage.

Beneficial Effects of Oral Contraceptives

In addition to providing almost 100% contraception, birth control pills have positive effects. These benefits include regularization of menses with less blood loss, less dysmenorrhea, less dysfunctional bleeding, less iron-deficiency anemia, few functional ovarian cysts, less premenstrual tension, less salpingitis (PID) with decreased risk of developing salpingitis in the presence of gonorrheal infection, less development of benign breast disease (fibroadenomata and benign cystic mastitis), less rheumatoid arthritis, and less endometrial and ovarian cancer.

How to Use Oral Contraceptives

If oral contraceptives are started on the fifth day of a menstrual cycle, effective contraception begins with that cycle. They may be started immediately following a first trimester therapeutic abortion and after 1 week in a second trimester abortion. In nonbreast-feeding postpartum women, pills may be started after 2 weeks, although if bromocriptine is used to suppress lactation, the pill must be started 5 days postpartum. Oral contraceptives decrease the quantity of breast milk in lactating women and appear in breast milk and are thus contraindicated until weaning.

If a pill is missed, it should be taken as soon as possible. If 2 successive pills are missed, that pill cycle should be stopped and a new pill cycle started in 7 days, with alternative contraception employed during that interval.

All combination oral contraceptives use a 21-day-on/7-day-off cycle. The 21-day package requires the patient to remember the pill-free week, and the 28-day packages provides 7 inert pills so that pill taking is continuous. Low-dose biphasic and triphasic pills cyclically vary the progestin or estrogen content, or both, to lower the total steroid dose administered during the pill cycle and decrease breakthrough bleeding.

There is no evidence that oral contraceptives cause permanent sterility; periodic pill-free intervals are unnecessary. Their use by teenage girls does not inhibit height or reproductive organ development. After stopping oral contraceptives, women do not have an increased rate of miscarriages or fetal anomalies. They may be used by DES daughters. There is no evidence that they cause pituitary tumors, but they may accelerate the growth of tumors already present.

Drug and Medical Interactions with Oral Contraceptives

Oral contraceptives have the potential to interact with a great many drugs because they alter the production of drug-binding plasma proteins and induce hepatic oxidative enzymes involved in drug metabolism; they are cholestatic and interfere with enterohepatic circulation. Despite this potential, clinical significance has been described only for rifampin (decreased contraceptive efficacy and increased breakthrough bleeding), warfarin, and anticonvulsants (especially phenobarbital) (increased seizure activity secondary to increased drug metabolism).

Combination oral contraceptives may interfere with the interpretation of endocrine, hepatic, and coagulation tests. They reduce the response to metyrapone; increase thyroid-binding globulin leading to increased protein-bound iodine, increase T_4 (by column or RIA), and decrease T_3 resin uptake; increase prothrombin and factors VII, VIII, IX, and X, decrease antithrombin 3, and increase norepinephrine-induced platelet aggregability.

PROGESTIN-ONLY MINIPILL

The minipill is a potent low-dose progestin that is taken daily and continuously. It exerts its action by interfering with cervical mucus quality, endometrial development, and possibly tubal motility—rather than through ovulation suppression. Without estrogen, however, progestins create an unstable endometrial lining that is subject to irregular shedding. The resulting breakthrough bleeding occurs in one-third of minipill users and is the primary cause of patient dissatisfaction. Breakthrough bleeding may be managed as for combination oral contraceptives (see above). The minipill may be indicated for women with absolute or relative contraindications to combination oral contraceptives or in whom estrogen usage may be hazardous. No serious or long-term side effects of minipill use have been demonstrated, although there are assertions that fetal deformities may result if the drug is administered during pregnancy.

INJECTABLE MEDROXYPROGESTERONE ACETATE

Injectable medroxyprogesterone is not approved as a contraceptive in the USA but has wide acceptance in other countries. Given as a 150-mg intramuscular injection every 3 months, it provides contraceptive efficacy equal to that of combination oral contraceptives. It exerts its action by altering the endometrium and the cervical mucus and by blocking the LH surge that induces ovulation. The majority of women become amenorrheic. Medroxyprogesterone is prescribed for women in whom estrogen or combination oral contraceptive use is contraindicated. However, its safety in regard to thromboembolic phenomena has not been proved in a controlled clinical study. Special advantages may include inhibition of sickling in sickle cell disease, patients in whom compliance is difficult (eg, mentally retarded patients), and lactating women (quantity of breast milk is not decreased; small concentration of the drug in breast milk with unknown effects). Side effects are breakthrough bleeding, weight gain, and mental depression. Breakthrough bleeding is common (one-third of patients in the first year) and is managed by the addition of exogenous estrogen as for combination oral contraceptives. The drug is not totally cleared for 6 months after the last injection, and the unwanted side effects may persist for months after treatment is discontinued.

POSTCOITAL CONTRACEPTION

High doses of estrogen given within 72 hours (preferably within 24 hours) of intercourse can prevent implantation even if fertilization has occurred. This method is highly effective but not acceptable for routine use because of the risks associated with high-dose steroid intake, estrogen side effects, and the risk of developmental anomalies in the fetus should the treatment fail (for this reason therapeutic abortion should be offered and discussed prior to treatment). An effective regimen is ethinyl estradiol/norgestrel (2 pills twice daily for 1 day).

RU 486

RU 486 (mifepristone) is a potent, long-acting progesterone antagonist that interferes with implantation and nidation. RU 486 can be used as a contraceptive when 10 mg is taken orally 1 week after ovulation and as an abortifacient when taken early in the first trimester.

INTRAUTERINE DEVICES (IUD)

Two different IUDs currently are available in the USA. The ParaGard T380A device is plastic wound with copper, while the Progestasert has a progesterone-releasing reservoir. The IUD is relatively inexpensive, does not require continued motivation, and is usually easily reversible. It is also associated with significant risks. Both IUDs are effective and appear to induce a limited foreign body inflammatory reaction. The resulting mobilization of leukocytes, or the enzymes they release, may immobilize or destroy spermatozoa, interfere with fertilization, exert a zygotoxic or blastotoxic effect, or prevent implantation. The addition of progesterone may affect the cervical mucus to inhibit sperm transport or may exert an additional anti-implantation effect by local progesterone effects on the endometrium. The incidence of cramping and bleeding may be reduced owing to the effect of local progesterone on the endometrial production of prostaglandins. The addition of copper may exert a direct metabolic effect on endometrial cells or may reduce sperm transport within the uterus. The Progestasert must be replaced annually, while the ParaGard needs replacement every 4 years. IUDs have their best application in multiparous married women who want to maintain their fertility.

Contraindications to IUD Use

1. Pregnancy or suspicion of pregnancy.
2. Distorted uterine cavity (leiomyomas, congenital müllerian abnormalities, distorted uterus secondary to in utero DES exposure).
3. Pelvic inflammatory disease or a history of repeated PID.
4. Postpartum endometritis or infected abortion in the last 3 months.
5. Known or suspected uterine or cervical malignancy including unresolved abnormal Pap smear.
6. Genital bleeding.
7. Cervicitis until infection is controlled.
8. Previous ectopic pregnancy.
9. Valvular heart disease.
10. Leukemia, chronic corticosteroid therapy, or any condition of decreased immunocompetence against infection.

Complications of IUDs

A. Pelvic Infection: A 2- to 5-fold increased risk of pelvic inflammatory disease occurs in women using IUDs, regardless of type, with an incidence of 1–4%. Risk factors include young age, nulliparity, multiple sexual partners, exposure to sexually transmitted infections, and low socioeconomic class. Actinomyces infection appears to be almost exclusively related to the existence of a foreign body, such as an IUD, in the uterine cavity. Actinomyces may be detected on a Papanicolaou smear which, in addition to a cervical culture, should be performed before the insertion of an IUD. Salpingitis can result in tubal damage and occlusion, thereby threatening future fertility. IUD use should be discouraged in nulliparous women who have the desire for future child bearing. Since recency of insertion appears to carry an increased risk of PID, close observation of patients during the first few cycles after IUD insertion is imperative. Symptoms of pelvic infection can include the new development of abnormal menstrual bleeding, vaginal discharge, abdominal or pelvic pain, dyspareunia, or fever. Cervical cultures for gonorrhea and chlamydia should be taken and doxycycline (100 mg orally twice a day) begun, with IUD removal within 24–48 hours if there is not marked clinical improvement. Signs or symptoms of peritonitis or adnexal mass require hospitalization and intravenous antibiotic therapy with penicillin, gentamicin, and clindamycin. Patients using an IUD should undergo a Papanicolaou smear evaluation at least once a year to detect the possible presence of Actinomyces. If Actinomyces is noted, removal of the IUD is indicated along with more aggressive therapy for symptomatic patients.

B. Pregnancy: Pregnancy with an IUD in place has an increased risk of septic abortion, septic shock, and death. The patient is at greatest risk in the second trimester. Initial symptoms may be insidious and not easily recognized but may include a flu-like syndrome, fever, abdominal cramping and pain, bleeding, and unusual vaginal discharge. If the pregnancy is unwanted, termination by suction curettage or dilation and evacuation may be performed. If pregnancy interruption is not desired, the risks of spontaneous abortion following IUD removal must be carefully weighed against the risks of septicemia with the IUD in place. Appropriate informed consent should be elicited for either course of action. In general, if the IUD string is visible, an atraumatic attempt at IUD removal should be made.

C. Ectopic Pregnancy: An IUD may increase the risk of ectopic gestation. Any patient with a delayed or unusual period, irregular vaginal bleeding, or pelvic/abdominal pain should be evaluated for ectopic pregnancy. Sensitive serum pregnancy tests and pelvic ultrasound should allow for early detection of an ectopic pregnancy prior to rupture.

D. Perforation: Perforation usually occurs at the time of insertion. Nulliparous women and patients who have been recently pregnant (after delivery or therapeutic abortion) are at increased risk. Migration of an IUD may be possible but it is rare. Suspected perforation may be evaluated best by pelvic ultrasound in the stable patient. Abdominal flat plate alone may not be diagnostic even though all IUDs are radioopaque. With known perforation, removal by an experienced laparoscopist is the procedure of choice.

BARRIER CONTRACEPTION & SPERMICIDES

Barrier contraception includes the diaphragm, condom, and cervical cap (not approved for use in the USA, but widely used in Great Britain). Maximal efficacy is achieved by simultaneous use of a spermicidal cream, jelly, foam, or suppository and is superior to the use of a spermicide alone. A spermicide-impregnated sponge (Today) is available. All require repeated use with each act of intercourse so that motivation and compliance are important factors in the use-efficacy of these methods. Contraindications, complications, and side effects are limited to allergic reactions to any of the spermicidal ingredients. Diaphragms and cervical caps require careful fitting, placement, and appropriate time of insertion in relation to coitus. Condoms and spermicides do not require a professional fitting and are widely and readily available. The active ingredient in all spermicides in the USA is the same—nonoxynol-9 in 2–12.5% concentration.

RHYTHM CONTRACEPTION

Rhythm contraception (natural family planning, Billing's method) requires periodic abstinence based on a woman's menstrual cycle. This method can be efficacious with good patient motivation and understanding of basic reproductive principles. The Billing's method depends on a woman's identification of a characteristic preovulatory vaginal discharge of cervical mucus. In general, the menstrual period is considered fertile, the ''dry'' days following the cessation of menses are infertile, and the interval from the beginning of the mucus discharge until 3 days after its disappearance is considered fertile. From the fourth day after disappearance of discharge until the next menstruation is considered infertile.

REFERENCES

Menopause and estrogen replacement therapy

Armstron BK: Oestrogen therapy after the menopause: Boon or bane? *Med J Aust* 1988;**148**:213.

Bush T, Castelli WP, Stampfer M: How ERT influences cardiovascular disease. *Contemp Obstet Gynecol* Nov:108, 1988.

Haney AF, Lobo RA, Schiff I: Options in estrogen replacement therapy. *Contemp Obstet Gynecol* 1988;**3:**190.

Miller PD: Advances in osteoporosis management. *Contemp Obstet Gynecol* Dec:31, 1988.

Omodei U, Speroff L: Outlook on continuous estrogen-progestin therapy. *Contemp Obstet Gynecol* Special Issue (Fertility) 1988.

Speroff L: Breast cancer and postmenopausal hormone therapy. *Contemp Obstet Gynecol* Jan:71, 1990.

Stampfer MJ et al: A prospective study of postmenopausal estrogen therapy and coronary heart disease. *N Engl J Med* 1985;**313:**1044.

The long-term effects of estrogen deprivation: A special report. *Postgrad Med* Sept 14, 1987.

Upton GV: Therapeutic consideration in the management of the climacteric. *J Reprod Med* 1984;**29:**71

Weinstein MC, Schiff I: Cost-effectiveness of hormone replacement therapy in the menopause. *Obstet Gynecol Surv* 1983;**38:**445.

Premenstrual syndrome

Keye WR: *The Premenstrual Syndrome.* Saunders, 1988.

Muse KN: Clinical experience with the use of GnRH agonists in the treatment of premenstrual syndrome. *Obstet Gynecol Surv* 1989;**44:**317.

Smith S, Schiff I: The premenstrual syndrome: Diagnosis and management. *Fertil Steril* 1989;**52:**527.

Infertility

Behrman SJ, Kistner RW, Patton GW: *Progress in Infertility,* Vol 3. Little Brown, 1988.

DeCherney AH, Polan ML, Lee RD, Boyers SP: *Decision Making in Infertility.* Decker, 1988.

Garcia CR et al: *Current Therapy of Infertility*—3. Decker, 1988.

Seibel MM: *Infertility: A Comprehensive Text.* Appleton & Lange, 1990.

Tanagho EA, Lue TF, McClure RD: *Contemporary Management of Impotence and Infertility.* Williams & Wilkins, 1988.

Wallach EE, Kempers RD: *Modern Trends in Infertility and Conception Control,* Vol 4. Yearbook, 1988.

Contraception

Diller L, Hembree W: Male contraception and family planning: A social and historical review. *Fertil Steril* 1977;**28:**1271.

Huggins GR, Zucker PK: Oral contraceptives and neoplasia: 1987 update. *Fertil Steril* 1987;**47:**733.

Kelly TM: Systemic effects of oral contraceptives. *West J Med* 1984;**141:**113.

Kessel E: Pelvic inflammatory disease with intrauterine device use: A reassessment. *Fertil Steril* 1989;**51:**1.

Nieman LK et al: The progesterone antagonist RU486, a potential new contraceptive agent. *N Engl J Med* 1987;**316:**187.

Rosenfield A: Update on oral contraceptives. *J Reprod Med* 1984;**29:**501.

Silvestre et al: Voluntary interruption of pregnancy with mifeprisone (RU486) and a prostaglandin analogue: A large scale French experience. *N Engl J Med* 1990;**327**:645.

Tatum HJ, Connell EB: Barrier contraception: A comprehensive overview. *Fertil Steril* 1981;**36**:1.

Upton GV: Lipids, cardiovascular disease, and oral contraceptives: A practical perspective. *Fertil Steril* 1990;**53**:1.

Secondary Amenorrhea

Alper MM, Garner PR: Premature ovarian failure: Its relationship to autoimmune disease. *Obstet Gynecol* 1985;**66**:27.

Baker ER: Menstrual dysfunction and hormonal status in athletic women: A review. *Fertil Steril* 1981;**36**:691.

Borson S, Katon W: Chronic anorexia nervosa: Medical mimic. *West J Med* 1981;**135**:257.

Friedman CI, Barrows H, Kim MH: Hypogonadotropic hypogonadism. *Am J Obstet Gynecol* 1983;**145**:360.

Neinstein LS: Menstrual dysfunction in pathologic states (clinical review). *West J Med* 1985;**143**:476.

Pepperell RJ: Prolactin and reproduction. *Fertil Steril* 1981;**35**:267.

Speroff L, Glass RH, Kase NG: *Clinical Gynecologic Endocrinology and Infertility.* Williams & Wilkins, 1989.

Menstrual cycle

Fritz MA, Speroff L: The endocrinology of the menstrual cycle: The interaction of folliculogenesis and neuroendocrine mechanisms. *Fertil Steril* 1982; **38**:509.

Knobil E: The neuroendocrine control of the menstrual cycle. *Recent Prog Horm Res* 1980;**36**:53.

Soules MR et al: The corpus luteum: Determinants of progesterone secretion in the normal menstrual cycle. *Obstet Gynecol* 1988;**71**:659.

Dysmenorrhea and endometriosis

Dawood MY: An update of dysmenorrhea. *Contemp Obstet Gynecol* June:73, 1984.

Henzl MR et al: Administration of nasal nafarelin as compared with oral danazol for endometriosis. *N Engl J Med* 1988;**318**:485.

Hill GA: Clinical experience in the treatment of endometriosis with GnRH agonist. *Obstet Gynecol Surv* 1989;**44**:305.

Hurst BS, Rock JA: Endometriosis: Pathophysiology, diagnosis, and treatment. *Obstet Gynecol Surv* 1989;**44**:297.

Schlaff WD: Treating myomas and endometriosis with GnRH analogs. *Contemp Obstet Gynecol* Feb:26, 1990.

Seibel, MM: Does minimal endometriosis always require treatment? *Contemp Obstet Gynecol* July:27, 1989.

Hirsutism

Azziz R: Determining the cause of hirsutism and anovulation. *Contemp Obstet Gynecol* May:126, 1988.

Azziz R, Zacur HA: 21-Hydroxylase deficiency in female hyperandrogenism: Screening and diagnosis. *J Clin Endocrinol Metab* 1989;**69:**577.

Barbieri RL, Smith S, Ryan KJ: The role of hyperinsulinemia in the pathogenesis of ovarian hyperandrogenism. *Fertil Steril* 1988;**50:**197.

Barnes RB et al: Pituitary-ovarian responses to nafarelin testing in the polycystic ovary syndrome. *N Engl J Med* 1989;**320:**559.

Barth JH, et al: Spironolactone is an effective and well tolerated systemic antiandrogen therapy in hirsute women. *J Clin Endocrinol Metab* 1989; **68:**966.

Case Records of the Massachusetts General Hospital, Case 22-1988. *N Engl J Med* 1988;**318:**1449.

Cummings DC, et al: Treatment of hirsutism with spironolactone. *JAMA* 1982; **247:**1295.

Daly DC, et al: A randomized study of dexamethasone in ovulation induction with clomiphene citrate. *Fertil Steril* 1984;**41:**844.

Guthrie GP, et al: Adrenal androgen excess and defective 11β-hydroxylation in women with idiopathic hirsutism. *Arch Intern Med* 1982;**142:**729.

Kuttenn F, et al: Late-onset adrenal hyperplasia in hirsutism. *N Engl J Med* 1985;**313:**224.

Loughlin T, et al: Adrenal abnormalities in polycystic ovary syndrome. *J Clin Endocrinol Metab* 1986;**62:**142.

Pang S et al: Hirsutism, polycystic ovarian disease and ovarian 17-ketosteroid reductase deficiency. *N Engl J Med* 1987;**316:**1295.

Schriock E, Martin MC, Jaffe RB: Polycystic ovarian disease. *West J Med* 1985;**142:**519.

Serafini P, Lobo RA: The effects of spironolactone on adrenal steroidogenesis in hirsute women. *Fertil Steril* 1985;**44:**595.

Sonino N: The use of ketoconazole as in inhibitor of steroid production. *N Engl J Med* 1987;**317:**812.

Diabetes Mellitus | 10

Mara Lorenzi, MD

Diabetes mellitus is a common metabolic disorder. In the USA, about 3% of the population has documented diabetes. Another 3% has glucose intolerance. About 1 in 600 schoolchildren requires insulin. Diabetes is progressively more common with advancing age; by the ninth decade, about 50% of the population has glucose intolerance. The enormous social impact of diabetes is mostly a consequence of its chronic complications: in the USA, 5000 new annual cases of blindness, 4000 cases of end-stage renal disease, and 80% of major amputations are attributable to diabetes. Manifestations of accelerated atherosclerosis represent the cause of death for three-quarters of North America's diabetics, whereas only one-third of the general population will die of an atherosclerotic disease.

The hallmark of diabetes is fasting and/or postprandial hyperglycemia. Hyperglycemia results from insufficient insulin effect due to either decreased availability (insulin deficiency) or interference with its action (insulin resistance).

Insufficient insulin effect also alters lipid and protein metabolism, as well as other hormones, neurotransmitters, and mineral homeostasis. Uncontrolled diabetes is thus a state of widespread metabolic derangement.

STRUCTURE & PHARMACOKINETICS OF INSULIN

Insulin is a polypeptide hormone consisting of 51 amino acids (MW 5734) arranged in 2 chains (A and B) connected by 2 disulfide bridges. The A chain consists of 21 amino acids and has a disulfide bridge between positions 6 and 11; the B chain consists of 30 amino acids.

Insulin is synthesized in pancreatic B cells as a prohormone, proinsulin, arranged in a single chain of 86 amino acids. The proinsulin molecule undergoes enzymatic cleavage of 2 dipeptides at 2 sites and yields insulin and a 31-amino-acid segment called C-peptide (connecting peptide). At the time of secretion into the portal circula-

---

SOME ACRONYMS USED IN THIS CHAPTER

CSII	Continuous subcutaneous insulin injection
CST	Contraction stress test
DKA	Diabetic ketoacidosis
FPG	Fasting plasma glucose
GABA	γ–Aminobutyric acid
GAD	Glutamic acid decarboxylase
GFR	Glomerular filtration rate
GLUT	Glucose transporter
HDL	High–density lipoprotein
HHNK	Hyperglycemic hyperosmolar nonketotic (state)
ICA	Islet–cell antibody
IDDM	Insulin–dependent diabetes mellitus
IGT	Impaired glucose tolerance
LDL	Low–density lipoprotein
NIDDM	Non–insulin–dependent diabetes mellitus
NK	Natural killer (cell)
NPH	Neutral protamine Hagedorn (insulin)
NST	Nonstress test
OGTT	Oral glucose tolerance test
VLDL	Very low density lipoprotein

---

tion, insulin and C-peptide are present in equimolar quantities, accompanied by only a small amount of intact proinsulin that has escaped cleavage. Because of its substantial uptake by the liver and other target tissues, insulin has a much shorter circulatory half-life (3–5 minutes) than C-peptide (10–11 minutes) and proinsulin (17 minutes). Thus, in the peripheral circulation, C-peptide is present in concentrations 5–10 times higher than insulin, and proinsulin accounts for up to 20% of circulating immunoreactive insulin. Proinsulin has less than 10% of the biologic activity of insulin, and no biologic role has thus far been attributed to C-peptide. Proinsulin and C-peptide are both catabolized mainly by the kidney, whereas approximately half of secreted insulin is taken up by the liver at first passage. Of the insulin reaching the general circulation, approximately 40% is cleared by the kidneys.

INSULIN SECRETION

Insulin is continuously secreted by the B cells: at basal rate in the postabsorptive state (6–12 hours after a meal), at a suppressed rate during prolonged fast, and in larger quantities upon ingestion of nutrients. **Stimulants of insulin secretion** are glucose, amino acids (in particular leucine and arginine), glucagon, vagal stimulation, sulfonylureas, β-adrenergic stimulation, and enteric hormones. **Inhibitors of insulin release** are somatostatin, α-adrenergic stimulation, and drugs such as diazoxide, phenytoin, β-adrenergic blockers, vinblastine, and L-asparaginase (mostly affecting synthesis).

Basal levels of serum insulin in normal, nonobese humans vary between 5 and 20 μU/mL in the peripheral circulation and are 2–3 times higher in the portal vein. A circadian variability of levels is needed to maintain euglycemia, the highest levels being needed between 4 and 8 AM. This **dawn phenomenon** has been observed in both normal and diabetic individuals.

Basal pancreatic production of insulin is about 23.6 U/d in a nondiabetic man (1.73 m^2). About 45% of this insulin is extracted by the liver, providing a basal systemic delivery rate of about 12.5 U/d.

Postprandial levels of serum insulin in normal nonobese individuals vary somewhat, depending on caloric composition and distribution of the meal. A typical pattern is depicted in Fig 10–1. These curves represent the mean plasma glucose and serum insulin levels in normal individuals after ingestion of a 520-calorie breakfast composed of 60 g of carbohydrate, 25 g of protein, and 20 g of fat.

The maximal postprandial glucose increment is 40–50 mg/dL and occurs 30–40 minutes after beginning the meal. Levels return to basal by 90–120 minutes. Systemic insulin levels peak at 30–40 minutes and

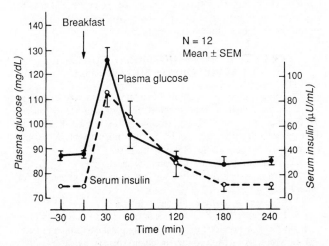

Figure 10–1. Plasma glucose and serum insulin following ingestion of a 520-kcal breakfast in normal nonobese individuals.

return to basal by 210–240 minutes. An early increment in portal insulin occurs only a few minutes after the entry of glucose into the duodenum and precedes by 5–10 minutes the increase in systemic levels. This early release of insulin depends on gastrointestinal factors and is crucial for the control of postprandial glucose levels.

The amount of insulin secreted in response to 3 daily meals in nondiabetic individuals is the equivalent of 30 U. Added to basal secretion, this brings the daily pancreatic production of insulin in the adult to approximately 50 U.

INSULIN RECEPTORS

The action of insulin is initiated through binding of the hormone to specific, high affinity receptors in the plasma membrane. The insulin receptor is composed of 2 identical α-subunits of 719 or 731 amino acids and 2 β-subunits of 620 amino acids. The α-subunits are extracellular and contain the insulin-binding site; the β-subunits span the plasma membrane and become phosphorylated when insulin binds to the α-subunits (autophosphorylation). The phosphorylated receptor has protein tyrosine kinase activity, ie, it phosphorylates endogenous proteins. This activity mediates most of insulin's biologic effects.

A characteristic of the insulin receptor that has a bearing on the altered carbohydrate metabolism of obesity and diabetes is the phenomenon of **down regulation**. Both in vivo and in vitro, exposure of cells to increasing concentrations of insulin results in time-dependent loss of insulin receptors, with a new steady-state being reached in 4–16 hours. Loss of insulin receptors is one mechanism leading to decreased insulin sensitivity and thus insulin resistance.

INSULIN ACTION & HORMONAL CONTROL OF CARBOHYDRATE METABOLISM

The crucial biologic function of insulin is to promote anabolism and inhibit catabolism. This action promotes storage of energy sources and building of structural tissue proteins. All tissues are therefore to some extent influenced by insulin, but the main targets of insulin action are the liver, muscle, and adipose tissue.

The **anabolic pathways** activated by insulin are

1. Glycolysis: glucose utilization and provision of precursors for fat and protein synthesis.

2. Glycogen synthetase: glycogen formation.

3. Lipoprotein lipase: hydrolysis of triglycerides carried by plasma lipoproteins to provide free fatty acids for uptake by adipose tissue.

4. Synthesis of triglycerides in adipose tissue and liver.

5. Ribosomal protein synthesis.

Table 10–1. Hormonal control of carbohydrate metabolism.

Decreases glucose

Insulin: Glucose transport across cell membranes, glucose metabolism, glycogen synthesis, lipogenesis, protein synthesis.

Growth hormone: Acute insulinlike action.

Somatostatin: Transient suppression of glucagon secretion.

Increases glucose

Growth hormone: Chronic decrease in glucose transport and metabolism. Enhancement of lipolysis, ketogenesis.

ACTH: Increase in glucocorticoids.

Glucocorticoids: Proteolysis, gluconeogenesis, lipolysis, ketogenesis, postreceptor insulin resistance.

Epinephrine and glucagon: Glycogenolysis, gluconeogenesis, lipolysis, ketogenesis.

Thyroxine: Glycogenolysis, gluconeogenesis.

Somatostatin: Decrease in insulin secretion.

The **catabolic pathways** inhibited by insulin are

1. Glycogenolysis (glycogen breakdown to yield glucose).

2. Gluconeogenesis (conversion of amino acids, lactate, and glycerol into glucose).

3. Lipolysis (mobilization of free fatty acids).

4. Oxidation of free fatty acids.

5. Formation of ketone bodies.

These catabolic pathways are instead stimulated by glucagon, the 29-amino acid polypeptide (MW 3485) synthesized and secreted by pancreatic A cells. It can thus be expected that at any time the relative concentrations of insulin and glucagon (the insulin:glucagon ratio) will govern the direction and net activity of these pathways. In the fasting state when provision of glucose must derive from the endogenous sources, the action of glucagon prevails. Glucagon represents the main defense of the body against hypoglycemia, which is in turn the main stimulus for glucagon secretion. In the fed state, secretion of insulin and postprandial hyperglycemia suppress glucagon secretion.

In addition to insulin and glucagon, several other hormones contribute to the modulation of carbohydrate metabolism. Most are insulin antagonists, and their mechanism of action and effects on circulating glucose levels are summarized in Table 10–1.

PHYSIOLOGY OF CARBOHYDRATE & FAT METABOLISM

Fasting State

The postabsorptive state (6–12 hours after a meal, overnight fast) is characterized by low insulin levels and sustained secretion of glucagon, growth hormone, and catecholamines. This hormonal milieu promotes fuel availability to tissues.

The peripheral insulin-sensitive tissues such as **fat and muscle** markedly diminish their glucose uptake (low insulin) and utilize as their main source of energy the circulating free fatty acids released from adipose tissue (growth hormone and catecholamine effects in presence of low insulin). Some of the free fatty acids reaching the liver are converted to ketone bodies. Ketogenesis depends on availability of free fatty acids and their rate of transport into mitochondria, which is regulated by carnitine acyltransferase (activated by the low insulin:glucagon ratio). Inside mitochondria, free fatty acids undergo β-oxidation and the acetyl-CoA molecules exceeding the capacity of the Krebs cycle are condensed to form β-hydroxybutyrate and acetoacetate. The third ketone body, acetone, derives from the non-enzymatic conversion of acetoacetate in the periphery. After an overnight fast, ketone bodies circulate in minute amounts (0.2–0.4 mmol/ L) and they are utilized mostly by muscle, although a minimal extraction by the brain has been observed.

For the **brain, other neural structures,** and **formed elements of the blood,** glucose uptake is insulin-independent and thus continues steadily in the fasting state. The amount of glucose utilized by these tissues is 1.1 mg/kg/min and represents 65–75% of the total basal glucose disposal rate, which amounts to approximately 1.6 mg/kg/ min. In order to maintain fasting glucose levels constant within the range of 70–100 mg/dL, the amount of glucose utilized is replaced to the circulating pool by the liver. Being endowed with the enzyme glucose-6-phosphatase, the liver is the only organ (in addition to the kidneys, whose role is quantitatively minor) able to release free glucose in the circulation. Hepatic glucose production is derived mostly from glycogenolysis (75%) and some from gluconeogenesis (25%); with prolonged fasting the relative contribution of gluconeogenesis progressively increases. The major driving force for hepatic glucose production is the low insulin:glucagon ratio.

Overall, basal levels of insulin serve a dual role: on one side they are sufficiently low to allow lipolysis, glycogenolysis, and gluconeogenesis to proceed; on the other their presence exerts a crucial restraining influence on the rate of these processes. In the absence of basal levels of insulin, hepatic glucose production and fat mobilization proceed beyond replacement rate and result respectively in fasting hyperglycemia and acceleration of ketogenesis.

Fed State

Upon ingestion of a carbohydrate meal, the hyperglycemia and prompt secretion of insulin inhibit growth hormone and glucagon secretion and suppress lipolysis and hepatic glucose production almost completely. The main circulating fuel is now glucose derived from ingested carbohydrates. This glucose serves the needs of insulin-independent tissues and is taken up for storage and oxidation by the insulin-sensitive tissues, especially muscle. Not all the absorbed glucose becomes available for peripheral tissues: approximately 30% is trapped by the liver, where it is used for glycogen synthesis, glyceride formation, and glycolysis. Overall, approximately two-thirds of a carbohydrate load is stored as fat and glycogen in hepatic and extra-hepatic tissues, and one-third is oxidized.

Glucose Transporters

Much of the physiology of glucose metabolism described above is regulated at the level of the plasma membrane. Being a polar molecule, glucose is transported across the lipid bilayer of the plasma membrane by special carriers: the Na^+-glucose cotransporter (brush border epithelial cells of the small intestine and proximal renal tubule) and the facilitative glucose transporters. Five isoforms of facilitative glucose transporters have been described: GLUT 1 (erythrocytes, other tissues), GLUT 2 (liver, pancreatic B cells), GLUT 3 (brain, other tissues), GLUT 4 (muscle, adipose tissue), and GLUT 5 (small intestine). GLUT 1 and 3 are ubiquitous and have a high affinity for glucose ($\simeq 1$ mmol/L); they probably mediate basal glucose uptake. In contrast, GLUT 4 is uniquely expressed in tissues (muscle and fat) responsible for insulin-mediated postprandial glucose uptake; accordingly it has a lower affinity for glucose ($\simeq 5$ mmol/L), and its translocation to the plasma membrane is greatly stimulated by insulin. GLUT 2 has an even lower affinity for glucose ($\simeq 15$ mmol/L), allowing pancreatic B cells to proportionately respond to increases in blood glucose levels and ensuring that at basal glucose concentrations glucose uptake is primarily into peripheral tissues rather than the liver.

DEFINITION & GENERAL PATHOPHYSIOLOGY OF DIABETES

The hallmark of diabetes is fasting hyperglycemia (plasma glucose > 140 mg/dL), postglucose hyperglycemia, or both. Within the natural history of the disease, hyperglycemia following a glucose load precedes the development of fasting hyperglycemia. Thus, if fasting hyperglycemia is not present, maximal diagnostic sensitivity is achieved by evaluation of the glycemic response to a pure glucose challenge (oral glucose tolerance test, OGTT). The sensitivity of OGTT is due to the fact that glucose uptake by fat and muscle (the major sites of disposal of an ingested glucose load) requires more insulin than that necessary for inhibition of hepatic glucose output (responsible for maintaining fasting glucose levels).

Thus, with mild insulin deficiency or resistance, plasma glucose may be elevated after a glucose load while fasting levels are still normal. With greater insulin deficiency or resistance, fasting plasma glucose will also become elevated but without significant increase in lipolysis (ie, no weight loss or ketosis). Finally, with severe insulin deficiency lipolysis, ketosis, and ultimately acidosis occur.

CAUSES OF DIABETES

The insufficient insulin action responsible for the hyperglycemia and metabolic derangement of diabetes may result from deficient production of insulin, resistance of target tissues to insulin's biologic effects, or both. Table 10–2 summarizes known causes of diabetes.

Idiopathic Destruction of Islet B Cells

Idiopathic destruction of pancreatic B cells is the basis of **type I insulin-dependent diabetes mellitus** (primary IDDM) not due to other causes. Type I diabetes is an autoimmune disease leading to the selective destruction of pancreatic B cells. Susceptibility is associated with the class II major histocompatibility complex, and the initial trigger may be viral or toxic injury to B cells.

A. Humoral Autoimmunity: Three main types of antibodies against islet-cell antigens are present at onset of primary IDDM and may precede clinical diabetes by several years, concomitant with a gradual loss of B-cell function. Islet-cell antibodies (ICAs) react to gangliosides in the cytoplasm of all islet cells. ICAs are present in up to 85% of type I diabetes at diagnosis, but their prevalence decreases with increasing duration of IDDM (20% positivity after 5 years) except when the disease is associated with other autoimmune endocrinopathies (Hashimoto's thyroiditis, Graves' disease, Addison's disease, ovarian failure, pernicious anemia). This finding has suggested the possibility of a purely autoimmune variant of diabetes that may account for 10–20% of all cases of primary IDDM. This form has distinct clinical and epidemiologic features: association with (and strong family history of) other autoimmune endocrinopathies, later mean age of onset (about 30 years), female preponderance, no seasonal variation in incidence. The prevalence of ICA is 0.5–1.7% in the population at large, 6–8% in nonobese diabetics treated with oral agents, and 3–12% in nonaffected first-degree relatives of patients with IDDM.

Highly selective against B cells, the 64K autoantibody reacts

Table 10–2. Causes of diabetes.

Deficient Insulin Production	Resistance to Insulin Action
Decreased islet B-cell mass	**Circulating insulin antagonists**
Pancreatic disease (pancreatectomy, relapsing pancreatitis, cystic fibrosis, hemochromatosis)	Counterregulatory hormone excess
	Antiinsulin receptor antibodies (type B syndrome with acanthosis nigricans)
Toxic destruction (streptozotocin, alloxan, rodenticide (Vacor), pentamidine)	Antiinsulin antibodies
Idiopathic destruction (autoimmune, ? virus, ? toxin, IDDM)	**Target tissue defects**
	Decreased number of insulin receptors (hyperinsulinism, obesity, type A syndrome with acanthosis nigricans)
Impaired islet B-cell secretion	
Hormonal (somatostatinoma, phechromocytoma)	Defects in insulin receptor function (genetic syndromes of extreme insulin resistance)
Drugs	Postreceptor defects (NIDDM, prolonged hyperglycemia; excess cortisol, growth hormone, progestins, estrogens)
Diuretics (thiazides, furosemide, chlortalidone, metolazone)	
Antihypertensives (clonidine, propranolol, diazoxide)	
Calcium channel blockers (occasionally)	
Phenothiazines	
Tricyclic antidepressants	
Diphenylhydantoin	
L-Asparaginase	
Isoniazid	
Genetic syndromes (hypothalamic and other central nervous system lesions, Chapter 1)	
Idiopathic (selective unresponsiveness to glucose; early IDDM and NIDDM)	
Abnormal B-cell secretory product	
Abnormal insulin molecule	
Incomplete conversion of proinsulin to insulin	

against a 64K B cell antigen, glutamic acid decarboxylase (GAD), involved in the synthesis of the inhibitory neurotransmitter (GABA). Only the pancreatic B cells and a subpopulation of central nervous system neurons express high levels of GAD; patients with the rare neurologic disease called stiff-man syndrome have high titers of autoantibodies against GAD and a high incidence of IDDM.

The third autoantibody, again highly selective against B cells, is an antibody to insulin, detected before initiation of insulin therapy.

B. Cellular Autoimmunity: Lymphocytes (NK or T cells) rather than autoantibodies are the primary agents of B-cell killing. The histology of the islets of Langerhans in patients who died soon after the onset of IDDM reveals a striking 'insulitis': inflammatory infiltrates consisting of macrophages, neutrophils, lymphocytes, and rare plasma cells.

C. Genetics and Environment: Type I (autoimmune) diabetes is more common in patients with particular cell-surface HLA antigens. These antigens are glycoproteins located on all cells except sperm and red blood cells. They allow the immune system to distinguish ''self'' from invading bacteria or viruses.

Several alleles at the contiguous DR and DQ loci of the HLA region are associated with IDDM. Haplotypes known to confer susceptibility to IDDM in Caucasians are DR4/DQw8 (formerly DQw3.2), DR3/DQw2, and DR1/DQw1.1. Common to the 3 DQ alleles is the fact that they have an amino acid other than aspartic acid at position 57 of the β-chain. In contrast, the haplotype DR2/DQw1.2 confers protection against IDDM, and the DQw1.2 allele has aspartic acid (a negatively charged amino acid) at position 57. The important role of the amino acid present at position 57 of the β-chain of the DQ molecule is attributed to its potential effect on the conformation of the cleft that binds antigen and, hence, on the presentation of antigen to T lymphocytes. The fact, however, that analysis for aspartic acid does not entirely account for susceptibility to IDDM, especially in non-whites, suggests that other alleles or genes outside the HLA region contribute to susceptibility.

Since concordance for IDDM is only 50% in identical twins as well as in siblings sharing HLA haplotypes, environmental factors must also play a role. Among viruses, mumps, rubella, and coxsackie B_4 have been associated with cases of IDDM. Environmental toxins have been postulated but as yet not identified.

D. Prevention of Type I Diabetes: The characteristics of type I diabetes (autoimmune disease preceded by an often long period of subclinical deterioration of B-cell function, predictable by immune-related markers in high-risk individuals such as first-degree relatives of type I diabetic patients) have prompted consideration of immune intervention therapy to halt or prevent B-cell destruction. The 1990 Position Statement of the American Diabetes Association recommends that intervention be attempted only in the context of defined clinical studies with Institutional Review Board oversight.

Selective Loss of B Cells Secretory Response to Glucose

This occurs while responses to nonglucose stimuli are intact or only partially diminished and is typical of mild **type II non–insulin-**

dependent diabetes mellitus (NIDDM). It also occurs in the early stages of diabetes of children who later develop the full picture of B-cell destruction and IDDM. It may represent an early sign of B-cell damage irrespective of the etiologic process.

Decreased Number of Insulin Receptors

This feature of hyperinsulinemic states (obesity, islet-cell adenoma) results from receptor down-regulation. Correction of the hyperinsulinemia (hypocaloric diet, tumor ablation) results in correction of the receptor defect.

A distinct syndrome of severe insulin resistance has been described in young women with ovarian dysfunction and virilization in addition to acanthosis nigricans (type A syndrome). These patients have no immunologic abnormalities—in contrast to type B—and the molecular basis for their reduced concentration of insulin receptors resides, at least in some cases, in point mutations that retard transport to the plasma membrane of insulin receptors.

Defects in Insulin Receptor Function

In genetic syndromes of extreme insulin resistance (type A syndrome, lipoatrophic diabetes, leprechaunism, Rabson-Mendenhall syndrome) mutations in the insulin receptor lead to decreased insulin binding, decreased tyrosine-specific protein kinase activity, or both.

Type II diabetic patients have decreased tyrosine kinase activity of the insulin receptor in liver, adipose tissue, and muscle. However, this defect is acquired and is largely reversible by effective antidiabetic treatment.

Postreceptor Defects

These account for most of the insulin resistance of type II diabetic patients, in whom the main abnormality of insulin-mediated glucose disposal is decreased muscle glycogen synthesis; this may precede overt carbohydrate intolerance. The severity of postreceptor defects can be lessened by effective antidiabetic treatment.

Abnormal B-Cell Secretory Products

These products are very rare causes of diabetes. An **abnormal insulin molecule** has been described in 6 families. In all cases, a single amino acid substitution within the receptor-binding region of the insulin molecule leads to very low binding potency (5% of normal). The disorder is inherited in an autosomal dominant pattern and results in mild diabetes with hyperinsulinemia but with normal sensitivity to exogenous insulin.

Incomplete conversion of proinsulin to insulin has been reported in 4 families. The clinical picture is normal or mildly abnormal carbohydrate tolerance and hyperinsulinemia (due to elevated levels of proinsulin cross-reacting in the assay) but with normal sensitivity to exogenous insulin.

Antiinsulin Receptor Antibodies

These antibodies have been found in patients with extreme insulin resistance, acanthosis nigricans, and other clinical (or laboratory) features of immunologic disease. It is called syndrome of insulin resistance and acanthosis nigricans, type B. In some patients, endogenous hyperinsulinemia is sufficient to maintain normal or only mildly impaired glucose tolerance; in others, clinical diabetes results. The resistance to insulin can be extraordinary: 15,000 U/h may fail to normalize glycemia. Treatment must be directed to the immune system.

Many of these causes of diabetes are not mutually exclusive but contribute in temporal sequence or in additive fashion to the clinical picture of diabetes. For these reasons the currently recommended classification of diabetes (see below) is based on clinical features more than on pathogenesis. However, the possible causes and aggravating factors must always be considered when approaching a diabetic patient.

CLASSIFICATION & CLINICAL FEATURES

The current classification of diabetes was formulated in 1979 by the National Diabetes Data Group of the NIH. The criteria guiding the classification are mostly clinical. The 6 recommended classes encompassing diabetes and other categories of glucose intolerance are summarized in Table 10–3.

Insulin-Dependent Diabetes Mellitus (IDDM, Type I)

Although it may occur at any age, this form of diabetes has its peak incidence at around puberty. The basic lesion is destruction of islet B-cells, and the clinical hallmark is insulin deficiency and proneness to ketosis.

A. Onset: The onset of illness in youngsters appears to be quite abrupt, with an average reported duration of symptoms of 3–4 weeks. The appearance of islet-cell antibodies and of selective unresponsiveness of B cells to glucose may precede by years the full picture of diabetes and the onset of symptoms.

B. Symptoms and Signs: The presenting symptoms and signs depend upon the severity and duration of insulin deficiency and thus intensity of ketosis. Full-blown ketoacidosis is common, especially in children: the patient is drowsy or unconscious, respiration is deep and sighing (Kussmaul breathing), the breath smells of acetone, there may be circulatory collapse due to dehydration, the skin and mucous membranes are dry, the face may be flushed, and the temperature may be low even in the presence of infection. Other signs of infection should be searched for, since the metabolic decompensation may be precipitated by an intercurrent illness.

In almost all patients it is possible to elicit a history of at least some weeks of polyuria, enuresis, polydipsia, weight loss, and fatigue. The polyuria results from the osmotic diuresis induced by glycosuria. Despite marked hyperglycemia and glycosuria the polyuria may not become dramatic until the onset of ketosis. When high levels of ketones accumulate in blood, they are excreted in the urine in large quantities, worsening the solute diuresis. When the onset is less acute, the above symptoms are milder and often accompanied by pruritus vulvae, balanitis, blurred vision due to osmotic changes in refraction, paresthesias and cramps in the legs, and skin infection.

C. Remission Phase: A few weeks after treatment is initiated, about 60–70% of patients newly diagnosed with IDDM experience a remission phase (honeymoon period) during which little or no insulin will be required. This phenomenon is probably due to a transient recovery of B-cell function and may persist for weeks or even months. Remissions lasting longer than 2 years cast doubts on the diagnosis of type I diabetes.

D. Extent of Insulin Deficiency: The extent of insulin deficiency tends to increase with time; although during the first few years of IDDM many patients have minimal but some residual insulin secretion, after 10 years almost all patients are completely insulin deficient.

Non–Insulin-Dependent Diabetes Mellitus (NIDDM, Type II)

Although NIDDM does occur in young people (autosomal dominant in families with "maturity onset diabetes of the young," youngsters of Indian- and Spanish-American background), this form of diabetes is most common in adults. Critical risk factors are obesity and NIDDM in a first-degree relative. The strong genetic contribution to NIDDM is documented by the 90% concordance between identical twins and by the estimate that 43% of first-degree relatives of patients with NIDDM will ultimately have the disease.

A. Onset: The onset of type II diabetes is generally gradual. The pathogenesis involves a combination of diminished insulin secretion and varying degrees of target tissue resistance to insulin action. These abnormalities, even when resulting in severe fasting hyperglycemia (300–400 mg/dL) do not routinely lead to ketosis. Thus, patients may be asymptomatic for years and discovered through a routine blood or urine test.

Table 10–3. Classification of diabetes.

Class	Former Terminology	Clinical Characteristics	Associated Factors	Pathology	Prevalence (% of All Diabetics)
Insulin-dependent diabetes mellitus (IDDM, type I)	Juvenile onset, ketosis-prone; brittle diabetes	Dependency upon exogenous insulin to prevent ketosis and preserve life.	Etiology based on combination of autoimmunity, genetic factors (HLA association, twin concordance 50%), environmental agents; 10–20% of cases have other autoimmune endocrinopathies.	Insulitis, destruction of islet B cells	10–20%
Non–insulin-dependent diabetes mellitus (NIDDM, type II)	Adult onset, ketosis-resistant, stable diabetes	Not insulin-dependent or ketosis prone under routine circumstances. Age at onset often > 40. Insulin levels may be high, normal, or low.	Strong genetic component not HLA associated, twin concordance > 90%, autosomal dominant inheritance in some families (former MODY: maturity-onset diabetes of the young).		80–90%
Nonobese NIDDM				Modestly reduced B-cell mass when compared with weight-	< 30% of NIDDM
Obese NIDDM			Obesity.		>70% of NIDDM

			matched controls
			Characteristic of primary condition
Diabetes associated with another condition or syndrome (pancreatic disease; hormonal; drug or chemical induced, insulin-receptor abnormality; genetic)	Secondary diabetes	Depending on etiology, may be IDDM or NIDDM.	Characteristic of primary condition.
Impaired glucose tolerance	Chemical diabetes; latent diabetes	Fasting glucose not diagnostic for diabetes, OGTT between normal and diabetic. ?Increased susceptibility to atherosclerotic disease.	Etiology unclear; may evolve in NIDDM or IDDM, remain stable for years, revert to normal.
Gestational diabetes	Gestational diabetes	Glucose intolerance that develops during pregnancy. Associated with ↑ perinatal complications and ↑ risk for DM within 5 years.	Failure to compensate for the insulin resistance that normally develops from second trimester of pregnancy.

(Continued)

Table 10–3. (cont'd) Classification of diabetes.

Class	Former Terminology	Clinical Characteristics	Associated Factors	Pathology	Prevalence (% of All Diabetics)
Previous abnormalities of glucose tolerance	Latent diabetes	Abnormalities of glucose tolerance secondary to pregnancy, obesity, trauma, stress, which have disappeared.			
Potential abnormalities of glucose tolerance	Prediabetes	Persons with normal glucose tolerance who are at risk of DM because of associated factors	↑ Risk for IDDM: positive ICA (islet cell antibody), identical twin with IDDM, HLA-haploidentical sibling with IDDM, offspring of an IDDM diabetic ↑ Risk for NIDDM: identical twin or first-degree relative with NIDDM, mother of a neonate weighing > 9 lbs, obese individuals, member of a racial group with higher prevalence of NIDDM.		

B. Symptoms and Signs: When symptoms and signs appear, they are subtle and may be attributed to other causes: dryness of the mouth, sense of fatigue, frequency due to polyuria, paresthesias, impotence, menstrual irregularities, and skin infections. A very common symptom especially in obese women is pruritus vulvae and candidal vulvovaginitis. In long-standing undiagnosed cases, patients may present with symptoms or signs of the chronic complications: cataract, vitreous hemorrhage due to retinopathy, glaucoma due to rubeosis, neuropathic lesions, foot lesions due to neuropathy or ischemia, claudication, and angina.

Although patients with type II diabetes are resistant to ketosis under normal circumstances, they may acutely decompensate upon intercurrent illness, trauma, or stress. Thus, on occasion, patients admitted to hospitals in ketoacidosis can later be successfully managed with diet and oral agents and thus be classified as having NIDDM.

The **severity of hyperglycemia** in untreated type II diabetes is highly variable. For NIDDM to become manifest, some disturbance in insulin secretion must have developed in addition to insulin resistance. This results first in abnormal glucose tolerance and then in modest fasting hyperglycemia (<180 mg/dL), which is readily responsive to maneuvers directed at increasing insulin sensitivity (caloric restriction, prudent diet, exercise) and, eventually, insulin secretion (small doses of sulfonylureas). If this stage goes untreated, hyperglycemia worsens and further exhausts insulin secretory capacity. The combination of protracted hyperglycemia and relatively low insulin exacerbates postreceptor defects in insulin action and hence insulin resistance. At this stage, fasting glucose levels are often greater than 300 mg/dL, and at least temporary insulin replenishment may be necessary to ameliorate the postreceptor defect and reestablish responsiveness to dietary intervention and sulfonylureas.

LABORATORY FEATURES

Circulating Glucose

The interpretation of glucose values for diagnostic purposes has been standardized for measurements performed in **venous plasma**. In practice, however, 2 parameters may differ: site of collection (venous, capillary, arterial) and type of specimen (plasma, serum, whole blood).

Table 10–4 summarizes the relationships among glucose measurement per unit volume (dL) in the respective specimen.

Capillary blood obtained by fingerstick is widely used. Although whole blood is applied to the surface of the strip, the strip creates an

Table 10–4. Glucose measurements in different specimen types.

Site of Collection	Type of Specimen	Difference from Venous Plasma	Reason for Difference
Venous	Plasma	**Standard**	
Venous	Serum	Same	
Venous	Whole blood	10–15% lower	Glucose distribution space is smaller owing to presence of red blood cell structural components
Arterial	Plasma	Same if fasting; 20–40% higher if postprandial	Increased glucose extraction by tissues widens arteriovenous difference
Capillary	Plasma	Same if fasting; 20–40% higher if postprandial	Glucose extraction by tissues ongoing

ultrafiltrate that results in only plasma actually coming into contact with the reagent.

The accuracy of glucose measurement in any type of specimen depends on prevention of the continuous utilization of glucose by red and other blood cells (7% decrease in glucose in 1 hour). Thus, whole blood glucose determinations must be performed promptly after specimen collection; plasma or serum from blood without preservative must be separated from the cells or the clot within a half-hour after the blood is drawn. Glycolysis can be prevented and glucose stabilized for up to 24 hours at room temperature by adding fluoride ions to the specimen (gray top vacutainers).

Chemical determinations of glucose in clinical laboratories are performed by enzymatic methods (hexokinase, glucose oxidase) that are highly specific for glucose. Glucose oxidase is the reagent present in the strips used for home monitoring.

The timing and circumstances of blood glucose measurement should be standardized in order to derive meaningful information.

For diagnosis of diabetes: fasting glucose and eventually OGTT.

For management: preprandial and 2 hours postprandial glucose.

A. Fasting Plasma Glucose: The measurement of fasting glucose yields information on the capability of basal levels of insulin to control glycogenolysis and gluconeogenesis and thus to prevent fasting hyperglycemia.

Determination of fasting plasma glucose is the first procedure to be performed when entertaining a diagnosis of diabetes. The patient is kept on usual average diet and, after an overnight fast (10–16 hours), blood is drawn in the morning.

Interpretation: Less than 115 mg/dL is normal.

Between 115 and 140 mg/dL may be *compatible with diabetes*; perform glucose tolerance test and determine glycosylated hemoglobin.

Greater than 140 mg/dL is *indicative of diabetes mellitus*; the test should be repeated once for confirmation (OGTT is contraindicated).

B. Oral Glucose Tolerance Test: This test is intended to measure insulin-mediated disposal of a glucose load, as a result of both adequate secretion and action of the hormone. Although 75 g of pure glucose do not mimic a balanced meal, the test is constructed to achieve maximal sensitivity, useful for diagnostic and epidemiologic purposes.

OGTT is indicated when (1) fasting plasma glucose is borderline (115–140 mg/dL), and (2) fasting plasma glucose is normal but patient has symptoms compatible with a complication of diabetes (retinopathy, neuropathy, hypertriglyceridemia).

OGTT is contraindicated when fasting plasma glucose values are 140 mg/dL or greater on more than one occasion, since they already establish the diagnosis of diabetes.

1. Patient preparation–After 3 days or more of a normal diet including at least 150 g of carbohydrates per day, in the morning after an overnight fast of between 10 and 16 hours, 75 g of an aqueous solution of glucose is given. The various commercially prepared cola-flavored carbonated test drinks are convenient to use and more palatable than a pure glucose solution.

Blood samples are drawn at 0, 30, 60, 90, and 120 minutes.

In pregnant women, the test dose is 100 g of glucose. Blood is drawn at 0, 1, 2, and 3 hours.

Some patients vomit after the test drink. The test is invalid and must be repeated.

2. Interpretation–(a) **Normal** (in nonpregnant adult): plasma glucose at 30, 60, and 90 minutes < 200 mg/dL *and* plasma glucose at 120 minutes < 140 mg/dL.

(b) **Indicative of impaired glucose tolerance (IGT)**: if at least one of the values at 30, 60, or 90 minutes is > 200 mg/dL *and* the value at 120 minutes is between 140 and 200 mg/dL. Glucose tolerance may fluctuate in this group, and there is a 1–5% annual progression to type II diabetes; cumulative progression is about 25%.

(c) **Indicative of diabetes mellitus**: if any one of the 30, 60, and 90 minute values *and* the value at 120 minutes is > 200 mg/dL.

The criteria for diagnosis of diabetes during pregnancy (**gestational diabetes**) are stricter than outlined above. During pregnancy, even mild diabetes becomes a significant risk factor for fetal morbidity and mortality. Thus, the OGTT is performed with 100 g of glucose, and it indicates gestational diabetes when 2 or more of the following values (in mg/dL) are reached or exceeded: fasting 105; 1 hour 190; 2 hours 165; 3 hours 145.

C. Preprandial and 2-Hour Postprandial Glucose: These determinations are crucial to optimize treatment in known diabetics. Most generally they are obtained by patients themselves through home-monitoring techniques. In healthy individuals, plasma glucose values have returned to baseline levels by between 90 and 120 minutes after a meal; thus both preprandial and 2-hour postprandial values are within the range of fasting values.

Glycosuria

Glycosuria appears when the blood glucose level exceeds the renal threshold for reabsorption of glucose. This normally lies between 150 and 170 mg/dL but may be lower in renal tubular disease or raised in diabetics to above 300 mg/dL, so that glycosuria may be absent in these patients despite markedly elevated blood glucose levels. Glycosuria not associated with hyperglycemia occurs in the following nondiabetic conditions: pregnancy, Fanconi's syndrome, renal glycosuria, and nephrotic syndromes.

Semiquantitative tests for glycosuria are based either on the reaction with glucose oxidase as in the dipsticks (Diastix, Keto-Diastix) or on the copper reduction methods as in the Clinitest tablets. Quantitative urinary glucose determinations are seldom necessary. High glucose concentrations increase urinary specific gravity and osmolality; if necessary, the glucose concentration can be determined and its contribution to osmolality calculated:

$$\text{(Glucose in mg/dL)/18} = \text{mOsm/L}$$

Measurements of urinary glucose in the management of the diabetic patient are being abandoned in favor of the more informative and accurate approach offered by blood glucose monitoring.

Glycosylated Hemoglobin (Glycohemoglobin, HbA₁)

During the 120-day life span of the red cell, hemoglobulin A becomes glycosylated owing to the nonenzymatic, largely irreversible attachment of a molecule of glucose to the N-terminal valine of the B-chain and to ϵ-amino groups of lysines of both A and B chains. The degree of glycosylation is directly proportionate to the level of glucose in the blood, and the amount of glycohemoglobin present in blood is a reflection of the average blood glucose level over the preceding 4–8 weeks. Thus, the periodic determination of glycosylated hemoglobin has become a useful adjunct in the monitoring of diabetic patients and it has been shown to result in sustained improvement of metabolic control.

Since glycohemoglobin levels are still normal when OGTT is frankly diabetic, glycohemoglobin represents a less sensitive approach to diagnosis and should definitely not be employed for detection of gestational diabetes. In nonpregnant adults with borderline fasting glucose (115–140 mg/dL), a glycohemoglobin measurement complements the information obtained with the OGTT by detecting the extent of hyperglycemia present under routine daily circumstances.

Measurement of glycohemoglobin is most accurately performed by means of **boronate affinity chromatography**. The procedure is based on the specific affinity of phenylboronic acid resins for *cis*-diol groups such as those found in glucose. If glucose is attached to a protein (eg, hemoglobin), the resin will separate glycosylated from nonglycosylated species.

This method avoids errors inherent in procedures based on charge (cation-exchange column chromatography). Sources of such errors include (1) temperature sensitivity, (2) exclusion of non–N-terminal glycosylation from the measurement, (3) inclusion instead of reversible glucose-hemoglobin adducts (labile fraction), (4) interference by hemoglobins having a charge similar to the glycosylated fraction (eg, HbF), and (6) underestimation of glycosylation of HbS and HbC, which, owing to their more positive charge, elute from the cation exchange resin with the main HbA peak rather than with the faster glycosylated hemoglobin.

Other techniques used to measure glycohemoglobin are electrophoretic separation based on isoelectric focusing and, rarely, colorimetric methods.

The result for glycohemoglobin is expressed as a percentage of total hemoglobin. Normal range is 5–7% (inquire about specific range in your laboratory); values at 8–10% call for optimization of metabolic control, and values above 10% require intensification of treatment.

Glycosylated Serum Proteins (Fructosamine)

Measurement of glycosylated serum proteins has been advocated for the monitoring of short-term changes in glycemic control and thus as a complement to glycohemoglobin. Because the half-life of serum proteins (average 17 days) is shorter than that of hemoglobin (average 60 days), fructosamine levels reflect glycemia over a shorter period of time (1–3 weeks). The colorimetric test for fructosamine is based on the ability of ketoamines (glucose-protein linkage) to reduce nitroblue tetrazolium at alkaline pH. Normal range is 1.5–2.7 mmol/L.

Despite the ease of analysis, the fructosamine assay has not become widely used. The only reliable guide for changes in treatment remains blood glucose monitoring, and the goal of obtaining an integrated picture of glycemia over time is well served by determination of glycohemoglobin.

Ketone Bodies & Anion Gap

The ketone bodies acetoacetate and β-hydroxybutyrate are produced by the liver from oxidation of circulating free fatty acids. Acetone results from the peripheral nonenzymatic conversion of acetoacetate. Extent of ketone body formation is modulated by the ratio of counterregulatory hormones and insulin levels, a high ratio being ketogenic. Thus, independent of the presence of diabetes, ketone bodies are formed during prolonged fasting, in acute febrile illness, in toxic states with vomiting and diarrhea, in cachexia, and following anesthesia and surgery. Only in severe insulin deficiency is hepatic formation of ketone bodies (which are strong organic acids) grossly excessive and results in diabetic ketoacidosis (DKA).

A. Determination Methods for Ketones: The most common method for estimating the degree of ketonemia and ketonuria involves the use of nitroprusside tablets (Acetest) or reagent strips (Ketostix) and can thus be performed at the bedside. With Acetest tablets, the test is performed by placing a drop of urine, serum, plasma, or whole blood on a tablet. The result is read after 30 seconds with urine, 2 minutes with plasma or serum, and 10 minutes with whole blood (remove clotted blood from tablet before comparing to color chart). The reaction is positive if the tablet develops a color varying from lavender to deep purple; in this case serial dilutions of the specimen must be performed until the highest dilution yielding a frankly positive reaction.

B. Misleading Ketone Results: False-positives are rarely of concern: sulfobromophthalein and phenylketones react with the reagents but they are uncommonly present; levodopa may, however, cause a false-positive result. The important pitfall of the nitroprusside reagent (false-negatives) is that it reacts best with acetoacetate (sensitive to 5–10 mg/dL), reacts much less with acetone (5–10 times less sensitive), and does not react with β-hydroxybutyrate. This is a potential source of problems. While under circumstances of mild ketosis (fasting, suboptimal insulin effect), the ratio of β-hydroxybutyrate to acetoacetate is about 2:1 and the latter ketone body is well represented, in situations of prolonged severe insulin deficiency (DKA) and poor tissue oxygenation (lactic acidosis complicating DKA), β-hydroxybutyrate will be the prevalent or exclusive ketone body present. The nitroprusside reaction may thus be only weakly positive or even negative in the presence of dangerous ketosis. Occasionally the positivity of tests for serum ketones may become stronger as the treatment of ketoacidosis is under way and the patient is improving. This paradox is explained by the fact that, as the acidosis is reduced, some β-hydroxybutyrate is converted to acetoacetate, which is readily detected by the nitroprusside reagent.

C. The Anion Gap—Ketoacidosis Versus Lactic Acidosis: The suspicion of ketoacidosis should arise if hyperglycemia is found with a low serum bicarbonate (HCO_3) and increased anion gap. The anion gap [$Na - (Cl + HCO_3)$] is normally 8–16 mEq/L; in significant ketoacidosis, it is often over 30 mEq/L. Although there are other causes of metabolic acidosis with increased anion gap—lactic acidosis, uremia, ingestion of toxins (salicylates, methanol, ethylene glycol, paraldehyde)—these are *not* accompanied by significant hyperglycemia (plasma glucose < 200 mg/dL) and have other differential clinical and laboratory features. In uncomplicated diabetic ketoacidosis, lactate levels—which normally are < 1.5 mmol/L or 13.5 mg/dL (mmol × 9)—may be mildly elevated to 2–4 mmol/L and correlate with the extent of volume contraction and the degree of acidosis, which prevents tissue conversion of lactate to pyruvate. Lactate levels characteristic of true lactic acidosis (more than 7 mmol/L) are encountered in ketoacidosis only upon presence of complicating factors such as severe hypotension, cardiac events, hepatic disease, and biguanide administration.

D. Quantitation of Ketosis: Although quantitation of ketone bodies cannot be precise, an approximation may be reached by knowing that the reagent is positive to 0.5–1 mmol/L of acetoacetate: thus, a positivity at 1:8 dilution will indicate approximately 5–6 mmol/L of acetoacetate. This will be multiplied by 3 to take into account the contribution of the unmeasurable β-hydroxybutyrate. Such rough estimate will be compared with the calculated anion gap to verify that the latter is in fact accounted for by ketone bodies. Although serum acetone concentrations are markedly elevated in patients with diabetic ketoacidosis, this ketone is not an acid and is readily excreted in breath and urine.

Proteinuria & Microalbuminuria

Excretion of total protein in urine of healthy individuals is about 100 mg/24 h, and albumin represents ≈10% of this amount. Diabetic patients excreting > 500 mg total protein per 24 hours are diagnosed to have clinical nephropathy. Their urine tests positive to commercial protein-testing sticks (eg, Albustix), and their albumin excretion rate is > 250 mg/24 h, corresponding to 50% of total urine protein excretion. Hence, diabetic renal disease leads not only to increased total protein excretion but also to a disproportionate increase in the filtration of albumin (a polyanion) versus other molecules. This reflects progressive loss of the fixed negative electrical charge of the glomerular membrane.

Sensitive immunoassays make it possible to document that patients without overt proteinuria may have excessive urinary albumin excretion (30–250 mg/24 h; microalbuminuria). Albumin may represent up to 22% of total urinary protein. Whether low levels of microalbuminuria predict clinical nephropathy is still debated; levels > 80 mg/24 h are associated with abnormal glomerular structure, thus reflecting early renal lesions.

Causes of proteinuria not related to diabetic glomerular disease are physical exercise, dehydration, stress, febrile illness, exposure to cold, posture (orthostatic proteinuria, occurs in 3–5% of healthy young adults), and tubular disease (renal tubular acidosis, Fanconi's syndrome, pyelonephritis). The possible presence of any such situation must be considered when interpreting the meaning of proteinuria in a diabetic patient. In particular, periodic follow-up should be performed when the patient is under basal conditions (not during hospitalization for intercurrent illness).

Insulin & C-Peptide

Determinations of circulating insulin and C-peptide levels are not warranted for the diagnosis or management of diabetes. However, they are useful tests in the diagnostic workup of hypoglycemia.

Antiinsulin Antibodies

Patients receiving insulin who appear to have insulin resistance (insulin > 100 U/d) may have developed significant IgG antibodies against insulin. These patients ordinarily have been receiving combined beef/pork or less well purified insulins. Determination of antiinsulin antibodies is generally not required, since the patient is ordinarily empirically switched to a human or purified pork insulin preparation.

Islet-Cell Antibodies (ICA)

These antibodies may herald islet B-cell destruction and insulin deficiency and thus be a marker for type I diabetes. The assay for ICA should be performed by standardized methodology and possibly calibrated by participation in a proficiency testing program.

TREATMENT OF DIABETES

The ultimate goal of treatment is prevention of the long-term complications of diabetes. The knowledge at hand suggests that these may result from the chronically abnormal metabolic milieu, well reflected in the severity of the hyperglycemia. Thus, the all-encompassing target is normalization of glucose levels, while avoiding frequent or profound hypoglycemia.

Achieving good metabolic control is possible only through constant input from the patient. The patient therefore requires knowledge about the disease and methods for monitoring glycemic responses to daily events and specific interventions. *Thus, every patient diagnosed with any form of diabetes should be offered comprehensive education, including the use of self-monitoring of blood glucose.* Intensive education is not an intrusion upon patient's time but rather an investment. Well-educated patients experience fewer acute hospitalizations and may avoid chronic complications.

EDUCATION & SELF-MONITORING OF GLUCOSE

The material should be taught at the level of patient's comprehension but in a dialectic fashion (ie, no monologs or mere distribution of pamphlets). The content should focus on the specific form of diabetes manifested by the patient. Diabetes education has 2 phases, the first aimed at stabilizing the metabolic status and the second at optimizing control.

Information for Initial Stabilization

1. General concepts of insulin deficiency or insulin resistance and their consequences, significance of ketones, testing for ketones in urine.

2. Concepts and specifics of caloric and carbohydrate content of meals (see below, under Diet) and importance of consistency from day to day in meal pattern.

3. Pharmacokinetics of insulin preparations chosen for therapy (see below, under Insulin Therapy). The timing of action is best demonstrated with simple graphs.

4. Techniques for self-administration of insulin. When two types of insulin are mixed in the same syringe, the short-acting (Regular) should be drawn first in order to avoid contamination of the vial with the absorption-retarding agent present in long-acting insulins. The site of injection should be rotated in order to prevent fibrosis or hypertrophy of the adipose tissue; the injection should be made subcutaneously (not intradermally, because it is painful and not absorbed, and not intramuscularly, because absorption is accelerated). Among the best insulin syringes is the B-D Ultrafine, providing the finest needles.

5. Self-monitoring of blood glucose. This procedure has replaced urine testing for all patients. The direct information derived from blood testing makes the patient aware of the relationship between blood glucose levels and symptoms and helps guide therapeutic adjustments.

Obtain a drop of blood from a fingertip (the sides are less painful than the center). The finger does not need to be disinfected; if this is done, the alcohol must be allowed to dry before the fingerstick to avoid dilution of blood and spuriously low glucose readings. The fingerstick is relatively painless when a small mechanical device (Autolet, Monoject, Penlet, ExacTech) fitted with disposable lancets is used. The drop of blood is placed on the reagent pad (glucose oxidase) of a strip and allowed to react for the appropriate time. Results are read either by visual comparison with a color chart or by meters providing a digital read-out. The latter are particularly useful for patients with failing sight. Table 10–5 provides a sample of the strips and meters most widely used.

During the period of stabilization, patients are requested to perform blood glucose monitoring 4 times a day: before breakfast, lunch, and dinner and at bedtime. This guides initial insulin adjustments, which should aim toward blood glucose levels of 80–140 at the above times of testing. The target blood glucose levels are increased if the patient has significant or frequent hypoglycemia.

Adjustments should be made by 1–2 U of insulin at a time, following guidelines from Table 10–7, but simplified for preprandial targets only. The patient should be encouraged to establish telephone contact if a problem or question arises.

6. Hypoglycemia. The patient should be familiar with symptoms and signs of hypoglycemia, triggering events, prevention, and treatment (see below, under Complications of Insulin Therapy).

Table 10–5. Blood glucose monitors.

Strip for Visual Reading (Manufacturer)	Meter (Manufacturer)
Chemstrips bG (Boehringer Mannheim)	Accu-Check bG (Bio-Dynamics)
Gucostix (Ames)	Glucometer II (Ames)
Diascan (Home Diagnostics)	Diascan S (Home Diagnostics)
Trend (British American Medical)	Beta Scan Audio* (British American Medical)
	ExacTech Pen Sensor† (Medisense)
	One Touch† (Life Scan)

*Audible read-out of test results.
†Procedure requires no timing, wiping, or blotting.

Information for Optimization of Diabetic Control

1. Exercise and its impact on glycemic control should be discussed (see below, under Exercise).

2. In insulin-dependent patients, the frequency of home monitoring may be increased to 7 times a day (preprandial and 2 hours postprandial) for 2–3 weeks in order to obtain a comprehensive pattern of daily glucose excursions and quantify the individual's response to various carbohydrates, physical activity, and daily stresses. This exercise results in fine-tuning of the overall regimen and invaluable self-knowledge.

TREATMENT OF TYPE I DIABETES

Diet

The aim is to achieve smooth glycemic control and to reduce the risk of cardiovascular disease. The general population has been advised to eat less fat and more unprocessed carbohydrates and these recommendations should be extended to diabetic patients.

When prescribing the diet for a diabetic patient, 3 aspects should be addressed: (1) caloric content, (2) proportion of basic nutrients and optimal sources, and (3) distribution of nutrients in daily meals.

A. Caloric Content: The theoretic daily caloric requirement is calculated on the basis of *ideal body weight*, obtained either through published height and weight tables (eg, Metropolitan Life Insurance Company) or by using approximative calculations.

The calculated theoretic daily caloric requirement is compared with the actual caloric intake of the patient, derived by dietary history (detailed recall of timing and specific composition of meals of 2–3 typical days). This maneuver serves 2 purposes: it provides insight into the patient's habits and identifies the type and magnitude of changes to be recommended.

B. Proportion of Basic Nutrients and Optimal Sources: The total daily caloric need will be provided by carbohydrate 50–60% (4 kcal to 1 g), fat 20–30% (9 kcal to 1 g), and protein 15–20% (4 kcal to 1 g). Among carbohydrates, glucose and sucrose should be restricted; favored instead are those providing fibers (whole-grain bread and cereals, starchy vegetables, and legumes). Raw vegetables and fruit are also good sources of dietary fibers. An increase in dietary fiber intake is recommended not only for the beneficial bulk effect but also because fibers slow the digestion and absorption of carbohydrates, thus decreasing the amplitude of postprandial hyperglycemia.

The total fat intake should ideally be less than 30% of total daily calories with less than 10% saturated fatty acids. The cholesterol content should be less than 300 mg/d.

The total intake of protein recommended for the adult individual is 0.8 g/kg body weight. An allowance of 15–20% of total daily calories in the form of protein will amply satisfy established need. The best sources of protein are the ones with little concomitant fat: skim or low-fat milk, poultry, fish, nonfat cheeses, and legumes.

C. Distribution of Nutrients in Daily Meals: In general, multiple smaller meals are preferable to a couple of large ones. A widely used schedule entails breakfast (about 25% of daily calories), a mid-morning snack (5–10%), lunch (25%), dinner (30%), bedtime snack (10%). The carbohydrate content of the meals is of crucial importance toward insulin need and overall glycemic control; it is estimated that in insulin-dependent patients every 10 g of dietary carbohydrates require for utilization 1–1.5 U of insulin, with the highest dose being needed for breakfast. Therefore, the carbohydrate content of each meal should be kept constant from day to day. Since the patient should be able to utilize a variety of foods, Exchange Group Systems have been developed. With these systems any food within a particular list can be substituted with the indicated amount of any other food on that list. It is helpful to provide 3 or 4 basic menus reflecting the desired caloric and carbohydrate composition of the daily meals. By following these menus for a couple of weeks, patients become familiar with portion size and changes in preparation procedures (less fat, simple dressings, no sucrose).

Moderate **alcohol** consumption should be permitted as long as the following aspects are understood: (1) Beverages to be preferred are the ones with low carbohydrate content (spirits, dry wines, dry sherries, low-calorie beers). (2) The caloric contribution of alcohol itself (7 cal to 1 g) should be computed in the total daily caloric intake. (3) Because alcohol potentiates or precipitates hypoglycemia through inhibition of gluconeogenesis, it is safest to drink during a meal.

Exercise

Regular physical activity should be encouraged. Exercise is crucial for (1) caloric balance and thus weight control, (2) improved cardiovascular performance, (3) antiatherogenic changes in plasma lipoproteins, and (4) a satisfied frame of mind and overall better self-image.

The exercising muscle increases its fuel consumption by 7–40 times. Such fuel is provided by free fatty acids mobilized from muscle and adipose tissue triglycerides, and by glucose mobilized from glycogen stores in muscle and liver.

In the insulin-dependent patient, 3 difficulties may arise:

1. The inability to decrease circulating insulin compromises hepatic glucose output and accelerates glucose disposal by muscle, thus possibly precipitating hypoglycemia. This should be prevented by (1) providing extra food before and during the activity (10 g of carbohydrate every 30 minutes of moderate exercise), or (2) decreasing the dose of the type of insulin anticipated to be particularly active at the time of exercise or decreasing (or discontinuing for short exercise) the rate of an insulin infusion.

2. The absorption of insulin injected in the exercising limb will be enhanced by the combination of increased temperature and increased blood flow, thus further contributing to possible hypoglycemia. This can be prevented by injecting the insulin in the subcutaneous tissue of the abdomen.

3. Some insulin activity remains necessary during exercise. In its absence, lipolysis and hepatic glucose production would be excessive. Thus, physical activity in the insulin-deficient state enhances hyperglycemia and ketogenesis. Exercise should be planned only with adequate basal insulinization.

It is best to ask the patient to determine blood glucose before and after a set duration and amount of exercise. The data reflect the individual's response and allow optimal adjustments in caloric intake and insulin doses.

The types and extent of physical activity will vary tremendously among patients on the basis of age, fitness, habits, and cardiovascular status. The only firm contraindication to exercise is recent vitreous hemorrhage. Patients with proliferative retinopathy should be warned against forms of exercise involving heavy lifting, head-low positions, and Valsalva-like maneuvers. Pulmonary function testing is also contraindicated in such patients. Patients with decreased sensation in feet and legs should avoid activities involving possible trauma. Otherwise, at least some form of benign activity (walking, calisthenics) should be encouraged even in the elderly and complicated patient.

Insulin Therapy

In clinical practice, insulin is still administered into the subcutaneous tissue, either as discrete injections or through continuous infusion. This method of insulin replacement is not physiologic, since it fails to achieve high portal concentrations of insulin or the brisk insulin release initiated by a meal. However, while awaiting clinical applicability of implantable intraperitoneal or intravenous devices coupled with implantable glucose sensors, the rational use of available insulin preparations and frequent self-monitoring of glucose permit fairly successful replacement regimens.

A. Goals of Insulin Replacement: In principle, the dose and modalities of insulin administration should aim in all patients at normalization of glycemia. In practice, however, it is necessary to establish slightly higher targets, weighing the expected long-term benefits (prevention of complications) against the dangers of hypoglycemia. In this regard, 2 categories of patients can be identified and target glucose levels set as initial guidelines.

	Target glucose levels (mg/dL)		
	Fasting	**Preprandial**	**2-Hour Postprandial**
1. Young and healthy (tight control)	80–120	80–120	80–140
2. Elderly and all ages with documented vascular complications, autonomic neuropathy, or history of seizures (acceptable control)	100–140	100–140	100–180

B. Insulin Preparations: Insulin preparations available in the USA and for the most part in Europe are listed in Table 10–6.

1. Source and purity–Bovine and porcine insulin is extracted from the respective animals' pancreas; human insulin is made either through recombinant DNA in *Escherichia coli* (biosynthetic) or by chemical substitution of the terminal alanine of the B-chain of the pork insulin with threonine, which converts pork insulin to human insulin (semisynthetic).

2. Immunogenicity–The insulins to be preferred are the least immunogenic: highly purified pork insulin (only 1 amino acid difference from human, in contrast to 3 amino acid difference in beef insulin) and human insulin. Definitive indications for these preparations are local or systemic insulin allergy, lipoatrophy, insulin antibody-mediated insulin resistance (see below, under Complications of Insulin Therapy), and intermittent insulin treatment (gestational diabetes, type II diabetics undergoing major stress, such as infection or surgery). The highly purified pork or human insulins are also indicated in all diabetics newly started on insulin in order to prevent the possible complications of insulin therapy mentioned above. Patients who are already using the standard insulin preparations (beef and pork, purity < 50 ppm proinsulin) and whose diabetic control is satisfactory need not be switched to the highly purified pork or human insulins.

3. Concentration–All the listed insulin preparations are available in U-100 concentration (ie, 100 U of insulin per milliliter). The Regular Iletin II (Lilly) is available also in U-500 strength. The less purified insulins are also available in U-40 concentration, occasionally useful for pediatric doses. The syringes employed must be appropriate for the insulin concentration.

4. Pharmacokinetics–The pharmocokinetics of the different insulins allow their classification in rapid- (and short-) acting, intermediate-acting, and long-acting. The mechanism whereby insulin is made into intermediate- or long-acting preparations is a decrease in the solubility of insulin at body pH that results in delayed absorption from the site of injection. The agents used to decrease insulin solubility are **protamine** in NPH and protamine-zinc insulins or a high concentration of **zinc** in Lente and Ultralente insulin preparations. Thus, although they are alike in action, Lente insulin has a potential for being less immunogenic than NPH insulin, since it is free from foreign modifying protein.

The average times of onset of action, peak, and duration of the various insulin preparations are summarized in Table 10–6. Additional information essential for appropriate and safe use of insulin follows:

(a) The action of Regular Insulin may sometimes last 16–20 hours owing to its interaction with insulin antibodies.

(b) Absorption from abdomen and buttock is faster than from deltoid or anterior thigh. Exercise of injected extremity, local massage, and increased ambient temperature all accelerate absorption.

(c) Solubility of Regular Insulin decreases when it is mixed with intermediate-acting insulin as the proportion of the latter increases and the time since mixing lengthens. Thus, proportion of NPH or Lente:Regular should not be greater than 3:1, and the mixture should be promptly injected.

C. Conventional Versus Intensive Insulin Regimens: Any insulin regimen that safely maintains near-normoglycemia is the appropriate regimen for a patient. However, insulin therapy as conventionally used (1–2 daily insulin injections, occasional self-monitoring of urine or blood glucose) is less likely than intensive insulin regimens (3 or more daily insulin injections or continuous subcutaneous insulin infusion, frequent self-monitoring of blood glucose) to achieve the goal of near-normoglycemia. In the ongoing Diabetes Control and Complications Trial (DCCT), the conventional treatment group has maintained over 3 years glycohemoglobin levels of $\approx 9\%$, whereas in the intensive treatment group glycohemoglobin has been stably lowered to 7%. Hence, motivated patients who fail to achieve satisfactory control with conventional treatment should be guided to more intensive insulin regimens.

1. Conventional insulin treatment–With the exception of patients with newly diagnosed IDDM and the elderly—who may require only partial insulin replacement (see below)—the total daily dose of insulin required is usually between 0.4 and 1 U/kg/d. Both nutrient-stimulated insulin secretion (prandial insulin) and continuous postabsorptive insulin secretion (basal insulin) must be replaced. In most cases, a rapid- and short-acting insulin (referred to as Regular) and an intermediate-acting insulin (referred to as NPH/Lente) is employed. The insulin dose is divided into 2 injections: two-thirds of the total dose is given 20–30 minutes before breakfast and one-third is given 20–30 minutes before dinner.

In the most widely used approach, each dose consists of 30–40% Regular and 60–70% of NPH/Lente. The morning Regular is meant to

Table 10–6. Insulin preparations.

Product (Manufacturer)	Class*	Species	Strength
Rapid-acting (onset 0.5–4 hours; duration 5–16 hours) Regular and Semilente			
Humulin R (Regular) (Lilly)	P	Recombinant DNA human	U-100
Novolin R (Regular) (Novo Nordisk)	P	Semisynthetic human	U-100
Velosulin (Regular) (Novo Nordisk)	P	Semisynthetic human	U-100
Iletin II Regular (Lilly)	P	Beef	U-100
Iletin II Regular (Lilly)	P	Pork	U-100, U-500
Purified Pork Regular (Novo Nordisk)	P	Pork	U-100
Velosulin (Regular) (Novo Nordisk)	P	Pork	U-100
Iletin I Regular (Lilly)	C	Beef/pork	U-40, U-100
Regular (Novo Nordisk)	C	Pork	U-100
Iletin I Semilente (Lilly)	C	Beef/pork	U-40, U-100
Semilente (Novo Nordisk)	C	Beef	U-100
Intermediate-acting (onset 1–4 hours; duration 16–18 hours) Lente and NPH			
Humulin N (NPH) (Lilly)	P	Recombinant DNA human	U-100
Humulin L (Lente) (Lilly)	P	Recombinant DNA human	U-100
Insulatard NPH (Novo Nordisk)	P	Semisynthetic human	U-100
Novolin L (Lente) (Novo Nordisk)	P	Semisynthetic human	U-100
Novolin N (NPH) (Novo Nordisk)	P	Semisynthetic human	U-100
Iletin II Lente (Lilly)	P	Beef	U-100
Iletin II NPH (Lilly)	P	Beef	U-100
Iletin II Lente (Lilly)	P	Pork	U-100

Iletin II NPH (Lilly)	P	Pork	U-100
Insulatard (NPH) (Novo Nordisk)	P	Pork	U-100
Purified Pork Lente (Novo Nordisk)	P	Pork	U-100
Purified Pork NPH (Novo Nordisk)	P	Pork	U-100
Iletin I Lente (Lilly)	C	Beef/pork	U-40, U-100
Iletin I NPH (Lilly)	C	Beef/pork	U-40, U-100
NPH (Novo Nordisk)	C	Beef	U-100

Long-acting (onset 4–6 hours; duration 36 hours) PZI and Ultralente

Humulin U (Ultralente) (Lilly)	P	Recombinant DNA human	U-100
Iletin II PZI (Lilly)	P	Pork	U-100
Iletin II PZI (Lilly)	P	Beef	U-100
Iletin I PZI (Lilly)	C	Beef/pork	U-40, U-100
Iletin I Ultralente (Lilly)	C	Beef/pork	U-40, U-100
Ultralente (Novo Nordisk)	C	Beef	U-100

Mixtures

Humulin 70/30† (Lilly)	P	Human	U-100
Mixtard Human 70/30† (Novo Nordisk)	P	Human	U-100
Novolin 70/30† (Novo Nordisk)	P	Human	U-100
Mixtard† (Novo Nordisk)	P	Pork	U-100

*The 2 recognized classes of insulins based on FDA standards of proinsulin content are conventional (C) with < 50 ppm and purified (P) < 10 ppm. Semisynthetic human insulin is derived from pork insulin, with the terminal amino acid of the B chain chemically changed to form the human insulin molecule.
†These insulins contain 70% NPH and 30% Regular.

cover breakfast and contribute to covering lunch; the evening Regular is meant to cover dinner and contribute to covering the bedtime snack. The morning NPH/Lente is meant to cover lunch and the interval between lunch and dinner. The evening NPH/Lente is meant to cover bedtime snack and the interval between bedtime snack and breakfast.

Diligent home glucose monitoring is necessary to guide adjustments of insulin dosage and caloric intake. The guidelines in Table 10–7 provide a framework for insulin-calorie adjustments. Changes in insulin doses are generally done by 1–2 U at a time; the choice between adjusting insulin dose or caloric intake depends on body weight goals.

The most common problem of the split-dose mixed insulin regimen is morning fasting hyperglycemia. This can be a reaction to nighttime hypoglycemia (Somogyi phenomenon). The patient should be carefully questioned about symptoms of hypoglycemia: nightmares, headache and nausea upon waking; and should perform a 2–3 AM fingerstick blood glucose determination. If nocturnal hypoglycemia is documented, a smaller dose of nighttime NPH/Lente should be tried. Smaller nighttime NPH/Lente doses may, however, fail to maintain an adequate insulinization until morning. The early morning hours (5–9 AM) are characterized by some resistance to insulin. This "dawn phenomenon" contributes to fasting morning hyperglycemia especially as the NPH/Lente insulin injected the previous evening is reaching its nadir. An effective maneuver to prevent fasting hyperglycemia is to delay the injection of the evening dose of NPH/Lente until bedtime, thus increasing to 3 the number of daily insulin injections.

2. Intensive Insulin Treatment–This offers 2 advantages: improved glycemic control and greater flexibility in timing of daily activities. These advantages can only be achieved through preventive/corrective adjustments in the doses of insulin to be injected, which in turn mandate frequent self-monitoring of blood glucose (at least before each meal and at bedtime). The most important complication of regimens aiming at near-normoglycemia is a 2- to 3-fold greater incidence of severe hypoglycemia. To prevent the occurrence of potentially catastrophic hypoglycemia, patients who have experienced more than 2 episodes of severe hypoglycemia during the preceding 2 years or more than one episode while awake but without warning, should not be committed to achievement of near-normoglycemia. A second effect to be monitored is weight gain. It is most striking in patients who exhibit the greatest improvement in glycemic control, indicating that reduction of glycosuria and lost calories is the main determinant.

Multiple insulin injections are the easiest approach to intensified treatment and should be tried first. Three widely used regimens are the following:

Table 10–7. Guidelines for insulin-caloric adjustments when using the Regular + Lente insulin regimen.

Event	Time	Action to Be Taken on Following Day
Hypoglycemia (symptoms or readings below 60 mg/dL)	Mid- to late-morning	Decrease AM Regular or increase mid morning snack
	Mid-to-late afternoon	Decrease AM NPH/Lente or add mid-afternoon snack
	Bedtime	Decrease PM Regular or increase dinner
	During the night	Decrease PM NPH/Lente or increase bedtime snack
Hyperglycemia (readings above target levels previously defined)	2 hours after breakfast but satisfactory or low prelunch	Increase AM Regular and decrease AM NPH/Lente or redistribute calories between breakfast and midmorning snack
	2 hours after breakfast and prelunch	Increase AM Regular or decrease breakfast
	2 hours after lunch and satisfactory or low predinner	Increase AM NPH/Lente and add a mid-afternoon snack or decrease lunch and add a midafternoon snack
	2 hours after lunch and predinner	Increase AM NPH/Lente or decrease lunch
	2 hours after dinner and satisfactory or low bedtime	Increase PM Regular and decrease PM NPH/Lente
	2 hours after dinner and bedtime	Increase PM Regular or decrease dinner
	Fasting before breakfast	Increase PM NPH/Lente

1. Regular and NPH/Lente before breakfast, Regular before dinner, NPH/Lente at bedtime (15–25% of total daily dose).

2. Regular before breakfast, lunch, and dinner, and NPH/Lente at bedtime. This regimen offers greater flexibility because it eliminates concern about the timing of NPH/Lente peak during the day, but it entails 4 injections.

3. Regular before breakfast and before lunch, and Regular mixed

with Ultralente before dinner. Generally 40% of the total daily insulin dose is given as Ultralente, which through its long action (36–96 hours) and relatively peakless kinetics, provides basal insulin requirements throughout the day. In view of the slow absorption of Ultralente insulin, several days are necessary to achieve steady-state. If hypoglycemia attributable to the action of Ultralente occurs, the dose should be completely omitted for 1 day and restarted at a reduced amount.

Continuous Subcutaneous Insulin Infusion (CSII)

CSII through portable pumps has 4 advantages over multiple injection regimens: (1) Only Regular insulin is employed with consequent elimination of the antigenicity characteristic of longer acting insulin preparations. (2) The continuous delivery of basal insulin is steadier than possibly achieved with NPH or Lente insulin. (3) The patient-activated preprandial boluses allow for greater flexibility in timing and composition of meals. (4) Preprogrammable devices allow for automatic changes in basal rate of insulin, which may be useful in counteracting the dawn phenomenon.

Disadvantages are the substantial cost, wearing of a mechanical appendix, risk of pump failure resulting in loss of control and ketoacidosis (there is no depot of long-acting insulin), possibility of accidental insulin overdosage, and risk of infections and allergic skin reactions at the site of continuous infusion. Pump therapy is a labor-intensive effort on the part of the patient, the physician, and paramedical personnel. It should be given consideration only if a trial period of multiple injections in a motivated patient has failed to achieve the desired glycemic control or if the patient prefers to use a pump. To be successful and safe CSII should be implemented under the care of physicians broadly experienced in the method and willing to provide patients with 24-hour access to expert advice.

To initiate pump therapy, the following steps are taken: (1) Contact representatives of pump manufacturers (eg, MiniMed Technologies, Sylmar, CA) for information on latest models, pricing, and modes of acquisition. (2) Choose a device preprogrammable for changes in basal delivery rates in the simplest possible manner. The device should have fail-safe features to signal malfunction, and it should come in the smallest possible size. (3) Arrange with the patient for 4–5 days of hospitalization.

Initiation of CSII treatment should ideally follow a careful attempt at optimizing treatment with insulin injections. This will indicate the approximate total daily insulin need for the individual patient, which will generally be between 0.4 and 1 U/kg/d. Initially, just 80% of the prior total daily insulin dose is given and is divided as follows: basal infusion 40%, prebreakfast bolus 20%, prelunch bolus 15%, predinner bolus 15%, and bedtime snack bolus 10%, with premeal boluses being given 20 minutes before the meal. Intensive blood glucose monitoring will dictate the size and direction of changes from this empirical approach. The magnitude of the dawn phenomenon is documented by measuring blood glucose at 3 AM and 7 AM on a constant basal rate. The extent of the blood glucose rise guides the programming of an automatic increase in basal rate, to be started at 4 AM. The patient wearing a pump must be knowledgeable about diabetes and pump protocol.

Syringe Alternatives

Infusers (eg, Markwell Medical Institute; Diabetes Center, Inc.) are needles to be inserted and taped in place (generally in subcutaneous tissue of the abdomen) for 48–72 hours that create ''portals'' for the injection of insulin. There is a high incidence of local infection. **Insulin pens** (eg, Novo Nordisk; Ulster) include an insulin cartridge (Regular or intermediate-acting or premixed insulin), a disposable needle, and a trigger button for selecting and injecting the dose. They are not expensive and are especially convenient for patients on multiple injections (less material to carry) and for patients with dexterity impairment. **Jet injectors** (eg, Derata; Medi-Jector EZ) use air pressure to propel insulin into subcutaneous tissue without a needle. Because insulin becomes finely dispersed, it is absorbed more rapidly into the blood stream and may provide more physiologic periprandial coverage. Jet injectors can deliver only one type of insulin at a time, are expensive, bulky, and somewhat complex to operate. They also may cause bruising, especially in thin patients. **Automatic injectors** (eg, Inject-Ease) hide the syringe and needle. The needle is injected by a spring released by push button; the patient then presses the plunger. They are useful for patients who fear needles.

Premixed Insulin

Instances in which the mixing may become an unsafe procedure are poor understanding or failing sight. In such instances, use of a premixed insulin preparation will at least ensure delivery of some regular insulin in addition to the longer-acting preparation. The available premixed insulins are reported on Table 10–6; they are constituted of 30% Regular and 70% NPH. This combination is generally used for prebreakfast and predinner doses, and can be administered through insulin pens or jet injectors.

Intercurrent Illnesses

If the patient is not vomiting and is able to maintain some caloric intake, guidelines can be as follows: continue usual NPH/Lente or Ultralente doses and adjust preprandial Regular insulin depending on preprandial blood glucose readings. In particular:

For blood glucose 150–200 mg/dL: add 2–3 U of Regular to usual dose

For blood glucose 200–250 mg/dL: add 3–5 U of Regular to usual dose

For blood glucose 250–300 mg/dL: add 4–6 U of Regular to usual dose

For blood glucose over 300 mg/dL: add 6–8 U of Regular to usual dose.

At the time of each blood glucose test, urine should be tested for ketones. If urine ketones are large and blood glucose is over 300 mg/dL, add 10–12 U of Regular. Fluids should be drunk in abundance; if blood glucose remains below 200 mg/dL, fluids may contain sugar, and if blood glucose is above 200–250 mg/dL, fluids should be sugar-free.

If the patient is vomiting, the dose of intermediate-and long-acting insulins should be decreased to two-thirds of usual (since some of that insulin is normally used to cover meals). Regular insulin is administered in multiple small doses (3–4 U) every 4–6 hours depending on blood glucose readings; this approach allows the additional coverage warranted by the illness to be spread over time and remain relatively constant, avoiding peaks of insulin activity in a situation of much decreased caloric intake. Attempts should be made to provide some caloric intake and salt (Na, K) replacement with continuous sipping of fluids: fruit juices, milk—eventually with added sucrose—tomato juice, broth, and vegetable soup. Urine testing for ketones is mandatory. Even in the absence of severe hyperglycemia (blood glucose < 300 mg/dL), if urine ketones are large the dose of regular insulin should be doubled. If ketonuria is not diminished within a few hours, the patient should be brought to the emergency room to be evaluated for ketoacidosis. Even in the absence of worrisome ketonuria, it is unsafe to continue home treatment of the patient with vomiting and diarrhea for longer than 48 hours. If the symptomatology is not resolving by then, the patient should be hospitalized in order to be evaluated and to ensure adequate intravenous hydration and calories.

It is always important to determine the cause of symptoms, particularly with unexplained deterioration of diabetic control. Such may be caused by bacterial or fungal infections of the urinary tract, ingrown toenails, or infection of foot ulcers in patients with the "anesthetic foot." Patients should be specifically questioned about these possibilities and evaluated without delay.

Honeymoon Period

Sixty to 70% of newly diagnosed type I diabetic patients experience a remission phase shortly after presentation and need substantially less insulin. The honeymoon period starts 2–4 weeks after diagnosis and may be protracted for several months. During this period total daily requirement for exogenous insulin may be as low as 0.1 U/kg, and the dose may then be administered in a single injection of NPH or Lente before breakfast. As the requirement increases above 0.3 U/kg, 2 doses, possibly containing some Regular insulin at least before breakfast, will provide a smoother pattern to the more extended coverage needed. Throughout this period, diligent home-monitoring is essential to promptly identify changing insulin needs.

The Elderly

Insulin-dependent diabetes may have its onset at any age, but generally the extent of insulin deficiency is less in older individuals. Very often such patients have responded for some time to oral agents, but over a period of months weight loss and mild ketosis develop, necessitating insulin replacement. Since the consequences of hypoglycemia may be magnified in the elderly by a diminished vascular supply to organs, it is safe—if the patient is metabolically stable—to start insulin therapy with "exploratory" doses. Start with a single morning dose of 0.2 U/kg of NPH/Lente insulin. Then increase the dose by 1–2 U/d toward achieving predinner blood glucose values between 100 and 140 mg/dL; attention is then moved to the fasting values. Frequent telephone contact with the physician should be encouraged. If the adequate replacement dose appears to exceed 0.3–0.4 U/kg, split doses are instituted.

Compromised Renal Function

The kidney plays a major role in the catabolism of insulin. In healthy individuals, about 50% of the insulin secreted daily reaches the peripheral circulation, and of this approximately 40% is cleared by the kidney through glomerular filtration, followed by near complete reabsorption and degradation at the proximal tubule. In the diabetic patient treated with subcutaneous insulin, the kidney accounts for catabolism of approximately half the daily insulin dose. Thus, nephropathy and declining glomerular filtration rate (GFR) compromise the clearance of circulating insulin with consequent prolongation of the half-life and biologic action of the injected dose. These changes start to be evident at GFR < 40 mL/min and become important at GFR < 10 mL/min. Some resistance to the action of insulin accompanies uremia. However, the total daily insulin dose needs to be significantly reduced to prevent severe hypoglycemic episodes due to prolonged insulin action and inefficient warning and counterregulating mechanisms caused by autonomic neuropathy.

A. Hemodialysis: For the patient newly started on hemodialysis, intensive glucose monitoring is warranted, since on the days of dialysis, insulin need may be somewhat decreased if the dialysate's glucose concentration is less than 100 mg/dL. Since insulin is not dialyzed, the same insulin would work on a reduced substrate and induce hypoglycemia.

To patients on chronic abdominal peritoneal dialysis (CAPD), insulin may be conveniently administered intraperitoneally along with dialysis solutions.

Protocols differ among centers, but they generally entail the addition of Regular insulin in a dose equal to one-quarter of the original total daily dose to each of the four bags used for the daily exchanges, with supplementation based on the glucose concentrations of the dialysate. The insulin dose is slightly reduced for the overnight exchange. Intensive self-monitoring of glucose for 7–10 days will help establish a satisfactory insulin regimen.

B. Renal Transplantation: Prednisone substantially increases the insulin requirement postoperatively, especially when very large doses are used to counteract acute rejection. In such situations, subcutaneous insulin is poorly effective, and to prevent severe hyperglycemia it may be necessary to administer continuous intravenous Regular insulin or small intravenous boluses of Regular insulin (4–6 U) before main meals, in addition to the subcutaneous regimen.

Elective Surgery

In normal humans, surgery and anesthesia induce a marked stress response characterized by increased levels of counterregulatory hormones, insulin resistance, and decreased insulin secretion. The degree of the resulting glycemic rise is proportionate to the severity of the operation. Severe hyperglycemia occurs in nondiabetic patients undergoing open-heart surgery. In the poorly insulinized diabetic patient, surgery may precipitate ketoacidosis.

A. Preoperative Management: Before **major surgery**, the patient should be brought under excellent control. If possible, patients are admitted 48 hours in advance and stabilized on their usual insulin regimen. Long-acting insulins (eg, Ultralente) are discontinued and replaced with appropriate doses of NPH/Lente insulin. The morning of surgery, blood glucose should be less than 150 mg/dL; the usual insulin dose is omitted and intravenous therapy initiated.

For **minor surgery**, patients who are known to be in good control may be admitted the night before or the morning of surgery.

B. Intraoperative Management: The goal is to maintain blood glucose between 100 and 200 mg/dL, and the key to this goal is to persuade the anesthesiologist to perform intraoperative measurements of blood glucose. An intravenous continuous infusion of insulin and glucose started in the early morning before surgery is the most effective and safest approach. The regimen consists in delivering 0.2 U of

Regular insulin per gram of glucose. Thus, if D5 is infused at 100 mL/h, the 5 g of glucose will call for 1 U of insulin/h. STAT blood glucose measurements are performed every 1–2 hours, and insulin dose is adjusted toward target glucose levels following this simple algorithm:

(Blood glucose in mg/dL)/150 = rate of intravenous insulin infusion (U/h)

In situations of severe insulin resistance (patients receiving high doses of glucocorticoids intraoperatively, infected patients, patients with gross obesity or liver cirrhosis), the initial insulin dose is increased to 0.4 U/g of glucose and the algorithm determining the rate of insulin infusion (U/h) for adjustments becomes

(Blood glucose in mg/dL)/100 = rate of intravenous infusion (U/hour)

These guidelines must be adapted to individual response.

The insulin for intravenous infusion is prepared by adding 50 U of Regular insulin to 500 mL of normal or half-normal saline (0.1 U/mL, 1 U/10 mL) and running at least 50 mL of the solution through the administration set before connecting to the patient. It is then administered through a pump at the desired rate. The glucose solution is delivered through an independent intravenous set. Modifying the 2 rates independently allows for greater flexibility and for the use of glucose infusion to correct declining glucose levels.

C. Postoperative Management: The goal is to maintain glucose levels between 100 and 200 mg/dL *and* to provide some caloric support. In order to provide some calories without excessive fluid intake, glucose may be given as D10, delivered at 100 mL/h (10 g glucose/h). Insulin is infused at a rate of 0.2 U/g of glucose with adjustments based on the algorithms previously described.

The intravenous infusion is continued until the patient is eating. After at least one well-tolerated meal, the insulin infusion is discontinued before the following meal. *Before* discontinuation of the infusion, the patient should receive a dose of subcutaneous insulin comparable with preoperative insulin doses. *Never discontinue an intravenous insulin infusion without first giving subcutaneous insulin.*

Patients who have undergone minor surgery are generally allowed to return to oral feeding within the day of surgery. Blood glucose is determined before the meal, and the subcutaneous insulin dose is decided based on (1) blood glucose level, (2) interval from previous dose, (3) time of day, and (4) caloric content of the meal. By the following day, patients generally resume their usual meals and insulin schedule.

Complications of Insulin Therapy

A. Hypoglycemia: Severe insulin-induced hypoglycemia can have catastrophic consequences. The brain is an avid glucose consum-

other organs, the brain does not derive energy from oxida-
~~e~~ fatty acids and utilizes ketone bodies only when circulating
.~~....~~ .~~..~~ very elevated, as in prolonged starvation. With excessive
insulin activity, not only do circulating levels of glucose fall, but
lipolysis and ketogenesis are also suppressed. This totally curtailed
fuel availability is perceived by hypothalamic and peripheral sensors
as warranting rapid restoration of euglycemia.

1. Counterregulatory response–Four hormones are involved in
the response to hypoglycemia: glucagon, epinephrine, growth hormone, and cortisol. **Glucagon** and **epinephrine** constitute the first-
line defense: they are briskly secreted upon a drop in plasma glucose
below 50 mg/dL and provide a rapid increase of glucose via glycogenolysis. In the absence of both glucagon and epinephrine, acute
restoration of euglycemia is severely compromised. **Cortisol** and
growth hormone are secreted with some delay after hypoglycemia
and antagonize insulin by interfering with its action and enhancing
lipolysis; hypercortisolism also enhances the glycogenolytic response
to glucagon and epinephrine.

When the above mechanisms are functional and hepatic glycogen
stores are adequate, insulin-induced hypoglycemia is usually mild,
transient, and easily overcome, since the prompt glucagon and epinephrine responses prevent progression to dangerous and symptomatic
levels. However, in patients with type I diabetes, the glucagon response to hypoglycemia is compromised. The extent of the compromise is partially related to duration of the disease, resulting after 10–12
years of diabetes in minimal or absent glucagon responses to hypoglycemia. By then the epinephrine response is also diminished and
recovery from hypoglycemia is delayed with consequently more prolonged and profound hypoglycemic episodes.

Thus, patients with recent onset of diabetes usually experience
only minimal and rapidly correctable hypoglycemic episodes, while
patients with long-standing diabetes can have severe life-threatening
hypoglycemia especially in the presence of autonomic neuropathy,
β-adrenergic blockers (which reduce the glycogenolytic effect of epinephrine), or renal failure (leading to prolonged insulin activity).
Poorly controlled diabetic patients experience symptoms of hypoglycemia at plasma glucose concentrations higher than those required
to produce symptoms in nondiabetic or well-controlled individuals.
Hypothyroidism, liver disease, and excessive alcohol consumption
may predispose the patient to more severe hypoglycemic episodes.

A common consequence of hypoglycemia is rebound hyperglycemia, often with ketosis. This is called the **Somogyi phenomenon**
and is caused by the hyperglycemic, lipolytic, and ketogenic effects of
the counterregulatory hormones persisting when the subcutaneous
depot of insulin is becoming depleted. It is especially important to

identify the possible role of this phenomenon in causing fasting hyperglycemia and ketonuria.

2. Treatment of hypoglycemia–Hypoglycemia must be treated promptly, as soon as warning signs develop (tingling of mouth and fingers, difficulty in concentrating, nervousness, tachycardia, perspiration). Every diabetic treated with insulin must have ready access to a source of 10–15 g of carbohydrates (eg, Dextro-Energens, Dextrosol tablets, graham crackers, Lifesavers, orange juice). If symptoms do not improve within 10 minutes, the patient should repeat the ingestion or preferably consume a snack containing complex carbohydrates and proteins. Should the patient become unconscious and thus not a candidate for oral treatment, 1 mg of glucagon should be administered intramuscularly or subcutaneously (through an insulin syringe). As the patient regains consciousness, oral treatment should be instituted to prevent recurrences. Patients may vomit after the glucagon injection.

B. Local and Systemic Reactions: Local and systemic reactions to insulin are becoming increasingly rare since current insulin preparations consist of less antigenic insulin molecules (porcine and human insulin; see Table 10–6) and contain negligible impurities (in particular proinsulin).

Patients allergic to insulin typically are allergic to other substances, especially penicillin, and have received intermittent insulin treatment. Allergic reactions to insulin are mediated by antiinsulin IgE antibodies.

1. Local reactions–Local reactions range from a burning and itching sensation at the site of injection to development of local erythema, induration, and wheal formation. The reaction may be immediate or delayed by 6–8 hours. It is important to review the patient's injection technique, to ensure that the insulin is being injected subcutaneously and not intradermally. Since bona fide local reactions are mostly due to impurities, over 80% of patients will improve if switched to highly purified pork or human insulin. Patients who do not respond are encouraged to tolerate the inconvenience for a few months, since the condition may improve spontaneously. Antihistamines may reduce the symptoms.

Few patients require **desensitization**. It is performed by first injecting 1/100 U subcutaneously and then doubling the dose every 30 minutes. A convenient Insulin Allergy Desensitization Kit with ready-made appropriate insulin dilution and detailed instructions is prepared by the Eli Lilly Company, Indianapolis, IN 46285, and supplied to physicians upon request on a complimentary basis. For the very few patients who fail to respond to all the above maneuvers, the use of dexamethasone mixed with the insulin has been advocated, with beginning doses of 0.04 mg in each insulin injection, not to exceed 0.50 mg/d.

2. Systemic reactions–Systemic allergic reactions to insulin may occur with or without local reactions. Manifestations include generalized pruritus, skin rash, purpura, serum sickness, bronchospasm, angioedema, and anaphylactic shock. Most systemic allergies are responses to the insulin molecule proper. Therefore, switching to the least antigenic insulins (ie, pork or human) may cure the problem. The switch to pork or human insulin is made through a standard desensitization procedure (described above).

Since the majority of patients with systemic insulin allergy are adult-onset and often obese, it is always important to critically assess their need for insulin therapy. Many such patients may in fact respond to a more careful diet with or without the addition of oral agents. The best course of action is to hospitalize such patients for a few days, assess their metabolic status while off insulin therapy and then decide whether desensitization to insulin is warranted. Desensitization lasts only as long as insulin is continued (at least twice daily is best).

Systemic allergic reactions to protamine (hypotension, bronchospasm) have been reported as a serious occurrence in patients who receive protamine to reverse heparin anticoagulation (vascular surgery, cardiac catheterization). Diabetic patients who have been treated with insulin preparations containing protamine (NPH and protamine-zinc insulins) are at increased risk, probably because they develop antiprotamine IgE antibodies.

C. Insulin Resistance: has traditionally been defined as a situation in which more than 200 U of insulin per day are necessary for treatment. However, daily insulin requirements above 1.5 U/kg indicate some degree of insulin resistance. The most common causes are obesity (loss of insulin receptors) and poorly controlled type II diabetes (postreceptor defects in insulin action). In these situations insulin resistance is obvious from the outset of treatment and will decrease if therapeutic measures are successful. On the other hand, insulin resistance that develops during insulin treatment suggests an underlying disorder requiring treatment, eg, chronic infection (often occult), overinsulinization leading to rebound hyperglycemia (Somogyi), or chronic increase in circulating levels of antiinsulin hormones (thyrotoxicosis, acromegaly, Cushing's syndrome, or treatment with glucocorticoids, progestins, or estrogens).

Immune insulin resistance is rare. Although practically all patients treated with insulin develop IgG antibodies against it, these antibodies only slightly modify the kinetics of circulating insulin. Only rarely do they bind insulin sufficiently to critically reduce the amount of insulin available for receptor binding. A laboratory determination of the insulin-binding capacity of the patient's serum can be obtained in support of the diagnosis. Patients with immune insulin resistance generally respond to highly purified pork or human insulin in doses smaller than those used to fight the insulin resistant state. For patients who fail to respond to pork or human insulin, a trial of glucocorticoids is indicated. Prednisone, 40–80 mg/d, may restore insulin sensitivity within a few days. Prednisone is given for no longer than 10–15 days and rapidly tapered upon a positive response. Patients need to be carefully monitored, since they may experience severe hypoglycemia from a large dose of insulin previously ineffective.

Immune insulin resistance has been reported in a small number of patients with monoclonal gammopathies. Patients are predominantly male and have chronic lymphocytic leukemia, lymphoma, multiple myeloma, or macroglobulinemia. The insulin resistance parallels the activity of the monoclonal gammopathy, suggesting that the proliferative clone produces an immunoglobulin against the insulin molecule.

Two other mechanisms of insulin resistance are exceedingly rare: excessive degradation of insulin at the site of subcutaneous injection and development of antiinsulin receptor antibodies.

D. Insulin Lipoatrophy: is due to impurities in the insulin preparation, leading to local immune-mediated fibrosis. The depressions at the site of insulin injections are more common in children and women and respond dramatically to highly purified pork or human insulin. Patients should inject the new preparations in the very areas of lipoatrophy. The local lipogenic effect of injected insulin will restore adipose tissue in the affected areas; the beneficial effect starts to be evident within a week. Once the excavated area has been filled in, patients should resume rotation of the injection site in order to prevent lipohypertrophy. In 15% of patients developing lipoatrophy, other local manifestations of insulin allergy are demonstrable.

E. Insulin Hypertrophy: (mounding at the site of insulin injections) may be due to impurities or the action of insulin itself. The most important cause of the condition is failure to rotate the injection site. Patients should therefore use only highly purified insulin preparations, rotate injection sites, and restrain from injecting in already hypertrophic areas.

Pancreatic and Islet Transplantation

The current rate of success of pancreatic transplants (defined as providing normoglycemia for at least 1 year) is 50%. Because the benefits must be weighed against the dangers of lifelong immunosuppression, pancreas grafting has mostly been performed in diabetic uremic patients receiving renal transplantation. A few centers accept patients with signs of nephropathy but still reasonably good excretory function (creatinine clearance > 60 mL/min) in the hope that successful pancreas grafting will stabilize renal function. Diabetic retinopathy of any severity is not currently an indication for pancreas transplantation.

Pancreatic transplantation between identical twins still requires immunosuppression because the donor pancreas transplanted to the diabetic twin develops the same lesions of insulitis that caused the diabetes. B-cell transplant without immunosuppression is not yet possible, but encouraging results have been obtained with islet grafting in diabetic animals.

TREATMENT OF TYPE II (NIDDM) DIABETES

Patients with type II diabetes have varying degrees of compromise in insulin secretion and tissue responsiveness to insulin action. The result is derangement in carbohydrate metabolism sufficient to cause hyperglycemia but not ketoacidosis. Thus, type II diabetics are not insulin *dependent*; ie, exogenous insulin is not required, under usual circumstances, for prevention of catabolism and acute preservation of life. However, type II patients become candidates for insulin treatment when (1) hyperglycemia is unresponsive to other maneuvers and becomes a major risk factor for chronic complications or (2) intercurrent stressful events increase the demand for insulin to an extent that cannot be met by endogenous reserve.

While IDDM is irreversible, being mediated by the destruction of islet B cells, NIDDM may range from being completely reversible (obesity, excess antiinsulin hormones, oral contraceptives, thiazide diuretics, gestational diabetes) to representing prodromic expression of progressive islet-cell damage eventually leading to serious insulin deficiency and thus type I diabetes. In addition to developing the characteristic microvascular complications, NIDDM patients are plagued by increased morbidity and mortality due to atherosclerotic vascular disease. Hence, the therapeutic approach to type II diabetes moves along 3 lines:

1. Correction of precipitating or exacerbating situations (most commonly obesity).

2. Management of the hyperglycemia with surveillance for acute or chronic development of insulin deficiency.

3. Prophylaxis and therapy for atherosclerotic vascular disease.

Obesity & Its Treatment

About 80% of patients with type II diabetes are obese, ie, at least 20% above ideal body weight. While not all obese individuals will develop diabetes, many are at high risk, particularly those with a family history of diabetes or truncal obesity. The sequence of events underlying the association of obesity and diabetes may be reconstructed as follows: caloric intake excessive for the degree of energy expenditure → prevailing hyperinsulinemia → decrease in insulin receptor number → resistance to insulin → increased demand on B cells → impaired B-cell function → overt hyperglycemia. When implemented soon after discovery of mild hyperglycemia, successful weight reduction is likely to restore insulin sensitivity sufficiently to correct the diabetic state. When fasting glucose reaches levels above 250 mg/dL suggesting additional pathologic processes (insulin deficiency, postreceptor defects), weight loss alone may not completely correct the diabetes. Nonetheless, weight loss remains a mainstay of therapy for the obese patient.

The approach to weight loss should take into account the degree of obesity: mild obesity (20–40% overweight) responds well to moderate caloric restriction, nutritional education, behavior modification, and increased physical activity; moderate obesity (41–100% over ideal body weight) and severe obesity (> 100% overweight) may necessitate more drastic nutritional measures (very low calorie diets) in addition to the other maneuvers. For morbidly obese patients, surgical treatment may be necessary.

Diet

Moderate caloric restriction is the best approach for individuals 20–40% overweight, who represent 90% of all obese patients. Its rate of success (ie, weight maintenance after weight reduction) is 20–30%. Because the rate of weight loss is directly related to the difference between energy intake and energy requirements, the latter must first be calculated, taking into account resting metabolic rate and activity level. Resting metabolic rate is computed as follows: for men, 900 + 10 × weight (kg); for women, 800 + 7 × weight (kg). This number is multiplied by the "activity factor": 1.2 for low activity level (sedentary life); 1.4 for moderate activity level, and 1.6 for high activity level (job requiring manual labor; regular daily exercise program). Diets aiming at moderate caloric restriction will provide calories below the energy requirement but above 800 kcal/d. These diets meet overall needs for protective nutrients such as protein, vitamins, and minerals. Implementation of such balanced diets can be achieved in various ways.

Detailed modification of usual diet constituents involves reduction in refined carbohydrates, alcohol, and saturated fats and conversely an increase in fibers, and reduction of portions across the board. This is not expensive and may induce long-lasting change toward healthy eating habits; it has the disadvantage of remaining highly palatable, representing a constant source of temptation.

Liquid diet formulas are generally well tolerated. Advantages are simplicity and reduction of temptation; however, the liquid formula is monotonous and low in bulk, with consequent problems of constipation. Addition of 1 tablespoon of bran to each liquid feeding is recommended.

The above diets are made more effective by being administered in multiple, spaced feedings (4–5/d). The likelihood of success is enhanced by supportive follow-up through diet clubs and a skilled nutritionist. Patients must have realistic expectations concerning rate of weight loss. The energy deficit needed to lose 0.45 kg (1 lb) of fat is about 3600 kcal (9 kcal to 1 g), which on an 800- to 1000-kcal diet will occur over 5–6 days. However, during the first 10–14 days of dieting, the loss of a high proportion of water accelerates the rate of weight loss (often 0.45 kg every 2 days). Patients must be aware of these different phases in order to avoid discouragement.

Very low calorie diets (also known as protein-sparing modified fast) provide less than 800 kcal/d, are unbalanced and somewhat risky, and so are indicated only for refractory cases of moderate-severe obesity. They have specific contraindications: atherosclerotic cardiovascular disease; history of cardiac arrhythmias; liver or kidney disease; treatment with diuretics, steroids, adrenergic stimulating agents; and significant systemic disease. Patients must be carefully screened before being started on the diet, which is continued for no longer than 12 weeks. At 1- to 2-week intervals, patients are evaluated for progress and side effects (ECG, complete blood count, chemistry panel).

The composition of very low calorie diets should take into account some basic needs. The Recommended Dietary Allowance (RDA) for protein is 0.8 g/kg/d, which may be increased to 1 g/kg/d to reduce protein catabolism. The caloric provision for a 70-kg man would be 280 kcal. Carbohydrates at 50 g/d (200 kcal) minimize ketosis and help maintain circulating levels of triiodothyronine. Addition of 10 g of essential fatty acids (90 kcal) would bring the total caloric intake to 570 kcal/d. These diets should be implemented under strict physician supervision.

While these diets can be successful (2- to 3-kg weight loss per week) and completely correct hyperglycemia in many obese diabetic patients, long-term maintenance of the weight loss is not better than with behavior modification.

Exercise

Regular physical activity should always accompany dietary restriction. Exercise increases energy expenditure and reduces the loss in lean body tissue induced by caloric restriction (from 25% to 5%). It also facilitates weight loss by offsetting the decline in basal metabolic rate induced by caloric restriction (basal metabolic rate can decrease by as much as 20% within 2 weeks of caloric restriction).

Obese persons are reluctant to exercise, so recommendations

should begin at the patient's level and be specific. Physical activity is gradually increased toward target levels: exercise at 70% of maximum heart rate (maximum heart rate = 220 − age in years) for at least 20 minutes 3 or more times per week. These targets apply in the absence of ischemic heart disease, peripheral vascular disease, and neuropathy.

Behavior Modification

Behavior modification helps overweight subjects gain control over the environmental situations surrounding their eating. Eating behavior is analyzed by taking into account the ABC: *a*ntecedents of eating (when, where, how, with whom, likes, and dislikes); *b*ehavior of eating (what, how frequently, how rapidly); *c*onsequences of eating (positive and negative rewards). On the basis of the analysis, specific changes are suggested so that patients learn individualized techniques for decreasing caloric intake.

Behavior modification has a rate of success greater than very low calorie diets and pharmacologic treatment in ensuring maintenance of weight loss over time. Hence, the combination of caloric restriction, increased physical activity, and behavior modification (preferably conducted by a trained professional) is the cornerstone of the treatment of moderate obesity.

Drug Therapy

Drug therapy for weight loss is not recommended, since it does not produce any more long-term weight loss than diet alone and it is accompanied by significant side effects. Drugs either increase metabolic rate or suppress appetite. The least risky and occasionally successful drugs are those suppressing appetite. Anorectic drugs may be classified on the basis of chemical structure as phenethylamines or nonphenethylamines.

A. Phenethylamine Derivatives: Amphetamine (Biphetamine), phenmetrazine (Preludin), diethylpropion (Tenuate, Tepanil), phentermine (Fastin, Ionamin, Adipex-P, others), fenfluramine (Pondimin), phenylpropanolamine. The latter is the only drug of this class available over the counter. Amphetamine and phenmetrazine have been abandoned as anorexics, since other derivatives are as effective and have fewer central nervous system and cardiovascular side effects.

B. Nonphenethylamine Derivatives: Mazindol (Mazanor, Sanorex).

These drugs are clearly more effective than placebo but only slightly if at all more effective than diet alone. Side effects are headache, nausea, constipation; insomnia with all except diethylpropion and fenfluramine; and depression and diarrhea often with fenfluramine.

Surgical Interventions

Diets, exercise, behavioral changes, and anorectic drugs have generally failed to modify severe obesity. Since these patients are at high risk for multiple reasons (diabetes, hypertriglyceridemia, increased cardiac work, hypoventilation with hypercapnia, hypertension, cholelithiasis, osteoarthritis), they are candidates for surgical procedures.

The procedure of choice is currently gastric bypass (partial or complete gastric exclusion, gastric transsection), which has proved more benign than jejunoileal bypass. The latter has allowed dramatic weight loss but has several serious complications: fluid and electrolyte imbalance, malnutrition, liver failure, cholelithiasis, bacterial overgrowth, arthritis, and calcium oxalate nephrolithiasis.

Bilateral subdiaphragmatic truncal vagotomy has recently been used in a small number of patients (less than 20 reported) with good success in suppressing appetite and allowing weight loss.

MANAGEMENT OF HYPERGLYCEMIA IN TYPE II DIABETES

The goal of therapy is to maintain fasting plasma glucose (FPG) below 120 mg/dL with normal glycohemoglobin levels. In elderly patients, FPG below 150 mg/dL is acceptable. Education, diet, and exercise are essential in all NIDDM patients. Recommended for all patients are changes in diet composition toward the prudent diet described for type I patients. However, because NIDDM patients are especially prone to potentially harmful effects of high-carbohydrate diets (increased triglyceride and VLDL levels, decreased HDL levels), these effects should be watched for and a partial replacement of carbohydrates with alternative sources of energy considered. Monounsaturated fat (eg, olive oil) does not untowardly increase triglycerides or VLDL or LDL cholesterol and may increase HDL cholesterol. Caloric restriction is mandatory in overweight patients.

In *untreated* type II diabetics on a stable diet and physical activity, FPG is remarkably stable and correlates well with changes in plasma glucose throughout the day. Fasting plasma glucose is thus the easiest way to assess severity of diabetes and make therapeutic choices.

Individuals with FPG less than 180 mg/dL do well for at least some time on diet and exercise. Individuals with FPG above 180 mg/dL should also be started on diet and exercise, but sulfonylureas or insulin may need to be added presently to achieve the desired lowering of FPG. A 2-month trial of diet and exercise is reasonable; however, patients presenting with FPG over 250 mg/dL must be closely monitored (home glucose- and weight-monitoring; weekly telephone contact) because their insulin secretory defect and insulin resistance may not respond to diet and exercise.

Oral Drug Therapy

A. Sulfonylureas: The mechanism of action of sulfonylureas is dual: increase in insulin secretion and improvement of insulin action at target cells. These drugs are a useful *adjunct* to therapy in patients whose hyperglycemia has not responded to diet and exercise.

The University Group Diabetes Program study reported in 1971 that a group of diabetic patients treated with tolbutamide had a statistically significant increase in cardiovascular mortality (2.5 times that of the diet-alone group). Since 1971, several independent reevaluations of this study have found weaknesses in the study's design and conduct. The tolbutamide group may have had greater cardiovascular risk factors at entry into the study. The finding occurred at only 4 centers; none of the treatment modalities (diet alone, fixed dose of tolbutamide, fixed dose of insulin, variable dose of insulin) resulted in correction of the hyperglycemia. In addition, 4 other controlled studies failed to confirm the findings of the University Group study. The FDA, while maintaining a label for warning, has changed its 1975 position that (for adult-onset diabetes) insulin treatment is always preferable to oral hypoglycemics.

The sulfonylureas currently available in the USA are classified as "first generation" (tolbutamide, tolazamide, chlorpropamide, acetohexamide) and "second generation" (glyburide, glipizide). The main difference between the 2 groups is the greater potency on a weight basis of the second-generation compounds. Because smaller doses may reduce the incidence of side effects, preference is currently given to second-generation sulfonylureas.

Contraindications for sulfonylurea drug treatment are (1) type I diabetes, (2) pregnancy, (3) major surgery, (4) history of adverse reactions or allergy to sulfonylureas or similar compounds, and (5) significant liver or kidney disease, because these patients are more susceptible to severe hypoglycemia.

1. Tolbutamide (Orinase, Oramide)–Tolbutamide is the shortest acting of the sulfonylureas; it has a plasma half-life of 4–5 hours and duration of hypoglycemic action of 6–12 hours. It is metabolized by the liver to completely inactive products, which are excreted, with the parent drug, in the urine. Effective daily dose ranges between 500 and 3000 mg, to be administered in 2–3 divided doses before meals. Tolbutamide has not been reported to cause water retention, but it has been associated with alcohol-induced flushing.

2. Tolazamide (Tolinase, Ronase, Tolamide)–Tolazamide is an intermediate-acting sulfonylurea. The plasma half-life is 7 hours and the duration of action 12–24 hours. It is metabolized by the liver to mostly inactive products; excretion is 85% through the kidneys. Daily dose ranges between 100 and 1000 mg, to be given either in one dose before breakfast (for doses up to 500 mg) or in 2 divided doses. It has not been associated with either water retention or alcohol-induced flushing.

3. Chlorpropamide (Diabinese)–Chlorpropamide is the longest acting, most powerful, and riskiest of the sulfonylureas. The plasma half-life is 36 hours and the duration of hypoglycemic action up to 60 hours. Liver metabolism is slow, and 60–80% of the active drug is excreted through the kidneys. Daily dose ranges between 100 and 500 mg, to be administered in a single dose. Chlorpropamide has been associated with water retention (inappropriate ADH → dilutional hyponatremia) and alcohol-induced flushing. In view of the very long half-life of the drug, chlorpropamide-induced hypoglycemia may be life-threatening when not promptly recognized and treated. Treatment may require sustained infusion of concentrated glucose solutions (10% dextrose) for days to prevent recurrent hypoglycemia. Patients unresponsive to 500 mg of chlorpropamide per day should be switched to insulin.

4. Acetohexamide (Dymelor)–Acetohexamide has characteristics similar to tolazamide, with the disadvantage that its hepatic metabolism yields products 2–3 times more potent than the parent drug. Since it offers no specific therapeutic advantage, it is rarely used.

5. Glyburide (DiaBeta, Micronase)–Glyburide may be considered a more benign counterpart to chlorpropamide. It is a powerful drug, with a duration of action of about 24 hours. It is metabolized by the liver to inactive products and is excreted by both the gut and kidneys. Daily dose ranges between 2.5 and 20 mg administered as a single daily dose. It has not been associated with water retention, and it may actually increase free water clearance. It is effective in moderate diabetes and relatively safe in the face of mild renal impairment. Because of its protracted and powerful hypoglycemic effect, it is contraindicated in elderly patients.

6. Glipizide (Glucotrol)–Glipizide is a short-acting sulfonylurea with a distinct insulinotropic effect. Most of the drug disappears from the plasma within 10 hours of administration; it is metabolized by the liver to inactive products excreted with the parent drug through the kidneys. Daily dose ranges between 2.5 and 40 mg, to be given in divided doses 30–40 minutes before meals. Successful treatment with a single larger dose before breakfast has been reported. In view of its rapid and short action, glipizide has been advocated for control of postprandial glucose excursions and prevention of B-cell desensitization to the action of sulfonylureas. Glipizide has not been associated with water retention and has a low incidence of alcohol-induced flushing. It is an effective and relatively benign drug with the disadvantage of usually requiring multiple daily doses and the contraindication of significant liver or kidney disease.

Drug interactions–Sulfonylureas are bound to some extent to plasma proteins, and most are metabolized by the liver. Other drugs with competing pharmacokinetics may therefore increase sulfonylurea effect. On this basis, the hypoglycemic effect of sulfonylureas may be potentiated by nonsteroidal antiinflammatory agents, sulfonamides, salicylates, dicumarol, chloramphenicol, monoamine oxidase inhibitors, and β-adrenergic blocking agents. Hypoglycemic action is also increased by probenecid, which reduces the urinary excretion of sulfonylureas and their metabolites. Drugs known to cause hyperglycemia (Table 10–2) antagonize the sulfonylurea effect.

Toxicity of sulfonylureas–Reported frequencies of side effects in large series are 3.2% for tolbutamide, 6% for chlorpropamide, and 1.5% for glyburide and glipizide. Most side effects appear within the first 2 months of treatment. They include blood dyscrasias; allergic skin reactions (including Stevens-Johnson syndrome); photosensitivity reactions; gastrointestinal disturbances (nausea, heartburn, abnormal liver function tests, jaundice); vasomotor phenomena (flushing, mostly with alcohol, headache, tachycardia); antidiuresis and dilutional hyponatremia (mostly induced by cholorpropamide); and hypoglycemia profound and prolonged (mostly induced by chlorpropamide, acetohexamide, large doses of glyburide).

B. α-Glucosidase Inhibitors (Acarbose, Miglitol): α-Glucosidase inhibitors have a high affinity for intestinal sucrase, glycoamylase, and maltase and act primarily to delay the digestion and absorption of complex carbohydrates. In some NIDDM patients, acarbose results in decreased postprandial blood glucose and triglyceride levels. Side effects are flatulence, nausea, and diarrhea. α-Glucosidase inhibitors may become useful adjuncts to sulfonylurea therapy, especially in overweight patients.

C. Biguanides (Phenformin, Metformin): Biguanides are currently not approved for use in the USA because of the risk of lactic acidosis. They are, however, widely used in Europe, Canada, and Australia. They have no effect on insulin secretion but increase glucose uptake by tissues. Metformin (glucophage) is begun in doses of 250–500 mg once daily added to ongoing glyburide administration. The dose is increased gradually to about 500 mg 2 or 3 times daily. Side effects include nausea, weight loss, increased gut motility, flatulence, metallic taste, occasional headache, and dizziness. These symptoms often improve with time. Metformin is most useful in obese patients. It should not be used in underweight patients and must be stopped in normal-weight patients who lose weight. Although Metformin may be less likely than Phenformin to produce lactic acidosis, cases have been reported in the presence of decreased liver or renal function. It should not be given to patients with serum creatinine > 1.5 mg/dL.

D. Insulin: Although type II diabetics can survive without insulin, its use is often necessary to attain control of hyperglycemia. Moreover, the introduction of highly purified pork and human insulins with their minimal antigenicity and lessened risk of immunization has expanded the confidence in situational, temporary use of insulin therapy.

Candidates are (1) patients who, on diet and sulfonylurea therapy, maintain FPG > 120 mg/dL and glycohemoglobin levels above the normal range. (2) Patients whose diabetes may still be responsive to sulfonylureas but who have developed renal or hepatic disease or become pregnant. (3) Patients who, normally controlled on diet and sulfonylureas, experience stressful events (severe infection, surgery, trauma, cardiovascular event).

Insulin treatment can be initiated with a single daily dose (0.2–0.3 U/kg) of an intermediate-acting (NPH or Lente) or long-acting (Ultralente) insulin given before breakfast or at bedtime to supplement basal insulin needs. Patients are requested to monitor their FPG; the dose is increased by 2–3 U at weekly intervals to achieve the desired FPG level. When doses above 30–40 U are needed, administration in 2 separate injections (before breakfast and at bedtime) reduces the risk of hypoglycemia at the time of peak action of the insulin preparation.

If the postprandial blood glucose concentration fails to return to basal before the next meal, regular insulin is added before one or more of the main meals to limit glycemic excursions. The daily insulin dose required to achieve euglycemia may vary from 12 U in lean patients compliant with diet and exercise to 300 U in obese, overfed patients.

An exciting feature of insulin therapy in type II patients is that restoration of euglycemia may be followed by sufficient improvement in insulin secretion and sensitivity to allow reduction in dosage and even discontinuation.

Patients with long-standing severe, untreated type II diabetes gain weight after initiation of insulin therapy. The initial (2 weeks) weight gain is partly due to sodium and fluid retention. However, if the overweight patient is to avoid further weight gain, caloric restriction must be reemphasized when initiating insulin therapy.

Prophylaxis of Atherosclerotic Vascular Disease

Diabetes accelerates cardiovascular disease dramatically in the presence of other risk factors (hypertension, elevated LDL cholesterol, decreased HDL cholesterol, and cigarette smoking). These risk factors must be treated aggressively after achieving good glycemic control. Atherosclerotic disease may be quantified with Doppler studies of the carotid and ileofemoral arteries. Patients with significant peripheral atherosclerosis have a high likelihood of having some coronary disease as well. In the patient already affected by atherosclerotic disease, aggressive lipid-improving measures are indicated (Chapter 12). Routine monitoring of symptoms, peripheral pulses, and feet will identify conditions amenable to medical treatment before they progress to debilitating stages.

HYPERGLYCEMIC EMERGENCIES

DIABETIC KETOACIDOSIS

Diabetic ketoacidosis (DKA) is a profound metabolic derangement caused by severe insulin deficiency. The hallmarks of DKA are **hyperglycemia** (plasma glucose > 300 mg/dL), **ketonemia** (serum ketones positive at a dilution of 1:2 or more), and **acidosis** (arterial pH < 7.3). Obvious concomitants are glycosuria and ketonuria. Additional elements of DKA are dehydration and subsequently elevated serum blood urea nitrogen and creatinine; depletion of total body potassium, phosphorus, and sodium; hyperosmolality; hyperlipidemia; mildly increased serum lactic acid; and increased serum amylase, creatinine phosphokinase, and transaminases.

Symptoms & Signs

Patients present with varying degrees of depressed sensorium (from drowsiness to coma), dehydration (from thirst to loss of skin turgor and postural hypotension with tachycardia), hyperventilation (from mild tachypnea to Kussmaul breathing), and they may complain of abdominal pain. The degree of altered mental status depends on the degree of hyperosmolality and central nervous system acidosis; hyperventilation depends on the degree of metabolic acidosis. Abdominal pain and nausea are common but should spark consideration of intra-abdominal problems that may have provoked the development of ketoacidosis.

The severity of clinical symptoms and biochemical abnormalities is a function of the degree and duration of insulin deficiency. The most serious disturbances are often encountered when ketoacidosis is the presenting manifestation of previously undiagnosed diabetes. Under these circumstances, patients are unaware of the significance of their worsening symptoms and may be brought to medical attention only when dramatic manifestations prompt concern from family or friends.

Pathophysiology & Implications for Treatment

Insulin deficiency allows unrestrained mobilization of energy stores. Since lipolysis, which provides free fatty acids for ketogenesis, is inhibited by very low levels of insulin (< 20 μU/mL), the degree of insulin deficiency must be severe to allow development of DKA. However, absolute insulin deficiency is rare, and additional factors often precipitate DKA, ie, counterregulatory hormones (glucagon, cortisol, growth hormone, catecholamines) and dehydration. Falling insulin levels allow increased glucagon secretion, which itself intensifies ketogenesis and hepatic glucose output. (Pancreatectomized diabetics have a delayed onset and milder degree of ketosis and hyperglycemia.) With progressive insulin deficiency, growth hormone and cortisol levels also rise and further accelerate catabolic processes (Table 10–1). With sustained hyperglycemia, osmotic diuresis and dehydration ensue; hypovolemia stimulates catecholamine secretion, which further reduces insulin delivery to tissues. In advanced DKA, dehydration reduces renal perfusion and total glycosuria, thus contributing to the hyperglycemia. Therefore, initiation of treatment with both insulin and hydration becomes urgent.

Illness increases secretion of antiinsulin hormones. Common precipitators of DKA are infections, even mild ones; vomiting and diarrhea; vascular events; and trauma. Thus, a history focusing on recent events, a careful physical examination, and appropriate x-ray and laboratory studies must be obtained while acute metabolic treatment is begun.

Hyperglycemia & Hyperosmolality

Correction of hyperglycemia is one of the goals of treatment of DKA and is achieved by fluid and insulin therapy. In rare cases, successful treatment may have a potentially fatal complication—**cerebral edema**. A proposed mechanism is the lowering of blood glucose causing an osmotic gradient between blood and brain and a shift of free water into brain tissue. This shift would occur because during sustained hyperglycemia the brain protects itself from dehydration by intracellular accumulation of osmotically active particles of unknown nature (idiogenic osmoles) that dissipate slowly upon correction of the hyperglycemia. Although clinically apparent cerebral edema is a rare complication of DKA treatment, subclinical brain swelling is common. It is recommended that circulating glucose concentrations be corrected gradually and not driven below 250 mg/dL. The target rate of decline in plasma glucose in patients with DKA is approximately 75–100 mg/dL/h, which is safely achieved with a continuous insulin infusion rate of 4–8 U/h.

Ketoacidosis & Bicarbonate

The measurement of ketone bodies, the anion gap, and lactic acidosis are described on pp 484–485.

The routine use of bicarbonate to correct acidosis is discouraged because it offers no advantages and may have untoward effects: (1) reduced tissue oxygenation (correction of the shift to the right of the oxyhemoglobin dissociation curve while 2,3 diphosphoglycerate levels in red blood cells remain depressed); (2) risk of severe hypokalemia; and (3) paradoxical central nervous system acidosis (a decrease in acidosis-driven hyperventilation will lead to an increase in pCO_2, which equilibrates rapidly across the blood-brain barrier while bicarbonate does not, thus causing central nervous system acidosis when the systemic pH is being corrected).

Nevertheless, when acidosis is so profound (pH 7 or less, bicarbonate < 5 mmol/L) that life-threatening arrhythmias and hypotension may ensue, bicarbonate should be exogenously provided. The target of alkali therapy is to raise the pH to 7.2 or the bicarbonate to 8–10 mmol/L. The amount of sodium bicarbonate required can be estimated by multiplying the desired increase in bicarbonate (mmol/L) times its volume of distribution (L), which is approximately 50% of body weight (kg). Thus, over the first hour of therapy, 1–2 ampules (44–88 mmol) of bicarbonate diluted in 1 L of 0.45% saline may be infused. Sodium bicarbonate should *never* be added to 0.9% saline lest a markedly hypertonic solution be produced that may worsen any degree of hyperosmolality already present.

Laboratory Abnormalities

A. Fluid & Sodium Losses: The osmotic diuresis from protracted hyperglycemia causes **dehydration**. Some degree of dehydration is always present. Severe dehydration causes sunken eyes, dry mucosa, loss of skin turgor, absence of axillary sweating, and hypotension. Such signs indicate that fluid loss approximates 6–10% of body weight. The fluid necessary over the first 24 hours ranges in the adult individual with DKA between 5 and 10 L. Two liters should be provided within the first 2 hours to reestablish urine flow (with the benefit of enhanced glycosuria) and to improve tissue perfusion; the remaining requirement can be more gradually provided.

Although losses of water are in excess of solute, a substantial sodium deficit is also generally present. Serum sodium is generally normal or reduced to 125–130 mEq/L, but some of the reduction is dilutional consequent to hyperglycemia and hyperlipidemia. See p 57.

Guidelines for fluid and sodium administration are the following: 0.9% saline is administered at 1L/h for the first 2 hours—with the exception that if bicarbonate is needed this should be diluted in 0.45%

saline; fluids are then switched to 0.45% saline infused at 300–400 mL/h; as soon as plasma glucose declines below 300 mg/dL, administration of 5% dextrose solution is initiated to maintain glycemia between 250 and 300 mg/dL.

B. Potassium: A deficit in total body potassium is a consistent feature of DKA as a result of the extensive catabolism of the lean body mass, of which potassium is an integral component, and of the enhanced aldosterone secretion that is triggered by hypovolemia. Potassium is mostly lost through the urine but also through the gastrointestinal tract if vomiting and diarrhea are present. Despite such total body deficit, serum levels may be normal or elevated, since the hypercatabolism and the metabolic acidosis maintain a continuous shift of potassium from the intracellular to the extracellular compartment. Any impairment in renal function, preexisting or due to hypovolemia, further contributes to the hyperkalemia often observed at presentation of DKA. Few patients in DKA present with hypokalemia, and their potassium deficits are severe and life-threatening.

As treatment for DKA is initiated, serum potassium levels decline through several mechanisms. Fluids expand volume and improve renal function, which augments potassium excretion. This mechanism accounts for the fact that during the treatment of DKA not only endogenous potassium but also up to 50% of the administered potassium is excreted in the urine. Insulin causes reentry of potassium into the cellular compartment both as a direct effect and as a consequence to the reduction of acidemia. If bicarbonate is administered, the latter effect will be magnified and greater potassium supplements will be necessary to avoid severe hypokalemia.

Patients who remain oliguric during treatment still need some potassium replacement because the cellular reentry mechanisms will be operative; replacement should be approximately 50% of usual owing to reduced renal potassium excretion. In general, if serum potassium is over 4 mEq/L at presentation, potassium replacement is initiated during the second hour of treatment at a rate of 10–30 mEq/h if the patient has adequate urine output. If the initial potassium is less than 4 mEq/L, replacement should be added to treatment immediately. A maximum of 60–80 mEq of potassium can be given per hour, but only rare patients will need acute replacement of this magnitude.

Potassium replacement is titrated on the basis of frequent monitoring of serum levels and of changes in the ECG. Hyperkalemia is suggested by flat P waves and high peaked T waves; hypokalemia by lowered QRS voltage, ST depression, low or inverted T waves, and appearance of U waves. While it is critical to maintain adequate serum potassium levels, it is also critical to avoid hyperkalemia. Full correction of the total body deficit need not be achieved within the short period of acute therapy but may await restoration of oral intake.

C. Phosphorus: Since phosphorus is an integral component of lean body mass, its behavior during ketoacidosis parallels that of potassium. Tissue catabolism and phosphaturia induce depletion of total body phosphorus, averaging 1 mmol/kg body weight. Yet at presentation, patients are generally hyperphosphatemic owing to the ongoing catabolic processes and to the impaired uptake of glucose by tissues, which would mediate phosphorus reuptake. As therapy with fluid and insulin is instituted, there is a decline in serum phosphate that may reach levels below 1 mg/dL by the fourth to sixth hour of therapy. When serum phosphate falls below 1 mg/dL, serious disturbances in tissue metabolism, central nervous system dysfunction, and rhabdomyolysis may occur. Since intravenous phosphorus replacement is hazardous (hypocalcemia and tetany) and since addition of phosphate to the standard therapy for DKA does not change the outcome, *intravenous phosphate replacement is not generally prescribed.* Exceptions are the rare patient with hypophosphatemia on presentation and patients with serum phosphate less than 1 mg/dL after the first 4–6 hours of treatment. In these cases, phosphate is provided at a rate not exceeding 3 mmol/h. This is given as potassium phosphate salt (Abbot stock solution, 5-mL vial containing 4 mEq K/mL and 3 mmol PO_4/mL). One-half of this vial (2.5 mL) added to 1 L of fluid infused at 300–400 mL/h will provide the desired rate of phosphate replacement. Additional KCl should be added to the fluid in order to achieve the desired rate of potassium administration (10–30 mEq/h). *Calcium levels should be carefully followed.*

Phosphorus replacement is contraindicated in patients with renal insufficiency.

D. Hyperlactacidemia and Lactic Acidosis: Hypoxia of any cause results in increased production of lactic acid by skeletal muscle, liver, and erythrocytes, with subsequent increase in blood levels. Normal lactate levels in venous blood are up to 1.5 mmol (mEq)/L or 13.5 mg/dL (mmol × 9). Concentrations above 7 mmol/L constitute lactic acidosis. In uncomplicated DKA, lactate levels may be mildly elevated to 2–4 mmol/L and correlate with the extent of volume contraction and the degree of acidosis that prevents tissue conversion of lactate to pyruvate. Lactate levels in the range of lactic acidosis are seldom encountered in ketoacidosis unless concomitant factors such as hypotension, cardiac events, and—until a few years ago—phenformin administration, are present. In view of the problems surrounding precise quantitation of keto acid concentrations, it is safe routine to obtain a determination of blood lactate in patients with severe ketoacidosis. In obtaining the sample, special precautions are taken to avoid spuriously elevated levels due to continuing glycolysis by red cells: blood is collected either directly in tubes containing a deproteinizing agent (perchloric acid) or in tubes containing sodium fluoride and potassium oxalate; separation of the plasma should be completed within 15 minutes.

E. Hyperlipidemia and Serum Enzyme Abnormalities: Most patients with DKA have significant lipemia. Depending on the severity, it may be readily detected at the time of blood drawing ("cream of tomato" appearance of blood), noticed in the laboratory, suspected because of significant hyponatremia or documented by measurement of triglycerides, which should routinely be obtained. Serum triglycerides may be elevated to 2000–20,000 mg/dL.

Hypertriglyceridemia of insulin deficiency is caused by the reduced synthesis of lipoprotein lipase in adipose tissue, with consequent impaired clearance of triglyceride-rich lipoproteins. Thus, the most severe hypertriglyceridemia occurs when the development of insulin deficiency is gradual so that the patient maintains regular food intake and accumulates alimentary chylomicrons. The hyperlipidemia is readily responsive to insulin therapy and does not require any additional acute treatment, but restriction of dietary fat for a few days may be necessary for complete correction.

Severe hypertriglyceridemia may produce pancreatitis. Although pancreatitis is generally associated with triglyceride levels above 2000 mg/dL, lower levels may be found if the patient has not eaten for a few days. Since patients with DKA often complain of abdominal pain and have a slight elevation of serum amylase (generally of salivary origin), the possibility of pancreatitis often arises. Because triglyceride-rich lipoproteins inhibit serum amylase activity, the amylase measurement should be performed on a diluted sample to avoid underestimation. In addition to careful assessment of clinical status, measurement of plasma lipase activity—usually not increased in uncomplicated DKA—is a useful diagnostic adjunct toward excluding pancreatitis.

Other serum enzymes are often increased in DKA: transaminases and creatinine phosphokinase. In the absence of other causes, the former may be attributed to hepatic enlargement; the latter may be related to subclinical rhabdomyolysis.

Protocol for Treatment of DKA

If the patient is comatose, routine measures are the following:

1. Establish airway.

2. Establish intravenous access, and obtain 30 mL of blood* for STAT laboratory studies (lytes, glucose, osmolality, renal and liver function, complete blood count).

3. Stabilize the cardiopulmonary system, and start ECG monitor.

4. Administer intravenously, 1 ampule of naloxone, 100 mg of thiamine, and 25 mL of 50% dextrose in water (½ ampule). The last will be therapeutic if the cause of coma is hypoglycemia and will not significantly alter the outcome if the cause is a hyperglycemic state, but see footnote*.

5. Place bladder catheter and nasogastric tube.

6. Obtain arterial blood gas.

7. Obtain urinalysis and chest x-ray.

Once the diagnosis of DKA is established, in the comatose as well as the conscious patient, treatment must begin. Take charge; enter all interventions and the patient's responses on an appropriate flow-sheet; monitor the patient's chemistries every 1–2 hours; inform the patient's family about the seriousness of the condition: for elderly patients mortality approaches 5–10%.

A. First Hour:

1. Fluids–Give 0.9% saline at 1000 mL/h unless bicarbonate is needed.

2. Potassium–Consider only if initial potassium is less than 4 mEq/L; in such case provide at 20 mEq/h (40 mEq/h if initial potassium is less than 3 mEq/L).

3. Bicarbonate–Consider only if initial pH is 7.0 or below and patient is very ill. The sodium bicarbonate (44–88 mEq; see above) should be diluted in 0.45% saline to be infused at 1000 mL/h. It should *not* be given as a bolus, since it may depress respiratory drive.

4. Insulin–Under no circumstance should initiation of insulin treatment be delayed. Give 10 U of Regular insulin intravenously as a bolus, and start continuous intravenous infusion at 0.1–0.15 U/kg/h depending on the severity of the DKA. The infusion bag is prepared by adding 50 U of Regular insulin to 500 mL of 0.45% or 0.9% saline (0.1 U/mL) and flushing at least 50 mL of the solution through the entire tubing system to saturate all binding of insulin to the plastic. If continuous intravenous infusion is impossible for any reason, give Regular insulin as discrete intramuscular injection at doses of 0.15 U/kg. The subcutaneous route is discouraged because of unreliable absorption.

Recheck blood glucose, electrolytes, and arterial pH after 1 hour of treatment. Begin treating underlying factors, if identified.

B. Second Hour:

1. Fluids–Continue 0.9% saline at 1000 mL/h unless bicarbonate administration needs to be repeated (pH still below 7.0).

2. Potassium–Begin KCl at 20 mEq/h in all patients unless serum potassium remains greater than 5.5 mEq. Use 10 mEq/h if patient is oliguric.

---

* Place a drop of the blood drawn on a reagent strip for glucose determination, and if urine has been obtained, test for glucose and ketones. This accelerates by 1 hour the diagnosis of a hyperglycemic emergency and avoids administration of glucose to a patient with coma due to DKA.

3. Bicarbonate–If pH remains below 7.0 and patient appears very ill, repeat protocol used during first hour.

4. Insulin–Continue intravenous infusion (or intramuscular injection) at same rates as during the first hour. If by the end of the first hour, the fall in plasma glucose was less than 10% of initial value, repeat intravenous bolus of 10 U of Regular insulin.

Recheck glucose, pH, and electrolytes.

C. Thereafter:

1. Fluids–Switch to 0.45% saline at 300–400 mL/h. When plasma glucose declines below 300 mg/dL, switch to 5% dextrose at the same rate, aiming at maintaining plasma glucose between 250 and 300 mg/dL.

2. Potassium–Continue replacement at 10–30 mEq/h.

3. Phosphate–Replacement is generally started by the third to fourth hour of treatment if serum levels have fallen below 1 mg/dL. Provide at a rate of 3 mmol/h as potassium phosphate, decreasing accordingly the content of potassium chloride in fluids. Monitor serum calcium.

4. Insulin–As blood glucose decreases, the rate of infusion is empirically adjusted on the basis of the following formula:

(Plasma glucose in mg/dL)/150 = Units of insulin/h

Recheck glucose and electrolytes every 2 hours.

The targets of treatment of DKA are correction of the acidosis (serum bicarbonate > 15 mmol/L) and of the hyperglycemia (plasma glucose stabilized at approximately 250 mg/dL). The latter goal is achieved earlier than the former (average time is 6 hours versus 11 hours for correction of the acidosis). *Intensive insulin therapy (intravenous or intramuscular) should continue until stable correction of the acidosis.* Only at that time can the transition be made to subcutaneous insulin therapy and to completion of electrolyte replenishment through the oral route with resumption of feeding. When interrupting intravenous delivery of insulin it should be remembered that the plasma half-life of insulin is only 3–5 minutes and the biologic half-life does not exceed 90 minutes. Thus, an appropriate crossover period should be allowed, and subcutaneous insulin should be started on the tail of the intravenous infusion.

By this time it should have been determined which precipitating or complicating factors had contributed to the development of ketoacidosis. Treatment of concurrent illnesses should be under way, and plans should be made to educate the patient in order to prevent future episodes.

HYPERGLYCEMIC HYPEROSMOLAR NONKETOTIC STATE

The hyperglycemic hyperosmolar nonketotic (HHNK) state is characterized by the following: (1) Severe hyperglycemia (plasma glucose > 500 mg/dL). (2) Hyperosmolality (serum osmolality > 330 mOsm/kg. (3) Profound dehydration. (4) Absence of ketonemia (serum ketones negative or positive only in undiluted serum). (5) Absence of acidosis (arterial pH > 7.3, and serum bicarbonate greater than 18 mEq/L—unless there is concomitant lactic acidosis). Additional elements include elevation in serum blood urea nitrogen and creatinine, often greater than in DKA owing to the more profound dehydration; depletion of total body potassium and phosphorus of lesser magnitude than in DKA owing to lack of acidosis; some degree of hyperlactacidemia depending on precipitating or accompanying illnesses; and varying degrees of hyperlipidemia.

Depressed sensorium, seizures, or focal neurologic findings may be present. The degree of mental obtundation correlates with serum osmolality: above an osmolality of 350 mOsm/kg, coma can be expected. Focal findings might represent a clue to the precipitating event (cerebrovascular accident) but may also be due to the metabolic encephalopathy of the hyperosmolar state. Hyperventilation and Kussmaul breathing are absent unless lactic acidosis is also present.

Patients are generally older than those presenting with DKA, are often not known to have diabetes, or may have had mild diabetes. Preexisting cardiac or renal disease is common (up to 80%), and patients may be taking medications such as thiazide diuretics, β-adrenergic blockers, phenytoin, chlorpromazine (all capable of reducing insulin secretion), or glucocorticoids. A careful drug history will often help identify the precipitating event, which may also be an infection, an acute cardiovascular event (silent myocardial infarction!), trauma, or surgery.

Pathophysiology & Implications for Treatment

The HHNK state results from a degree of insulin deficiency sufficient to impair peripheral glucose utilization and to promote excessive hepatic glucose output but not sufficient to allow lipolysis and ketogenesis. These patients have lesser insulin deficiency than patients with DKA.

In a mild diabetic, the HHNK state may be initiated by dehydration (diuretics, gastrointestinal upset, poor nutritional status), which leads to hyperosmolality and to impaired insulin secretion.

The search for precipitating events must be as prompt and exhaustive as in patients with DKA. Neurologic abnormalities are common but are usually a consequence of the hyperosmolar state. Lethargy or coma, hallucinations, aphasia, homonymous hemianopia, hemisensory deficits, hemiparesis, unilateral hyperreflexia, Babinski's signs, myoclonic twitches, vestibular dysfunction, hyperpnea, hyperthermia, and meningeal signs and seizures have all been reported in patients. Such manifestations usually improve with correction of the hyperosmolar state.

A. Hyperglycemia, Dehydration, and Hyperosmolality: Patients who are unaware of having diabetes may further aggravate their hyperglycemia by consuming large volumes of sugar-containing drinks to quench their thirst. Such patients may nevertheless be protected from becoming severely hyperosmolar, since the continuous oral intake of fluids compensates for the osmotic diuresis and dilutes other osmotically active particles, particularly sodium chloride. The patients most likely to become hyperosmolar (prompted by hyperglycemia, dehydration, and hypernatremia) are those with poor oral intake (elderly, confused, bedridden patients) with protracted gastrointestinal losses or with inappropriate absence of thirst. Such severe hyperosmolar states are uncommon in patients with DKA, since the acidosis produces symptoms well before the development of extreme dehydration.

The aggressiveness of fluid therapy depends upon the degree of dehydration. In the HHNK state, larger quantities of fluids are necessary than in DKA, generally 2–3 L over the first 2 hours and 6–12 L throughout the period of intensive treatment. During the first 2 hours, 0.45% saline should be used to correct the hyperosmolar state as well. Only if the patient is hypotensive should fluid therapy be started with 0.9% saline. As serum osmolality and sodium fall, 0.9% saline is used, and when plasma glucose levels decline below 300 mg/dL, 5% dextrose solutions are administered. Because patients presenting with HHNK syndrome are generally elderly and often have some cardiovascular or renal compromise, it is best to monitor central venous pressure during the intensive phase of fluid replacement.

While the main metabolic abnormalities underlying DKA (ketonemia and acidosis) can only be reversed by insulin therapy, the main abnormalities of the HHNK state (dehydration and hyperosmolality) are responsive to fluid replacement. The hyperglycemia should be treated with insulin. Generally, the overall amount of insulin required is smaller than in DKA because patients are less completely insulin-deficient, and as the hyperosmolar state is corrected, endogenous insulin secretion may improve. Since patients are generally profoundly dehydrated at presentation, insulin is administered either intravenously (the preferred route) or intramuscularly. *Subcutaneous insulin should not be used*. The plasma glucose response should be monitored hourly for the first 2–3 hours in order to individualize rates of insulin administration. Occasional patients may be highly resistant to insulin; they should be treated with continuous intravenous infusion at rates sufficient to induce a decrement in plasma glucose of 70–100 mg/h.

B. Electrolyte Disturbances: Protracted osmotic diuresis causes depletion of *total body* sodium, potassium, and phosphorus. Such deficits are milder in the HHNK state than in DKA owing to a lesser degree of tissue catabolism and lack of acidosis.

The circulating levels of electrolytes in the HHNK state also differ from those in ketoacidosis: serum sodium is generally elevated (more severe dehydration), and serum potassium and phosphorus are usually normal or only slightly elevated (lesser shift to the extracellular compartment owing to absence of acidosis). Since with hydration and insulin therapy, circulating potassium will fall, potassium replacement may be necessary from the beginning of treatment. The rate of replacement should take into account kidney function and urine production. As in DKA, acute phosphate therapy does not appear to alter the immediate outcome. However, if patients are severely hypophosphatemic at presentation or if the phosphate level declines during therapy to less than 1 mg/dL, conservative phosphate replacement (3 mmol/h) is implemented as for DKA. Calcium levels must be carefully monitored to prevent hypocalcemia. In the severely phosphorus-depleted patient (weakness, osteomalacia), replacement should be continued through the oral route.

Protocol for Treatment of HHNK State

If the patient is comatose, routine measures are as for ketoacidosis (see p 522).

A. First Hour:

1. Fluids–Give 0.45% saline at 1000–1500 mL/h depending on severity of dehydration. If patient is hypotensive, use 0.9% saline at 1000 mL/h.

2. Potassium–If initial potassium is less than 5 mEq/L, add 10–20 mEq KCl to each liter of fluids.

3. Insulin–Give 10 U of Regular insulin as an intravenous bolus, and start continuous intravenous infusion at 0.1–0.15 U/kg/h depending on severity of presentation. The infusion bag is prepared as described above under Treatment of DKA. If electing to use discrete intramuscular insulin injections instead of continuous infusion, give 0.15 U/kg.

Recheck glucose and electrolytes toward the end of the first hour of treatment.

B. Second Hour:
1. Fluids–Continue same protocol as for first hour.
2. Potassium–Begin (or continue) replacement at 20 mEq/h unless serum potassium value remains greater than 5.5 mEq/L. Reduce dose by 50% if patient is oliguric.
3. Insulin–Continue intravenous infusion or discrete intramuscular injections at same doses as during first hour.
Recheck glucose and electrolytes.
C. Thereafter:
1. Fluids–Continue 0.45% saline at 400–700 mL/h depending on state of hydration. If serum sodium declines below 130 mEq/L or when serum osmolality declines below 320 mEq/L in the absence of hypernatremia, fluids should be switched to 0.9% saline.
When glucose declines below 300 mg/dL, switch to 5% dextrose in 0.45% or 0.9% saline.
2. Potassium–Continue replacement on the basis of serum values.
3. Phosphate–Replace only if serum phosphorus is less than 1 mg/dL. Run potassium phosphate at a rate of 3 mmol/h while decreasing accordingly the content of potassium chloride in other fluids.
4. Insulin–As glycemia is falling, the rate of infusion should be empirically adjusted on the basis of the following formula:

(Plasma glucose in mg/dL)/150 = Units of insulin/h

If intramuscular injections are used, doses should range between 10 and 20 U of Regular insulin every 4 hours.
Recheck glucose, osmolality, and electrolytes every 2–3 hours until patient is stable.
The targets of treatment of the HHNK state are correction of the hyperosmolality (to < 315 mOsm/kg) and of the hyperglycemia (to plasma glucose < 250 mg/dL). Intensive insulin therapy should continue until these goals are achieved.
Many patients presenting with the HHNK syndrome, once the acute decompensation is corrected, will not need chronic insulin therapy. It is recommended, however, that they be observed in the hospital for several days prior to discharge. During this time, diabetic control is optimized; drugs and other factors that may have precipitated the event are eliminated or treated, and the patient and family are educated to prevent future episodes.
The mortality rate of HHNK coma is 10–20% of cases, a much larger figure than for DKA. This reflects the older age of these patients and the frequent presence of other serious medical problems.

CHRONIC COMPLICATIONS OF DIABETES

CHARACTERISTIC FEATURES

Diabetes of several years' duration damages most organs and systems. The most disabling long-term effects are due to the lesions of small and large blood vessels (micro- and macroangiopathy) and of the peripheral nervous system (neuropathies). (See Table 10–8.)

Microangiopathy causes retinopathy, nephropathy, and foot ischemia.

Macroangiopathy is an acceleration of widespread atherosclerosis.

Neuropathy can be manifested as (1) focal mononeuropathy and radiculopathy, (2) symmetrical sensorimotor neuropathy that may be associated with disabling pain and depression, and (3) autonomic neuropathy.

PATHOGENESIS & THERAPEUTIC IMPLICATIONS

That the presence of clinical diabetes is necessary for the appearance of organ damage is supported by 3 lines of evidence: the nondiabetic identical twins of patients with diabetes do not suffer from

Table 10–8. Guidelines for detection and monitoring of diabetic complications.

At each visit:	Blood pressure (and pulse) supine and upright
	Examination of lower legs (edema)
	Examination of feet (hygiene, lesions)
Twice yearly:	Complete urinalysis
	Serum creatinine, electrolytes, cholesterol, triglycerides
	Visual acuity (macular edema often not detected on fundoscopic examination)
	Fundoscopic examination
	Peripheral pulses
	Neurologic examination
Yearly:	Comprehensive physical examination
	Chemistry panel (protein, enzymes, thyroid) and complete blood count with indices
	Ophthalmologic consultation
	Podiatrist consultation
	ECG

diabetic complications, patients with diabetes due to pancreatitis or toxic B-cell destruction develop the characteristic lesions of microangiopathy, and normal kidneys transplanted to diabetic patients develop the same pathologic features found in diabetic nephropathy. Thus, complications of long-term diabetes are due to the metabolic derangement of the disease rather than a closely linked genetic disorder.

It should therefore be possible to prevent complications with tight glycemic control from the onset of diabetes. Studies in experimentally diabetic dogs have shown that this is the case. However, prolonged restoration of near-normoglycemia does not appear to arrest progression of even incipient stages of diabetic retinopathy, although it can halt progression of some renal abnormalities (increased glomerular and mesangial volume; microalbuminuria). Functional improvements have been observed: decreased exercise-induced microalbuminuria, increased nerve conduction velocity, improved Valsalva ratio.

A prospective approach to the question of whether near-normalization of blood glucose can prevent, arrest, or reverse vascular lesions is currently under way in the Diabetes Control and Complications Trial (DCCT). This multicenter clinical study has randomized 1441 IDDM patients to intensive versus conventional insulin therapy and demonstrated satisfactory glycemic separation between the 2 groups. Pending the results of the trial (it will end in 1993), current information indicates that tight metabolic control should afford its greatest impact when initiated shortly after the onset of diabetes.

Among the many metabolic abnormalities of diabetes, hyperglycemia is likely to play a critical role in the development of microangiopathy and neuropathy. High glucose activates the polyol pathway, resulting in intracellular accumulation of sorbitol (hypertonicity), depletion of myoinositol, and altered intracellular redox state; it also induces nonenzymatic glycosylation of proteins leading to cross-link formation (advanced glycosylation end products). Inhibitors of aldose reductase (the enzyme responsible for conversion of glucose to sorbitol) have proved unable to prevent retinopathy in dogs or to arrest its progression in humans but have improved neuropathologic lesions of diabetic neuropathy. Inhibitors of protein–cross-link formation (eg, aminoguanidine) are in early stages of investigation.

Duration of Diabetes

The duration of diabetes is a major determinant of all complications, especially in IDDM patients, in whom prevalence of retinopathy is 2% after 2 years but 90% after 15 or more years of diabetes. The prevalence of proliferative retinopathy is 20% after 15 years and 60%

after 30 years. Nephropathy is present in 15% of patients after 15 years and 40% after 30 years. Neuropathy is present in 15% of patients after 15 years and 70% after 30 years.

Some rare patients with over 50 years of diabetes are free from complications. Although they may have had better metabolic control than others, substantial differences are not easily documented.

Genetic characteristics therefore appear to endow refractoriness or susceptibility to diabetic complications. The HLA DR4 and DR3 phenotypes may be associated with proliferative retinopathy and a predisposition to hypertension with nephropathy.

Other Risk Factors

In juvenile diabetics, the severity of retinopathy, nephropathy, and coronary artery disease are significantly related to hypertension, which must therefore be aggressively treated. Hyperlipidemia and smoking accelerate the rate of atherosclerosis in the diabetic as well as in the nondiabetic population. Since regular vigorous exercise has been demonstrated to reduce atherosclerotic risk in primates, a safe exercise program should be prescribed and tailored to the individual diabetic patient.

OCULAR LESIONS (See Table 10–9.)

Almost all patients with over 15 years of diabetes exhibit background or nonproliferative retinopathy. This is not associated with visual impairment unless there is macular edema, but in 3% of patients each year there will be progression to proliferative retinopathy that carries a high risk of blindness. Because in both IDDM and NIDDM the severity of retinopathy is related to duration of diabetes, higher glycosylated hemoglobin, and higher blood pressure, glycemic and blood pressure control should be implemented as early as possible in the course of the disease. A beneficial effect of aspirin in slowing progression of background retinopathy was found in a study in Europe but not in one in the USA. The treatment of proliferative retinopathy is panretinal photocoagulation, which preserves useful vision in 7 out of 10 patients who would otherwise become blind.

In older-onset patients, proliferative retinopathy may be present after a short (known) duration of diabetes (20% prevalence after 5 years), indicating the need for careful ophthalmologic evaluation shortly after diagnosis.

Table 10-9. Ocular lesions in diabetes mellitus (DM).

Structure	Abnormality	Pathogenesis	Reversibility	Treatment
Lens	Changes leading to short-sightedness (often at diagnosis of DM)	Dehydration.	Yes	Diabetic control (initially may result in hyperopia lasting 2–3 weeks).
	Subcapsular cataract in young patients (posterior pole opacities rapidly progressing)	Associated with severe hyperglycemia.	±	Diabetic control, surgical removal.
	Accelerated typical senile cataract	Acceleration in DM due to polyol accumulation and glycosylation of crystallin proteins.	No	Surgical removal.
Iris	Iritis or impairment of pupil reaction to light and accommodation	Glycogen infiltration of pigment epithelium of sphincter and dilator muscles.	Yes	Diabetic control.
	Rubeosis iridis and resultant neovascular glaucoma	New vessel proliferation on anterior iris and at the angle of anterior chamber (may occur after cataract extraction).	Rarely	Panretinal photocoagulation to decrease stimulus for new vessels; diagnose and treat glaucoma; cryoablation of ciliary body is last resort.

Retina				
	Increased fluorescein leakage into vitreous (detected by vitreous fluorophotometry	Increased permeability of pigment epithelium and retinal capillaries.	Yes	Diabetic control, blood pressure control.
	Background diabetic retinopathy: microaneurysms, hard yellow exudates, hemorrhages, retinal edema, focal maculopathy	Loss of supporting cells (pericytes), lesion of capillary endothelium, increased vascular permeability.	±	Diabetic control, blood pressure control, focal laser treatment for macular edema.
	Preproliferative retinopathy: soft white exudates (infarcted nerve fibers), venous beading, intraretinal microvascular abnormalities (IRMA), areas of capillary closure, diffuse maculopathy	Obliteration of vessels, ischemia.	±	Diabetic control, blood pressure control, grid laser treatment around macula for macular edema (not very effective).
	Proliferative retinopathy: neovascular proliferation, glial proliferation, retinal elevation, vitreous hemorrhage	Ischemia leads to local production of angiogenic factors. New vessels may hemorrhage into vitreous; glial proliferation and vitreo-retinal traction may cause retinal detachment.	Yes (by PRP), but abruptly tightened control may exacerbate it.	Panretinal photocoagulation (PRP) to decrease stimulus for angiogenic factor; vitrectomy after repeated vitreous hemorrhage; repair of retinal tears; blood pressure control.

RENAL MANIFESTATIONS (See Table 10–10.)

Diabetic nephropathy, defined as proteinuria > 0.5 g total protein/24 h, is a progressive condition that leads to end-stage renal failure or premature mortality due to cardiovascular disease. No genetic markers of susceptibility to nephropathy are firmly established, but patients at risk can be identified early in the course by repeated measurements of microalbuminuria, which precedes overt proteinuria. The initial phase of microalbuminuria is closely related to poor metabolic control; its progression is related to both poor glycemic control and rise in blood pressure. In overt diabetic nephropathy, the rate of decline of GFR can be substantially reduced by effective antihypertensive treatment and possibly by a reduction in protein intake.

Diabetic patients are particularly susceptible to renal damage induced by **x-ray contrast dyes**. This renal tubular damage causes oliguria-anuria and rising creatinine. The rise in serum creatinine is usually transient, peaking at 48–96 hours after the procedure and returning to baseline within 1–4 weeks. Occasionally, acute renal failure develops. Predisposing factors for this complication are older age, dehydration, preexisting renal impairment, and liver disease. In patients with florid nephrotic syndrome or serum creatinine > 3 mg/dL, the diagnostic yield of the x-ray procedure should be very carefully weighed against the risk of precipitating permanent renal insufficiency.

In order to reduce this possible complication of dye studies, diabetic patients should be appropriately hydrated before the procedure. Hydration should be continued after the procedure with detailed monitoring of fluid balance (acute fluid overload is a real risk if renal function declines acutely) and serum creatinine checked at 12-hour intervals until a pattern is identified.

DIABETIC NEUROPATHIES (See Tables 10–11 and 10–12.)

Focal neuropathies (mononeuropathy and radiculopathy) tend to be acute in onset, to be asymmetrical, and to resolve spontaneously. Patients with foot-drop due to peroneal palsy should be splinted and have physical therapy to prevent contractures.

Peripheral sensorimotor polyneuropathy tends to be gradual in onset, to be symmetrical, and to mostly affect feet and legs in a stocking distribution. Damage to large sensory fibers produces decreased position and light touch sensation, and damage to small fibers produces decreased pain and temperature sensation. Deep tendon reflexes (especially the Achilles tendon) are diminished or absent. Symptoms may be absent, may reflect the predominant deficit (impaired balance, numbness, recurrent trauma due to loss of pain and temperature sensation), or be manifested as pain (contact paresthesia, tingling, burning, shooting, stabbing, tearing). Disabling pain (reflecting small-fiber regeneration) may occur in the absence of striking neurologic defects and of impaired conduction velocity. An especially severe form of painful neuropathy is part of the syndrome of "diabetic neuropathic cachexia" described mostly in elderly male diabetics. These patients manifest neuropathic pain, depression, anorexia, impotence, leg muscle wasting (amyotrophy), and severe weight loss. Patients with these symptoms will spontaneously regain weight and completely recover.

Peripheral polyneuropathy is probably related to the abnormal metabolic milieu and it is treated with attempts at optimizing diabetic control. Although this may not resolve the neuropathy entirely and may, at the outset, even worsen the pain, it generally produces long-term amelioration. Treatment with drugs that prevent accumulation of sorbitol and depletion of myoinositol within the nerve (aldose-reductase inhibitors) is still experimental. Treatment of pain usually begins with amitriptyline in gradually increasing doses; ordinarily 75 mg at bedtime will suffice. At higher doses, postural hypotension, urinary retention, and drowsiness may become disabling side effects. In cases not responding sufficiently to amitriptyline, fluphenazine (1 mg 3 times daily) may be added. Topical analgesic treatment with capsaicin cream is effective in some patients.

The most severe and irreversible degrees of autonomic neuropathy are generally found in patients with long-standing type I diabetes.

HEART & VASCULAR DISEASE

Heart disease is a major cause of morbidity and mortality in diabetics. Coronary artery atherosclerosis is 2–3 times more common in diabetics of all ages when compared with age-matched control groups. Acute myocardial infarction in the diabetic patient is followed by shorter 5-year survival than in the nondiabetic and is complicated by a greater incidence of shock, silent infarction, and congestive heart failure. Heart failure may, however, be independent from coronary artery disease and stem instead from diabetic cardiomyopathy, characterized by cardiomegaly, nonspecific electrocardiographic changes, and echocardiographic evidence of decreased left ventricular function in the absence of angiographic evidence of coronary artery disease. Pathologically there is interstitial fibrosis and accumulation of PAS-positive material (glycoproteins). The increased risk imparted by diabetes for both coronary artery disease and heart failure is greater in women than in men.

Table 10-10. Renal lesions in diabetes.

Structure	Abnormality*	Pathogenesis*	Reversibility	Treatment
Glomerulus	Hypertrophy, hyperfiltration (GFR > 120 mL/min)	Hyperglycemia, excess growth hormone	Yes	Diabetic control.
	Microalbuminuria (30–250 mg/24 h, NV < 14)	Increased glomerular permeability secondary to altered hemodynamics and basement membrane composition	±	Diabetic control, blood pressure control.
	Persistent proteinuria (> 0.5 g/24 h)	Same	±	Blood pressure control, ?diabetic control.
	Decreased GFR, rapidly progressing toward renal failure	Obliteration of critical mass of glomeruli by mesangial expansion (Kimmelstiel-Wilson nodules, diffuse glomerulosclerosis)	No	Blood pressure control, reduced protein intake, hemodialysis, peritoneal dialysis, transplantation.
	Hypertension	Blood volume expansion secondary to decreased GFR	No	Salt restriction. Drugs‡: thiazide diuretics, loop diuretics, angiotensin-converting enzyme inhibitors, calcium-channel blockers.

Juxtaglomerular apparatus	Syndrome[†] of hyporeninemic hypoaldosteronism (chronic renal insufficiency, hyperkalemia, hyperchloremic acidosis)	Lesion of juxtaglomerular cells secondary to hyalinization of afferent arterioles	No	If K > 5.5, consider Furosemide.
Medulla	Acute form of renal tubular acidosis following DKA; acute tubular necrosis following x-ray contrast	?Osmotic changes secondary to severe hyperglycemia and ketonemia	Yes	Diabetic control, hydration.
	Necrotizing papillitis	Complication of pyelonephritis hyperglycemia	No	Antibiotics; watch for hydronephrosis.
	Acute/chronic pyelonephritis	Renal involvement from often asymptomatic urinary tract infections common in diabetics	±	Surveillance for asymptomatic urinary tract infection, antibiotics.

*GFR = Glomerular filtration rate.

[†]This syndrome may also be consequent to impaired renin release due to autonomic neuropathy and/or to production of inactive renin of large molecular weight.

[‡]See also treatment of hypertension in diabetic patients.

537

Table 10–11. Neuropathies in diabetes.

Type	Affected Structure	Pathogenesis	Clinical Manifestations	Reversibility	Treatment
Mononeuropathy	Mixed spinal or cranial nerve	Vascular	*Common:* 3rd, 4th, or 6th cranial nerve palsy (ptosis, diplopia, ophthalmoplegia), 7th cranial nerve (Bell's palsy), ulnar palsy, peroneal palsy (foot drop).	Yes (1–8 months)	None
Radiculopathy	Nerve root	?Vascular	Acute onset of pain and sensory loss in the dermatome distribution of a spinal cord nerve root; *Thoracic:* pressure or sharp pain in lower chest/upper abdomen; *Lumbar:* pain in hips, anterior	Yes (6–20 months)	Nerve block; amitriptyline

			...thigh, knee, calf. Perform EMG to substantiate diagnosis.		
Polyneuropathy	Somatosensory nerve fibers and terminals (Schwann cell abnormalities and segmental demyelination)	Metabolic (sorbitol accumulation, myoinositol depletion)	*Lower extremities* generally involved bilaterally; pain and paresthesias most common at night; diminished sensation to touch, temperature, pain, vibration; loss of reflexes. *Upper extremities*: atrophy of intrinsic hand muscle, sensory impairment.	±	Diabetic control.* For relief of pain: amitriptyline†, 25–200 mg, ± fluphenazine, 1 mg 3 times a day; topical capsaicin cream.
Autonomic neuropathy	Parasympathetic fibers, sympathetic ganglion cells and post-ganglionic fibers	Metabolic	See Table 10–12.	±	Diabetic control and specifics in Table 10–12.

*Initially pain may be transiently exacerbated by improved control.
†Amitriptyline may cause postural hypotension and urinary retention.

Table 10–12. Autonomic neuropathy in diabetes.

System Involved	Abnormality	Pathogenesis	Clinical and Diagnostic Features	Treatment
Cardio-vascular	Persistent resting tachycardia	Compromised vagal innervation of the heart	Heart rate >90 beats/min; subclinical denervation can be detected by: overshoot bradycardia during Valsalva's maneuver ↓ heart rate variation during deep breathing ↓ beat-to-beat variation in heart rate.	
	Orthostatic hypotension	Postganglionic lesions of sympathetic nerve fibers	A fall in systolic blood pressure > 30 mm Hg upon standing.	Slow change of position; leg compression (Jobst stockings); fludrocortisone (start with 0.05 mg/d); somatostatin analogs.)*
	Neuropathic edema	Sympathetic denervation →vasodilation + arteriovenous shunting →venous pooling	Gross edema of ankle and foot.	Diuretics; support stockings; ?ephedrine 30 mg 4 times a day.
	Neuropathic arthropathy (Charcot's joint)	As above, leading to bone resorption; insensitivity to pain	Painless or mildly painful swelling of ankle and foot (bilateral in 25% of cases); x-ray to document osteo-lysis.	Prevent weight-bearing on the affected joint for 3–6 months.
Sweat glands	Severe nocturnal sweating		Mostly truncal and unrelated to hypoglycemia.	
	Gustatory sweating	Possible aberrant vagal connection with denervated sympathetic sweat glands	Appears seconds after starting to chew food (cheese, pickles, alcohol, fruits); involves head, neck, shoulders, and upper chest.	A trial of anticholinergics.

Gastro-intestinal	Altered esophageal motility	Compromised vagal innervation; changes in smooth muscle	Heartburn, dysphagia; perform barium swallow.	Metoclopramide.
	Gastroparesis	Same as above	Unexplained poor diabetic control, nausea, fullness after meals, vomiting of undigested food; perform emptying study with isotopic technique.	Metoclopramide, 10 mg 4 times a day; erythromycin, 250 mg three times a day; evaluate for bezoar.
	Diarrhea	Compromised intrinsic innervation + bacterial overgrowth	Profuse watery diarrhea usually intermittent and worse at night.	Tetracycline, 250 mg 4 times a day for 10 days; Lomotil; paregoric and/or kaopectate.
	Constipation	Colonic atony	May follow diarrhea.	Laxatives to include lactulose, magnesium citrate; watch electrolytes!
Urogenital	Cystopathy (neurogenic paralytic bladder or bladder/sphincter dyssynergism)	Peripheral and autonomic neuropathy	Increased interval between voidings; urinary retention; infection of bladder with risk of ascending pyelonephritis. Cystometry: increased capacity with lack of sensation.	If infection present: drainage of bladder and antibiotics; Chronic: voiding every 3 hours aided by manual pressure; eventually bethanecol. Possible surgery: bladder neck resection (will not lead to incontinence but may induce retrograde ejaculation).
	Impotence†	Impairment of the pelvic parasympathetic nerves (nervi erigentes)	Absence of spontaneous nocturnal erections; absence of testicular sensitivity (normal in psychogenic impotence); often abnormal cystometrogram.	Consider possible causative role of drugs (antihypertensives); penile injections of papaverine and phentolamine; external ring device; implant of penile prosthesis.

* Experimental.

† May also be caused by peripheral vascular disease.

Peripheral vascular disease is also accelerated by diabetes, which represents a powerful risk factor in addition to hypertension and cigarette smoking. Clinical manifestations of peripheral vascular disease include ischemia of the lower extremities, cerebrovascular accidents, and impotence.

The mechanisms underlying the atherogenic-thrombotic potential of diabetes are multiple and include both lipid and platelet abnormalities.

The consumption of fish oils derived from certain fish (eg, herring, salmon, mackerel) and containing omega-3 fatty acids has been associated with protection against coronary artery disease. Although these fatty acids can decrease plasma lipids, blood pressure, and platelet aggregation, the clinical effectiveness and safety of dietary supplementation with fish oils have not yet been adequately evaluated. In fact, in NIDDM patients such supplementation may lead to rapid (but reversible) deterioration of glycemic control.

THE DIABETIC FOOT (See Table 10–13.)

The frequency and severity of foot lesions in diabetic patients originate from a combination of several factors. **Sensory neuropathy** with loss of sensation (the anesthetic foot) leads to deformities and, in combination with skin atrophy due to **microangiopathy**, enhances the likelihood of inadvertent trauma and pressure point ulceration, which remain asymptomatic and often become infected. **Macrovascular peripheral disease** compromises blood flow and thus the spontaneous healing process. The functional sympathectomy of **autonomic neuropathy** leads to arteriovenous shunting, abnormal distribution of blood flow with high venous pressures that may cause bone demineralization, disruption of the midfoot (Charcot's joint), and intractable edema. Purely vascular lesions are less common; they are characterized by the sudden development of painful distal foot lesions, usually secondary to trauma and generally associated with findings of peripheral vascular disease (decreased pulses, dependent rubor, and pallor with elevation).

MUSCULOSKELETAL & SKIN PATHOLOGY (See Table 10–14.)

Certain musculoskeletal and skin changes are common in diabetes. Dupuytren's contracture and carpal tunnel syndrome may require hand surgery.

Muscle cramps (commonly nocturnal and while recumbent) are common. Muscle cramps usually improve with quinine sulfate, one 260-mg tablet at bedtime; the dose may be increased to include one tablet at dinner. Side effects are unusual and include rash and tinnitus. Hemolysis may occur in patients with glucose-6-phosphate dehydrogenase (G-6-PD) deficiency. Quinine is poorly absorbed in the presence of aluminum-containing antacids. The drug slows metabolism of digoxin, neuromuscular blocking agents, and warfarin. Urinary alkalinizing agents such as sodium bicarbonate and acetazolamide may increase quinine levels.

HYPERTENSION

Conservative Management

Obese subjects with hypertension display a 2-fold increase in circulating plasma norepinephrine levels compared to nonobese hypertensive subjects. This may be due to overfeeding. Caloric restriction is the first line of therapy, since it normalizes plasma norepinephrine and lowers blood pressure (1 mm Hg systolic and 0.5 mm Hg diastolic for each 0.45 kg of weight loss). Patients in poor glycemic control tend to have slightly higher systolic blood pressure than patients in good control; improvement of metabolic status ameliorates blood pressure levels. Limitation of dietary sodium intake (no added salt) is a useful first approach and will augment the effectiveness of diuretic regimens.

Medical Management

For the hypertensive diabetic patient without renal insufficiency, the first line of therapy is angiotensin-converting enzyme inhibitors or calcium channel blockers. Angiotensin-converting enzyme inhibitors have 3 major advantages: selective normalization of intraglomerular pressure through dilation of the efferent arteriole, documented efficacy in reducing proteinuria even in normotensive diabetic patients, and absence of adverse effects on glucose tolerance and lipid levels. A dry cough is a side effect that frequently limits treatment. Calcium channel blockers are a reasonable alternative, especially in patients with coronary ischemia; they have no adverse impact on plasma lipids and have been associated with impaired glucose tolerance only occasionally.

Thiazide diuretics are no longer recommended as first-line therapy, especially in NIDDM patients, because of their metabolic side effects (decreased insulin secretion and glucose tolerance only partially mediated by hypokalemia; increased plasma triglycerides and LDL cholesterol). The effects of thiazides on lipids are detected early in the course of treatment, and patients should be switched promptly to

Table 10–13. Prevention of diabetic foot lesions.

Patient Education

Patients should be taught to

Inspect both feet daily, using a mirror to look at the bottom of the feet.

Keep feet clean; bathe them daily in warm (**not hot**) water; dry carefully including between the toes; apply lanolin or petrolatum.

Wear clean socks or stockings every day, avoiding those with seams or mends.

Before wearing, inspect shoes on the inside for nail point, torn lining, etc.

Use soft leather shoes, and buy comfortable size. Avoid pointed and open-toed shoes.

Never walk barefooted; this includes the beach and when getting up at night.

Avoid extremes of temperature; instead of using hot water bottles, heating pads, etc, to warm feet, wear wool socks.

Cut toenails straight across and not too short; for treatment of corns and calluses, see a podiatrist.

Avoid use of any chemicals on feet.

Report injuries promptly.

Give up smoking to preserve good circulation.

Monitoring at Office Visits

At each visit

Obtain a history of foot problems since last visit.

Document if the patient is compliant with the above rules for hygiene (footwear, cleanliness, nails, corns, calluses).

Examine in detail for deformities, skin lesions, and ulcers, noting presence or absence of pain or infection.

At appropriate intervals, depending on patient, but at least yearly

Check peripheral pulses: dorsalis pedis, popliteal, tibial, femoral.

Check for bruits.
Check sensation in toes and feet.

Interventions

Three goals

1. **Prevention or relief of maldistribution of pressure and its inherent risk of ulceration.** Thus, if bony deformities or superficial ulcers are observed, the patient should be referred to podiatrist/orthopedist for fitting of pressure-relieving devices or for conventional orthopedic procedures (bunionectomy, claw and hammer-toe revision, tendon release, etc).

2. **Prompt treatment of infections.** Determine by physical examination, Gram stain, and x-ray the nature and extension of the infection (capsule, tendons, bone, ?gas). Obtain material for aerobic and anaerobic cultures, and institute antibiotic treatment and bed rest. Unless very superficial, infections should be treated with intravenous antibiotics. While cultures and sensitivities are pending, treatment is started with cefoxitin (effective in vitro against most bacteria associated with foot infection, including *B fragilis*), a wide-spectrum cephalosporin combined with metronidazole (to cover *B fragilis*), or a combination of aminoglycoside and semisynthetic penicillin. For deep infections, debridement is often necessary both for therapeutic reasons and in order to obtain a meaningful sample for cultures. Diabetic control should be maintained as tight as possible.

3. **Documentation and possible correction of vascular insufficiency.** If symptoms and signs of ischemia develop, studies of tissue viability (transcutaneous oxygen diffusion) and blood supply (noninvasive Doppler) are performed.

If attempts at revascularization are considered, arteriography may need to be performed, and the possibility of angioplasty during arteriography should be discussed. The potential nephrotoxicity of repeated x-ray contrast administration should be anticipated. In diabetics, peripheral vascular disease is often diffuse and small vessel disease coexists; attempts at revascularization do not have a high success rate. The epithelialization of poorly granulating extremity ulcers may be improved with hyperbaric oxygen or even with surface oxygen delivered into a loosely fitted bag around the ulcer.

Table 10–14. Musculoskeletal and skin manifestations in diabetes.

Abnormality	Clinical Features
Soft-tissue periarthritis	Shoulder stiffness; shoulder-hand syndrome.
Dupuytren's contracture	Found in 3–21% of individuals with diabetes.
Carpal tunnel syndrome	Found in 5–17% of individuals with diabetes.
Diabetic cheirarthropathy	Found in type I diabetics. Finger stiffness and periarticular swelling with waxy thickened skin (resembling scleroderma).
Diabetic dermopathy	Shin spots: darkly pigmented flat circumscribed patches on legs caused by minor trauma.
Necrobiosis lipoidica diabeticorum	Initially red papules that coalesce into round areas; mature lesion: yellow depressed plaque with a waxy appearance. Central atrophy may produce ulceration. Most common on legs; may occur in any location.
Yellowing of skin	In > 10% of patients; prominent on palms and soles, nasolabial folds, forehead, and chin. Presumably due to carotenemia.
Eruptive xanthomas	Crops of small reddish-yellow papules, sometimes pruritic. Caused by elevated triglycerides in uncontrolled diabetes.
Candida infections	Thrush and angular cheilitis; paronychia; intertrigo.
Muscle cramps	Particularly nocturnal in legs; resolve with quinine treatment.

another class of drugs. The lowest effective dose of hydrochlorothiazide (12.5–25 mg/d) should be used.

When more than one agent is necessary for control of hypertension, an angiotensin-converting enzyme inhibitor and a calcium channel blocker may be combined or combined with a thiazide diuretic.

In patients with established nephropathy, the antihypertensive regimen generally requires a diuretic. When serum creatinine is greater than 2 mg/dL or GFR is below 25% of normal, loop diuretics (furosemide) are more effective than thiazide diuretics and work well in combination with angiotensin-converting enzyme inhibitors or calcium channel blockers. It must be noted that angiotensin-converting enzyme inhibitors may induce hyperkalemia and worsen azotemia, necessitating discontinuation of this class of drugs, and that the impact of calcium channel blockers (vasodilators that may increase glomerular hyperfiltration) on the natural history of diabetic nephropathy has not been established.

Adrenergic blockers and peripheral vasodilators such as hydralazine should be used sparingly because their side effects may greatly magnify abnormalities already present in diabetic patients.

α-Blockers (prazosin, clonidine, α-methyldopa) can cause and aggravate postural hypotension and impotence. β-Blockers can compromise the perception of—and recovery from—insulin-induced hypoglycemia, in addition to having adverse effects on plasma lipids, insulin secretion, and peripheral vascular disease. Hydralazine causes reflex tachycardia, which may not be readily tolerated by patients who already have an elevated heart rate (autonomic neuropathy) or who are not candidates for the addition of a β-blocker.

DIABETES & PREGNANCY

Poorly controlled diabetes during pregnancy is a major cause of serious complications. Table 10–15 lists the incidence of major complications affecting infants of diabetic mothers.

INFANT COMPLICATIONS

Congenital Malformations
Complications for infants of diabetic mothers are due to the abnormal maternal metabolic milieu, possibly to hyperglycemia itself. Congenital malformations are 2–4 times more frequent in diabetic pregnancies. Dysmorphogenesis occurs at the initial stages of gestation when women are often unaware of their pregnancy and may be paying minimal attention to diabetic control. In particular, the most common congenital anomalies in infants of diabetic mothers (caudal regression syndrome, spina bifida, hydrocephalus and other central nervous system defects, anencephalus, heart anomalies, anal/rectal atresia, renal anomalies, situs inversus) are all determined before the

Table 10–15. Complications in infants when diabetes in mothers is poorly controlled.

Time of Gestation	Complication	Rates
Early:	Congenital malformations	5–15%
Late:	Macrosomia	16–40%
	Hypoglycemia	16–76%
	Hypocalcemia	8–22%
	Polycythemia	10–45%
	Hyperbilirubinemia	19–35%
	Respiratory distress	2–9%

seventh gestational week. Maintenance of near-normoglycemia (glycosylated hemoglobin levels within 4–6 SD of the normal mean) from the time of conception substantially decreases the incidence of congenital malformations. Diabetic women must be forewarned to conceive only after excellent diabetic control is established and documented for 3–4 months.

Women who are found at an early prenatal visit to have an elevated glycosylated hemoglobin level, especially if within the high-risk category (> 12 SD above the normal mean), should be studied immediately for the presence of fetal malformations. Ultrasound scanning at 12–14 weeks, combined with a determination of α-fetoprotein level in maternal serum (a sensitive indicator of neural tube defects; values > 100 μg/L are abnormal), helps in deciding whether to continue the pregnancy.

Late Complications

The developing fetus is completely dependent on the mother for fuel supply. Fetuses exposed to chronic maternal hyperglycemia develop hyperinsulinism that causes excessive fat deposition and organomegaly resulting in **macrosomia**, ie, birth weight above the 90th percentile for gestational age. Macrosomia is associated with a higher risk of difficult labor, shoulder dystocia, and neonatal asphyxia. The sudden withdrawal of maternal glucose at birth, in the presence of fetal hyperinsulinism, results in **neonatal hypoglycemia** (blood glucose < 30 mg/dL). The **erythremia** (hematocrit > 65%) often observed in infants of diabetic mothers is attributed to the elevated erythropoietin levels associated with a state of relative hypoxia in utero. **Hyperbilirubinemia** (bilirubin > 12 mg/dL) is at least partly due to the erythremia. **Neonatal hypocalcemia** (serum calcium < 7 mg/dL) is due to functional hypoparathyroidism. The **respiratory distress syndrome** is due to delayed maturation of the enzymatic machinery for synthesis of lung phospholipids. All are associated with poor control of maternal diabetes during pregnancy.

NORMAL GESTATIONAL CHANGES IN FUEL METABOLISM

Changes in maternal metabolism parallel the growth of the conceptus and are therefore especially prominent during the second half of pregnancy. The continuous fetal siphoning of glucose and gluconeogenic precursors leads in the fasting state to maternal hypoglycemia and hypoalaninemia and tendency to starvation ketosis. In the fed state, the antiinsulin action of placental hormones [human placental lactogen (chorionic somatomammotropin), estrogens, and progesterone] and of increased levels of bound and free cortisol induces a state of insulin resistance. In the nondiabetic, euglycemia is maintained by a 40% increase in maternal insulin secretion as well as by the increased glucose utilization of the growing fetus. However, when additional mechanisms of insulin resistance (eg, obesity) are operative or when insulin secretory reserve is borderline, the "metabolic stress test" of pregnancy results in the development of maternal diabetes (gestational diabetes). The severity of established diabetes also worsens during the second half of pregnancy, necessitating increased insulin dosage.

DIAGNOSIS OF GESTATIONAL DIABETES

Gestational diabetes (carbohydrate intolerance of variable severity with onset or first recognition during pregnancy) complicates 2–3% of pregnancies in the USA and identifies a group of women at high risk of becoming diabetic later in life (60% in the 16 years following pregnancy).

Testing for gestational diabetes on the basis of the established risk factors (Table 10–16) identifies no more than half of gestational diabetics. It is therefore currently recommended that *all pregnant women be screened for gestational diabetes*.

The screening test is performed at 24–28 weeks of gestation and consists of a 50-g oral glucose load administered without regard to the time of the last meal. Venous plasma glucose is measured 1 hour later. A value of 140 mg/dL or greater indicates the need for a complete OGTT, performed with 100 g of glucose. The complete OGTT should also be given to all women who are obese (weight > 120% of normal for height). Gestational diabetes is diagnosed if 2 or more of the following venous plasma glucose concentrations are met or exceeded: fasting, 105 mg/dL; 1 hour, 190 mg/dL; 2 hours, 165 mg/dL; 3 hours, 145 mg/dL. Women with an abnormal screening test and only one abnormal value on 3-hour OGTT should have the OGTT repeated at week 32. High-risk women should be screened at the first prenatal

Table 10–16. Risk factors for gestational diabetes.

Diabetes in a first-degree relative
Previous abnormality of glucose tolerance
Obesity (> 20% over ideal body weight)
Advanced maternal age
Poor obstetric history:
   Large babies for gestational age (past or present)
   Unexplained stillbirths
   Congenital anomalies
   Polyhydramnios (past or present)

visit; if the screening test is normal, it should be repeated at weeks 24–28.

Measurement of glycosylated hemoglobin is not a sufficiently sensitive test for the diagnosis of gestational diabetes.

METABOLIC GOALS IN PREGNANCY COMPLICATED BY DIABETES

The management of pregnancy complicated by maternal diabetes should aim at 4 goals:

(1) Attainment of optimal weight gain: 10–12 kg (22–26.4 lb).

(2) Control of plasma glucose: fasting and preprandial, 70–100 mg/dL; 1-hour postprandial, < 140 mg/dL; 2-hour postprandial, < 120 mg/dL; glycosylated hemoglobin within the normal range.

(3) Avoidance of hypoglycemia.

(4) Absence of fasting ketonuria. Ketone bodies cross the placenta and may jeopardize the neuropsychological development of the infant.

The following steps help achieve these goals: appropriate nutrition, frequent home-monitoring of blood glucose and urine ketones with proper changes in insulin dosage, office follow-up every 2 weeks and weekly after the 30th gestational week, monthly determinations of glycohemoglobin. Office follow-up is particularly efficient when performed jointly by the team of specialists caring for the pregnant woman with diabetes: obstetrician, diabetologist, nutritionist.

NUTRITION IN PREGNANCY

The generally recommended dietary allowances for pregnancy include the following:

Daily total calories: 30 kcal/kg ideal body weight in the first trimester and 38 kcal/kg ideal body weight in the second and third trimesters after increase in appetite is established. Total daily calories are distributed as follows: 50–60% carbohydrate, 20–30% protein, less than 30% fat.

Protein: 1.5–2 g/kg ideal body weight daily.

Iron: 30–60 mg supplemental elemental iron daily.

Calcium: 400 mg supplemental elemental calcium daily.

Folic acid: 400–800 µg supplemental folic acid daily.

The iron, calcium, and folic acid recommended are generally contained in one tablet of ''prenatal vitamins.''

Although pregnancy is not the time for weight loss, excessive weight gain is firmly discouraged. Generally, 1500–1700 kcal/d in overweight patients allows for appropriate fetal growth without risk of starvation ketosis. Total calories should be divided into meals and snacks: breakfast, midmorning snack, lunch, midafternoon snack, dinner, bedtime snack. The last is essential to prevent fasting ketonuria and should contain both carbohydrate and protein.

MANAGEMENT OF GESTATIONAL DIABETES

Gestational diabetes can often be managed by simply educating patients on proper nutrition: daily caloric allowance, sources, distribution. If dietary compliance does not maintain glycemic levels within the desired range (see above), or if such levels are attained at the expense of fasting ketonuria or suboptimal weight gain, insulin therapy should be instituted. It is important to employ the least antigenic insulin preparations (purified pork or human), since these patients are likely to need insulin therapy only intermittently for a number of years (pregnancy, severe illness). The insulin dose will be dictated by home-monitoring data: in some instances, the only problem is represented by the level of fasting glucose, in which case an injection of NPH or Lente before the bedtime snack may be sufficient. Nocturnal hypoglycemia should be watched for and prevented by modification of dose and timing of insulin injection, carbohydrate content and timing of evening snack, or both. In some cases of gestational diabetes, supplementation of both basal and preprandial insulin is required; thus, multiple-component regimens may need to be instituted.

MANAGEMENT OF ESTABLISHED DIABETES DURING PREGNANCY

Type I Patients

During the first trimester of pregnancy, the insulin dose needs either no adjustment or occasionally a slight decrease to compensate for the increasing glucose consumption by the developing fetus and placenta. As placental production of antiinsulin hormones becomes established, insulin requirements progressively increase. On average, from about 0.7 U/kg required up to 10 weeks' gestation, the insulin dose reaches about 1 U/kg by the time of delivery. Multiple-injection regimens (see above) provide the best coverage of prandial glycemic excursions and the greatest flexibility. A practical scheme is as follows:

Two-thirds of total dose before breakfast (one-third Regular, two-thirds intermediate-acting)

One-sixth of total dose before dinner (all Regular).

One-sixth of total dose before bedtime snack (all intermediate-acting).

Administration of intermediate-acting insulin at bedtime instead of before dinner reduces the risk of hypoglycemia in the middle of the night and ensures better fasting glucose levels.

Dietary recommendations should aim at the targets previously discussed and follow the pattern of 3 meals and 3 snacks. Occasionally, if dinner is a relatively early meal, 2 snacks may be prescribed for the evening hours, to be consumed at 3-hour intervals. This will reduce the length of the nocturnal fasting period and prevent the tendency to both hypoglycemia and starvation ketosis. Home-monitoring should be performed 4 times a day (before the main meals and at bedtime) with 2-hour postprandial values measured during 1–2 days each week. The first morning urine specimen should be tested for ketones. Patients should be taught how to modify insulin doses.

Type II Patients

In patients with type II diabetes, the chances for prepregnancy counseling are not often available; being milder, the disease may have gone undiagnosed or been minimally cared for. These women are thus at particularly high risk of carrying the first few months of pregnancy in a hyperglycemic environment. Because oral antidiabetic agents are contraindicated during pregnancy, most type II diabetics need insulin therapy. The majority of type II patients are overweight and thus insulin-resistant; the added effects of placental hormones increase the requirement for insulin, which may reach 2.5 U/kg/d during the second half of pregnancy. Multiple-component insulin regimens are necessary to attain the desired target blood glucose levels. In these patients, hypoglycemia is a rare occurrence. Dietary recommendations should follow the discussed guidelines and allow for the desired weight gain.

MANAGEMENT OF PREGNANT DIABETICS WITH MICROVASCULAR DISEASE

Retinopathy

Diabetic retinopathy is not a contraindication to pregnancy, nor does it affect the prognosis for a favorable maternal and fetal outcome. However, close follow-up by an experienced ophthalmologist is essential during pregnancy. Background retinopathy is not accelerated by pregnancy but may progress as part of its own evolution or as a result of abrupt institution of tight metabolic control; proliferative retinopathy despite prior photocoagulation may always recur. Active retinal neovascularization at the end of pregnancy is an indication for elective caesarean section in order to minimize the risk of hemorrhages due to the increased intravascular pressure during the second stage of labor.

Nephropathy

Diabetic nephropathy without azotemia is not a contraindication to pregnancy. Patients without hypertension and with a serum creatinine below 1.5 mg/dL have the best prognosis for having an uncomplicated pregnancy and a healthy baby. The presence of hypertension or a serum creatinine level above 2 mg/dL involves an increased risk of preeclampsia and of prematurity. Rarely will a woman with a prepregnancy serum creatinine in excess of 3 mg/dL complete a normal pregnancy. Pregnancy itself does not accelerate loss in renal function but may greatly worsen proteinuria and edema during the third trimester. In most instances, proteinuria returns to prepregnancy levels after delivery.

Women with established nephropathy (serum creatinine > 1.5 mg/dL) should be carefully counseled and evaluated prior to conception. Baseline studies should include serum blood urea nitrogen, creatinine, uric acid, and 24-hour urine collection for creatinine clearance and quantitative proteinuria. Hypertension should be brought under satisfactory and stable control. In view of potential teratogenicity of angiotensin-converting enzyme inhibitors, patients should be preventively or promptly switched to other classes of antihypertensives. Calcium channel blockers, α-methyldopa, hydralazine, clonidine and β-adrenergic blockers are widely used in pregnancies complicated by maternal hypertension, but adverse effects should be watched for. Diuretics may be used, but fluid balance should be strictly monitored, since volume depletion may decrease placental perfusion and endanger the pregnancy. Salt content of the diet is carefully limited and surveillance is established for asymptomatic urinary tract infections. Baseline laboratory studies are repeated at 2- to 3-month intervals or more often if new problems arise. Good control of diabetes remains of the utmost importance; insulin requirements tend to be smaller (owing to prolonged half-life of insulin from decreased renal clearance) and risk of severe hypoglycemia greater.

Pregnancies in women with chronic renal failure who are on hemodialysis are possible but rarely fully successful; there is a very high risk of spontaneous abortion and multiple congenital malformations.

Recipients of renal transplants have completed successful pregnancies. The chances for a favorable outcome are best if (1) the patient has had 2 years of stable good health after renal transplantation, (2) recent serum creatinine is less than 2 mg/dL, and there is no significant hypertension; and (3) good allograft function is maintained on a dose of prednisone of 15 mg/d or less and of azathioprine no greater than 3 mg/kg/d. The experience with cyclosporine is still limited, but uncomplicated pregnancies have been reported in renal transplant recipients receiving cyclosporine, 450 mg/d.

Possible complications of pregnancies in renal transplant recipients are occurrence of rejection episodes, mechanical interference with urinary flow, hypertension, proteinuria, transmission of HbsAg to the fetus who becomes antigen carrier, granulocytopenia, and lymphopenia in the infant possibly due to maternal immunosuppressive therapy. The rate of congenital anomalies does not appear increased. The shortened life-expectancy of the mother is a major consideration. Thus, these pregnancies should be planned only after extensive counseling sessions in which the problems are clearly presented to the prospective mother and father.

TIMING & MANAGEMENT OF LABOR & DELIVERY

Meticulous control of maternal diabetes, modern obstetric technology, and repeated testing for fetal well-being and lung maturity make it possible to carry most diabetic pregnancies to term and deliver viable infants.

Assessment of fetal well-being assists in timely identification of the fetus in jeopardy and in need of delivery, and conversely, in reassuring that delivery can be postponed until full maturity. Tests are performed by monitoring, through a Doppler transducer applied to maternal abdomen, the fetal heart rate during a nonstress test (NST) or a contraction stress test (CST). In the NST, which is the preferred screening test, fetal heart acceleration of 15 beats/min and lasting 15 seconds in concomitance with fetal movements is considered indicative of fetal well-being. A reactive NST appears to be predictive of fetal well-being for 1 week; thus, it should be repeated weekly while awaiting spontaneous labor. If the NST is suspicious or nonreactive, a CST should be performed. The CST consists of an intravenous oxytocin challenge titrated to produce 3 uterine contractions in a 10-minute interval: the absence of persistent late decelerations of the fetal heart rate after uterine contractions indicates fetal well-being. Conversely, the recording of delayed fetal heart decelerations during the CST should prompt immediate assessment of fetal lung maturity in consideration of early delivery.

Assessment of fetal lung maturation is particularly important in diabetic pregnancies because documentation of maturity allows a planned delivery early enough to avoid the late-pregnancy stillbirths previously so common in diabetes. The evaluation is accomplished by performing amniocentesis and studying the phospholipid pattern of amniotic fluid. In normal pregnancies, a lecithin:sphingomyelin (L:S) ratio of 2 or above is considered indicative of fetal lung maturity and thus of minimal risks of respiratory distress syndrome and hyaline membrane disease. In diabetic pregnancies, obstetricians feel more confident with an L:S ratio above 2.5. The presence of 3% or more phosphatidylglycerol (PG) in the amniotic fluid is considered the most reassuring indicator of fetal lung maturity.

Women with mild gestational diabetes are generally allowed to reach term and enter spontaneous labor. However, if delivery does not occur by the 40th gestational week, an NST is performed at weekly intervals, and pregnancy is not permitted to progress beyond the 42nd week, since fetal postmaturity is associated with an increased risk of uterine fetal demise.

In women with type I or II diabetes, weekly or twice weekly NSTs are initiated at 32 weeks' gestation; at 38 weeks, ultrasonography and amniocentesis are performed to assess fetal lung maturity. The optimal time for delivery and the desirability of inducing labor are based on the combined results of lung maturation studies and documentation of fetal well-being.

Diabetic management during labor and delivery should aim at maintaining plasma glucose between 70 and 120 mg/dL in order to prevent neonatal hypoglycemia, which may occur upon sudden withdrawal from a hyperglycemic milieu that has caused increased fetal insulin secretion. Tight glycemic control is best achieved by continuous insulin infusion coupled with glucose delivery in order to meet the energy expenditure of active labor. Insulin is administered at a rate determined by the following equation:

$$\text{[Blood glucose values (mg/dL)]}/150 = \text{Units/h of insulin}$$

in order to bring blood glucose within the desired range. At that point, glucose infusion (5% dextrose) is started at a rate of 125 mL/h and insulin infusion adjusted as above on the basis of glycemic values obtained by blood glucose meter (usual range 0.5–2 U/h). Insulin administration should be stopped immediately after delivery of the placenta, while glucose infusion should be continued until resumption of oral feeding. The immediate postpartum period is characterized by a sharply decreased insulin requirement, which may last 48–72 hours. During this time, small doses of Regular insulin (4–8 U) administered before meals are the safest course of action. By the third day after delivery, patients may generally be restarted on insulin doses approximating the prepregnancy ones.

Women with diabetes are encouraged to breast-feed. Caloric adjustments are made as for nondiabetic women, and insulin dose may require a slight reduction.

REFERENCES

Physiology of Carbohydrate Metabolism

Bell GI et al: Molecular biology of mammalian glucose transporters. *Diabetes Care* 1990;**13**:198.

Felig P, Bergman M: Integrated physiology of carbohydrate metabolism. In: *Diabetes Mellitus Theory and Practice*, 4th ed. Rifkin H, Porte D (editors). Elsevier, 1990.

Olefsky JM: The insulin receptor: A multifunctional protein. *Diabetes* 1990;**39**:1009.

Polonski KS, Rubenstein AH: C-peptide as a measure of the secretion and hepatic extraction of insulin. *Diabetes* 1984;**33**:486.

Rosen OM: After insulin binds. *Science* 1987;**237**:1452.

Thiebaud D et al: The effect of graded doses of insulin on total glucose uptake, glucose oxidation, and glucose storage in man. *Diabetes* 1982;**31**:957.

Causes & Classification of Diabetes

Baekkeskov S et al: Identification of the 64K autoantigen in insulin-dependent diabetes as the GABA-synthesizing enzyme glutamic acid decarboxylase. *Nature* 1990;**347**:151.

Baisch JM et al: Analysis of HLA-DQ genotypes and susceptibility in insulin-dependent diabetes mellitus. *N Engl J Med* 1990;**322**:1836.

Bogardus, C, Lillioja S: Where all the glucose doesn't go in non-insulin-dependent diabetes mellitus. *N Engl J Med* 1990;**322**:262.

Bottazzo GF et al: In situ characterization of autoimmune phenomena and expression of HLA molecules in the pancreas in diabetic insulitis. *N Engl J Med* 1985;**313**:353.

Eriksson J et al: Early metabolic defects in persons at increased risk for non-insulin-dependent diabetes mellitus. *N Engl J Med* 1989;**321**:337.

Flier JS, Kahn CR, Roth J: Receptors, antireceptor antibodies and mechanisms of insulin resistance. *N Engl J Med* 1979;**300**:413.

Haneda M et al: Familial hyperinsulinemia due to structurally abnormal insulin: Definition of an emerging new clinical syndrome. *N Engl J Med* 1984;**310**:1288.

Leahy JL: Natural history of β-cell dysfunction in NIDDM. *Diabetes Care* 1990;**13**:992.

Mac Laren NK, Rossini AA, Eisenbarth GS: International research symposium on immunology of diabetes. *Diabetes* 1988;**37**:662.

National Diabetes Data Group: Classification and diagnosis of diabetes mellitus and other categories of glucose intolerance *Diabetes* 1979;**28**:1039.

Shulman GI et al: Quantitation of muscle glycogen synthesis in normal subjects and subjects with non-insulin-dependent diabetes by ^{13}C nuclear magnetic resonance spectroscopy. *N Engl J Med* 1990;**322**:223.

Taylor SI et al: Mutations in insulin-receptor gene in insulin-resistant patients. *Diabetes Care* 1990;**13**:257.

Ziegler AG et al: Predicting type I diabetes. *Diabetes Care* 1990;**13**:762.

Laboratory Tests

Baker JR et al: Serum fructosamine concentration as measure of blood glucose control in type I (insulin dependent) diabetes mellitus. *Br Med J* 1985;**290**:352.

Chavers BM et al: Glomerular lesions and urinary albumin excretion in type I diabetes without overt proteinuria. *N Engl J Med* 1989;**320**:966.

Fluckiger R, Woodtli T, Berger W: Quantitation of glycosylated hemoglobin by boronate affinity chromatography. *Diabetes* 1984;**33**:73.

Garlick RL et al: Characterization of glycosylated hemoglobins. *J Clin Invest* 1983;**71**:1062.

Halperin ML et al: Selected aspects of the pathophysiology of metabolic acidosis in diabetes mellitus. *Diabetes* 1981;**30**:781.

Larsen ML, Horder M, Mogensen EF: Effect of long-term monitoring of glycosylated hemoglobin levels in insulin-dependent diabetes mellitus. *N Engl J Med* 1990;**323**:1021.

Oh MS, Carroll HJ: The anion gap. *N Engl J Med* 1977;**297**:814.

Treatment of Type I Diabetes

Campbell PJ et al: Pathogenesis of the dawn phenomenon in patients with insulin-dependent diabetes mellitus. *N Engl J Med* 1985;**312**:1473.

Hirsch IB, McGill JB: Role of insulin in management of surgical patients with diabetes mellitus. *Diabetes Care* 1990;**13**:980.

Jenkins DJA, Taylor RH, Wolever TMS: The diabetic diet, dietary carbohydrates and differences in digestibility. *Diabetologia* 1982;**23**:477.

Krzentowski G et al: Glucose utilization during exercise in normal and diabetic subjects. *Diabetes* 1981;**30**:983.

Nathan DM: Modern management of insulin-dependent diabetes mellitus. *Med Clin North Am* 1988;**72**:1365.

Rabkin R, Simon NM, Steiner S, Colwell JA: Effect of renal disease on renal uptake and excretion of insulin in man. *N Engl J Med* 1970;**282**:182.

Westphal SA, Goetz FC: Current approaches to continuous insulin replacement for insulin-dependent diabetes: Pancreas transplantation and pumps. *Adv Intern Med* 1990;**35**:107.

Zinman B: The physiologic replacement of insulin: An elusive goal. *N Engl J Med* 1989;**321**:363.

Complications of Insulin Therapy

Galloway JA, Bressler R: Insulin treatment in diabetes. *Med Clin North Am* 1978;**62**:663.

Gerich JE: Glucose counterregulation and its impact on diabetes mellitus. *Diabetes* 1988;**37**:1608.

Kumar D et al: Immunoreactivity of human insulin of recombinant DNA origin. *Diabetes* 1983;**32**:516.

Lorenzi M, Karam JH: Human insulin in the treatment of insulin allergy. *West J Med* 1985;**143**:387.

Lorenzi M et al: Duration of type I diabetes affects glucagon and glucose responses to insulin-induced hypoglycemia. *West J Med* 1984;**141**:467.

Schade DS, Duckworth WC: In search of the subcutaneous-insulin-resistance syndrome. *N Engl J Med* 1986;**315**:147.

Weiss ME et al: Association of protamine IgE and IgG antibodies with life-threatening reactions to intravenous protamine. *N Engl J Med* 1989;**320**:886.

Treatment of Obesity and Type II Diabetes

Bray GA, Gray DS: Obesity. 2. Treatment. *West J Med* 1988;**149**:555.

Garg A et al: Comparison of a high-carbohydrate diet with a high-monounsaturated-fat diet in patients with non-insulin-dependent diabetes mellitus. *N Engl J Med* 1988;**319**:829.

Garvey WT et al: The effect of insulin treatment on insulin secretion and insulin action in type II diabetes mellitus. *Diabetes* 1985;**34**:222.

Glauber H et al: Adverse metabolic effect of omega-3 fatty acids in non-insulin-dependent diabetes mellitus. *Ann Intern Med* 1988;**108**:663.

Henry RR et al: Metabolic consequences of very-low-calorie diet therapy in obese non-insulin-dependent diabetic and nondiabetic subjects. *Diabetes* 1986;**35**:155.

Lebovitz HE: Oral hypoglycemic agents. In: *Diabetes Mellitus Theory and Practice*, 4th ed. Rifkin H, Porte D (editors). Elsevier, 1990.

Reaven GM: Dietary therapy for non-insulin-dependent diabetes mellitus. *N Engl J Med* 1988;**319**:862.

Reaven GM: Role of insulin resistance in human disease. *Diabetes* 1988;**37**:1595.

Exercise and NIDDM. [Technical Review.] *Diabetes Care* 1990;**13**:785.

Hyperglycemic Emergencies

Feig PU, McCurdy DK: The hypertonic state. *N Engl J Med* 1977;**297**:1444.

Fulop M: Serum potassium in lactic acidosis and ketoacidosis. *N Engl J Med* 1979;**300**:1087.

Gerich JE, Martin MM, Recant L: Clinical and metabolic characteristics of hyperosmolar nonketotic coma. *Diabetes* 1971;**20**:228.

Kebler R, McDonald FD, Cadnapaphornchai P: Dynamic changes in serum phosphorus levels in diabetic ketoacidosis. *Am J Med* 1985;**79**:571.

Kreisberg RA: Diabetic ketoacidosis: New concepts and trends in pathogenesis and treatment. *Ann Intern Med* 1978;**88**:681.

Lever E, Jaspan JB: Sodium bicarbonate therapy in severe diabetic keto-acidosis. *Am J Med* 1983;**75**:263.

Maccario M: Neurological dysfunction associated with nonketotic hyper-glycemia. *Arch Neurol* 1968;**19**:525.

Marliss EB et al: Altered redox state obscuring ketoacidosis in diabetic patients with lactic acidosis. *N Engl J Med* 1970;**283**:978.

Winegrad AI, Kern EFO, Simmons DA: Cerebral edema in diabetic keto-acidosis. *N Engl J Med* 1985;**312**:1184.

Chronic Complications of Diabetes

Aspects of diabetic autonomic neuropathy. *Ann Intern Med* 1980;**92**(2 **Suppl, part 2**):289.

Bastron JA, Thomas JE: Diabetic polyradiculopathy. *Mayo Clin Proc* 1981;**56**:725.

Bilous RW et al: The effects of pancreas transplantation on the glomerular structure of renal allografts in patients with insulin-dependent diabetes. *N Engl J Med* 1989;**321:**80.

Brownlee M, Cerami A, Vlassara H: Advanced glycosylation end products in tissue and the biochemical basis of diabetic complications. *N Engl J Med* 1988;**318:**1315.

Cagliero E, Maiello M, Boeri D, Roy S, Lorenzi M: Increased expression of basement membrane components in human endothelial cells cultured in high glucose. *J Clin Invest* 1988;**82:**735.

Colwell JA, Lopes-Virella MF: A review of the development of large-vessel disease in diabetes mellitus. *Am J Med* 1988;**85(Suppl 5A):**113.

Damad Study Group: Effect of aspirin alone and aspirin plus dipyridamole in early diabetic retinopathy. *Diabetes* 1989;**38:**491.

Diabetes Control and Complications Trial (DCCT): Update. *Diabetes Care* 1990;**13:**427.

Edmonds ME: The diabetic foot: Pathophysiology and treatment. *Clin Endocrinol Metab* 1986;**15:**889.

Ellenberg M: Diabetic neuropathic cachexia. *Diabetes* 1974;**23:**418.

Engerman RL: Pathogenesis of diabetic retinopathy. *Diabetes* 1989;**38:**1203.

Godine JE: The relationship between metabolic control and vascular complications of diabetes mellitus. *Med Clin North Am* 1988;**72:**1271.

Greene DA, Lattimer SA, Sima AAF: Sorbitol, phosphoinositides, and sodium-potassium-ATPase in the pathogenesis of diabetic complications. *N Engl J Med* 1987;**316:**599.

Hoeldtke RD, O'Dorisio TM, Boden G: Treatment of autonomic neuropathy with a somatostatin analogue SMS-201-995. *Lancet* 1986;**2:**602.

Janssens J et al: Improvement of gastric emptying in diabetic gastroparesis by erythromycin. *N Engl J Med* 1990;**322:**1028.

Kennedy WR et al: Effects of pancreatic transplantation on diabetic neuropathy. *N Engl J Med* 1990;**322:**1031.

Klein R et al: The Wisconsin epidemiologic study of diabetic retinopathy. 2 parts. *Arch Ophthalmol* 1984;**102:**520 and 527.

Mangili R et al: Increased sodium-lithium countertransport activity in red cells of patients with insulin-dependent diabetes and nephropathy. *N Engl J Med* 1988;**318:**146.

Mogensen CE: Prediction of clinical diabetic nephropathy in IDDM patients. *Diabetes* 1990;**39:**761.

Orchard TJ et al: Prevalence of complications in IDDM by sex and duration. *Diabetes* 1990;**39:**1116.

Parfrey PS et al: Contrast material–induced renal failure in patients with diabetes mellitus, renal insufficiency, or both: A prospective controlled study. *N Engl J Med* 1989;**320:**143.

Parving HH et al: Effect of captopril on blood pressure and kidney function in normotensive insulin dependent diabetics with nephropathy. *Br Med J* 1989;**299:**533.

Pollare T, Lithell H, Berne C: A comparison of the effects of hydrochlorothiazide and captopril on glucose and lipid metabolism in patients with hypertension. *N Engl J Med* 1989;**321:**868.

Ramsey RC et al: Progression of diabetic retinopathy after pancreas transplantation for insulin-dependent diabetes mellitus. *N Engl J Med* 1988;**318:**208.

Rand LI et al: Multiple factors in the prediction of risk of proliferative diabetic retinopathy. *N Engl J Med* 1985;**313:**1433.

Reddi AS, Camerini-Davalos RA: Diabetic nephropathy: An update. *Arch Intern Med* 1990;**150:**31.

Report and recommendations of the San Antonio conference on diabetic neuropathy. [Consensus Statement.] *Diabetes* 1988;**37:**1000.

Sorbinil Retinopathy Trial Research Group: A randomized trial of sorbinil, an aldose reductase inhibitor, in diabetic retinopathy. *Arch Ophthalmol* 1990;**108:**1234.

Diabetes & Pregnancy

Greene MF et al: First-trimester hemoglobin A1 and risk for major malformation and spontaneous abortion in diabetic pregnancy. *Teratology* 1989;**39:**225.

Hollingsworth DR: *Pregnancy, Diabetes, and Birth: A Management Guide.* Williams & Wilkins, 1984.

Kitzmiller JL et al: Diabetic nephropathy and perinatal outcome. *Am J Obstet Gynecol* 1981;**141:**741.

Landon MB, Gabbe SG: Diabetes and pregnancy. *Med Clin North Am* 1988;**72:**1493.

Ogburn PL et al: Pregnancy following renal transplantation in class T diabetes mellitus. *JAMA* 1986;**255:**911.

Phelps RL et al: Changes in diabetic retinopathy during pregnancy: Correlations with regulation of hyperglycemia. *Arch Ophthalmol* 1986;**104:**1806.

Hypoglycemia | 11

Mara Lorenzi, MD

DEFINITION & PATHOPHYSIOLOGY

A plasma glucose value below 45 mg/dL (or blood glucose below 40 mg/dL) identifies hypoglycemia. Hypoglycemic disorders are characterized by the Whipple triad of (1) hypoglycemia, (2) symptoms and signs of hypoglycemia, and (3) reversibility of symptoms by glucose administration.

Abnormally low glucose levels are a consequence of defective hepatic glucose production or of exaggerated peripheral glucose utilization or of both. Under usual circumstances, hypoglycemia is prevented in the normal individual by precisely integrated neural and hormonal mechanisms. Upon ingestion of a mixed meal, the increase in peripheral insulin levels is concomitant with the increase in the circulating glucose and other nutrients. Abnormal kinetics of glucose absorption or of insulin secretion lead to **hypoglycemia in the fed state** (reactive hypoglycemia).

Approximately 4–8 hours after ingestion of a meal, absorption and utilization of exogenous nutrients is complete; further fuels come from endogenous sources. The 2 mechanisms for continuous replenishment of circulating glucose in the postabsorptive state are hepatic glycogenolysis and gluconeogenesis. Hepatic glycogen stores (80–100 g) are depleted after 12–18 hours of fasting. After this time, glucose is provided only by gluconeogenesis. Genetic or acquired conditions interfering with such mechanisms compromise hepatic glucose production and lead to **fasting hypoglycemia**. When fasting hypoglycemia is caused by excess insulin, an additional mechanism contributing to hypoglycemia is increased glucose uptake by peripheral tissues.

Normal individuals usually do not manifest hypoglycemia, but in 3 physiologic situations (pregnancy, strenuous exercise, and prolonged fasting) blood glucose levels may decline into the hypoglycemic range. During pregnancy, the maternal level of fasting plasma glucose declines as a result of the siphoning of glucose and gluconeogenic precursors by the growing fetus. During prolonged strenuous exercise, the rate of gluconeogenesis may not sufficiently

---

SOME ACRONYMS USED IN THIS CHAPTER

ACTH	Adrenocorticotropic hormone
GH	Growth hormone
hCG	Human chorionic gonadotropin
IGF	Insulinlike growth factor
MEN	Multiple endocrine neoplasia
OGTT	Oral glucose tolerance test

---

match the vastly increased utilization of glucose by skeletal muscle. Prolonged fasting leads to hypoglycemia especially in women. While after 72 hours of fasting, normal men maintain their plasma glucose above 50 mg/dL, in women plasma glucose levels may fall below 30 mg/dL. A possible reason for such sex differences is a lesser release of gluconeogenic substrates in women, either because of their smaller muscle compartment or because the greater degree of ketosis they develop during starvation may inhibit gluconeogenesis.

When hypoglycemia occurs in the normal individual, it is both transient and asymptomatic owing to 3 lines of response:

(1) Hypoglycemia itself, increased sympathetic activity, and epinephrine release all suppress insulin secretion by stimulating α-adrenergic receptors on pancreatic B-cells. This effect is critical in the prevention of progressive hypoglycemia since it not only arrests further uptake of glucose by insulin-dependent tissues, but also permits increased liver gluconeogenesis and ketogenesis.

(2) Enhanced secretion of epinephrine, glucagon, and cortisol stimulates various steps of gluconeogenesis. Enhanced secretion of growth hormone—in concert with epinephrine, glucagon, and cortisol—stimulates lipolysis and ketogenesis.

(3) The increased circulating levels of ketone bodies provide an important, albeit not optimal, fuel for the brain that is endowed with the enzymes necessary for their oxidation. Although the access of ketones to the brain normally is limited by the blood-brain barrier (whose permeability to ketones is not homogeneous), at elevated circulating levels they are transported across the barrier in sufficient amounts to satisfy the brain's energy needs and thus prevent overt symptomatology.

CLINICAL FEATURES

The manifestations of hypoglycemia depend on 3 factors: (1) the rate of fall of plasma glucose; (2) the severity of the hypoglycemia;

and (3) preexisting structural abnormalities of the vasculature serving the central nervous system.

A rapid fall of plasma glucose, as occurs when peripheral glucose uptake is greatly enhanced by excess insulin action (an overdose of Regular insulin, a burst of insulin secretion by a pancreatic B-cell tumor, reactive hypoglycemia), leads—if the autonomic nervous system is intact—to a sudden and substantial adrenergic discharge. Thus, symptoms include manifestations of abrupt neuroglycopenia (headache, blurred vision, inappropriate affect) and those caused by elevated levels of epinephrine (nervousness, anxiety, tremor, palpitations, perspiration, and hunger).

Hypoglycemia evolving more slowly is characteristic of conditions that impair adequate hepatic glucose output without inducing rapid and excessive peripheral glucose utilization. This occurs with long-acting insulins or sulfonylureas, with steadily secreting B-cell tumors, with nonpancreatic tumors secreting insulinlike factors, and with all the other conditions compromising hepatic glucose output. This more chronic hypoglycemia fails to activate a massive sympathoadrenal discharge, and the prevailing symptomatology is that of neuroglycopenia. Difficulty in concentrating, amnesia, disorientation, confusion, and bizarre behavior often lead to psychiatric diagnoses.

Irrespective of the modalities of development of hypoglycemia, if the counterregulatory response or exogenous glucose supply fails to correct or interrupt the blood glucose decline, profound central nervous system dysfunction ensues with lethargy, seizures, coma, and eventually death.

Focal neurologic changes may occur in all patients but more often in patients with preexisting structural vascular abnormalities resulting in relative ischemia of specific cerebral areas. When glycemic levels are low, such areas are at the highest risk of severe energy curtailment.

CLASSIFICATION & CAUSES

A classification of the common causes of hypoglycemia is presented in Table 11–1. It is critical to document hypoglycemia and identify whether it occurs in the fasting state. Fasting hypoglycemia (occurring 5 or more hours after a meal) often results from organic causes, and a correct diagnosis can lead to specific treatment. Hypoglycemia occurring solely in the fed state [1–5 hours after a meal or an oral glucose tolerance test (OGTT)] is most generally functional and does not pose a threat to the health of a patient.

Table 11–1. Causes of hypoglycemia.

Fasting hypoglycemia with hyperinsulinism
Insulin overdose (iatrogenic or surreptitious)
Sulfonylurea overdose (iatrogenic or surreptitious)
Pentamidine treatment (may occur acutely)
Pancreatic B-cell tumor
Insulin autoimmune syndromes (autoantibodies to insulin or to the insulin receptor)

Fasting hypoglycemia without hyperinsulinism
Severe diffuse hepatocellular damage
Severe renal insufficiency
Inanition
Overwhelming sepsis
Ethanol ingestion
Glucocorticoid deficiency (primary or secondary to pituitary insufficiency)
Growth hormone deficiency
Nonpancreatic tumors

Childhood presentation
Ketotic hypoglycemia of childhood
Genetic deficiency of hepatic enzymes (aglycogenosis, glycogen storage disease, fructose-1,6-bisphosphatase deficiency)
Induced by leucine (leucine hypersensitivity)
Induced by galactose (galactosemia)
Induced by fructose (hereditary fructose intolerance)

Nonfasting (reactive) hypoglycemia
Alimentary (postgastrectomy)
Occult diabetes (hypoglycemia 4–5 hours into an abnormal OGTT)
Functional (observed during OGTT, rarely with mixed meals)

Childhood presentation
Induced by leucine (leucine hypersensitivity)
Induced by galactose (galactosemia)
Induced by fructose (hereditary fructose intolerance)

FASTING HYPOGLYCEMIA (See Fig. 11–1.)

Fasting Hypoglycemia with Hyperinsulinism

Fasting hypoglycemia with hyperinsulinism (ie, insulin levels that are inappropriately elevated for the concomitant blood glucose level; see below for diagnostic ratios) is diagnostic of insulin-mediated hypoglycemia. If insulin or sulfonylurea administration in the diabetic patient is excluded, the most common cause of this form of hypoglycemia is an islet B-cell tumor (insulinoma).

Insulinomas are generally benign, small (less than 2 cm in diameter), solitary tumors without predilection for any part of the pancreas. They occur more often in women and in the later decades of life. Because the symptomatology may be intermittent, variable, and suggestive of a variety of neuropsychiatric disorders, the diagnosis may be delayed by many years. Although symptoms are more common in the morning before breakfast and in the late afternoon, they may occur at various times during the day but generally several hours after any meal. Only 20% of patients will report a history of weight gain. About 10% of patients may have multiple tumors or diffuse islet-cell disease (hyperplasia, nesidioblastosis), in which case there is a high likelihood of associated other endocrine neoplasias (multiple endocrine adenomatosis, type I). Insulinomas exhibit malignant behavior in 10–20% of cases: malignancy may be suggested by increased frequency and severity of the hypoglycemic attacks, but the diagnosis rests chiefly on the demonstration of metastases (mostly occurring in the liver), since the histologic appearance of benign and malignant insulinomas is similar.

Surreptitious or malicious administration of insulin or sulfonylureas occurs but is rare. It should be considered in the differential diagnosis of fasting hypoglycemia with hyperinsulinism in individuals who have familiarity with the medical profession and exposure to the drugs. Several tests are available to confirm the diagnosis of such intentional hypoglycemias (see below).

Insulin Autoimmune Syndromes

Insulin autoimmune syndromes are exceedingly rare causes of hypoglycemia. **Insulin antibodies** only rarely develop in the absence of any exposure to exogenous insulin. These patients have a combination of carbohydrate intolerance and fasting/reacting hypoglycemia. The hypoglycemia is probably caused by release of free hormone from a large pool of antibody-bound insulin. Characteristic of this condition are elevated titers of antiinsulin antibodies that bind both human and beef/pork insulin but fail to bind bovine and porcine proinsulin and C-peptide. As a result of the interference of insulin antibodies with radioimmunoassay, serum insulin assay determinations are spuriously high (double-antibody assay) or low (single-antibody precipitation assay).

Insulin receptor antibodies in most cases cause severe insulin resistance and diabetes. However, in some patients a transition may occur from severe diabetes to fasting hypoglycemia, whereas in others fasting hypoglycemia may be the first and only manifestation. Antiinsulin receptor antibodies usually occur along with other signs of autoimmunity and have also been described in Hodgkin's disease. Plasma insulin levels may remain detectable during hypoglycemia, but plasma levels of proinsulin are not elevated, in contrast to those of the typical patient with insulinoma.

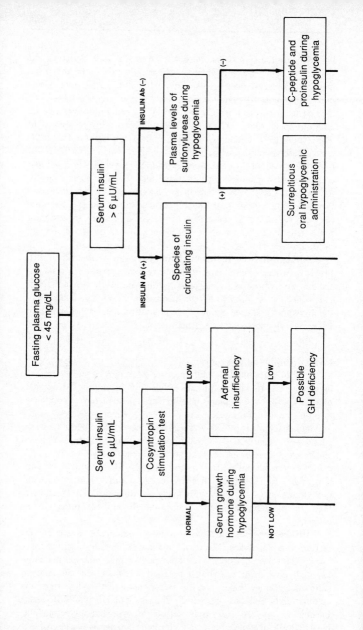

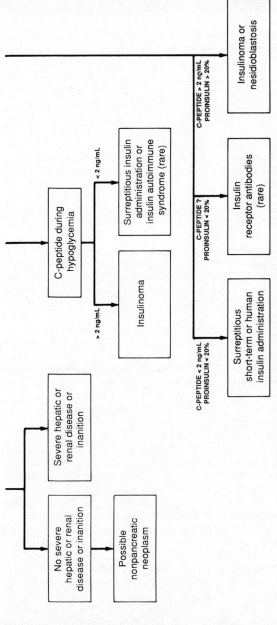

Figure 11-1. Differential diagnosis of fasting hypoglycemia in adults.

Fasting Hypoglycemia Without Hyperinsulinism

Fasting hypoglycemia without hyperinsulinism (ie, with circulating insulin levels that are appropriately suppressed at the time of hypoglycemia) is caused by inadequate hepatic glucose output. Diffuse hepatic disease such as may occur in viral hepatitis or toxic necrosis compromises hepatic cellular components involved in glycogenolysis and gluconeogenesis; severe renal disease and extreme inanition (anorexia nervosa, chronic starvation) limit the supply of substrates for gluconeogenesis.

Ethanol ingestion precipitates hypoglycemia if superimposed on an insufficient caloric intake; after depletion of glycogen stores, hypoglycemia ensues because alcohol oxidation impairs the oxidation of substrates for gluconeogenesis. It is of interest that marked inhibition of gluconeogenesis is observed with concentrations of alcohol between 10 and 20 mg/dL, levels that can be produced in humans after drinking only 1–2 ounces of whisky.

Glucocorticoid deficiency (primary or secondary to ACTH deficiency) induces fasting hypoglycemia by compromising multiple steps in gluconeogenesis and by facilitating insulin action on the liver and peripheral tissues. Hypoglycemia due to cortisol deficiency is accentuated by concomitant malnutrition and made very severe by ethanol ingestion.

Growth hormone deficiency may cause hypoglycemia in the fasting state and 5–6 hours after a meal. This is due to heightened sensitivity to insulin, resulting in an increase in peripheral glucose utilization and a decrease in lipolysis, provision of gluconeogenic substrates (glycerol), and hepatic glucose output.

Nonpancreatic tumors of mesodermal, ectodermal, or endodermal origin may cause fasting hypoglycemia in adults. Tumor types that have been associated with severe fasting hypoglycemia are adrenocortical carcinoma, malignant pheochromocytoma, neurilemmoma, hypernephroma, lymphoma, hepatoma, hemangiopericytoma, mesothelioma, fibrosarcoma, leiomyosarcoma, and rhabdomyosarcoma. Those of mesodermal origin are often situated in the retroperitoneum. These tumors are generally low-grade malignancies and thus reach noticeable size by the time that they cause symptoms. The mechanism of the hypoglycemia is heterogeneous; both increased glucose utilization and decreased hepatic glucose production have been documented. In some cases, there may be excessive glucose consumption by the large tumor mass itself. In other cases, elevated plasma concentrations of insulinlike growth factors (IGFs) may contribute to the hypoglycemia. IGF-like material has been found particularly elevated in patients with hemangiopericytomas, whereas most patients with lymphomas have low values. Although IGFs have a low affinity for the insulin receptor, when their concentration increases to a critical level, they bind and activate a sufficient number of receptors to exert biologic actions similar to those of insulin. Serum immunoreactive insulin is not elevated.

Ketotic Hypoglycemia

Ketotic hypoglycemia may be precipitated by fasting in infants and children who have some deficiency of the gluconeogenic substrate alanine, or it may be due to genetic deficiency of hepatic enzymes involved in glycogen synthesis, glycogenolysis, and gluconeogenesis (aglycogenosis, glycogen storage disease, fructose-1,6 bisphosphatase deficiency). Children who are fasting before surgery should always be given intravenous 5% dextrose.

REACTIVE HYPOGLYCEMIA

Reactive hypoglycemia (that occurring 1–5 hours after food intake) is usually caused by abnormal kinetics of glucose absorption, insulin secretion, or both.

Alimentary Hypoglycemia

Alimentary hypoglycemia occurs in patients who have undergone surgical procedures that accelerate gastric emptying (gastrectomy, gastrojejunostomy, pyloroplasty). In these cases, the rapid transit time of the hypertonic alimentary content leads to enhanced secretion of insulinotropic gut factors and to a rapid and excessive rise in blood glucose. This combination in turn results in excessive insulin release. Hypoglycemia generally occurs within 90–180 minutes of food intake. Since the rate of glucose decline is very rapid, it is accompanied by adrenergic symptoms. In these patients, the symptoms of hypoglycemia may be difficult to distinguish from the symptoms of the ''dumping'' syndrome (gastric discomfort, nausea, palpitations, diaphoresis, weakness).

Hypoglycemia As Manifestation of Occult Diabetes

Reactive hypoglycemia as an early manifestation of occult diabetes is seldom a clinical problem, since only occasional patients will have symptoms after regular meals. The abnormality is well documented during a 5-hour OGTT. The OGTT is abnormal, indicative of carbohydrate intolerance or diabetes, and hypoglycemia occurs not earlier than 3–5 hours into the OGTT. The principal defect in these patients, who are often obese and have a strong family history of diabetes, is a delay in the insulin secretory response, allowing an excessive and protracted rise in blood glucose that eventually results in late, excessive secretion of insulin, whose biologic activity continues when glucose absorption from the gut is ending. Since the decline in blood glucose is less precipitous or severe than in alimentary hypoglycemia, the symptoms are generally milder.

Functional Hypoglycemia

Functional (idiopathic) hypoglycemia is the form of hypoglycemia most often claimed but rarely documented. Subjects presenting with this complaint are generally young, most often women, with an anxious and compulsive personality. Their medical history is otherwise benign, and they seek physician's advice for ill-defined symptoms of lightheadedness, weakness, tremulousness, and diaphoresis generally occurring 2–4 hours after a meal. When these patients are tested with an OGTT, the proportion manifesting chemical hypoglycemia is similar to that of asymptomatic controls (10–25%), and when they are tested with mixed meals, chemical hypoglycemia is very seldom documented despite the claim or manifestation of symptoms. Since a role for hypoglycemia in this syndrome has not been established, it has been suggested that the disorder be termed **idiopathic postprandial syndrome**.

Hypoglycemia Due to Leucine Hypersensitivity

Leucine hypersensitivity is a common cause of hypoglycemia in infancy, generally appearing within the first 2 years of life. This form of hypoglycemia follows ingestion of dietary proteins with a high content of L-leucine, which in turn triggers exaggerated insulin secretion. Whatever the reason for the increased B-cell sensitivity to leucine, it disappears spontaneously into childhood. Since these infants often manifest fasting hypoglycemia as well, additional problems with gluconeogenesis are likely to be present. Leucine hypersensitivity as a cause of hypoglycemia in adults is extremely rare.

Hypoglycemia Due to Galactosemia and Hereditary Fructose Intolerance

Galactosemia and hereditary fructose intolerance cause hypoglycemia that is classified as reactive because it only occurs if the diet contains the poorly tolerated nutrient (galactose or fructose). However, it is often manifested as fasting hypoglycemia. Galactose-induced hypoglycemia occurs owing to deficiency of galactose 1-phosphate uridyl transferase, which impairs the capability to metabolize dietary galactose. Galactose accumulation in the liver—as well as in other organs—compromises gluconeogenesis. This syndrome should be suspected in infants showing melituria not due to glucose; prompt recognition and elimination of lactose from the diet prevents severe sequelae and allows normal development. Patients with the autosomal recessive disorder of hereditary fructose intolerance lack the hepatic enzyme fructose 1-phosphate aldolase. Upon eating fructose-containing food, these individuals develop protracted vomiting and hypoglycemia lasting several hours. The latter is probably caused by inhibition of hepatic glycogenolysis and gluconeogenesis owing to accumulation of fructose 1-phosphate, which cannot be transformed into glucose because of the enzymatic defect. The therapeutic approach to this disorder is exclusion of fructose from the diet.

DIAGNOSTIC WORK-UP OF ADULTS

HISTORY & PHYSICAL EXAMINATION

History should focus on (1) description of symptoms, (2) time of their occurrence in relationship to meals and alcohol intake, (3) response of symptoms to food, and (4) duration of the symptomatology (months, years). Although the same patient may experience different types of symptoms during different episodes of hypoglycemia, in most patients the same symptoms tend to recur, and the presence or absence of adrenergic discharge is helpful toward delineating the pathogenesis of hypoglycemia. Inquiries about the timing of episodes in relationship to food intake must be detailed and specific in order to identify whether hypoglycemia occurs in the fasting state or exclusively postprandially. The 2 pictures may co-exist in some patients with B-cell tumors whose insulin secretion is not completely autonomous, in patients with factitious hypoglycemia, and in the rare patient with spontaneous antiinsulin antibodies. A temporal relation of symptomatology with alcohol intake incriminates the latter as a precipitating factor but does not exclude other more serious causes of hypoglycemia. Most patients with recurrent hypoglycemia have learned that food ingestion alleviates the symptoms; thus, such information gives further credit to the likelihood of hypoglycemia. A few patients may, however, have failed to recognize the therapeutic role of food. The length of time over which the symptomatology has recurred is important information; periods of years are almost pathognomonic for a benign insulinoma.

Physical examination will detect acanthosis nigricans or features of an autoimmune disease in patients with autoantibodies to the insulin receptor and stigmata of malnutrition, liver or kidney disease, or glucocorticoid deficiency. Tumor masses must be searched for, since nonpancreatic tumors producing hypoglycemia have generally achieved noticeable size by the time they produce symptoms.

DOCUMENTATION OF HYPOGLYCEMIA

There are circumstances in which the history is sufficiently vague and the symptomatology sufficiently nonspecific to cast doubts on the diagnosis of hypoglycemia. It is cost-effective in such cases to attempt a documentation of hypoglycemia on an outpatient basis before scheduling costly hospitalization. Patients are asked to perform a fingerstick and obtain a blood glucose reading whenever symptoms occur. The best reagent strips to be used for this purpose are Chemstrips bG, since they can be read visually quite accurately and the reacted strip is stable for at least 3 days, thus allowing verification by the physician.

FASTING HYPOGLYCEMIA

If the combination of history, symptoms, and chemical data indicates fasting hypoglycemia, a thorough diagnostic work-up is initiated. The first step is to document that in fact hypoglycemia occurs in the fasting state and to explore whether it is accompanied by hyperinsulinemia. To this end the most specific and benign test is the prolonged fast.

Prolonged Fast

This can be considered a "suppression test" for insulin secretion, insofar as the decline in blood glucose levels normally occurring during fasting and the concomitant increase in adrenergic activity are powerful inhibitors of insulin secretion. The relationship between circulating immunoreactive insulin (IRI) and glucose (G) levels can be expressed as the ratio.

$$[IRI (in \ \mu U/mL)]/[G (in \ mg/dL)]$$

which in normal nonobese individuals is maintained below 0.25 (in obese patients, it may be slightly greater but is not accompanied by hypoglycemia) or by the amended ratio

$$[IRI (in \ \mu U/mL) \times 100]/[G (in \ mg/dL) - 30]$$

which is normally below 49 (it may be slightly greater in obese patients but is not accompanied by hypoglycemia), or it can be assumed that during hypoglycemia insulin levels should be no greater than 6μU/mL. This cutoff point sometimes offers greater diagnostic accuracy than the above ratios.

Patients undergoing a prolonged fast should be hospitalized and kept under careful supervision. After an overnight fast, a sample for plasma glucose and insulin is obtained; there is a high likelihood of observing values in the hypoglycemic range. If this is not the case, the fast is prolonged until chemical or symptomatic hypoglycemia occurs. Throughout this period, samples for plasma glucose and insulin are obtained at 2- to 3-hour intervals and at the onset of symptoms. In most patients with insulin-producing tumors, the interval between the last meal and onset of symptomatic hypoglycemia ranges between 6 and 60 hours—in 75% of patients, symptoms occur within 24 hours; by 48 hours, 98% of patients will be hypoglycemic; and by 72 hours practically all patients will be hypoglycemic. The occurrence of symptomatic hypoglycemia may be accelerated by a short bout of physical exercise, with plasma glucose and insulin samples obtained before and at the end of exercise. Whenever symptoms develop, they should be treated by oral feeding or intravenous glucose administration, depending on the severity.

Intravenous Tolbutamide Test

Since the prolonged fast has an excellent diagnostic yield in identifying patients with fasting hypoglycemia mediated by hyperinsulinism, several provocative tests routinely used in the past have been abandoned. In cases in which the insulin/glucose relationship during fasting is not clearly diagnostic and yet the clinical suspicion of an insulin-producing tumor remains high, an intravenous tolbutamide test is performed. Sodium tolbutamide, 1g, is infused intravenously over 2 minutes, and samples for glucose and insulin are drawn at intervals. Two protocols may be used.

The most benign protocol involves a **short tolbutamide test**, during which insulin levels are measured every 5 minutes after the beginning of the bolus for a 15-minute period—insulin levels in excess of 195 μU/mL are diagnostic of insulinoma. This protocol is safe, not allowing profound hypoglycemia to develop and persist, but it has a high rate of false-negative results.

The **long tolbutamide test** (3 hours) encompasses the most discriminating portion of the test, which occurs between 120 and 180 minutes. Samples for glucose and insulin are drawn at 30-minute intervals. In normal subjects, insulin levels have returned to basal by 60 minutes after the tolbutamide injection and plasma glucose by 120 minutes is over 55 mg/dL. Patients with insulinoma manifest persistent hyperinsulinemia at 120–180 minutes with glucose values below 55 mg/dL and often in the frank hypoglycemic range. The best separation of normals and insulinoma patients has been obtained by calculating the difference between the plasma glucose value and one-half the insulin value at 150 minutes after tolbutamide injection—control subjects have differences greater than 43 and insulinoma patients have differences less than 43. Although the long tolbutamide test is sensitive and specific, it may be uncomfortable and hazardous in view of the prolonged hypoglycemia. One may choose a stepwise diagnostic strategy—attempt to obtain the most information through the fasting test, not hesitating to repeat it several times—and if further testing is indicated, perform a short tolbutamide test. Only if the combination of the 2 tests is still equivocal, additional benign tests (insulin antibodies, C-peptide) are not diagnostic, and the clinical suspicion is high for insulinoma, proceed with the long tolbutamide test.

Fasting Hypoglycemia with Hyperinsulinism

If fasting hypoglycemia with hyperinsulinism is diagnosed, the source of insulin must be identified. An insulin-producing tumor is most likely, but the possibility of surreptitious administration of insulin or ingestion of sulfonylureas should be entertained and the syndrome of hypoglycemia due to insulin autoantibodies, albeit exceedingly rare, needs to be excluded. A simple test that can assist in the differential diagnosis is the measurement of insulin antibodies that are expected to be negative in patients with insulinoma.

If insulin antibodies are detected, 3 possibilities exist: (1) surreptitious insulin administration sufficiently frequent and prolonged to have led to immunization (at least 4 weeks), (2) insulin autoimmune syndrome, (3) development of an insulinoma in a patient who has previously received insulin treatment. The possibility of surreptitious insulin administration can be documented by (1) determination of the species of circulating insulin through chromatography or amino acid analysis (this maneuver would assist in diagnosing surreptitious administration of porcine or bovine but not human insulin) and (2) measurement of serum C-peptide (index of endogenous insulin secretion) during a spontaneous hypoglycemic episode or an insulin tolerance test. Normally, C-peptide levels are suppressed during hypoglycemia to less than 2 ng/mL. If the patient harbors an autonomously secreting insulinoma, C-peptide levels will not be suppressed. In the very rare patient with insulin autoantibodies, C-peptide levels should normally be suppressed by hypoglycemia, but the presence of complexes between autoantibodies and proinsulin (which contains insulin and C-peptide within its structure) may impair the possibility of precisely correlating circulating C-peptide levels and B-cell secretory response.

If the patient's serum is negative for insulin antibodies, the insulin autoimmune syndrome is excluded but not factitious hypoglycemia. Surreptitious administration of insulin may have been taking place for too short a period, or hypoglycemia may be due to ingestion of sulfonylureas. The latter possibility is easily documented by obtaining a plasma level of the more common sulfonylureas.

An additional test useful for diagnosis of insulinoma is measurement of **circulating proinsulin**—frequently patients with an insulinoma have an increased proportion of proinsulin in plasma (more than 20% of total immunoreactive insulin), even when the insulin level is not markedly elevated. High levels of circulating proinsulin are encountered also in the rare patient with familial hyperproinsulinemia due to defective conversion of proinsulin to insulin.

Localization of an Insulinoma

If the appropriate combination of diagnostic tests yields biochemical data pointing to an insulinoma, then and only then are localization procedures undertaken. Preoperative real-time sonography of the pancreas detects 60% of solitary insulinomas. CT scanning detects about 50%, and intraoperative high-frequency sonography visualizes 86% of solitary insulinomas. Intraoperative sonography is especially valuable to detect small intrapancreatic insulinomas that are not palpable and to determine the relationship of the insulinoma to pancreatic and bile ducts, thereby facilitating safe enucleation. Arteriography and transhepatic portal venous pancreatic sampling (the latter only available at specialized centers and subject to possible interpretative difficulties) are generally not required. Labeled somatostatin analogs may detect certain endocrine tumors and their metastases owing to the fact that they have a higher density of somatostatin receptors than surrounding healthy tissue. However, a substantial proportion of insulinomas express few or no somatostatin receptors.

When the biochemical diagnosis is firmly established, the patient becomes a candidate for exploratory laparotomy even in the absence of radiologic evidence of tumor. In the hands of experienced surgeons, a tumor is found in over 80% of patients with a well-established biochemical diagnosis of insulinoma.

The suspicion of malignant insulinoma is raised by increased frequency and severity of the hypoglycemic episodes. Nonspecific tumor markers such as hCG or its subunits (α-hCG, β-hCG) are elevated in about 50% of patients with malignant insulinoma but in none of the patients with benign tumors. The hCG determination, although not a sensitive discriminatory test, can identify some of the malignant tumors and be used to follow effectiveness of treatment. Staging of the tumor is obtained preoperatively by CT scanning.

In patients with insulinoma, the possibility of multiple endocrine neoplasia (MEN I) is explored by at least obtaining a careful family history (the disorder is autosomal dominant) and serum calcium and phosphorus levels, since primary hyperparathyroidism is the most common manifestation of the syndrome. Patients with MEN I have multiple, small insulinomas that can rarely all be localized and excised. Subtotal pancreatectomy may need to be performed in these patients.

Fasting Hypoglycemia Without Hyperinsulinism

If fasting hypoglycemia is not accompanied by hyperinsulinism, the underlying disorder is often diagnosed on the basis of physical examination and routine laboratory data (diffuse hepatocellular damage, renal insufficiency, inanition, ethanol ingestion). The 2 important etiologies to be investigated are glucocorticoid deficiency and nonpancreatic tumors. A simple screening test for glucocorticoid deficiency is the **cosyntropin (ACTH) stimulation test**, which, if positive, should be followed by a thorough work-up of pituitary-adrenal function. Since the nonpancreatic tumors associated with hypoglycemia are generally of very large size, the presenting symptoms may include those due to mass effect in addition to hypoglycemia. These tumors are often detected by careful physical examination and simple radiographic procedures (chest x-ray, flat films of abdomen, gastrointestinal series, intravenous pyelogram, CT scans).

A **glucagon stimulation test**, which can be considered a test of hepatic reserve, is often helpful in documenting the pathogenesis of nonhyperinsulinemic fasting hypoglycemia. Normally, 30 minutes after the intravenous bolus administration of 1 mg of glucagon, plasma glucose levels increase by about 40 mg over basal owing to brisk glycogenolysis. An absent or minimal glycemic rise indicates nonexistent or depleted glycogen stores (severe hepatic or renal disease, inanition, glucocorticoid deficiency, occasional nonpancreatic tumors). A normal or exaggerated response in patients with nonpancreatic tumors is compatible (although nondiagnostic) with production of insulinlike factors promoting hepatic glucose storage and antagonizing physiologic glucose release. Administration of glucagon may induce nausea and vomiting.

Documentation of insulinlike factors in the serum of patients with nonpancreatic tumors associated with hypoglycemia is not required for diagnosis or treatment.

REACTIVE HYPOGLYCEMIA

Since conditions causing reactive hypoglycemia may also cause fasting hypoglycemia (insulinomas not completely autonomous, insulin antibodies) the work-up for reactive hypoglycemia starts after exclusion of fasting hypoglycemia. This is easily accomplished by home measurement of blood glucose and, if suspicion arises, by repeated determinations on an outpatient basis of plasma glucose and insulin levels after an overnight fast. If fasting hypoglycemia is excluded, the etiologic diagnosis of reactive hypoglycemia is simple.

The diagnosis of alimentary hypoglycemia is based on a history of surgical interventions that accelerate gastric emptying and on the documentation of hypoglycemia at the time of symptoms. This is particularly important, since in these patients the symptomatology occurring 1–2 hours after food ingestion may be entirely due to the "dumping" syndrome. In the rare patient who manifests symptoms and mild hypoglycemia 3–5 hours after meals, a 5-hour OGTT with insulin levels can be obtained. The OGTT is likely to show carbohydrate intolerance or diabetes with a delayed and then exaggerated insulin response causing late hypoglycemia.

In individuals with ill-defined symptomatology occurring 2–4 hours after food intake, any work-up is contingent on documentation of hypoglycemia during a mixed meal. Most often such documentation will not be forthcoming, and there is therefore no indication for further work-up and in particular for an OGTT. The latter might well result in hypoglycemic values, but so it does in 10–25% of asymptomatic normal individuals.

MANAGEMENT OF HYPOGLYCEMIC DISORDERS

INSULINOMA

The treatment of choice for insulinoma is surgical excision.

Before Surgery

Three pieces of information must be on hand. (1) *Presence or absence of metastatic disease.* Only 10% of insulinomas are malignant, but such information drastically affects the surgical indication and strategy. (2) *Rate of glucose infusion needed to maintain euglycemia.* This is established in advance of surgery using a 5% or 10% dextrose infusion for 4–6 hours and will prevent dangerous hypoglycemia throughout the often long surgical procedure. (3) *Responsiveness of hypoglycemia to oral diazoxide or verapamil.* Diazoxide is a benzothiadiazine with a potent inhibitory effect on insulin secretion. Generally, patients respond to 200–600 mg/d, although occasional patients may require up to 1 g/d. The drug is an antidiuretic that may cause sodium retention treatable with a diuretic; it may also cause hirsutism. The calcium antagonist verapamil in doses of 80 mg three times a day is effective in lowering insulin levels and reducing the frequency and severity of hypoglycemic attacks in patients with insulinoma. A therapeutic trial of these drugs is important in planning the surgical approach. In patients who respond to and tolerate diazoxide or verapamil, a negative pancreatic exploration (observation and palpation) need not be followed by blind pancreatic surgery (two-thirds distal pancreatectomy, progressive sectioning of the pancreas from tail to head), since medical therapy can be continued indefinitely. In contrast, in patients whose hypoglycemia does not respond to drugs, the attainment of a surgical cure becomes more critical and thus justifies blind resections. The success rate of blind partial pancreatectomy is 25–34%.

During Surgery

During surgery, the patient must be infused with glucose at the rate previously determined to maintain euglycemia, and blood glucose values must be checked frequently. Since in 10% of cases tumors may be multiple, the entire gland must be carefully palpated even after detection of one discrete mass. Shortly after removal of all hypersecreting tissue, glycemia tends to rise, and this is a favorable sign to be watched for.

After Surgery

If surgery has been successful, patients may remain hyperglycemic for a few days. This is probably a consequence of the protracted suppression of normal B-cell function by the prevailing hypoglycemia. Only severe hyperglycemia needs to be corrected (by administration of small doses of Regular insulin); otherwise some degrees of hyperglycemia may be a beneficial stimulus for resumption of normal insulin secretion.

In 10–20% of cases, hypoglycemia persists postoperatively despite extensive surgery. These situations are generally due to persistent disease (adenoma, nesidioblastosis) in the head of the pancreas, which is the most difficult area to explore and the most complicated to resect. These patients may be managed with diazoxide or verapamil; if these drugs are ineffective or poorly tolerated, frequent feeding containing complex carbohydrates is recommended. Weight gain may become a real problem. Total pancreatectomy represents the last resort in view of operative morbidity, chronic exocrine insufficiency, and insulin-requiring diabetes.

Metastatic islet-cell carcinoma generally responds to the cytotoxic drug streptozocin with or without fluorouracil. Patients experience remission of hypoglycemia and tumor regression lasting for several months and occasionally years. The most serious side effect of streptozocin is nephrotoxicity manifested as renal tubular damage. Because patients with malignant pancreatic endocrine tumors are at risk of developing elevation of a second or third hormone and related symptoms (eg, hypergastrinemia and gastrointestinal bleeding), regular biochemical and clinical surveillance should be continued for life.

Somatostatin analog (octreotide; Sandostatin) has also been effective in some cases of benign or metastatic islet cell tumor, including insulinoma. For insulinoma, octreotide plus verapamil may have an additive effect. Some patients treated with octreotide may experience worse hypoglycemia, so close monitoring is necessary.

INSULIN AUTOIMMUNE SYNDROMES

Hypoglycemia associated with antibodies to the insulin receptor has been reported to respond promptly (2–3 days) to prednisone therapy (80–120 mg/d). After 2–3 months of therapy, the titer of antireceptor antibodies may fall sufficiently to allow discontinuation of the drug.

No specific therapy is available for patients with hypoglycemia caused by antiinsulin autoantibodies. Recognition of the syndrome and a sufficiently frequent intake of dietary carbohydrates appears to be the best treatment we can offer today.

NONPANCREATIC TUMORS

The hypoglycemia caused by these tumors is unresponsive to diazoxide. Supportive therapy with frequent feedings is the course of action while more definitive measures are addressed to the primary neoplasm.

ALIMENTARY HYPOGLYCEMIA

This condition is secondary to surgical procedures that accelerate gastric emptying and is first approached with dietary measures—more frequent but smaller meals containing complex carbohydrates, fiber, fat, and proteins and avoidance of rapidly absorbed sugars. Anticholinergic drugs may be added (propantheline bromide, 7.5–15 mg orally, 30 minutes before meals).

LATE REACTIVE HYPOGLYCEMIA

When secondary to occult diabetes, this condition responds to weight reduction and dietary modifications in obese patients. Elimination of refined carbohydrates and sufficiently small, spaced meals will ameliorate both the diabetic state and the late hypoglycemia. Small doses of a sulfonylurea may be added to restore the early phase of insulin release.

FUNCTIONAL (IDIOPATHIC) HYPOGLYCEMIA

Anticholinergic drugs may be helpful in the rare instances of functional (idiopathic) hypoglycemia in which chemical hypoglycemia is documented, especially if combined with a mild sedative. Patients with the distressing symptomatology of ''idiopathic postprandial'' syndrome but in whom genuine hypoglycemia cannot be documented during regular meals, may benefit from measures aimed at relieving tension and anticipation—regular exercise programs, psychologic counseling, mild tranquilizers. Modification of the diet toward smaller and more frequent meals in which refined sugars are substituted by complex carbohydrates is worth prescribing but is rarely successful.

LEUCINE-INDUCED REACTIVE HYPOGLYCEMIA

This condition is almost exclusively encountered in childhood. Restriction of leucine in the diet is not safely accomplished because leucine is necessary for normal growth and development. Patients are generally managed with diazoxide and conservative measures, since the disease is self-limited.

REFERENCES

Bauman WA, Yalow RS: Hyperinsulinemic hypoglycemia. *JAMA* 1984; **252:**2730.

Berger M et al: Functional and morphologic characterization of human insulinomas. *Diabetes* 1983;**32:**921.

Charles MA et al: Comparison of oral glucose tolerance tests and mixed meals in patients with apparent idiopathic postabsorptive hypoglycemia. *Diabetes* 1981;**30:**465.

De Marinis L, Barbarino A: Calcium antagonists and hormone release. 1. Effects of verapamil on insulin release in normal subjects and patients with islet-cell tumor. *Metabolism* 1980;**29:**599.

Doppman JL et al: Localization of islet cell tumors. *Gastroenterol Clin North Am* 1989;**18:**793.

Glaser B et al: Chronic treatment of a benign insulinoma using the long-acting somatostatin analogue SMS 201-995. *Isr J Med Sci* 1990;**26:**16.

Goldman J et al: Characterization of circulating insulin and proinsulin-binding antibodies in autoimmune hypoglycemia. *J Clin Invest* 1979;**63:**1050.

Gorden P et al: Hypoglycemia associated with non-islet-cell tumor and insulin-like growth factors. *N Engl J Med* 1981;**305:**1452.

Gorman B et al: Benign pancreatic insulinoma: Preoperative and intraoperative sonographic localization. *AJR* 1986;**147:**929.

Insulinoma. (Case Records of the Massachusetts General Hospital.) *N Engl J Med* 1988;**318:**1523.

Lamberts SWJ et al: Somatostatin receptor imaging in the localization of endocrine tumors. *N Engl J Med* 1990;**323:**1246.

Lev-Ran A, Anderson RW: The diagnosis of postprandial hypoglycemia. *Diabetes* 1981;**30:**996.

Marks V: Diagnosis and differential diagnosis of hypoglycemia. *Mayo Clin Proc* 1989;**64:**1558.

Martensson H et al: Localization and surgical treatment of occult insulinomas. *Ann Surg* 1990;**212:**615.

Merimee TJ, Tyson JE: Stabilization of plasma glucose during fasting. *N Engl J Med* 1974;**291:**1275.

Mozell E et al: Functional endocrine tumors of the pancreas: Clinical presentation, diagnosis and treatment. *Curr Probl Surg* 1990;**27:**301.

Pun KK et al: The use of glucagon challenge tests in the diagnostic evaluation of hypoglycemia due to hepatoma and insulinoma. *J Clin Endocrinol Metab* 1988;**67:**546.

Rizza RA, Cryer PE, Gerich JE: Role of glucagon, catecholamines, and growth hormone in human glucose counterregulation. *J Clin Invest* 1979;**64:**62.

Rothmund M et al: Surgery for benign insulinoma: An international review. *World J Surg* 1990;**14:**393.

Service FJ et al: Insulinoma: Clinical and diagnostic features of 60 consecutive cases. *Mayo Clin Proc* 1976;**51:**417.

Shapiro ET et al: Tumor hypoglycemia: Relationship to high molecular weight insulin-like growth factor II. *J Clin Invest* 1990;**85:**1672.

Stehouwer CD et al: Aggravation of hypoglycemia in insulinoma patients by the long-acting somatostatin analogue octreotide (Sandostatin). *Acta Endocrinol (Copenh)* 1989;**121:**34.

Stehouwer CD et al: Malignant insulinoma: Is combined treatment with verapamil and the long-acting somatostatin analogue octreotide (SMS 201-995) more effective than single therapy with either drug? *Neth J Med* 1989;**35:**86.

Taylor SI et al: Hypoglycemia associated with antibodies to the insulin receptor. *N Engl J Med* 1982;**307:**1422.

Walters EG et al: Hypoglycemia due to an insulin-receptor antibody in Hodgkin's disease. *Lancet* 1987;**1:**241.

Wynick D, Williams SJ, Bloom SR: Symptomatic secondary hormone syndromes in patients with established malignant pancreatic endocrine tumors. *N Engl J Med* 1988;**319:**605.

Lipid Metabolism | 12

Philip H. Frost, MD, & Thomas P. Bersot, MD, PhD

The disorders of lipid metabolism are characterized by abnormalities of circulating lipoproteins or their concentrations. Elevations of lipoproteins such that the total cholesterol or triacylglycerol content is above a defined limit are designated the **hyperlipidemias**. Clinical interest in these disorders results from evidence linking abnormalities in lipoprotein concentrations to the development of **atherosclerotic cardiovascular disease** and in the case of marked increases in the triacylglycerol-rich lipoproteins with **pancreatitis**. Marked deficiencies in circulating lipoproteins, the **hypolipidemias**, occur infrequently but have multiple clinical consequences.

PLASMA LIPIDS

The plasma lipids of major clinical significance are triacylglycerols and cholesterol. Others, such as phospholipids, glycolipids, and sphingolipids, have important physiologic roles, but there are no known metabolic disorders in which abnormal metabolism of these minor plasma lipid components cause accelerated atherosclerotic cardiovascular disease. The lipids in the blood are primarily in transit from one organ to another. However, certain lipids may perform specific intravascular functions. For example, plasma phospholipids may provide arachidonic acid as a substrate for prostaglandin (prostacycline) synthesis by platelets and endothelial cells.

Triacylglycerols (Triglycerides)*

Triacylglycerols are composed of 3 long-chain fatty acids esterified to a glycerol backbone. Plasma triacylglycerol concentrations must be measured in the fasting state, and normal values range from

---

*According to the current standardized terminology of the International Union of Pure and Applied Chemistry (IUPAC) and the International Union of Biochemistry (IUB), the monoglycerides, diglycerides, and triglycerides are to be designated monoacylglycerols, diacylglycerols, and triacylglycerols, respectively. The older terminology may be used occasionally in this book.

25 to 250 mg/dL. The triacylglycerols in plasma arise from 2 sources: the small intestine and liver. They are synthesized in the epithelial cells of the small intestine, after absorption of dietary fat. These triacylglycerols are then incorporated into chylomicrons that have been secreted from the intestinal epithelial cells. The chylomicrons leave the intestine through the lymphatic system and ultimately reach the blood circulation via the thoracic duct. Triacylglycerols transported by chylomicrons have been designated as exogenous fat because of their dietary origin.

Endogenous triacylglycerols in the blood are synthesized in the liver from accumulated fatty acids too numerous for the liver's metabolic requirements. These triacylglycerols are incorporated into very low density lipoproteins (VLDLs), which transport the triacylglycerols out of the liver.

Control of triacylglycerol synthesis in both the intestine and the liver is primarily a function of fatty acid (substrate) availability. In the liver the fatty acids may be synthesized de novo or may enter the liver as nonesterified fatty acids bound to albumin. These nonesterified fatty acids arise from the hydrolysis of adipose tissue triacylglycerols, exit the adipocyte, and are then bound to albumin. The metabolic fate of lipoprotein triacylglycerols is discussed below.

Cholesterol

Cholesterol is a ubiquitous substance that is synthesized by most cells and is used for a variety of purposes. It is a structural component of the plasma membrane and other intracellular membranes. It is also an important precursor of steroid hormones (the adrenal gland uses more plasma cholesterol per unit weight than any other tissue in the body). Cholesterol is also the precursor of bile acids produced in the liver.

About two-thirds of the blood cholesterol is esterified to a long-chain fatty acid at the C_3 position of the A ring of the cholesterol molecule. The effect of esterification is to decrease the solubility of the cholesterol molecule in water.

LIPOPROTEINS & APOLIPOPROTEINS

The plasma lipoproteins are for the most part spherical pseudomicelles composed of (1) nonpolar lipids—triacylglycerol and cholesteryl ester, (2) amphipathic lipids—phospholipid and unesterified cholesterol, and (3) specific apolipoproteins. These spherical lipoproteins are of varying diameter and are organized such that the water-insoluble triacylglycerols and cholesteryl esters are located in the interior of the complex (core) and the unesterified cholesterol, phospholipids, and apolipoproteins are situated on a thin (2.1 nm) surface. The apolipoproteins, phospholipids, and unesterified cholesterol have both a water-soluble and lipid-soluble face; thus, these compounds function as detergents. It is assumed that the structure of the lipoproteins is not static. Components, both hydrophobic and hydrophilic, are constantly being added to and removed from the lipoproteins as they traverse the plasma compartment.

At least 15 apolipoproteins are associated with the several classes of plasma lipoproteins, and many of these apolipoproteins have functions in addition to solubilizing lipids (Table 12–1). Two apolipoproteins, apo B-100 and apo E, serve as ligands that bind specific lipoproteins to cell surface receptors. There are 2 well-characterized lipoprotein receptors, the apo B,E (LDL) receptor and the apo E (chylomicron remnant) receptor. The binding of apo B-100– and apo E–containing lipoproteins to the apo B,E receptor or the binding of apo E–containing lipoproteins to the apo-E receptor permits these lipoproteins to enter those cells that possess these receptors. Whereas the apo B,E receptor is present on almost all cells, including the liver parenchymal cells, the chylomicron remnant receptor is predominantly or exclusively localized to the liver parenchymal cells. This receptor-mediated uptake of lipoproteins is a primary process that governs the concentrations of lipoproteins in the plasma and, ultimately, the plasma concentrations of cholesterol and triacylglycerols.

Lipoprotein Nomenclature

Plasma lipoproteins have been named on the basis of the techniques employed to separate and isolate them. The first technique employed was electrophoresis. The current nomenclature (chylomicron, VLDL, IDL, LDL, HDL) is based on the separation of these

Table 12–1. Apolipoproteins with major identified functions in lipoprotein metabolism*.

Apolipo–protein	Lipoprotein Associated With	Synthesis Site	Function
A–1	Lymph chylomicrons, HDL	Intestine >>liver	Removal of cholesterol from tissues and incorporation into HDL Activator of LCAT
B-100	VLDL, IDL, LDL	Liver	Ligand for binding LDL to apo B,E(LDL) receptor Structural protein of VLDL, IDL, LDL
E	Chylomicrons, VLDL, IDL, HDL	Liver	Ligand for binding chylomicron and VLDL remnants and HDL-with-apo-E to the apo B,E(LDL) and apo E (chylomicron remnant) receptors
C-II	Chylomicrons, VLDL, HDL	Liver	Cofactor for LPL

*HDL = high-density lipoprotein; LCAT = lecithin:cholesterol acyltransferase; VLDL = very low density lipoprotein; IDL = intermediate-density lipoprotein; LDL = low-density lipoprotein; apo = apolipoprotein; HDL-with-apo-E = a cholesterol-rich subclass of high-density lipoprotein that contains apo E; LPL = lipoprotein lipase.

classes of lipoproteins by ultracentrifugation. Less frequently they are described in terms of their apolipoprotein constituents, size, or chemical composition. Characteristics of the primary lipoproteins are summarized in Table 12–2. Fig 12–1 summarizes the origins and metabolic fates of the apo B–containing lipoproteins.

Chylomicrons

The chylomicrons are microscopic particles that are large enough to scatter light and render plasma turbid. Chylomicrons are buoyant in water; their mean hydrated density of 0.93 gm/mL accounts for their flotation (ie, chylomicrons form a creamlike layer at the top of a tube of plasma that has stood overnight in a refrigerator at 4°C). Dietary and biliary lipids provide the raw material from which chylomicrons are synthesized in the epithelial cell lining of the small intestine. After absorption, dietary triacylglycerol, fatty acids, and monoacylglycerols are resynthesized into triacylglycerols in the smooth endoplasmic reticulum of the enterocytes. The chylomicron phospholipids are derived primarily from biliary lysolecithin that is reabsorbed and then esterified. The chylomicron apolipoproteins that are synthesized by the

Table 12–2. Size and chemical composition of human plasma lipoproteins.

Class	Chylomicrons	VLDL	IDL	LDL	HDL-2	HDL-3
Diameter Å	800–5000	300–800	250–350	216	100	75
Density (g/mL)	0.93	0.95–1.006	1.006–1.019	1.019–1.063	1.063–1.125	1.125–1.210
Mobility (electro-phoresis)	Origin	Pre-β	Slow pre-β	β	α	α
Major apolipoproteins	B-48, C, E	B-100, C, E	B-100, E	B-100	A-I, II, C, E	
% Composition						
Surface						
Proteins	2	8	19	22	40	55
Phospholipids	7	18	19	22	33	25
Unesterified cholesterol	2	7	9	8	5	4
Core						
Cholesteryl esters	3	12	29	42	17	13
Triacylglycerols	86	55	23	6	5	3
% Surface	11	33	47	52	78	84
% Core	89	67	52	48	22	16

* Adapted, with permission, from Havel RJ, Goldstein JL, Brown MS: Lipoproteins and lipid transport. Page 398 in: *Metabolic Control and Disease*, 8th ed. Bondy PK, Rosenberg LE (editors). Saunders; 1980.

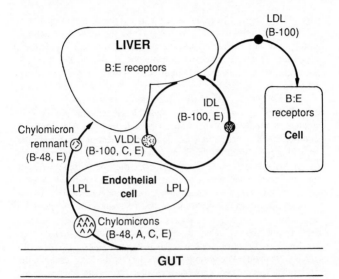

Figure 12–1. Origins and metabolic fates of apo B–containing lipoproteins. B:E receptors = LDL receptors; B-48, B-100, A, C, E = apolipoproteins; IDL = intermediate-density lipoprotein; LDL = low-density lipoprotein; LPL = lipoprotein lipase; VLDL = very low density lipoprotein.

intestine are apo A-I, A-IV, and B-48. The adult small intestine synthesizes apo B-48. Although apo B-48 and apo B-100 are the products of a single gene, apo B-48 alone is synthesized by the intestine secondary to the organ-specific introduction of a stop codon to the messenger RNA. Apo B-48 is integral to chylomicron secretion, and its determination marks the presence of the native particle or its remnant.

After chylomicrons are released into the lymph and enter the plasma, their apolipoprotein constituents are altered. The chylomicrons acquire a complement of E and C apolipoproteins and they lose the A apolipoproteins, which then are found in association with HDL. The apo C-II is a cofactor of lipoprotein lipase, the enzyme on the surface of vascular endothelial cells that hydrolyzes chylomicron tricylglycerols.

Hydrolysis of chylomicron triacylglycerols makes the triacylglycerol fatty acids available for use by the various tissues that possess lipoprotein lipase (adipose tissue, skeletal muscle, myocardium, mammary gland, lung). After chylomicron triacylglycerol hydrolysis occurs, the liberated fatty acids are taken up by the tissue in which the hydrolysis occurs. In adipocytes, the chylomicron fatty acids are reincorporated into triacylglycerols for storage; in the breast, they are incorporated into milk fat; and in striated muscle, they are used for energy.

After the lipoprotein lipase–mediated removal of a substantial portion of its triacylglycerol, the chylomicron remnant is relatively enriched in cholesterol. The remnant particle then detaches from the endothelial cell surface and acquires a complement of apo E from the circulating pool of apo E that is associated with HDL. The remnants have a half-life of only about 20 minutes because of their efficient removal from the plasma via a hepatic receptor that specifically recognizes and binds apo E (ie, the chylomicron remnant receptor). Loss of triacylglycerol from the chylomicron is accompanied by loss of some of its surface constituents, phospholipids, and C apolipoproteins. These become incorporated into the pool of circulating HDL.

Since chylomicron cholesterol is derived primarily from dietary sources, the uptake of chylomicron remnants by the liver results in the delivery of this dietary cholesterol to the liver. The liver uses the cholesterol primarily for the synthesis of bile acids and membranes.

Very Low Density Lipoprotein (VLDL)

VLDLs are the triacylglycerol-rich lipoproteins in fasting plasma. Individuals with defined elevations in VLDL often have other associated findings, most frequently a decrease in the concentration of HDL and an apparent modification of LDL such that they are smaller and relatively dense. If elevated sufficiently to cause hypercholesterolemia, the VLDL are thought to be atherogenic. Whether this property is directly related to the increased concentration of VLDL or to associated abnormalities is not clear. The massive hypertriacylglycerolemia that precipitates pancreatitis is usually due to concomitant increases in the concentration of both chylomicrons and VLDLs. Most commonly the accumulation of chylomicrons follows the saturation of the removal process by an increased concentration of VLDL (Fig 12–1). Saturation occurs frequently when VLDL triglycerides approach 1000 mg/dL.

VLDL is synthesized in the liver. The production of VLDL is thought to be stimulated primarily by the accumulation of long-chain fatty acids in the liver. These fatty acids may be derived from the uptake of free fatty acids bound to albumin, from chylomicron triacylglycerols, or from de novo fatty acid synthesis. Irrespective of the source, the fatty acids are synthesized into triacylglycerols and incorporated into the VLDL particle along with phospholipids, apolipoproteins, and cholesterol. Nascent VLDL is assembled in the hepatocyte with apo B-100 as its integral protein. In the Golgi apparatus, the apolipoproteins undergo glycosylation before being packaged into secretory vesicles and transported to the hepatocyte surface for secretion into the circulation.

Newly released VLDL is processed in a manner similar to that of chylomicrons. Apo C-II is donated by HDL, and triacylglycerol hydrolysis proceeds by the action of lipoprotein lipase located on the surface of vascular endothelium. In this manner, triacylglycerol fatty acids are made available for use peripherally with the resulting particle a VLDL remnant.

Intermediate-Density Lipoprotein (IDL)

IDLs (VLDL remnants) are products of the hydrolysis of VLDL with cholesterol now the major lipid (Table 12–2). Apo B-100 and apo E are the major apolipoproteins with several copies of apo E on each IDL. IDL has 2 metabolic fates: either it is removed intact by the apo-B,E receptor in the liver or it is further processed to LDL. Normally IDL is present only in small amounts, but it accumulates in apo-B,E receptor deficiency states or when apo E with normal receptor binding properties is absent (dysbetalipoproteinemia). IDL is thought to be atherogenic.

Low-Density Lipoprotein (LDL)

LDLs are the major cholesterol-bearing lipoproteins in normal plasma, and high concentrations of LDL correlate directly with the incidence of coronary heart disease. The concentration of LDL is a function of LDL production from IDL and removal by apo-B,E receptor–dependent and –independent pathways. Apo-B,E receptor activity plays a central role both in regulating LDL production and in removal (Fig 12–1). Apo-B,E receptor activity is reduced with delivery of dietary cholesterol to the liver in the form of chylomicron remnants. An increase in the number of apo-B,E receptors can be achieved by increasing demand for hepatic bile acid synthesis (eg, when patients are treated with bile acid sequestrants) or by inhibiting hepatic cholesterol synthesis with an HMG-CoA reductase inhibitor. The disease known as familial hypercholesterolemia is typified by elevated LDL levels resulting from an inherited deficiency or lack of functional receptors (see below).

High-Density Lipoprotein (HDL)

HDLs are a heterogeneous group of lipoproteins that vary in size, density of flotation, and apolipoprotein constituents. HDL-2 is larger than HDL-3 (Table 12–2). HDL-2 is present in higher concentrations in premenopausal women than in men and is thought to confer protection from coronary heart disease. The major apolipoprotein constituents of HDL are apo A-I and apo A-II. Apolipoprotein A-I is synthesized primarily by the intestine and secondarily by the liver and is thought to participate in the removal of cholesterol from cells [in part as an activator of LCAT (see below)]. Apolipoprotein A-II is synthesized by the liver; its precise metabolic role is unclear.

The process by which unesterified cholesterol is incorporated into HDL, esterified, and transported to the liver or other tissues for use is called **reverse cholesterol transport**. About two-thirds of the plasma cholesterol in humans is esterified to long-chain fatty acids, predominantly linoleate. These cholesteryl esters arise from the action of lecithin:cholesterol acyltransferase (LCAT), an enzyme synthesized and secreted by the liver and found in plasma associated with HDL. The process of reverse cholesterol transport is initiated with incorporation of unesterified cholesterol into an HDL complex containing apo A-I, LCAT, and lecithin. LCAT catalyzes the transfer of long-chain fatty acids from the 2-position of lecithin to cholesterol, and the cholesterol, now esterified, moves to the core of the HDL. Cholesteryl ester is transported to "acceptor lipoproteins" (chylomicrons, VLDL, and LDL) by cholesteryl-ester transport protein for recycling.

Lipoprotein(a) [Lp(a)]

Lp(a) is a macromolecular complex found in human plasma that combines structural elements from the lipoprotein and blood clotting systems. It is assembled apparently from LDL and a large hydrophilic glycoprotein called apolipoprotein(a) [apo(a)]. After simple disulfide reduction, Lp(a) dissociates into LDL and apo(a).

Apo(a) has a high degree of homology to plasminogen with several isoforms distinguishable ranging in apparent molecular weight from approximately 400,000 to 700,000. Lp(a) differs from LDL in protein composition, larger particle size (diameter 23.6–25.5 nm), higher buoyant density (1.055–1.085 g/mL), and pre-β electrophoretic mobility. Chemical composition is 3% triglycerides, 33% cholesterol esters, 9% unesterified cholesterol, 22% phospholipids, and 33% proteins. It is frequently labeled the "sinking pre-β" lipoprotein.

Plasma Lp(a) concentrations vary 1000-fold between individuals and represent a continuous quantitative genetic trait. This variation is under genetic control with about 40% of the variability in Lp(a) concentration explained by the measured variability at the apo(a) locus. Lp(a) concentrations are significantly increased in familial hypercholesterolemia heterozygotes, and the interaction of apo(a) alleles with defective LDL-receptor genes explains a large fraction of the variability of plasma Lp(a) concentration.

While many aspects of its metabolism and function remain unknown, it has been confirmed that increased Lp(a) concentration is a strong and independent risk factor for coronary disease. Reliable assays are not yet available for quantification of Lp(a). When they are available, Lp(a) should be determined in patients considered at increased risk for atherosclerotic cardiovascular disease on the basis of family history or abnormalities of other established risk factors.

Lamellar Lipoproteins

Lamellar lipoproteins are found in plasma in cholestasis, following chronic intravenous infusion of Intralipid, and in LCAT deficiency. These abnormal lipoproteins consist of lipid bilayers composed predominantly of a 1:1 molar mixture of unesterified cholesterol and phospholipid (mainly lecithin). Two predominant species are described: (1) vesicles varying in size from 30 to 60 nm with a composition by weight of 30% unesterified cholesterol, 65% phospholipids, 3% proteins, and less than 2% triacyglycerols and cholesteryl esters, and (2) disks 19 to 4.4 nm in size with a composition by weight of 29% unesterified cholesterol, 45% phospholipid, 21% protein, 4% triacylglycerols, and 1% cholesteryl esters. The former are called lipoprotein X (LP-X), the lipoprotein of cholestasis, and the latter are predominant in LCAT deficiency. The presence of LP-X should be considered in a clinical setting of hypercholesterolemia and possible cholestasis. While LP-X may be present without icterus, alkaline phosphatase is invariably elevated. Suspicion of LP-X can be confirmed by electron microscopy and an increased ratio of plasma unesterified to total cholesterol (> 0.4). These determinations are available in specialized lipid laboratories.

LIPID DISORDERS

Several systems for classifying the lipid disorders are in common use. Abnormalities in circulating lipoproteins occur both primarily and secondarily to other medical disorders. A descriptive nomenclature that identifies the lipoprotein abnormality, determines whether it is primary or secondary to another metabolic process, defines aggravating factors, and seeks genetic determinants is useful. Family study provides information important for treatment decisions and for identification of other affected family members.

HYPERTRIACYLGLYCEROLEMIAS

Elevations of VLDL alone (not accompanied by elevations of LDL) can predispose to myocardial infarction, and this occurs commonly when HDL is also low or when the individual is a member of a family with combined hyperlipoproteinemia (see below). It is unclear whether the VLDL itself is atherogenic or whether the atherogenicity is related to low HDL or to an associated abnormality. Many people with elevated blood triacylglycerols and normal concentrations of blood cholesterol present with atherosclerotic cardiovascular disease and need treatment. Treatment should be considered in individuals at risk for atherosclerosis for elevations of VLDL with or without elevations of LDL when the arithmetic difference between total cholesterol and HDL cholesterol (the non-HDL cholesterol) is repeatedly in excess of 200 mg/dL. Individuals with chronic, marked elevations of triacylglycerols (>1000 mg/dL), a result of chylomicronemia alone or more commonly elevated VLDL and accumulated chylomicrons, frequently present with pancreatitis. Hypertriacylglycerolemia with repeated fasting levels about 1000 mg/dL requires immediate attention. Primary and secondary causes of the hypertriacylglycerolemias are given in Table 12–3.

Familial Hypertriacylglycerolemias

These patients usually present in the third or fourth decade of life with increased concentrations of VLDL and in severe cases with mixed elevations of chylomicrons and VLDL. The occurrence of multiple cases in a kindred is evidence for considering this disorder familial, with current evidence suggesting an interaction of multiple genetic factors for clinical expression. Because both VLDL and chylomicrons are competing substances for the same lipolytic pathway, saturation of the removal mechanism with VLDL may lead to rapid accumulation of the gut-derived chylomicrons. Therefore, as the se-

Table 12–3. Causes of hypertriglyceridemia.

Primary	Secondary
Familial hypertriacylglycerolemia	Obesity
Familial combined hyperlipidemia (also increased cholesterol)	Diabetes mellitus
	Acute stress (eg, myocardial infarction)
Familial lipoprotein lipase deficiency	Uremia
Hereditary apo C-II deficiency	Nephrotic syndrome
Dysbetalipoproteinemia	Hypothyroidism
	Chronic alcohol use
	Cushing's syndrome
	Lipodystrophies
	Glycogen storage diseases
	Dysglobulinemias
	Systemic lupus erythematosus
	Waldenström's macroglobulinemia
	Drugs (thiazides; β-blockers; estrogens; oral contraceptives; glucocorticoids)

verity of the endogenous lipemia increases, a mixed lipemia often results. Most patients have evidence of an increase in VLDL production and a decrease in the capacity for triacylglycerol removal. Factors that increase VLDL production, such as increased caloric intake, alcohol use, or estrogen administration, may lead to marked hypertriacylglycerolemia and subsequently pancreatitis.

Familial Combined Hyperlipidemia

About 11% of myocardial infarction patients below age 60 have familial combined hyperlipidemia. ''Combined'' refers to the occurrence of elevated levels of different lipoproteins within the same kindred. In any given family member there may be an elevation of VLDL and LDL, VLDL alone, or LDL alone. Thus, multiple lipoprotein phenotypes (IIa, IIb, and IV in the Fredrickson classification system) may coexist within the same family. The minimal criterion for this diagnosis in small families is the presence of hypercholesterolemia and hypertriacylglycerolemia in family members and at least one family member with blood cholesterol above the 95th percentile in the absence of hypertriacylglycerolemia. Elevation of apolipoprotein B is characteristic. Although the mode of inheritance of familial combined hyperlipidemia is thought to be autosomal dominant, proof awaits discovery of the underlying metabolic defect.

Patients with elevated VLDL levels due to familial combined hyperlipidemia often have lower HDL and smaller, denser LDL when compared to their normotriacylglycerolemic family members. No physical findings are characteristic.

Familial Lipoprotein Lipase Deficiency

Lipoprotein lipase deficiency is a rare autosomal recessive disorder characterized clinically by massive accumulation of chylomicrons (occasionally VLDL), repeated episodes of abdominal pain, recurrent pancreatitis, eruptive cutaneous xanthomas and hepatosplenomegaly. The severity of symptoms is a function of the degree of chylomicronemia, which in turn is related quantitatively to the intake of dietary fat.

The diagnosis is often made in early childhood, but cases have been recognized late in adult life with the patient having learned to avoid dietary fat. With adequate restriction of dietary fat, these patients grow and develop normally and avoid episodes of pancreatitis. Patients with this disorder do not have an increased incidence of atherosclerotic vascular disease. Dietary fat restriction to less than 20 g/d may be required with maximal restriction necessary in the event of pregnancy; additional fat calories can be supplied by providing patients with medium-chain triacylglycerol because these fatty acids of 12 carbons or less are absorbed directly into the portal circulation rather than being incorporated into chylomicrons.

Lipoprotein lipase is normally present in the vascular endothelial cells of extrahepatic tissue and is responsible for the hydrolysis of chylomicron and VLDL triacylglycerols. The enzyme is released into the blood by heparin and can be assayed in postheparin plasma. Diagnosis is based on a finding of low or absent enzyme activity in an assay system that excludes other lipolytic activities and contains a source of apolipoprotein C-II, a necessary cofactor for maximal enzyme activity. This assay can be performed only in selected lipid research laboratories.

Hereditary Apolipoprotein C-II Deficiency

Deficiency of normally functioning apo C-II is a rare disorder that causes an increase in chylomicron and VLDL concentrations in the plasma. Since apo C-II is a cofactor of lipoprotein lipase, its absence severely impairs lipoprotein triacylglycerol clearance. Features that distinguish apo C-II deficiency from lipoprotein lipase deficiency include a later onset of pancreatitis and the relative absence of eruptive xanthomas and hepatomegaly. Inheritance is as an autosomal recessive disorder. Diagnosis is based an assay of lipoprotein lipase activities with and without the addition of a source of normal apolipoprotein C-II.

Dysbetalipoproteinemia

Both the plasma triacylglycerol and cholesterol concentrations are elevated in dysbetalipoproteinemia, which is also referred to as type III hyperlipoproteinemia. Because patients with this condition respond to the same therapeutic measures used for hypertriacylglycerolemias, dysbetalipoproteinemia is included among the primary hypertriacylglycerolemias. The frequency of this disorder in a patient with cardiovascular disease below age 60 is estimated to be 0.2–1%.

The underlying metabolic defect in dysbetalipoproteinemia is the inheritance of one of several mutant alleles of the gene that codes for apo E. These mutant genes code for altered isoforms of apo E that bind poorly to both the apo B,E (LDL) receptor and the hepatic apo E receptor. As a consequence, cholesterol-rich chylomicron and VLDL remnants accumulate in the plasma.

There are 3 alleles for apo E in the human population. Each allele codes for an isoform of apo E that varies from the others by single amino acid substitutions, as follows:

Isoforms	Sites of Amino Acid Substitution (Residue Number)		Receptor Binding Activity
	112	158	
E3 (most common; parent form)	Cysteine	Arginine	Normal
E2 (associated with dysbetalipoproteinemia)	Cysteine	Cysteine	Abnormal
E4 (variant; unknown metabolic significance)	Arginine	Arginine	Normal

Most patients with dysbetalipoproteinemia are homozygous for the allele that codes for apo E-2. This isoform exhibits abnormal binding to the hepatic apo E receptor and the apo B,E receptor. Most commonly, the diminished lipoprotein binding is due to the substitution of cysteine for arginine at amino acid 158. The positive charge of the ϵ-amino group at residue 158 is critical for normal binding of apo E to its receptors (other receptor-defective variants associated with dysbetalipoproteinemia have also been identified). Thus, normal clearance of chylomicron remnants does not take place in patients with the E2/2 phenotype, and the altered metabolism of VLDL results in the accumulation in the plasma of cholesteryl ester–rich particles at density < 1.006 g/mL. These d<1.006 lipoproteins that accumulate in patients with dysbetalipoproteinemia have β-electrophoretic mobility rather than the typical pre-β mobility of normal VLDL and are termed β-VLDL.

Although the E2/2 phenotype (or other rarer apo E phenotypes) is a requisite for the development of dysbetalipoproteinemia, more than this structural abnormality of apo E is required in many cases to produce the hyperlipidemia. Not all individuals who have E2/2 phenotype become hyperlipidemic, and occurrence of the hyperlipidemia is age-dependent. About 1% of the population are E2/2 homozygotes; however, the incidence of dysbetalipoproteinemia is only a fraction of 1%. In addition, the occurrence of the hyperlipidemia in dysbetalipoproteinemia almost never occurs before age 20 despite the existence of the E2/2 phenotype from the time of conception. Other factors that may precipitate or aggravate the hyperlipidemia in E2/2 homozygotes include obesity, hypothyroidism, and menopause.

Patients with dysbetalipoproteinemia come to medical attention initially because of xanthomas, the onset of symptomatic atherosclerotic vascular disease, or both. The xanthoma that distinguishes dysbetalipoproteinemia from all other plasma lipoprotein disorders is the palmar crease xanthoma [xanthoma striatum palmare (yellow deposits in the creases of the palms of the hands)]. Tuberoeruptive xanthomas of the elbows, palmar and dorsal aspects of the hands, and knees are also common. Extensor tendon xanthomas occur in only about 10% of patients. Hyperglycemia and hyperuricemia are also frequently encountered, but clinical diabetes mellitus and gout are rare.

The presence of tuberoeruptive xanthomas or palmar xanthomas should be taken as a strong indication that a patient may have dysbetalipoproteinemia. However, about half of patients have no xanthomas. In these patients, the disorder must be suspected on the basis of nearly equal elevations of plasma triacylglycerol and cholesterol concentrations. Once the question has arisen, the diagnosis can be made by isoelectric focusing of the VLDL apolipoproteins to confirm that the patient has the E2/2 phenotype. However, this procedure must be done in a lipid research laboratory and is not routinely available. Ultracentrifugal fractionation of the plasma lipoproteins into VLDL, LDL, and HDL can also be used to establish the diagnosis. If the ratio of the VLDL cholesterol concentration to the total plasma triacylglycerol concentration exceeds 0.3, it is usually possible to say with confidence that a patient has dysbetalipoproteinemia.

Secondary Hypertriacylglycerolemias

Elevated VLDL concentrations occur commonly in individuals with obesity, diabetes mellitus, chronic renal failure, nephrotic syndrome, hypothyroidism, and chronic alcohol use. Cushing's syndrome and several of the glycogen storage diseases are also associated with elevation of the VLDL concentration. Dysgammaglobulinemia syndromes (as seen in systemic lupus erythematosus or Waldenström's macroglobulinemia) may also rarely cause hypertriacylglycerolemia if the paraprotein forms a complex with VLDL and retards VLDL catabolism. Drugs such as thiazide diuretics, certain β-blockers (propranolol, atenolol), estrogens, oral contraceptives, and glucocorticoids also elevate the VLDL concentration (see Table 12–3).

HYPERCHOLESTEROLEMIAS

As noted above, hypercholesterolemia is a consequence of moderate to marked elevations of the triacylglycerol-rich lipoproteins as well as elevations of LDL or rarely marked elevations of HDL.

Hypercholesterolemia & Atherosclerosis

Atherosclerosis is the leading cause of death and disability in the USA. Coronary heart disease was responsible for about 513,000 deaths in the USA in 1987. Five percent of all heart attacks occur in people under age 40 and more than 45% in people under age 65.

For coronary heart disease events alone, the estimated direct health costs (hospital and nursing home services, physician and nursing services, and medications) currently are $34.8 billion and lost productivity an additional $6.8 billion. These astronomical figures do not begin to convey the toll in human suffering. The disease is so common that many people, physicians included, look upon the development of atherosclerosis as a natural progression in human life. However, the results of studies from a variety of scientific fields provide strong evidence that lowering plasma cholesterol concentrations can prevent atherosclerosis and subsequent myocardial infarction.

Metabolic ward studies have shown a relationship between diet and plasma cholesterol levels. Reduction in the saturated fat and cholesterol content of the diet is a key maneuver in lowering blood cholesterol levels. Clinical trials employing diet alone and diet plus drugs have shown that lowering cholesterol levels prevents coronary heart disease. Together, these trials suggest that for each 1% reduction in cholesterol level, there is a reduction of 2% in the incidence of coronary disease. Thus, normalizing the cholesterol level of individuals at high risk (those with cholesterol levels above the 90th percentile) would reduce the incidence of coronary heart disease in this group by as much as 50%.

Hypercholesterolemia associated with premature coronary disease usually occurs as a consequence of one of 3 mechanisms. The most common is diet-related, induced by consumption of excessive amounts of saturated fat and cholesterol. A second mechanism is genetic; about 20% of patients below age 60 are estimated to have one of several genetically determined disorders of plasma lipoprotein metabolism. A third common cause is disorders that result in secondary hyperlipidemia, eg, diabetes mellitus and hypothyroidism.

Primary hypercholesterolemia can take a number of forms: familial hypercholesterolemia, familial combined hyperlipidemia, and polygenic hypercholesterolemia. The primary and secondary causes are summarized in Table 12–4.

Table 12–4. Causes of hypercholesterolemia.

Primary	Secondary
Increased HDL cholesterol	Hypothyroidism
Familial hypercholesterolemia	Nephrotic syndrome
Familial combined hyperlipidemia	Dysglobulinemias
Polygenic hypercholesterolemia	Hepatoma
	Acute intermittent porphyria
	Cushing's syndrome
	Cholestasis
	Hepatic failure
	Anorexia nervosa

Familial Hypercholesterolemia

Familial hypercholesterolemia is one of the most common genetically determined disorders of lipid metabolism. Heterozygous familial hypercholesterolemia occurs in 1 of 500 individuals and is transmitted as an autosomal dominant trait. The homozygous form of this disorder is much rarer (1/1,000,000).

A reduction in the number of functional apo B,E (LDL) receptors is the fundamental defect. Heterozygotes display half the number of receptors that normal subjects do in assays of apo B,E receptor number performed upon fibroblasts in tissue culture. Fibroblasts of homozygous patients have no more than 2% of the normal complement of receptors. Because of the lack of receptor-mediated clearance of LDL in these patients, cells in many of their tissues synthesize excessive cholesterol. In the liver, this may cause an increase in the synthesis of VLDL. The lack of receptor-mediated clearance of IDL is thought to be the primary mechanism by which the apo-B,E receptor defect leads to an increased production of LDL. Increased production and decreased catabolism results in increased LDL concentrations. Triacylglycerol levels may occasionally be increased because of the overproduction of VLDL, but the plasma cholesterol concentration always exceeds the triacylglycerol level in this disorder. The cholesterol concentration of heterozygotes almost always exceeds 280 mg/dL, and homozygotes usually have cholesterol levels above 500 mg/dL.

The diagnosis of familial hypercholesterolemia can be made at birth by measuring the cord blood cholesterol concentration; it is usually above 90 mg/dL in affected infants. The first sign of this disease in homozygotes is the appearance of xanthomas by age 5 with the same common by the third decade of life in heterozygotes. Clinically evident coronary heart disease in heterozygotes is usually evident by age 45 in men and 55 in women. The homozygous patient usually has coronary disease before age 10 and often dies before reaching 20.

The most common physical finding in these patients is the extensor tendon xanthoma of the hands or Achilles tendon. Premature arcus lipoides corneae is also common. The diagnosis depends on assays of LDL binding to fibroblasts from skin biopsies of suspected patients. However, this procedure is not commonly available, and usually the diagnosis is based on the finding of an elevated total cholesterol concentration secondary to an elevated LDL level, of tendon xanthomas, and of a family history of accelerated coronary atherosclerosis.

Familial Combined Hyperlipidemia

Certain members of kindreds with familial combined hyperlipidemia have elevated levels of LDL, with or without elevated VLDL concentrations. The pathophysiology underlying the hyperlipidemia is unknown. Clinically, it is not possible to distinguish patients with LDL elevations due to familial combined hyperlipidemia from those with LDL elevations due to familial hypercholesterolemia. However, the course of the disease is different. The patient with familial combined hyperlipidemia does not become hyperlipidemic until the second decade of life, and tendon xanthomas, common in familial hypercholesterolemia, are highly unusual. Fibroblasts of patients with familial combined hyperlipidemia display normal numbers of apo B,E receptors. In a given patient, these criteria may suggest the diagnosis of familial combined hyperlipidemia. Proof requires testing all family members and demonstrating the existence of elevated concentrations of many different lipoproteins.

Polygenic Hypercholesterolemia

Polygenic hypercholesterolemia is another disorder associated with premature coronary disease and elevated LDL concentrations. Hereditary factors mediated by genes and environmental factors are thought to combine to cause elevation of LDL levels. Diet may play a significant role in the induction of hypercholesterolemia in such patients. Assignment of this diagnosis requires that the patient have a large extended family willing to undergo exhaustive screening that reveals a continuous distribution of cholesterol concentrations in the family, as opposed to the bimodal distribution in kindreds with familial hypercholesterolemia. No physical findings can be used to distinguish these patients from kindreds affected by familial combined hyperlipidemia. However, treatment is the same as for familial hypercholesterolemia or familial combined hyperlipidemia. It is not necessary to make the diagnosis to be able to treat patients effectively.

Secondary Hypercholesterolemias

Frequenty encountered secondary hypercholesterolemias include hypothyroidism and the lamellar lipoproteins of cholestasis (Table 12–4). Many of the medical conditions listed under the secondary hypertriacylglycerolemias in Table 12–3 can elevate LDL as well. Treatment is directed at correction of the primary disorder.

HYPOLIPIDEMIAS

Although the presentation of a patient with marked deficiencies in circulating lipoproteins occurs infrequently, the finding of a blood cholesterol level < 110 mg/dL or a triacylglycerol level < 25 mg/dL in an adult should be investigated.

LDL Deficiency: Familial Hypobetalipoproteinemia & Recessive Abetalipoproteinemia

Patients heterozygous for familial hypobetalipoproteinemia present with moderately low levels of total cholesterol with LDL cholesterol concentrations approximately 50% of normal and normal HDL cholesterol concentrations. They are usually asymptomatic. Individuals homozygous for this disorder share features with those afflicted with the recessively inherited abetalipoproteinemia. In these situations, all forms of apo B are absent, leaving HDL as the only lipoprotein. Clinical features include long-chain fatty acid malabsorption, acanthocytes, progressive degeneration of the central nervous system, and retinal degeneration. Treatment includes administration of fat-soluble vitamins to normalize plasma levels. Early diagnosis and vitamin supplementation may limit progression of central nervous system degeneration.

Normotriacylglycerolemic Abetalipoproteinemia

VLDL and LDL are absent from plasma, but fat absorption proceeds normally. The underlying disorder appears to be an inability to produce apo B-100, whereas secretion of the B apolipoprotein of chylomicrons, B-48, proceeds normally. Clinical features may include ataxia, minimal stomatocytosis of red cells, and tocopherol deficiency.

Severe HDL Deficiency

Severe HDL deficiency not occurring in the presence of severe hypertriacylglycerolemia or LCAT deficiency occurs rarely (Table 12–5). In the homozygous state of affected families, the HDL cholesterol is frequently less than 5 mg/dL. In **Tangier disease**, in addition to the HDL abnormality, affected individuals have low LDL and VLDL cholesterol and best fit the description of hypolipidemia with a low total cholesterol. **Familial apolipoprotein A-I and C-III deficiency**, **HDL deficiency with planar xanthomas**, and **fish-eye disease** have the very low HDL levels but a total cholesterol that is either normal or elevated. Blood triacylglycerol levels may be normal or elevated to around 500 mg/dL; in those individuals with absent apolipoprotein C-III, the triacylglycerol concentration is often normal. With severe HDL deficiency, corneal opacification is prominent and progresses to limit vision in fish-eye disease. Premature coronary artery disease occurs except in fish-eye disease.

Apolipoprotein A-I Variants

At least 12 apolipoprotein A-I variants have been identified with a charge shift observed on isoelectric focusing gel analysis and differing from normal apolipoprotein A-I by a single amino acid substitution.

Table 12–5. Primary HDL deficiency states and selected clinical features.

Disease	Corneal Opacification	Reticulo-endothelial Cell Deposition	Premature Coronary Artery Disease	Typical serum HDL-Cholesterol in mg/dL
Familial apo A-I and C-III deficiency (homozygous)	+	±	+ +	2
Tangier disease (homozygous)	+	+	+	2
HDL deficiency with planar xanthomas	+	+	+ +	3
Fish-eye disease	+ + +	–	–	7
Apo A-I (Milano heterozygote)	–	–	–	11
Familial hypo-alpha-lipopro-teinemia	–	–	+ + +	26

Individuals with **apolipoprotein A-I Milano** are thought to be descended from a family living in a small Northern Italian community in the 18th century. Heterozygotes have low HDL with low concentrations of a dense HDL-3 and nearly absent HDL-2, variable hypertriacylgcerolemia, and a low prevalence of atherosclerotic vascular disease. The abnormality is a cysteine-for-arginine substitution at residue 173. Only a small number of other identified variants are associated with low HDL. Apolipoprotein A-I serves as a cofactor for LCAT; 2 variants have decreased cofactor activity.

Familial Hypoalphalipoproteinemia

The finding of low HDL cholesterol is fairly common and may be the only apparent risk factor in many cases of premature coronary heart disease. Low levels of HDL cholesterol should be interpreted in the context of the habitual diet, taking into account that vegetarians and individuals on a very low fat diet have a lower HDL cholesterol than those with a higher saturated fat intake. In individuals with increased concentrations of triacylglycerol-rich lipoproteins, triacylglycerol exchanges with cholesterol as an inverse logarithmic function of the triacylglycerol level, causing an apparent decrease in HDL as determined by cholesterol content.

Familial hypoalphalipoproteinemia is thought to be transmitted as autosomal dominant with affected family members having an HDL cholesterol 50% of normal, normal cholesterol, and normal or mildly elevated triacylglycerols. No abnormality in apolipoprotein A-I has been identified. The finding of an HDL in this range is common among normocholesterolemic survivors of coronary disease. A low HDL cholesterol is an important determinant in assessing the need for treatment to control coronary artery disease.

LCAT Deficiency

LCAT deficiency is associated with low levels of HDL. The diagnosis of this recessive disorder is most often made in early adult life with clinical findings of corneal opacities and proteinuria. Hyperbilirubinemia and peripheral neuropathy may be present. Deposits of unesterified cholesterol and phospholipid in renal microvasculature lead to progressive loss of renal function. Lipoprotein abnormalities are complex, with triacylglycerols that are often elevated; a low normal to high cholesterol, only a small fraction of which is esterified; and the presence of abnormal vesicular lipoproteins in the LDL and HDL density ranges.

Secondary Hypolipidemias

Hypolipidemia may be secondary to a number of disorders including those characterized by cachexia, massive hepatic parenchymal disease, and elevations of specific immunoglobulins.

EVALUATION OF LIPID ABNORMALITIES

Evaluation of the individual with a lipid abnormality begins with defining the disorder as primary or as secondary to another medical problem. Factors that may aggravate the lipoprotein abnormality need to be identified and a careful family history, often supplemented with family screening, completed to define genetic contributions, case identification, and clinical expression of vascular disease in the family or origin.

The common secondary causes of the hyperlipidemias (Tables 12–3 and 12–4) should be excluded by an evaluation that includes urinalysis, complete blood count, serum TSH, glucose, alkaline phosphatase, and albumin.

Aggravating factors include obesity, alcohol use, diabetes control, cigarette smoking, stress, and several common pharmaceutical agents including estrogens, androgens, corticosteroids, β-adrenergic receptor blocking agents, and diuretics.

LABORATORY FEATURES

Clinical evaluation of lipoprotein levels can be accomplished in most cases by measurement of total cholesterol, triacylglycerols, and HDL cholesterol in fasting serum (or plasma). Visual inspection of chilled serum will reveal significant hypertriacylglycerolemia. Standardization of the laboratory is extremely important, and the relationship of determined values to standard methodology should be defined. Serum refrigerated overnight will appear increasingly opalescent with serum triacylglycerol concentrations of more than a few hundred. Chylomicrons float under these conditions, VLDL do not. If the triacylglycerol concentration is < 400 mg/dL and no chylomicrons (or increased IDL) exist, then LDL can be estimated from the following formula: LDL = serum cholesterol − [HDL cholesterol + (serum triacylglycerol/5)]. Serum triacylglycerol/5 is a good estimate of VLDL cholesterol given the above reservations. Serum lipoproteins are frequently quantitated in terms of their cholesterol content, and that convention is used for the most part in the following sections. Ultracentrifugal studies (and in some instances analyses of the apolipoproteins) may be necessary for the diagnosis of dysbetalipoproteinemia and some rare disorders. These studies are available in a laboratory specializing in lipoprotein analysis.

CHOLESTEROL SCREENING & TREATMENT RECOMMENDATIONS

The schema presented by the Adult Treatment Panel of the National Cholesterol Education Program (NCEP) for follow-up based on total cholesterol measurement is summarized in Table 12–6. A "desirable" cholesterol level is < 200 mg/dL, "borderline-high-risk" 200–239 mg/dL, and "high-risk" > 240 mg/dL. Further evaluation including a lipoprotein analysis on fasting plasma is recommended in the high-risk and borderline-high-risk categories if coronary disease is present or if 2 other risk factors are identified. Such risk factors include male sex, family history of premature coronary disease (before age 55), cigarette smoking, low HDL cholesterol (< 35 mg/dL), diabetes mellitus, hypertension, cerebrovascular or peripheral artery disease, and severe obesity (> 30% overweight). An additional risk factor that should be considered in treatment decisions is the presence of Lp(a) with an apo(a) concentration of 30 mg/dL being significant. Classification is further defined in terms of LDL cholesterol, with a "desirable" LDL cholesterol being < 130 mg/dL, "borderline-high-risk" 130–159 mg/dL, and "high-risk" > 159 mg/dL.

Table 12–6. National Cholesterol Education Program:
Recommended follow-up based on total cholesterol.

Total Cholesterol	Recommended Follow-Up
< 200 mg/dL	Repeat cholesterol measurement within 5 years.
200–239 mg/dL	
Without definite coronary artery disease or 2 other coronary artery risk factors (one of which can be male sex)	Provide dietary information, and recheck cholesterol level annually.
With definite coronary artery disease or 2 other coronary artery risk factors (one of which can be male sex)	Perform lipoprotein analysis; further action based on LDL cholesterol level.
≥ 240 mg/dL	Perform lipoprotein analysis; further action based on LDL cholesterol level.

Table 12–7 summarizes the NCEP recommendations for treatment based on LDL cholesterol. In this schema, treatment decisions are based on LDL cholesterol (repeated and confirmed) in concert with the other risk factors named above. Current NCEP guidelines do not recommend treatment to prevent atherosclerosis in individuals with hypertriacylglycerolemia and elevations of cholesterol secondary to elevations of VLDL cholesterol alone. As for hypertriacylglycerolemias, treatment should be considered in individuals for elevations of VLDL with or without elevations of LDL when the arithmetic

Table 12–7. National Cholesterol Education Program:
Treatment decisions based on LDL cholesterol.

Therapeutic Approach	LDL Cholesterol (mg/dL)	
	For Initiation of Therapy	Minimum Goal of Therapy
Dietary treatment		
Without coronary artery disease or 2 other risk factors	≥ 160	< 160
With coronary artery disease or 2 other risk factors	≥ 130	< 130
Drug treatment		
Without coronary artery disease or 2 other risk factors	≥ 190	< 160
With coronary artery disease or 2 other risk factors	≥ 160	< 130

difference between total cholesterol and the HDL cholesterol (the non-HDL cholesterol) is repeatedly in excess of 200 mg/dL. This risk assessment tool, a non-HDL cholesterol > 200 mg/dL, can be accommodated into the NCEP treatment guidelines schema appropriately as a substitute for an LDL cholesterol of 160 mg/dL (Table 12–7). Many established clinicians would approach the patient with manifest coronary artery, cerebrovascular, or peripheral vascular disease more aggressively than the NCEP and actively attempt to establish optimal lipoprotein levels in these individuals.

Individuals with chronic, marked elevations of triacylglycerols (> 1000 mg/dL), a result of chylomicronemia alone or more commonly elevated VLDL and accumulated chylomicrons, are at significant risk for pancreatitis. Hypertriacylglycerolemia with repeated fasting levels above 1000 mg/dL requires immediate attention to prevent pancreatitis.

TREATMENT OF LIPID ABNORMALITIES

Treatment strategy is the successive use of diet modification, removal of aggravating factors, and correction of secondary causes of hyperlipidemia (Tables 12–3 and 12–4) when possible, followed as necessary by administration of one or several pharmacologic agents. Smoking cessation also has a positive effect on HDL cholesterol levels, regular exercise promotes the achievement and maintenance of ideal body weight, and stress reduction has beneficial lipoprotein effects in some individuals.

DIET

An effective diet prescription balances caloric consumption with expenditure to achieve and maintain normal body weight and additionally limits intake of saturated fat, total fat, and cholesterol for maximal lipid lowering. Alcohol restriction often reduces VLDL and less commonly LDL. A 2- to 4-week period of abstinence is useful as a test to assess response.

Table 12–8 summarizes the composition for the 2-step dietary program proposed by the Adult Treatment Panel of the NCEP. The Step-One Diet calls for reduction of the major and obvious sources of saturated fats and cholesterol in the diet; the Step-Two Diet requires careful attention to the whole diet to further reduce the intake of saturated fats and cholesterol.

Table 12–8. National Cholesterol Education Program:
Dietary therapy for hypercholesterolemia.

Nutrients	Recommended Intake*	
	Step-One Diet	Step-Two Diet
Total fat	< 30% of cal	< 30% of cal
Saturated fatty acids	< 10% of cal	< 7% of cal
Monounsaturated fatty acids	10–15% of cal	10–15% of cal
Polyunsaturated fatty acids	< 10% of cal	< 10% of cal
Carbohydrates	50–60% of cal	50–60% of cal
Protein	10–20% of cal	10–20% of cal
Cholesterol	< 300 mg/d	< 200 mg/d
Total calories	To achieve and maintain desirable weight	

*Cal = caloric intake.

The American Heart Association recommends a diet administered in 3 phases, with phase I restricting fat to 30%, phase II to 25%, and phase III to 20% of calories with cholesterol intake less than 300, 250, or 150 mg/d, respectively. Patients with chylomicronemia (eg, lipoprotein lipase deficiency) may need restriction of fat to 10–15 g/d, 5 g of which should be vegetable-oil rich in essential fatty acids and supplemented with fat-soluble vitamins. Practical guidelines for altering the diet by reducing the amount of saturated fat and cholesterol consumed are given in Table 12–9. Response to diet modification is variable; group data suggest a maximal effect in those with higher initial values. Diet is particularly effective in control of the triacylglycerol-rich lipoproteins and may be particularly dramatic in those individuals with a primary hypertriacylglycerolemia aggravated by type II diabetes mellitus.

Table 12–9. Guide to the low-saturated-fat, low-cholesterol diet.*

The purpose of this diet is to lower the blood cholesterol, particularly the LDL-cholesterol. Blood cholesterol has 2 sources: the cholesterol in the diet and that which is synthesized in the body. In most individuals, the blood cholesterol can be lowered by consumption of fewer saturated fats, less dietary cholesterol, and less total fat.

General guidelines and recommendations
- Use oils and margarines high in mono- and polyunsaturated fats in place of butter, lard, or shortening. Oils high in monounsaturated fats are olive and canola. Safflower, sunflower, and sesame oils are also good choices. The first ingredient listed on a margarine label should be liquid oil instead of hydrogenated or partially hydrogenated oil.
- Trim off all visible fat and skin from meat and poultry before cooking.
- Use low-fat cooking methods such as broiling, baking, stewing, stir frying, or steaming.

(continued)

Table 12–9. (Continued)

- Have red meat no more than once or twice a week, and in its place use fish, poultry, legumes, and beans. Limit portion size to 5 oz/d cooked fish or poultry.
- Have high-fat sweets, snacks, and desserts no more than once a week.
- Read labels carefully. Avoid hydrogenated oils, partially hydrogenated oils, lard, butter, shortening, and tropical oils.
- If fat is listed among the first 3 ingredients on a product, consider the product to be high in fat.
- Limit visible fat intake to no more than 4 tsp/d (visible fat includes cooking oil, margarine, mayonnaise, and salad dressing).
- Have no more than 2 tsp/wk nut butters. Buy natural nut butters.
- Limit nuts and seeds to once a week (portion size 2 tbs). Good choices are almonds, pecans, and walnuts.
- Use nonfat dairy products, and choose cheeses low in fat (< 5 g/serving).
- Limit egg yolks to 1–2 per week, including yolks used in casseroles or baked goods.

Food to choose more often

Fish: All fish. Oily fish (trout, salmon, sardines, mackerel) are high in omega-3 fatty acids, which have been shown to be especially beneficial in lowering plasma triacyglycerol levels.

Poultry: Chicken, squab, turkey, and Cornish hens (discard skin before cooking).

Meat (limit to once or twice a week): All meat trimmed of fat and skin.
Beef: Chuck (pot roast, steak, or ground), flank steak, loin (porterhouse, sirloin, T-bone, tenderloin, top loin, or top sirloin steak), round (roast, steaks, ground, or cubed), and shank (center cut or cross cut).
Lamb: Leg (roast, whole shank, center, and sirloin chop), loin (chop or roast), rib (chop or roast), shank, and shoulder.
Pork: Leg (fresh ham), whole, rump, center, and shank.
Other meats: Veal, rabbit, and venison.

Milk: Skim milk, nonfat dry milk, nonfat yogurt, buttermilk made from nonfat milk or 1% low-fat milk, 1% low-fat milk.

Cheese: Skim-milk cheese, part-skim-milk mozzarella cheese, nonfat cottage cheese, ricotta, sapsago, dry curd cottage cheese, and specially prepared low-fat cheese that has < 5 g fat per 3-oz portion.

Fat: See above.

Eggs: Egg whites or egg substitutes as desired.

Bread products: White, whole wheat, sour, rye, oatmeal, and bagels. Cereals and grain (wheat and rice) products without added fats. Dry grains and legumes. Crackers made without fats, pretzels, and homemade waffles, pancakes, rolls, low-fat muffins, and corn bread.

Fruits: All fresh, frozen, and canned fruits and juices.

Vegetables: All fresh and raw vegetables. All canned and frozen plain vegetables. Avocados and olives are high in monounsaturated fats and total fat; limit to once a week.

Soups and sauces: Clear soups, fat-free and skimmed-fat soups, and sauces made with allowable fats and milks.

(continued)

Table 12–9. (Continued)

Desserts and sweets: Nonfat frozen yogurt, ice milk, fruit ice, sorbet, angel food cake, pudding made with skim milk, and baked goods if made with allowable fats and no egg yolks. Cocoa powder, hard candies, jams, jellies, honey, gelatin desserts, and icings made with egg yolk or saturated fats. Nonfat baked goods.

Snacks: Pretzels, bagels, air-popped popcorn, rice cakes, popcorn cakes, fruits, vegetables, nonfat yogurts (fruit flavored), break sticks without seeds.

Food to limit
Fish: Fish roe or fish supplements.

Poultry: Goose, duck, and poultry skins.

Meat: Beef, lamb, and pork that is marbled or high in fat. Luncheon meats, hot dogs, sausage, bacon, regular ground beef, fast-food restaurant meats, canned pork and beans, canned meats in gravy sauces or meat mixtures, frozen or packaged dinners, salt pork spare ribs, and organ meats.

Milk: Whole milk, cream, half and half, yogurts made from whole milk (low-fat yogurt in moderation), sour cream, eggnog, malted milk, chocolate milk, canned whole milk, and powdered creamers.

Cheese: All cheeses made from cream, hard cheeses (eg, cheddar and jack), creamed cottage cheese, and processed cheese.

Fat: Butter, lard, hydrogenated oils and margarines, shortening, salt pork, chicken fat, coconut oil, or palm oil. These oils are solid at room temperature.

Eggs: Egg yolks limited to 1 or 2 a week.

Bread products: Commercial baked products with fat, eg, sweet rolls, biscuits, muffins, waffles, cookies, popovers, doughnuts, and pastries. Fried potatoes and potato chips.

Fruits: None to avoid.

Vegetables: Those to which butter or cream sauces have been added.

Soups and sauces: Creamed soups and sauces made from saturated fats or creams.

Desserts and sweets: Chocolate, ice cream, puddings, custards, milk shakes, all the commercial or homemade desserts of unknown ingredients, cake or cookie mixes with added fats, candy bars, and granola bars.

Snacks: Potato chips, taco or corn chips, candy bars.

Nuts and nut butters: No more than 2 tbs/wk. Almonds, pecans, and walnuts are preferred over peanuts, cashews, and macadamias. No more than 2 tsp/wk nut butters.

*Prepared by Raksha Shah, MS, RD, and Susan Shattuck, RD, University of California, San Francisco.

Omega-3 Fatty Acids

Patients with elevated VLDL concentrations may benefit from the regular consumption of oily fish (eg, trout, salmon, sardines, mackerel) that are rich in ω3 fatty acids. Ingestion of these oils reduces VLDL synthesis and also reduces platelet aggregation, an effect independent of serum lipid levels that also protects against coronary disease.

DRUG THERAPY

Indications for pharmacologic treatment of the hyperlipidemias are discussed above and those proposed by the NCEP summarized in Table 12–7. Clinical judgment is required in applying these guidelines; some clinicians suggest a more conservative approach to drug treatment in older women and a more aggressive approach in those with manifest coronary disease.

Abnormalities in lipoprotein concentrations often occur together. Elevations in LDL cholesterol are often associated with abnormalities in HDL cholesterol or VLDL cholesterol; elevated VLDL cholesterol frequently tracks with low HDL cholesterol and less frequently with elevated LDL cholesterol. The term dyslipidemia accounts for the inclusion of low HDL cholesterol to the constellation of the hyperlipoproteinemias. All the lipid-affecting agents have multiple lipoprotein effects, which should be considered in prescribing for the individual patient. The major lipoprotein effects, side effects, laboratory adverse effects, and relative contraindications are summarized in Table 12–10. Recommended drug(s) for the treatment of the primary hyperlipoproteinemias are listed in Table 12–11.

Elevated LDL Cholesterol

A. Bile Acid Sequestrants: The initial drug usually employed for reduction of LDL cholesterol is either cholestyramine (8–24 g/d) or colestipol (10–30 g/d). Each cholestyramine preparation (packet, scoop, or bar) contains 4 g and each colestipol preparation (packet or scoop) contains 5 g of the active preparation. The cholestyramine preparations contain a significant number of calories. These products are hydrated with water or juice. If the patient can tolerate a psyllium product in water, colestipol can be added, masking the graininess of colestipol and providing useful dietary fiber. Patients are started on one-third of the maximal dose taken with meals, and the dose is increased over a period of weeks as tolerated. Gastrointestinal complaints such as nausea, bloating, and constipation occur in some patients but usually subside after several months. The concomitant use of other medications may lead to binding of the second drug by the bile acid sequestrant. For example, bile acid sequestrants interfere with the

Table 12–10. Lipoprotein effects of lipid-lowering agents.

CHOLESTYRAMINE/COLESTIPOL

Lipoprotein effects

VLDL—variable (often increased in patients with preexisting hypertriacylglycerolemia or familial combined hyperlipidemia).
LDL—moderate reduction.
HDL—negligible.

Side effects

Constipation, heartburn, flatulence, nausea, diarrhea; malabsorption of vitamins A, D, and K and folic acid.
Increased incidence of gallstones in obese patients.
Dry skin.

Laboratory abnormalities

Elevated alkaline phosphatase, SGOT.

Contraindications

Avoid or give lower doses if inflammatory bowel disease or diverticulosis is present.
Give other drugs (except niacin, lovastatin, or gemfibrozil) 1 hour before or 4 hours after the resin.

NIACIN (NICOTINIC ACID)

Lipoprotein effects

VLDL—Moderate reduction.
LDL—Moderate reduction.
HDL—Moderate increase.

Side effects

Flushing.
Itching, rash, dry skin.
Acanthosis nigricans.
Nausea, abdominal discomfort.
Arrhythmias, toxic amblyopia (rare).

Laboratory abnormalities

Elevated SGOT, SGPT, alkaline phosphatase.
Elevated FBS, uric acid.

Contraindications/warnings

Significant liver or kidney dysfunction; severe acid-peptic disease. Use with caution or avoid in type II diabetes, in patients with significant ventricular arrhythmias, and in patients with a history of gout.

GEMFIBROZIL/CLOFIBRATE

Lipoprotein effects

VLDL—moderate reduction.
LDL—variable
HDL—variable increase.

Side effects

Nausea, gastric distress, diarrhea (uncommon).
Myositis (uncommon).
Rashes (uncommon).

(continued)

Table 12–10. (Continued)

Laboratory abnormalities
   Elevated SGOT, alkaline phosphatase.
   Elevated CPK.
   Elevated BUN.
   Decreased WBC, HCT (rare).

Contraindications/warnings
   Low serum albumin; liver disease; women likely to become pregnant.
   Reduce dose of oral anticoagulants by 30–50% at onset of therapy
      with fibrates.

LOVASTATIN (MEVINOLIN)
   Lipoprotein effects
   VLDL—moderate reduction.
   LDL—moderate to marked reduction.
   HDL—small increase.

   Side effects
   Myopathic syndrome (rare).
   Rash (uncommon), gastrointestinal symptoms.
   Insomnia (questionable).

   Laboratory abnormalities
   Elevated SGOT, SGPT.
   Elevated CPK.

   Contraindications/warnings
   Liver dysfunction.
   Women likely to become pregnant.
   Reduce dose and monitor closely if given with cyclosporine, fibrates,
      erythromycin, niacin.

PROBUCOL
   Lipoprotein effects
   VLDL—variable.
   LDL—modest reduction.
   HDL—modest reduction.
   Potent antioxidant effect on lipoproteins.

   Side effects
   Prolonged QT interval, syncope, ventricular arrhythmias, sudden
      death.
   Diarrhea, nausea, heartburn (uncommon).

   Contraindications/warnings
   Prolonged QT interval or concomitant use of drugs that may prolong
      QT interval (including tricyclic antidepressants, class I and III
      antiarrhythmics, and phenothiazines).
   Hypokalemia or hypomagnesemia.
   Severe bradycardia due to intrinsic heart disease or drug effects on
      the atrial rate or atrioventricular block.

BUN = blood urea nitrogen; CPK = creatine phosphokinase; FBS = fasting
blood sugar; HCT = hematocrit; SGOT = serum glutamic-oxaloacetic transaminase; SGPT = serum glutamic-pyruvic transaminase; WBC = white blood
count.

Table 12-11. Drug treatment of the primary hyperlipoproteinemias.*

	Single Drug	Drug Combination
Primary chylomicronemia (familial lipoprotein lipase or cofactor deficiency) Chylomicrons and VLDL increased	(Dietary management)	
Familial hypertriacylglycerolemia Severe Chylomicrons and VLDL increased	Niacin, gemfibrozil, clofibrate	Niacin plus gemfibrozil, clofibrate
Moderate VLDL ± chylomicrons increased	Gemfibrozil, clofibrate, niacin	
Familial combined hyperlipidemia (Multiple type hyperlipidemia) VLDL increased	Niacin, gemfibrozil, clofibrate	
LDL increased	Niacin, lovastatin	Niacin plus resin or lovastatin
VLDL and LDL increased	Niacin, gemfibrozil, lovastatin	Niacin plus resin or lovastatin; Gemfibrozil plus resin
Familial dysbetalipoproteinemia VLDL remnants and chylomicron remnants increased	Clofibrate, gemfibrozil, niacin, lovastatin	
Familial hypercholesterolemia Heterozygous LDL increased	Resin, lovastatin, niacin	Two or three of the single drugs
	If some receptor function:	
Homozygous LDL increased	Probucol	Resin plus niacin, plus lovastatin; Probucol plus agents above
Lp(a) hyperlipoproteinemia Lp(a) increased	Niacin	

*Single-drug therapy should be evaluated before drug combinations are used.

absorption of thyroid hormone, warfarin, and digitalis preparations. Thus, such drugs should be taken at least 1 hour before or 3–4 hours after a dose of bile acid sequestrant. When employed in combination therapy for LDL reduction, the bile acid sequestrants are taken concomitantly with niacin, lovastatin, or fibric acid derivatives (gemfibruzil and clofibrate).

After the sequestrant is taken, hepatic bile acid synthesis increases, creating a demand for additional cholesterol. This demand for cholesterol causes increased numbers of apo-B,E (LDL) receptors to be expressed by the liver and secondarily additional hepatic uptake of LDL. VLDL synthesis is stimulated by these agents and may lead to higher blood triacylglycerols in susceptible individuals. Mean response in compliant patients is a 22% decrease in LDL cholesterol and a 5–10% increase in HDL cholesterol. In primary prevention trials, cholestyramine reduced the incidence of myocardial infarction.

B. Nicotinic Acid (Niacin): Pharmacologic doses (3–6 g/d) of nicotinic acid are used alone or in combination with a bile acid sequestrant in patients whose cholesterol concentrations fail to normalize with the bile acid sequestrant alone. The drug causes itching, flushing, and gastric irritation, and it may elevate the uric acid, glucose, or hepatic transaminase levels. Therefore, nicotinic acid should not be employed in patients with gout, diabetes mellitus, or peptic ulcer disease. Itching and flushing can be controlled by beginning with low doses (eg, 100 mg 3 times a day) and gradually (every 2–7 days) increasing each dose by 100 mg. Taking the drug after meals and taking an aspirin about 30 minutes before the nicotinic acid also help diminish side effects. Regular niacin preparations should be used. Timed-release preparations produce less flushing but lead to an increased incidence of gastric irritation and hepatotoxicity. A change in brands, particularly from a regular to a timed-release preparation, has been followed by elevated hepatic transaminases, hypocholesterolemia, nausea, and occasionally vomiting. Blood glucose, uric acid, and hepatic transaminases should be monitored closely at the inception of nicotinic acid therapy and afterward at 3- to 4-month intervals.

In male myocardial infarction survivors, niacin reduced the incidence of nonfatal myocardial infarction and with prolonged surveillance was associated with improved survival.

C. HMG-CoA Inhibitors: In 1987, lovastatin, the first of several inhibitors of HMG-CoA (hydroxymethylglutaryl–coenzyme A) reductase being evaluated in humans was released for marketing. These agents inhibit the rate-limiting enzyme in cholesterol biosynthesis and increase hepatic apolipoprotein B,E (LDL) receptors. Lovastatin is administered in doses of 20–80 mg/d with dinner or as a twice-a-day regimen. Reductions in LDL cholesterol up to 40% have been reported with concomitant reductions in VLDL cholesterol up to

25% and elevations in HDL cholesterol up to 8%. Lovastatin is well tolerated. Drug-related adverse events leading to the withdrawal of lovastatin in study populations have included abnormalities in hepatic transaminases and a myopathy syndrome manifested by muscle weakness or pain, marked elevation of creatine kinase, and the rare event of rhabdomyolysis leading to acute renal failure. In populations taking lovastatin alone, these findings were dose related. In individuals taking 80 mg/d, a 3-fold elevation of transaminases occurred with a frequency of $< 1.2\%$, and the myopathy syndrome occurred with a frequency of $< 0.3\%$. Concomitant use of lovastatin in patients on immunosuppressive agents, including cyclosporine, or the lipid-lowering agents gemfibrozil and niacin have resulted in a significantly increased incidence of the myopathy syndrome, and for this reason these agents should be used concurrently only with great care. No long-term, placebo-controlled clinical studies are available for assessing safety or effect on cardiovascular disease risk.

D. Probucol: Probucol therapy (0.5–1 g/d) usually reduces LDL-C by about 10%, but there is an associated reduction in HDL-C of up to 30%. Preliminary information indicates that probucol may inhibit the oxidation and tissue deposition of LDL. Probucol is generally well tolerated with most frequently reported symptoms being diarrhea or loose stools, flatulence, nausea, and indigestion. Probucol has caused fatal cardiac arrhythmias in monkeys fed a diet high in cholesterol and saturated fat, but no adverse effects were observed in monkeys fed a low-fat diet with doses of probucol up to 30 times the human dose. Premonitory syncope was frequently observed in these animals and was associated with pronounced prolongation of the QT interval. Prolongation of the QT interval also is seen with probucol therapy in humans. Probucol is contraindicated in individuals with evidence of recent or progressive myocardial damage, a finding suggestive of serious ventricular arrhythmias, unexplained syncope or syncope of cardiovascular origin, a prolonged QT interval or the addition of drugs that prolong the QT interval (including tricyclic antidepressants, class I and III antiarrhythmics, and phenothiazines), or severe bradycardia due to intrinsic heart disease or drug effects on the atrial rate (β-blockers) or atrioventricular block (digoxin). Patients should be advised to adhere to a low-cholesterol, low-fat diet throughout treatment, and an ECG should be obtained before therapy, 6 months later, and annually. No extensive, long-term clinical studies are available for assessing safety or effect on cardiovascular disease risk in humans.

Elevation of VLDL Cholesterol & Blood Triacylglycerols

Gemfibrozil, (0.6–1.2 g/d) is approved for the treatment of hypertriacylglycerolemia severe enough to cause pancreatitis and for dysbetalipoproteinemia. Gemfibrozil acts by increasing the activity of lipoprotein lipase, decreasing VLDL production, and raising HDL levels. In patients with elevated blood triacylglycerols, LDL cholesterol may increase with the decrease in VLDL. Gemfibrozil is well tolerated, with the most common problem being gastrointestinal cramps. In the Helsinki Heart Study, where subjects were selected for a non-HDL cholesterol level > 200 mg/dL, gemfibrozil decreased the incidence of myocardial infarction by 34% in the total group and significantly in the 28% of participants with elevations of VLDL and LDL cholesterol. Subgroup analysis suggests primary benefit for those with the lowest HDL cholesterol and also suggests benefit for those who qualified on the basis of elevated VLDL cholesterol alone. Because gemfibrozil and warfarin compete for binding sites on serum proteins, the dose of warfarin must be reduced by 50% or more when a patient is taking both drugs. Gemfibrozil may lead to an increased incidence of cholelithiasis. It is the preferred agent in patients having type II diabetes mellitus or gout when there is a relative contraindication to niacin use.

A. Clofibrate: Clofibrate, like gemfibrozil, is a fibric acid derivative and is the older of the 2 agents. It is used primarily for the control of hypertriacylglycerolemia to reduce the risk of pancreatitis. Its effects and side effects are similar to those described above for gemfibrozil. It is used less frequently than gemfibrozil because of reports of long-term toxicity in clinical trials.

B. Nicotinic Acid (Niacin): Nicotinic acid is discussed above. Smaller doses (1.5–4.5 g/d) can be employed to treat the hypertriacylglycerolemias than for LDL cholesterol elevations. The side effects of hyperuricemia and hyperglycemia must be closely monitored because of the high incidence of gout and diabetes in this population.

REFERENCES

Austin MA: Plasma triglyceride as a risk factor for coronary heart disease: The epidemiologic evidence and beyond. *Am J Epidemiol* 1989;**129:**249.

Blankenhorn DH et al: Beneficial effects of combined colestipol-niacin therapy on coronary atherosclerosis and coronary venous bypass grafts. *JAMA* 1987; **257:**3233.

Bradford RH et al: Expanded clinical evaluation of lovastatin study results: Efficacy in modifying plasma lipoproteins and adverse event profile in 8245 patients with moderate hypercholesterolemia. *Arch Intern Med* 1991;**151:**43.

Breslow JL: Genetic basis of lipoprotein disorders. *J Clin Invest* 1989;**84:**373.

Brown G et al: Regression of coronary artery disease as a result of intensive lipid-lowering therapy in men with high levels of apolipoprotein B. *N Engl J Med* 1990;**323:**1289.

Canner PL et al: Fifteen-year mortality in Coronary Drug Project patients: Long-term benefit with niacin. *J Am Coll Cardiol* 1986;**8:**1245.

Cashin-Hemphill LC et al: Beneficial effects of colestipol-niacin on coronary atherosclerosis: A 4-year follow-up. *JAMA* 1990;**264:**3013.

Committee on Diet and Health, Food and Nutrition Board, Commission on Life Sciences, National Research Council: *Diet and Health: Implications for Reducing the Risk.* National Academy Press, 1989.

Frick MH et al: Helsinki Heart Study: Primary-prevention trial with gemfibrozil in middle-aged men with dyslipidemia: Safety of treatment, changes in risk factors, and incidence of coronary heart disease. *N Engl J Med* 1987; **317:**1237.

Gordon DJ et al: High-density lipoprotein cholesterol and cardiovascular disease: Four prospective American studies. *Circulation* 1989;**79:**8.

Grundy SM et al: The place of HDL in cholesterol management: A perspective from the National Cholesterol Education Program. *Arch Intern Med* 1989; **149:**505.

Havel RJ: Lowering cholesterol, 1988: Rationale, mechanisms, and means. *J Clin Invest* 1988;**81:**1653.

Joven J et al: Abnormalities of lipoprotein metabolism with the nephrotic syndrome. *N Engl J Med* 1990;**323:**579.

Kane JP, Malloy MJ: Treatment of hyperlipidemia. *Annu Rev Med* 1990; **41:**471.

Lipid Research Clinics Program: The Lipid Research Clinics Coronary Primary Prevention Trial Results. 1. Reduction in incidence of coronary heart disease. *JAMA* 1984;**251:**351.

Malloy MJ et al: Complementarity of colestipol, niacin, and lovastatin in treatment of severe familial hypercholesterolemia. *Ann Intern Med* 1987; **107:**616.

Report of the National Cholesterol Education Program Expert Panel on detection, evaluation, and treatment of high blood cholesterol in adults. *Arch Intern Med* 1988;**148:**36.

Schaefer EJ: Clinical, biochemical, and genetic features in familial disorders of high density lipoprotein deficiency. *Arteriosclerosis* 1984;**4:**303.

Seed M et al: Relation of serum lipoprotein(a) concentration and apolipoprotein(a) phenotype to coronary heart disease in patients with familial hypercholesterolemia. *N Engl J Med* 1990;**322:**1494.

Task Force on Cholesterol Issues: The cholesterol facts: A summary of the evidence relating dietary fats, serum cholesterol, and coronary heart disease. *Circulation* 1990;**81:**1721.

Utermann G: The mysteries of lipoprotein(a). *Science* 1989;**246:**904.

Appendix

Testing Protocols & Normal Laboratory Values

The testing protocols and normal laboratory values listed here were derived principally from the Clinical Laboratories Manual of the University of California, San Francisco (1989).

Factors used for converting conventional units to Système International (SI) units were derived mainly from those provided by Endocrine Sciences (Calabasas Hills, California). Conversion factors (CF) may be found in parentheses and are used as follows:

Conventional units × CF = SI units
SI units ÷ CF = Conventional units

Normal ranges vary among laboratories.

Testing Protocols & Normal Laboratory Values

Test	Collection Procedure	Common Units (Conversion Factor → SI)	Système International (SI) Units
Acetoacetate			
Semiquantitative	Serum or plasma (fluoride/oxalate)	Negative (< 3 mg/dL)	Negative (< 0.3 mmol/L)
	Urine	Negative	Negative
Acetone			
Semiquantitative	Serum or plasma (oxalate)	Negative (< 3 mg/dL)	Negative (< 516 µmol/L)
Quantitative		0.3–2 mg/dL (CF - 172)	60–344 µmol/L
Semiquantitative	Urine	Negative	Negative
Acid phosphatase See Phosphatase, acid.			
Adrenocorticotropic hormone (ACTH)	Plasma: collect in plastic syringe with 100 U heparin/5 mL blood. Ice immediately. Deliver to lab within 1 h. Cold centrifuge in plastic tubes. Freeze at −60°C.	20–100 pg/mL (CF - 0.222)	4.4–22 pmol/L
ACTH $_{1-24}$ **stimulation test** (rapid test). Dose: 250 µg cosyntropin IV or IM. Standardized as AM test	Plasma (EDTA) or serum baseline and 60 min after stimulation.	Cortisol increment after co-syntropin: > 7 µg/dL Cortisol peak after 1 h: > 16 µg/dL (RIA or HPLC) Cortisol peak after 1 h: > 18 µg/dL (fluorometric)	Cortisol increment after co-syntropin: > 0.2 µmol/L Cortisol peak after 1 h: > 0.45 µmol/L (RIA or HPLC) Cortisol peak after 1 h: > 0.5 µmol/L (fluorometric)
ADH See Antidiuretic hormone.			

(cont'd.)

Testing Protocols & Normal Laboratory Values (cont'd.)

Test	Collection Procedure	Common Units (Conversion Factor → SI)	Systeme International (SI) Units
Albumin	Serum	g/dL	g/L
		0–1 mo: 2.9–5.5	29–55
		1 mo–1 yr: 2.8–5.0	28–50
		1–4 yr: 3.9–5.1	39–51
		4–18 yr: 3.8–5.4	38–54
		18+ yr: 3.3–5.7	33–57
		Average about 0.3 g/dL, higher in ambulatory individuals	Average about 3 g/L, higher in ambulatory individuals
	Urine (24-h)	< 100 mg/d	< 100 mg/d
Aldosterone	Serum or plasma (Separate cells within 30 min. Freeze at −20°C.)	Normal sodium diet (100–200 mEq Na/d):	ng/dL	pmol/L
		7 AM fasting, recumbent	3–9	80–250
		9 AM upright (2 h)	4–30	110–830
		Adrenal vein	200–400	5500–11000
		Low sodium diet (< 20 mEq Na/d)		
		7 AM fasting, recumbent	12–36	330–1000
		9 AM upright (2 h)	17–137	470–3800
			(CF - 27.7469)	
	24 h urine (preservative, 1 boric acid tablet. Refrigerate while collecting. Freeze 200 mL at −20°C.)	Note: levels during pregnancy are 3–4 times higher.		
		Normal sodium diet (100–200 mEq Na/d)	μg/24 h	nmol/d
		Low sodium diet (< 20 mEq Na/d)	2–19	5.5–53
			10–40	28–111
			(CF - 2.7747)	

Alkaline phosphatase *See* Phosphatase, alkaline.

Alpha-fetoprotein (alpha-fetoglobulin) for malignancy	Serum (avoid hemolysis)	Adult males and nonpregnant females: < 5.0 ng/mL	
Aluminum	Plasma (special handling)	3–10 μg/L (levels > 100 associated with osteomalacia)	
	Dialysis fluid	< 10 μg/L (10–15 tolerable)	
Amylase	Serum (no anticoagulants)	20–110 U/L	
	Urine (timed, no preservative)	< 500 U/L or < 14 U/h	
	Note: Normal ranges vary considerably depending on type of units used.		

Androstanediol glucuronide　Serum

	ng/dL	pmol/L
Adult male:	260–1600	5550–34,150
Adult female:	60–810	1280–17,290
	(CF - 21.3447)	

Androstenedione (A or Δ⁴)　Serum

Age	Male	Female	Male	Female
	ng/dL	ng/dL	nmol/L	nmol/L
< 6 yr	7.1–19	9.6–22.9	0.25–0.66	0.34–0.80
6–8 yr	10.4–24.8	11.5–27.4	0.36–0.86	0.40–0.96
8–10 yr	13.1–31.3	21.6–47.4	0.45–1.09	0.75–1.66
10–12 yr	30.7–65.2	41.7–100	1.07–2.28	1.46–3.49
12–14 yr	44.9–98.7	79.8–190	1.57–3.45	2.69–6.63
> 14 yr	48.2–140	77.2–224	1.68–4.89	2.70–7.82
Adult	40.0–230	40.0–230	1.39–8.02	1.39–8.02
Postmenopause		30–80		1.05–2.79
	(CF - 0.0349)			

Angiotensin I	Peripheral venous plasma (EDTA)	11–88 pg/mL (CF - 0.7716)
		8.5–67.9 pmol/L
Angiotensin II	Plasma (EDTA)	24 ± 12 pg/mL Venous: 50–75% of arterial (CF - 0.956)
		Arterial: 22.9 ± 11.5 pmol/L Venous: 50–75% of arterial

(cont'd.)

Testing Protocols & Normal Laboratory Values (cont'd.)

Test	Collection Procedure	Common Units (Conversion Factor → SI)	Système International (SI) Units
Angiotensin-converting enzyme	Serum	Male: 12–35 mU/mL Female: 11–29 mU/mL	12–35 U/L 11–29 U/L
Anion gap [NA − (Cl + CO$_2$)]	Plasma (heparin)	5–15 mEq/L	
Antidiuretic hormone (ADH, vasopressin, arginine vasopressin, AVP)	Plasma (EDTA). Iced tubes. Freeze plasma within 2 h at −70°C.	Plasma (mOsmol/kg) < 290 ≧ 290	pg/mL < 2 2–12	pmol/L < 1.9 1.9–11.1

Note: The assay for AVP is difficult and infrequently useful clinically. During dehydration, serum levels of between 1 and 18 pg/mL have been noted in normals owing to individual differences in sensitivity to AVP.

Test	Collection Procedure	Common Units (Conversion Factor → SI)	Système International (SI) Units
Antidiuretic hormone-water deprivation test (Miller-Moses test)	Serum (6 AM) and hourly urine for osmolality; when urine osmolality plateaus after fluid restriction, measure serum osmolality and ADH.	Maximum urine osmolality before vasopressin administration > serum osmolality; at end of test, serum osmolality < 300 mOsm/kg; urine osmolality > 500 mOsm/kg; ADH levels, see table under ADH: 1 h after vasopressin administration < 5% increase in urine osmolality over previous specimen. (See Chapter 1.)	
Antimicrosomal antibodies *See* Thyroid antibodies.			
Antithyroglobulin antibodies *See* Thyroid antibodies.			
Atrial natriuretic peptide (ANP)		ng/mL (CF · 0.3247)	pmol/L

Test	Specimen	Reference range (conventional)	Reference range (SI)
Base excess	Whole blood (heparin)		Newborn: (−10)−(−2) mmol/L Infant: (−7)−(−1) mmol/L Child: (−4)−(+2) mmol/L Adult: (−3)(+3) mmol/L
Bicarbonate See Carbon dioxide, total.			
Blood urea nitrogen (BUN) See Urea nitrogen.			
C-peptide	Serum or plasma. Separate cells quickly. Freeze at −20°C within 8 h, fasting.	Fasting: 0.5–3.0 ng/mL Stimulated: 1.5–9.0 ng/mL (CF - 0.331)	0.17–1.0 nmol/L 0.5–3.0 nmol/L
		Increases with pregnancy, decreases with age.	
Calcitonin (CT)	Plasma (heparin) iced tubes. Unstable at room temperature. Process immediately.	Male: ≤ 91 pg/mL Female: ≤ 71 pg/mL (CF - 0.2926)	≤ 27 pmol/L ≤ 21 pmol/L
Note: Normal ranges vary considerably with the particular assay being used.			
Calcitonin-pentagastrin stimulation test. Dose: 0.5 μg/kg IV over 10–15 sec. NPO after midnight. Stimulation unnecessary if fasting CT > 500 pg/mL on more than one occasion.	Plasma. Samples collected baseline and after administration of pentagastrin at intervals of 1.5, 5, and 10 min.	Peak level: Male: < 190 pg/mL Female: < 80 pg/mL Note: Normal peak levels vary with the particular CT assay being used.	< 56 pmol/L < 23 pmol/L
Calcitonin-calcium infusion stimulation test. Dose: 15 mg Ca (as gluconate)/kg, IV infusion/4 h in 500 mL saline.	Serum or plasma (heparin); fasting, 3 and 4 h for CT.	Peak level: Male: < 210 pg/mL Female: < 140 pg/mL	Male: < 61 pmol/L Female: < 41 pmol/L
Calcium, ionized (iCa)	Serum, plasma, or whole blood (heparin)	Adults: 3.9–5.4 mg/dL at pH 7.4, 37°C	1.0–1.4 mmol/L

(cont'd.)

Testing Protocols & Normal Laboratory Values (cont'd.)

Test	Collection Procedure	Common Units (Conversion Factor → SI)	Système International (SI) Units
Calcium, total	Serum	mg/dL 0–6 yr: 9.4–10.8 6–20 yr: 9.1–10.6 > 20 yr: 8.5–10.5	mmol/L 2.35–2.7 2.28–2.65 2.13–2.63
	Urine (24-h)	mg/d Ca in diet Ca free: 5–40 Low to average: 50–150 Average: 100–300	mmol/d 0.13–1.0 1.25–3.8 2.5–7.5
Carbon dioxide, total (T$_{co_2}$)	Serum or plasma (heparin)	mmol/L Cord: 14–22 Newborn: 17–24 Child: 20–28 Adult: 24–32	
β-Carotene	Serum. Protect from light.	μg/dL Infant: 20–70 Child: 40–130 Adult male: 50–300 Adult female: 90–410	μmol/L 0.37–1.30 0.74–2.42 0.93–5.60 1.68–7.65
Catecholamines, fractionated	Urine (24 h) (preservative, 25 mL 6 N HCl)	Norepinephrine μg/d 1–4 yr: 0–29 4–10 yr: 8–65 10–15 yr: 15–80 Adult: 0–100 (CF - 5.91)	nmol/d 0–171 47–384 89–472 0–591

Test	Specimen/Method	Conventional Units	SI Units
Catecholamines, total	Urine (24-h) (preservative, 25 mL 6 N HCl)	Epinephrine µg/d 1–4 yr: 0–6.0 4–10 yr: 0–10.0 10–15 yr: 0.5–20 Adult: 0–15 (CF - 5.4615) Dopamine µg/d 1–4 yr: 40–260 4 yr–adult: 65–400 (CF - 6.5359)	Epinephrine nmol/d 0–33 0–55 2.7–109 0–82 Dopamine nmol/d 261–1700 425–2614
	Urine, timed (daylight hours) Urine, random	< 115 µg/d (CF - 5.677) 1.4–7.3 µg/h ≤ 18 µg/dL ≤ 135 µg/g creatinine (CF - 0.6422)	< 653 nmol/d 7.9–41 nmol/h ≤ 102 nmol/dL ≤ 87 nmol/mmol creatinine
Catecholamines, fractionated (high-pressure liquid chromatography)	Urine (24-h) (preservative, 25 mL 6 N HCl; pH should be between 2 and 3.)	µg/d Norepinephrine: 15–56 Epinephrine: 0–15 Dopamine: 100–440	nmol/d 89–331 0–82 654–2876
Catecholamines, free plasma	Plasma. Cold centrifuge. Freeze at −80°C.	pg/mL Epinephrine, random: < 88 (CF - 5.4615) Norepinephrine, random: 104–548 (CF - 5.91) Dopamine, random: < 136 (CF - 6.5359)	pmol/L < 481 615–3239 < 889

(cont'd.)

Testing Protocols & Normal Laboratory Values (cont'd.)

Test	Collection Procedure	Common Units (Conversion Factor → SI)		Système International (SI) Units
Catecholamines, total plasma	Plasma on ice. Process immediately. Cold centrifuge. Freeze at −80°C.	Norepinephrine: 100–500	pg/mL	pmol/L
		Epinephrine: 50–250		591–2955
		Dopamine (supine, resting 20-yr-old): < 150		273–1365
		Increases 3 pg/mL (20 pmol/L) yearly.		< 980
		Standing 5 min: 50–200% increase		
Chloride	Serum or plasma (heparin)	102–115 mmol/L (mEq/L)		
	Urine (24-h)	mmol/d		
		Infant: 2–10		
		Child: 15–40		
		Thereafter 170–250 (vary greatly with Cl intake)		
Cholesterol, total	Serum or plasma (EDTA). No heparin. Overnight fast recommended.		mg/dL	mmol/L
		Desirable:	< 200	< 10.3
		Borderline:	200–400	10.3–12.4
		High risk:	> 240	> 12.4
Cholesterol, HDL (high-density lipoprotein)	Serum or plasma (EDTA, not heparin)		mg/dL	mmol/L
		Cord blood:	5–50	0.13–1.29
		Male mean:	45	116
		Female mean:	55	142
		Desirable:	> 45	> 116
		Borderline risk:	35–45	0.90–116
		Higher risk:	< 35	< 0.90

Cholesterol, LDL (low-density lipoprotein)

Serum or plasma (EDTA, not heparin)

	mg/dL	mmol/L
Desirable:	< 130	< 3.4
Borderline risk:	130–159	3.4–4.1
High risk:	> 159	> 4.1

LDL is calculated by formula: (HDL cholesterol + Triglycerides/5). The calculation is not valid if triglycerides exceed 400 mg/dL.

Chorionic gonadotropin, β-subunit (β-hCG)

Serum or plasma (EDTA) (may cross-react with LH)

Males and nonpregnant females: not detectable

Female postconception
$$\text{IU/L}$$
7–10 d: > 2.0
30 d: > 100
40 d: > 2000
10 wk: 50,000–100,000
14 wk: 10,000–20,000
Trophoblastic disease: > 100,000

Results < 5 mIU/mL may reflect cross-reactivity with high levels of LH

Cobalamin See Vitamin B_{12}

Corticosterone (compound B)

Serum or plasma (heparin, EDTA, or oxalate)

0.13–2.3 μg/dL
(CF - 28.86)

3.75–66 nmol/L

Cortisol (HPLC method)

Serum or plasma (heparin)

8 AM 5–20 μg/dL
8 PM ≤ 50% of 8 AM
(CF - 27.5862)

138–552 nmol/L
Fraction of 8 AM: ≤ 0.50

(cont'd.)

Testing Protocols & Normal Laboratory Values (cont'd.)

Test	Collection Procedure	Common Units (Conversion Factor → SI)	Système International (SI) Units
Cortisol, free (unconjugated)	Urine (24-h) (preservative, 8 g boric acid or 10 mL 6 N HCl)	μg/d Child: 2–27 Adolescent: 5–55 Adult: 20–100 (CF - 2.7586)	nmol/d 5.5–74 14–152 27–276
	AM 1-h (7–8 AM) specimen	50–210 μg/g creatinine	15.6–65.5 nmol/mmol creatinine
	PM 1-h (10–11 PM) specimen	5–45 μg/g creatinine	1.6–14.0 nmol/mmol creatinine
	24-h specimen	25–95 μg/g creatinine (CF - 0.3121)	7.8–29.6 nmol/mmol creatinine
Cosyntropin stimulation test *See* ACTH₁₋₂₄ stimulation test.			
Creatinine	Serum or plasma	mg/dL 0–5 yr: 0.2–0.5 5–6 yr: 0.2–0.6 6–7 yr: 0.3–0.7 7–8 yr: 0.3–0.8 8–9 yr: 0.4–0.9 9–10 yr: 0.4–1.0 > 10 yr: 0.6–1.4	μmol/L 18–44 18–53 26–62 26–71 35–80 35–89 53–124
		Note: Ketone bodies falsely increase results. Special assay procedure required in presence of ketosis.	
	Urine (24-h)	Adult male: 1.0–2.0 g/24 h Adult female: 0.8–1.8 g/24 h (CF - 8.842)	0.9–1.8 mmol/24 h 0.7–1.6 mmol/24 h

Creatinine clearance	Urine (24-h) or timed, submit with serum	70–140 mL/min ("corrected") (give weight and height of patient if corrected clearance is needed)		
Cyclic AMP (cAMP)	Plasma (EDTA)	Male: 17–33 nmol/L Female: 11–27 nmol/L		
	Urine	1000–11,500 nmol/d < 6000 nmol cAMP/g creatinine		
Cystine or cysteine Qualitative	Urine, random	Negative		
Quantitative	Urine (24-h)	10–100 mg/d		

Dehydroepiandrosterone DHEA — Serum

	ng/dL			nmol/L	
	Male	Female		Male	Female
< 6 yr:	26.3–71.7	19.4–42.1		0.91–2.48	0.67–1.46
6–8 yr:	29.1–66.0	72.6–165		1.01–2.29	2.52–5.72
8–10 yr:	53.3–135	74.4–180		1.85–4.68	2.58–6.24
10–12 yr:	183–383	234–529		6.34–13.3	8.11–18.3
12–14 yr:	240–520	224–611		8.32–18.0	7.76–21.2
> 14 yr:	307–835	282–771		10.6–28.9	9.77–26.7
Postmenopause:		30–450			1.0–15.6
(CF - 0.3467)				83–830 µmol/d (Negative)	

(cont'd.)

Testing Protocols & Normal Laboratory Values (cont'd.)

Test	Collection Procedure	Common Units (Conversion Factor → SI) μg/dL		Système International (SI) Units μmol/L	
		Male	Female	Male	Female
Dehydroepiandrosterone sulfate (DHEAS)	Serum or plasma				
		Newborn: < 30,000	< 30,000	< 780	< 780
		1–8 yrs: 6.1–14.5	6.1–14.5	0.17–0.39	0.17–0.39
		8–10 yrs: 34.3–53.9	34.3–53.9	0.93–1.47	0.93–1.47
		10–12 yrs: 24.5–42.5	53.3–136	0.67–1.16	1.45–3.70
		12–14 yrs: 75.9–138	70.1–169	2.17–3.76	1.91–4.60
		14–16 yrs: 138–234	138–234	3.76–6.38	3.76–6.37
		Adults: 199–334	82–338	5.41–9.09	2.23–9.20
		Postmenopause*:	17–77		0.46–2.10
		Pregnancy (term):	23–117		0.63–3.18
			(CF - 0.02721)		

*Normal laboratory values from *N Engl J Med* 1986;**314**:43. Reported normal ranges may vary.

Test	Collection Procedure	Common Units (Conversion Factor → SI)	Système International (SI) Units
11-Deoxycortisol (compound S) Nonspecific. See *also* Metyrapone stimulation test.	Plasma (heparin, EDTA, or oxalate) On ice. Process immediately.	Without metyrapone < 2 µg/dL	< 60 nmol/L
		After metyrapone > 7 µg/dL	> 200 nmol/L
Specific (postextraction) for evaluation of adrenogenital syndrome	Serum	ng/dL	pmol/L
		Cord blood: 295–554	8516–15,993
		Premature infants: 48–579	1386–16,715
		Full-term infants:	
		3 days: 13–147	375–4244
		1–12 months: < 156	< 4503
		Prepubertal child (1–10 yr, 0800 h): 20–155	577–4475
		Adults (0800 h): 12–158	346–4561
		(CF - 28.8684)	

Test	Specimen	Conventional	SI
11-Deoxycorticosterone (DOC)	Serum or plasma (heparin, EDTA, or oxalate)	Ad lib diet, 8 AM: 4.3–12.3 ng/dL (CF - 30.2572)	130–372 pmol/L
Dexamethasone 1-mg overnight suppression test Dose: 1-mg PO at 11 PM (screening test for hypercortisolism (see Chapter 1)	Serum or plasma (EDTA) for cortisol at 8 AM following dexamethasone	Cortisol ≤ 5 μg/dL	Cortisol ≤ 138 nmol/L
Dexamethasone 8-mg overnight suppression test Dose: 8 mg PO at 11 PM	Serum or plasma (EDTA) for cortisol at 8 AM baseline and again at 8 AM following dexamethasone	Cortisol < 50% baseline in Cushing's disease	Cortisol < 0.50 baseline in Cushing's disease
(Helps distinguish cause of hypercortisolism; ie, Cushing's disease versus ectopic ACTH or adrenal neoplasm; see Chapter 1; see also ACTH).			
Dexamethasone low-dose (standard) suppression test Dose: adult, 0.5 mg every 6 h × 8; children, 5 μg/kg every 6 h	Serum 8 AM cortisol baseline and on 2nd and 3rd day of test	Suppressed cortisol ≤ 5 μg/dL	≤ 138 nmol/L
	Urine 24-h baseline and on 2nd day of receiving dexamethasone (17-OHCS preferable to 17-KGS)	Free cortisol < 20 μg/d; 17-OHCS < 4.5 mg/d; 17-KGS < 7.5 mg/d	Free cortisol < 55.2 nmol/d; 17-OHCS < 12.4 μmol/d; 17-KGS < 26 μmol/d
(Helps determine presence of hypercortisolism; see Chapter 1; see also Cortisol, urine free)			
Dexamethasone high-dose (standard) suppression test Dose: adult, 2 mg every 6 h × 8; children, 20 μg/kg every 6 h	Serum 8 AM cortisol baseline and on 2nd and 3rd day of test	Suppressed cortisol < 50% baseline in Cushing's disease	Suppressed cortisol < 0.50 baseline in Cushing's disease
	Urine 24-h baseline and on 2nd day of receiving dexamethasone (17-OHCS preferable to 17-KGS)	Free cortisol, 17-OHCS (or 17-KGS) < 50% baseline in Cushing's disease	Free cortisol 17-OHCS (or 17-KGS) < 0.50 baseline in Cushing's disease
(Helps distinguish cause of hypercortisolism; ie, Cushing's disease versus ectopic ACTH or adrenal neoplasm. See Chapter 1; see also ACTH.)			

(cont'd.)

Testing Protocols & Normal Laboratory Values (cont'd.)

Test	Collection Procedure	Common Units (Conversion Factor → SI)		Système International (SI) Units	
Dihydrotestosterone (DHT)	Serum	Prepubertal male: < 3–13 ng/dL		103–448 pmol/L	
		Prepubertal female: < 3–10 ng/dL		103–344 pmol/L	
		Adult male: 30–100 ng/dL		1033–3444 pmol/L	
		Adult female: 6–33 ng/dL		207–1136 pmol/L	
		(CF - 34.4353)			
1,25 Dihydroxyvitamin D See Vitamin D.					
Epinephrine See Catecholamines, fractionated.					
Erythropoietin	Serum	4–26 mIU/mL			
Estradiol (E₂)	Serum or plasma	pg/mL		pmol/L	
		Male	Female	Male	Female
		< 10.0	< 7.0	< 36.7	< 25.7
	Prepubertal:				
	8–12 yr:		8.2–17.8		30.1–65.3
	12–14 yr:		16.0–34.0		58.7–125
	14–16 yr:		20.0–68.0		73.4–250
	Adult:	20–50		73.4–184	
	Early follicular:		20–100		73.4–367
	Midcycle:		100–500		367–1835
	Luteal:		50–240		184–880
	Postmenopausal:		10–30		37–110
			(CF - 3.67)		

Estriol (E_3) (predominant estrogen in pregnancy)	Serum	Pregnancy (wk): ng/mL	nmol/L
		30–32: 2–12	7–42
		33–35: 3–19	10–66
		36–38: 5–27	17–94
		39–40: 10–30	35–104
		Male and nonpregnant female: < 2	< 7
		(CF - 3.4674)	
Estrone (E_1)	Serum	pg/mL: Female / Male	pmol/L: Female / Male
		Follicular: 30–100	111–370
		Ovulatory: > 150	> 555
		Luteal: 90–160	333–592
		Postmenopausal: 20–40	74–148
		Male: 10–50	Male: 37–185
		(CF - 3.6982)	
Ferritin	Serum (Hemolyzed specimens may give false elevations.)	ng/mL	μg/L
		Newborn: 25–200	25–200
		1 mo: 200–600	200–600
		2–5 mo: 50–200	50–200
		6 mo–15 yr: 7–142	7–142
		Adult male: 10–273	10–273
		> 66 yr: 39–399	39–399
		Adult female: 5–99	5–99
Fetoglobulin (alpha-fetoprotein)	Serum (avoid hemolysis)	Males and nonpregnant females: < 11 ng/mL; < 11 μg/L	
Fluoride	Random urine. Store in plastic, not glass.	≤ 1 mg/L Toxic level usually > 10 mg/L	

(cont'd.)

Testing Protocols & Normal Laboratory Values (cont'd.)

Test	Collection Procedure	Common Units (Conversion Factor → SI) ng/mL		Système International (SI) Units mIU/mL or IU/L	
		Male	Female	Male	Female
Follicle-stimulating hormone (FSH)	Serum or plasma (heparin)				
	Age				
	0–8 yr:	0.3–1.3	0.6–0.8	1.1–4.9	2.3–3.0
	8–12 yr:	0.8–1.1	1.2–2.4	3.0–4.2	4.6–9.1
	12–14 yr:	1.4–2.0	1.7–2.8	5.3–7.6	6.5–10.6
	14–16 yr:	2.0–3.0	2.2–3.0	7.6–11.4	8.4–11.4
	> 16 yr:	2.0–3.0	2.2–2.9	7.6–11.4	8.4–11.0
	Adult:	0.5–4.5		2–17	
	Premenopause:		1.1–5.3		4–20
	Midcycle peak:		2.6–24		10–90
	Pregnancy:		low or undetectable		
	Postmenopausal:		11–66		40–250
Free thyroxine index (FT$_4$I)	The serum total thyroxine level adjusted for the ability of the serum to bind thyroxine (see Thyroid resin uptake). Provides a better estimation of "free" (active) thyroxine but may not be an accurate estimate of free thyroxine in certain clinical situations (see Table 5–1).	6.5–12.5			
Free triiodothyronine (FT$_3$) *See* Triiodothyronine, free.					

Gastrin	Serum. Overnight fast recommended. No heparin.	Age: < 60 yr: < 200 pg/mL Age: > 60 yr: upper 15%. 100–800 pg/mL	< 95 pmol/L Upper 0.15 fraction of population, 48–380 pmol/L
Gastrin secretin stimulation test IV dose: 5 U secretin/kg	Serum, fasting, at 15-min intervals for 1 h	No response or slight suppression. Zollinger-Ellison syndrome: increase > 110 pg/mL if base level 80–500 pg/mL.	
GGT (gamma-glutamyl transpeptidase)		Male: 9–85 U/L. Female: 6–58 U/L.	
Glucagon	Plasma (heparin or EDTA) Collect in iced tube with 1/10 volume 0.5 M benzamidine. Prepare immediately. Cold centrifuge.	50–200 pg/mL (CF - 0.29)	16–58 pmol/L
Glucose (fasting)	Serum or plasma (EDTA)	mg/dL Cord: 45–96 Premature: 20–60 Neonate: 30–60 Newborn (1 d): 40–60 > 1 d: 50–80 Child: 65–130 Adult: 65–115 > 60 yr: 65–125 Adult: 60–105	mmol/L 2.5–5.4 1.1–3.4 1.7–3.4 2.2–3.4 2.8–4.5 3.6–7.3 3.6–6.4 3.6–7.0 3.3–5.8
	Whole blood (heparin)	(CF - 0.056)	

Note: prolonged fasting (> 12 h) may result in serum glucose levels as low as 50 mg/dL (2.8 nmol/L) in some normal women.

(cont'd.)

Testing Protocols & Normal Laboratory Values (cont'd.)

Test	Collection Procedure	Common Units (Conversion Factor → SI)	Système International (SI) Units
Glucose, 2-h postprandial	Serum or plasma (EDTA)	< 120 mg/dL Diabetes: see Glucose tolerance test, oral.	< 6.7 mmol/L
Glucose, urine quantitative (enzymatic) (nonpregnant)	Urine (random). Recommended collection with preservative (toluene).	< 120 mg/24 h	< 0.67 mmol/24 h
Glucose tolerance testing, oral (OGTT) standard oral test (nonpregnant) Dose: 75 g or 1.75 g/kg ideal body weight (IBW) liquid glucose	Serum or plasma (EDTA)	mg/dL Fasting: < 115 < 130 in child 30 min: < 200 1 h: < 200 90 min: < 200 2 h: < 140	mmol/L < 6.4 < 7.3 in child < 11.2 < 11.2 < 11.2 < 7.8
Glucose loading screen (used to screen pregnant women for gestational diabetes mellitus. Draw serum 1 h after 50 g liquid glucose PO.)	If fasting If not fasting	mg/dL < 140 < 130	mmol/L < 7.8 < 7.3

Patients having a positive screening test are tested with the standard 100-g oral test (see below).

Standard oral test (pregnant)
Dose: 100 g liquid glucose

	First trimester		Second trimester		Third trimester	
	mg/dL	mmol/L	mg/dL	mmol/L	mg/dL	mmol/L
Fasting:	< 85	< 4.7	< 85	< 4.7	< 90	< 5.0
1-h:	< 165	< 9.2	< 190	< 10.5	< 205	< 11.7
2-h:	< 145	< 8.0	< 155	< 8.6	< 195	< 10.8
3-h:	< 125	< 6.9	< 135	< 7.5	< 160	< 8.9

Note: Test fasting fingerstick or plasma glucose before giving oral glucose. A glucose level greater than 140 mg/dL (7.8 mmol/L) makes the OGTT unnecessary. The standard OGTT is performed with the patient seated after a 10- to 16-h fast, preceded by 3 days of normal physical activity and a diet containing at least 150 g carbohydrate daily. Interpret OGTT conservatively. An abnormal value indicates impaired glucose tolerance. The diagnosis of *diabetes* demands a fasting glucose of > 140 mg/dL (> 7.8 mmol/L) on more than one occasion *or* a level of > 200 mg/dL (> 11.1 mmol/L) both at 2 h and at some earlier interval between 0 and 2 h. The diagnosis of diabetes in children demands the presence of all 3 abnormalities if made on chemical grounds alone. Longer OGTTs for the diagnosis of reactive hypoglycemia are not warranted, since glucose levels may fall to < 40 mg/dL (< 2.2 nmol/L) 3–5 h after a glucose load and be associated with hypoglycemic symptoms in normal individuals.

Glycohemoglobin (glycosylated hemoglobin, HgbA, including HgbA₁c)

Blood (heparinized or EDTA; *do not* centrifuge)

3.9–6.9%

Note: Elevated fetal hemoglobin gives falsely high results. See text for other influencing factors.

Gonadotropins See Pregnancy tests; Chorionic gonadotropin; β-subunit; FSH; LH.

Growth hormone (GH, somatotropin) baseline

Serum or plasma

	ng/mL	pmol/L
Cord:	10–50	465–2325
Newborn:	15–40	698–1860
Child:	1–10	47–465
Adult:	< 8	< 372

Pregnancy: High values may be reported owing to cross-reaction of the assay with human placental lactogen. Evaluation for GH excess or deficiency usually necessitates functional testing described below.

Note: GH values fluctuate widely, and baseline levels must be interpreted critically.

(cont'd.)

Testing Protocols & Normal Laboratory Values (cont'd.)

Test	Collection Procedure	Common Units (Conversion Factor → SI)	Système International (SI) Units
Growth hormone (GH) suppressed (acromegaly, gigantism) Dose: 100 g PO, fasting	Serum or plasma 60 min after glucose	Male: < 2 ng/ml Female: < 5 ng/ml	Male: < 93 pmol/L Female: < 233 pmol/L
Growth hormone (GH) TRH test (acromegaly, gigantism) Dose: TRH, 500 mg IV	Serum or plasma baseline and at 15-min-intervals for 1 h after TRH	No increase in normals. An increase is observed in most patients with acromegaly or gigantism.	
Growth hormone stimulation tests (GH deficiency) (1) Exercise (2) Sleep (3) Arginine (dose: 0.5 g/kg IBW (up to 20 g) over 30 min, IV (4) L-Dopa (dose: 125 mg to 15 kg) 250 mg to 35 kg; 500 mg over 35 kg IBW. PO) (5) Insulin hypoglycemia See Insulin tolerance test. (6) Glucagon (dose: 1 mg, IV)	Serum baseline and 15 min after vigorous exercise, 90 min after onset of sleep, 30-min intervals for 2 h after arginine or insulin and for 3 h after L-dopa or glucagon	Normal: peak > 7 ng/mL or rise of > 5 ng/mL above baseline	Normal: peak > 326 pmol/L or rise of > 233 pmol/L above baseline

Note: Tests may be run simultaneously. Ten to 20% of normal children have a low response to any one test. Two or three tests help document a deficiency. Short children with normal GH stimulation testing may nevertheless have low baseline GH secretion. Administer propranolol (0.75 mg/kg up to 40 mg) 90 minutes before stimuli to increase the response. See also Chapter 3.

hCG See Chorionic gonadotropin.

Hemoglobin A₁c See Glycohemoglobin.

High-density lipoprotein See Cholesterol, HDL.

β-Hydroxybutyric acid	Serum or plasma	< 0.3 mmol/L

17-Hydroxycorticosteroids (17-OHCS)

Urine (24-h) (preservative, 5 mL 6 N HCl or 8 g boric acid)

	mg/d	μmol/d
0–1 yr:	0.5–1	1–3
Child:	1–6	3–17
Adult, M:	3–15	8–41
F:	2–12	6–33

(CF - 2.7586)

or 3–7 mg/g (CF - 0.3121) creatinine

or 0.9–2.2 mmol/mol creatinine

18-Hydroxycorticosterone (18-OHB)
For distinguishing cause of hyperaldosteronism

Plasma. High sodium intake (> 120 mEq/d).

Normal or adrenal hyperplasia: < 85 ng/dL
Adrenal neoplasm: > 85 ng/dL

5-Hydroxyindole acetic acid (5-HIAA)

Qualitative — Fresh random urine — Negative

Quantitative — Urine (24-h) (preservative, 10 mL 6 N HCl) Refrigerate during collection. — 2–8 mg/d (CF - 5.2301) — 10.5–42 μmol/d

Note: > 50 mg/d (262 μmol/d) is diagnostic of carcinoid. For 48 h before collection and during specimen collection, avoid alcohol, nuts, avocados, bananas, plantains, red-blue plums, red plums, berries, tomatoes, pineapple, and juices made from the above (falsely high results). Phenothiazines give falsely low values.

(cont'd.)

Testing Protocols & Normal Laboratory Values (cont'd.)

Test	Collection Procedure	Common Units (Conversion Factor → SI)	Système International (SI) Units
17-Hydroxyprogesterone (17-OHP)	Serum, fasting preferred.	ng/dL Newborn, 1–8 d: < 160 Child, up to 1 yr: < 230 Prepubertal male: < 120 Prepubertal female: < 160 Adult male: 30–220 Adult female: Follicular: < 90 Luteal: < 210 Postmenopausal: < 60 (CF - 0.03026)	nmol/L < 4.8 < 7.0 < 3.6 < 4.8 0.9–6.7 < 2.7 < 6.4 < 1.8
Hydroxyproline	Urine (24-h) (preservative, 25 mL 6 N HCl)	Total: 25–77 mg/d Free: ≤ 2 mg/d	190–586 µmol/d ≤ 15 µmol/d
Insulin (12-h fasting)	Serum. Cold centrifuge.	µU/mL Newborn: 3–20 Adult: 5–25 > 60 yr: 6–35 (CF - 7.175)	pmol/L 22–144 36–180 43–252
Insulin and glucose (72-h fasting)	Serum, every 6–12 h	> 50 mg glucose/dL during a 72-h period of fasting (water is permitted) with values slightly lower in females. Insulin: < 4 µU/mL or undetectable. Normal fasting insulin-glucose ratio: < 0.3.	> 2.8 mmol glucose/L during 72-h period of fasting with values slightly lower in female. Insulin: < 29 pmol/L or undetectable. Normal fasting insulin-glucose ratio: < 39.

				pmol/L
Insulin with oral glucose tolerance test (OGTT)	Serum			50–172
				179–1653
				129–197
				114–119
				29–272

		Insulin, μU/mL	ng/mL
	0 min:	7–24	0.3–1.0
	30 min:	25–231	1.0–9.2
	1-h:	18–276	0.7–11.0
	2-h:	16–166	0.6–6.6
	3-h:	4–38	0.2–1.5

Insulin tolerance test (ITT)
Dose: Regular insulin 0.15 U/kg IV.
Add 0.1 U/kg for type II diabetes, acromegaly, Cushing's syndrome. Subtract 0.05 U/kg for suspected hypopituitarism.

Serum baseline and every 15 min for 90 min. For glucose and desired hormone levels.

See Growth hormone; Cortisol; Prolactin.
Glucose levels should fall to < 40 mg/dL (< 2.3 nmol/L) or < 50 mg/dL (< 2.8 nmol/L) with definite symptoms of hypoglycemia.

Note: Patients ordinarily develop symptomatic hypoglycemia 20–40 minutes after insulin administration. Physician attendance is required. For severe symptoms, administer 25 mL of 50% dextrose. Do not use in patients with seizures, heart disease, or older than 60 years.

Insulin antibodies	Serum	Never insulin-treated: undetectable
		Insulin-treated: ratio bound:free < 1.0 or < 200 μU/mL
		(includes antibodies to human, beef, and pork insulin)

Insulinlike growth factor See Somatomedin C.

			μmol/L
Iron	Serum	μg/dL	
	Draw without hemolysis.	Newborn: 100–250	17.90–44.75
		Infant: 40–100	7.16–17.90
		Child: 50–120	8.95–21.48
		Adult Male: 50–160	8.95–28.64
		Adult Female: 40–150	7.16–26.85

Iron—liver biopsy	Submit at least 0.5 × 5 mm piece of tissue in metal-free container.	530–900 μg Fe per gram dry weight liver

(cont'd.)

Testing Protocols & Normal Laboratory Values (cont'd.)

Test	Collection Procedure	Common Units (Conversion Factor → SI)		Système International (SI) Units
Iron-binding capacity, total (TIBC)	Serum			μmol/L
		Infant: 100–400		17.90–71.60
		Thereafter: 250–400		44.75–71.60
Iron saturation	Serum	16–60%		Fraction saturation 0.16–0.60
17-Ketogenic steroids (17-KGS) Less specific than 17-OHCS; do not confuse with 17-KS. Used to screen for adrenal carcinoma.	Urine (24-h)	mg/d		μmol/d
		01–yr:	< 1.0	< 3.5
		1–10 yr:	< 5	< 17
		11–14 yr:	< 12	< 42
		Adult male:	5–23	17–89
		Adult female:	3–15	10–52
		> 70 yr male:	3–15	10–52
	(CF - based on DHEA, MW 288)	> 70 yr female:	3–13	10–45
Ketone bodies				
Qualitative	Serum	Negative		Negative
	Urine, random	Negative		Negative
Quantitative	Serum	0.5–3.0 mg/dL		5–30 mg/L
17-Ketosteroids (17-KS), total Zimmerman reaction	Urine (24-h) (preservative, 10 mL 6 N HCl or 8 g boric acid)	mg/d		μmol/d
		14 days–2 yr:	< 1	< 3.5
		2–6 yr:	< 2	< 7
		6–10 yr:	1–4	3.5–14
		10–12 yr:	1–6	3.5–21
		12–14 yr:	3–10	10–35

Chromatography

Urine (24-h)

14–16 yr: 5–12
Adult male: 9–22
Adult female: 5–15
(CF – 3.4674)

17–42
31–76
17–52

Decreases with age

17–42
10–35

Lactic acid

Blood (on ice), venous

5–18 mg/dL

0.5–2.0 mmol/L

Lipid profile
See Cholesterol (total, HDL, LDL), Triglycerides.

Serum or plasma (no heparin)
Fasting 14 h (water permitted)

Adult male: 5.0–12.0
Adult female: 3.0–10.0
(Conversion factor based on DHEA, MW 288)

Low-density lipoprotein See Cholesterol, LDL.

Luteinizing hormone (LH)

Serum or plasma (heparin)

Age	ng/mL		IU/L	
	Male	Female	Male	Female
0–8 yr:	1.0–1.2	0.7–0.9	9.5–11.4	6.7–8.6
8–12 yr:	1.4–1.7	0.9–1.4	13.3–16.2	8.6–13.3
12–14 yr:	1.5–1.7	0.9–1.3	14.3–16.2	8.6–12.4
14–16 yr:	1.6–1.8	1.5–1.9	15.2–17.1	14.2–18.1
> 16 yr:	1.6–1.8	1.7–3.0	15.2–17.1	16.1–28.5
Adult:	0.4–1.9		4–18	
Premenopause:		0.5–2.6		5–25
Midcycle peak:		4.2–15.8		40–150
Pregnancy:		Variable		Variable
Postmenopause:		3.2–21.1		30–200
		(CF – 9.5)		

(cont'd.)

Testing Protocols & Normal Laboratory Values *(cont'd.)*

Test	Collection Procedure	Common Units (Conversion Factor → SI)	Système International (SI) Units
Note: Measures both LH and hCG. High hCG levels found in pregnancy or trophoblastic disease cross-react in most assays causing falsely elevated LH levels.			
Magnesium	Serum	1.6–2.7 mg/dL or 1.5–2.5 mEq/L	0.8–1.3 mmol/L
Metanephrine, total with creatine	Urine (24-h) or "spot." No preservative required. Compatible with 6 N HCl used for catecholamines.	μg/mg creatinine < 2 yr: < 4.3 2–10 yr: < 2.8 10–15 yr: < 1.6 15+ yr: < 0.7	mmol/mol creatinine < 2.5 < 1.6 < 0.9 < 0.4
Metanephrines, total	Urine (24-h)	< 900 μg/24 h (CF - 5.2576)	< 24,900 nmol/24 h
Metyrapone stimulation test Single dose test. Dose: 30 mg/kg PO at midnight with snack (usually 2.5 g in adults)	Serum at 8 AM following morning for 11-deoxycortisol and cortisol	11-Deoxycortisol (compound S): > 7 μg/dL Cortisol: < 5 μg/dL	(> 200 nmol/L) < 138 nmol/L
Note: Nausea occurs frequently. The cortisol level is obtained to ensure that adrenal cortisol secretion is adequately suppressed.			
Microsomal antibodies, thyroid *See* Thyroid antibodies.			
Norepinephrine *See* Catecholamines, fractionated.			
Osmolality	Plasma (preferred) or serum Urine, random	Child, adult: 275–293 mOsm/kg water Note: Osmolality is increased by hyperglycemia, azotemia, and alcohol. P_{OSM} (mOsm/Kg) - 1.86 × Na (mEq/L) +	

$$\frac{\text{Glucose (mg/dL)}}{18} + \frac{\text{BUN (mg/dL)}}{2.8}$$

Osmolality ratio, urine/serum	Urine (24-h)	50–1400 mOsm/kg, depending on fluid intake After 12-h fluid restriction: > 850 mOsm/kg ≅ 300–900 mOsm/kg
	Urine and serum	1.0–3.0; > 3 after 12-h fluid restriction
Oxalate	Urine. Acidify to pH < 3 with HCl. Refrain from ingesting nuts, rhubarb, spinach, tea, chocolate, and vitamin C for 48 h before collection.	8–40 μg/mL; < 41 mg/24 h	90–445 μmol/L; < 446 μmol/24 h
Oxytocin	Plasma (EDTA)	< 3.2 μU/mL	< 3.2mU/L
Pancreatic polypeptide	Plasma, fasting	< 350 pg/mL (CF - 0.246)	< 86 pmol/L
Parathyroid hormone (PTH) (Simultaneous assay for calcium albumin, phosphorus, magnesium, and creatinine recommended)	Serum. Fasting preferred. Process immediately in refrigerated centrifuge.	Normal ranges vary considerably with laboratory and assay used. Intact molecule: 11–54 pg/mL (1.16–5.69 pmol/L) Midregion assay: < 40 μEq/mL. N-terminal assay: < 240 pg/mL (< 25.3 pmol/L). (CF - 0.1053)	
Pentagastrin stimulation test See Calcitonin.		

(cont'd.)

Testing Protocols & Normal Laboratory Values (cont'd.)

Test	Collection Procedure	Common Units (Conversion Factor → SI)	Système International (SI) Units
pH	Whole blood (heparin), arterial (must correct for body temperature)	7.35–7.45	H+ concentration: 36–44 nmol/L
	Urine, random	Newborn: 5–7 Thereafter: 4.5–8	0.1–10 μmol/L 0.1–32 μmol/L
Perchlorate thyroid discharge test Dose: 10 μCi ¹²³I (IV) After 1st 2-h uptake, give 0.5 g perchlorate (KClO₄) PO	Thyroid ¹²³I uptake 2 h after ¹²³I 2 hr after KClO₄ 4 hr after KClO₄	Normal individuals without thyroid organification defects show a decline in radioactivity of < 10% after KClO₄	
Phosphatase, acid (prostatic) Note: Thymolphthalein phosphate method measures primarily prostatic acid phosphatase	Serum. No anticoagulants Separate and buffer within 1 h of drawing. Buffer with 1 drop (20 μL) buffer to 2 mL serum	≤ 0.9 IU/L (thymolphthalein) < 3.0 ng/mL (prostatic, RIA)	≤ 0.9 IU/L < 3.0 μg/L
Phosphatase, alkaline	Serum. No anticoagulants.	Male U/L 0–2 yr: 132–423 2–10 yr: 163–328 10–17 yr: 98–391 17–19 yr: 56–266 19+ yr: 41–133	Female U/L 132–423 240–530 107–433 49–164 41–133
Note: Isoenzymes of alkaline phosphatase are unreliable. Obtain serum GGT to distinguish bone from liver enzyme if source of elevation is unclear.			
Phosphorus, inorganic	Serum, fasting	mg/dL 0–6 yr: 4.0–7.2 6–12 yr: 4.0–6.2 12–20 yr: 3.3–6.3 > 20 yr: 2.5–4.5	mmol/L 1.3–2.3 1.3–2.0 1.1–2.0 0.8–1.4
Note: Serum levels decrease with carbohydrate ingestion and rise with phosphate ingestion.			

Test / Specimen	Normal Value (conventional)	Normal Value (SI)
Urine (24-h) (with 10 mL of 6 N HCl)	Adults on diet containing 0.9–1.5 g P and 10 mg Ca/kg. On restricted diet: 0.4–1.3 g/d. < 1 g/d.	Adults on diet containing 29–48 mmol P and 0.25 mmol Ca/kg: < 32 mmol/d. On restricted diet: 13–42 mmol/d.

Placental lactogen (hPL)

Serum
Males and nonpregnant females

	μg/mL	mg/L
Males and nonpregnant females:	< 0.5	< 0.5
Weeks of gestation		
6–27:	< 4.6	< 4.6
28–31:	2.4–6.1	2.4–6.1
32–35:	3.7–7.7	3.7–7.7
36–40:	5.0–8.6	5.0–8.6

Potassium

Serum or plasma (preferred)
Avoid hemolysis
Urine (24-h)

0–2 weeks: 4–6 mEq/L or mmol/L
> 2 weeks: 3.5–5 mEq/L or mmol/L
2.5–125 mmol/d, varies with diet

Pregnancy tests See also Chorionic gonadotropin.

Semiquantitative
(routine pregnancy screen)

Serum or urine

Negative. In pregnancy can be detected at time of missed menses.

Note: Proteinuria and phenothiazines may cause false positives.

Pregnanediol

(Rarely indicated. Use serum progesterone.)

Urine (24-h)

	mg/24 h	μmol/d
Males and prepubertal females:	< 1.8	< 5.6
Proliferative phase:	0.3–2.3	0.9–7.2
Luteal phase:	1.5–6.6	4.7–20.6
Postmenopausal:	0.1–0.8	< 2.5
	(CF – 3.1201)	

(cont'd.)

Testing Protocols & Normal Laboratory Values *(cont'd.)*

Test	Collection Procedure	Common Units (Conversion Factor → SI)	Système International (SI) Units
Pregnanetriol	Urine (24-h). No preservative.	mg/24 h	µmol/d
		0–3 yr: ≤ 0.2	≤ 0.6
		3–12 yr: ≤ 1.0	≤ 3.0
		12 + yr: ≤ 2.0	≤ 5.9
		(CF - 2.9718)	
Progesterone *See also 17-OHP.*	Serum	ng/mL	nmol/L
		Male, pubertal	
		stage I: 0.11–0.26	0.35–0.83
		Adult: 0.12–0.3	0.38–1
		Female, pubertal	
		stage I: 0–0.3	0–1
		II: 0–0.46	0–1.5
		III: 0–0.6	0–1.9
		IV: 0.05–13.0	0.16–41
		Follicular: 0.3–0.8	1.0–2.5
		Luteal: 4.0–20.0	12.7–63.6
		(CF - 3.1797)	
Proinsulin	Serum	< 30% of total immunoreactive insulinlike material, or < 0.2 ng/mL	Fraction of immunoreactive insulinlike material: < 0.30, or < 0.2 µg/L
Prolactin (PRL)	Serum	ng/mL	nmol/L
		Newborn: < 500	< 20
		1–5 mo: 6.2–13.8	0.25–0.55
		Childhood: 4.0–8.2	0.16–0.33
		Adult male: < 15	< 0.6

Prolactin-insulin tolerance test (ITT) *See ITT for protocol.* Serum

Adult female: Follicular: < 20
Luteal: < 40
Pregnancy: 1st trimester: < 80
2nd trimester: < 160
3rd trimester: < 400
(CF · 0.04)

< 0.8
< 1.6
< 3.2
< 6.4
< 16.0

Prolactin-thyrotopin releasing hormone *See TRH for protocol.*

Peak PRL values: 1.4–19 × baseline within 35–75 min following stimulation

3- to 5-fold rise above baseline (decreasing with age)

Protein, total Serum

	g/dL	g/L
0–1 mo:	4.4–7.6	44–76
1 mo–1 yr:	4.2–7.4	42–74
1–4 yr:	5.6–7.2	56–72
4–18 yr:	5.9–7.7	59–77
18+ yr:	6.0–8.5	60–85

Note: About 0.5 g/dL (5 g/L) higher in ambulatory patients than in recumbent patients.

Radioactive iodine uptake (RAIU) *See Thyroid RAIU.*

Renin activity (measured as angiotensin I) Plasma (EDTA). On ice.

Normal sodium diet (75–150 mEq Na/d):
30-min supine: 0.2–2.3 ng/mL/h (0.2–1.8 nmol/L/h)
4-h upright: 1.3–4.0 ng/mL/h (1–3.1 nmol/L/h)
Low sodium diet (< 30–75 mEq Na/d):
4-h upright: 4.1–7.7 ng/mL/h (3.2–5.9 nmol/L/h)
(CF · 0.77)

Nonambulatory hospitalized patients have a higher upper limit than normal supine patients. Reference ranges are derived from peripheral blood samples and may not apply to samples

(cont'd.)

Testing Protocols & Normal Laboratory Values (*cont'd.*)

Test	Collection Procedure	Common Units (Conversion Factor → SI)	Système International (SI) Units
		obtained during catheterization. Discontinue diuretics, estrogens, and oral contraceptives for 2 weeks and nondiuretic antihypertensives for several days before testing. Maintain dietary Na for at least 3 days before testing.	
Resin T₃ uptake (RT₃U) *See* Thyroid resin uptake.			
Resin T₄ uptake (RT₄U) *See* Thyroid resin uptake.			
Reverse triiodothyronine (rT_3)	Serum	ng/dL 1–5 yr: 15–71 5–10 yr: 17–79 10–15 yr: 19–88 Adult: 30–80	nmol/L 0.23–1.1 0.26–1.2 0.29–1.36 0.46–1.23
	Note: Normal range varies with the assay used. rT_3 is elevated in cord serum and amniotic fluid.		
Schilling test (intrinsic factor test) Dose: 0.5–1 μCi ^{58}Co-vitamin B_{12}	Urine (24-h) Note: Some patients with vitamin B_{12} deficiency have a normal Schilling test.	> 7.5% of dose	Fraction of dose: > 0.075
Semen analysis (sperm count)	Ejaculate (AM specimen) Abstain for 3 d prior to test. Room temperature. Process immediately.	Volume: 2–5 mL. Sperm count: > 20 million/mL. Motility: > 60% at 2 h. Morphology: > 60% normal forms. Note: sperm count varies considerably.	
Serotonin *See also* 5-HIAA.	Whole blood. Preserve with 75 mg ascorbic acid (process and freeze immediately).	46–319 ng/mL (CF - 0.0057)	0.26–1.82 μmol/L
Sodium	Serum or plasma (heparin). Hemolysis produces falsely low results.	135–145 mEq/L (mmol/L)	
	Urine (24-h)	40–220 mEq/d and > 20 mEq/L (mmol/L). Varies with diet.	

Somatomedin C (Sm-C, IGF-I)

Serum.
Freeze at −20°C.

Age	ng/mL Male	ng/mL Female	nmol/L Male	nmol/L Female
0–3 yr:	14–56	14–60	1.8–7.3	1.8–7.3
3–6 yr:	13–81	18–97	1.7–10.6	1.7–12.7
6–10 yr:	29–108	34–137	3.8–14.1	3.8–17.9
10–13 yr:	102–182	104–374	13.3–23.8	13.3–48.9
13–16 yr:	98–319	192–347	12.3–41.7	25.1–45.4
16–18 yr:	136–293	132–305	17.8–38.3	17.3–39.9
18 + yr:	43–178	24–153	5.6–23.3	3.1–20.0

(CF · 0.1307)

Note: Results with plasma are 10–15% higher.

Somatotropin See Growth hormone.

Specific gravity

Urine, random	Adult: 1.002–1.030
	After 12-h fluid restriction: > 1.025
Urine (24-h)	1.015–1.025

Testosterone, total

Serum

	ng/dL Male	ng/dL Female	nmol/L Male	nmol/L Female
Prepubertal:	8–14	5–13	0.28–0.49	0.17–0.45
Pubertal:	84–180	9–24	2.81–6.25	0.31–0.83
Adult:	300–1000	30–70	10.4–34.7	1.04–2.43

(CF · 0.0347)

Testosterone, free*

Serum

pg/mL		pmol/L	
Adult male: 80–280		Male	Female
Adult female: 3–13		277–971	
		10.4–45.1	

Reported normal ranges vary.

(CF · 3.4674)

Testosterone (free and weakly bound to sex hormone–binding globulin)

Serum

ng/dL	nmol/L
Male: 150–560 (36–80% of total)	Male 5.2–19.4
Female: 4–23 (12–50% of total)	Female 0.1–0.8

(cont'd.)

Testing Protocols & Normal Laboratory Values (cont'd.)

Test	Collection Procedure	Common Units (Conversion Factor → SI)	Système International (SI) Units
Tetrahydrocortisol (THF)	Urine (24-h)	Adult: 0.5–1.5 mg/d	Adult: 1.4–4.1 µmol/d
Tetrahydrodeoxycortisol	Urine (24-h)	< 1000 µg/d	< 2.9 µmol/L
Thyroglobulin	Serum	Normal: < 40 ng/mL	< 40 µg/L
		After total thyroidectomy:	
		on T_4: < 5 ng/mL	< 5 µg/L
		off T_4: < 10 ng/mL	< 10 µg/L
	Note: Serum is first screened for antithyroglobulin antibodies, the presence of which may falsely lower the thyroglobulin level.		
Thyroid antibodies			
Microsomal antibodies		Titer < 100 (dilutions)	
Thyroglobulin antibodies		Titer < 10 (dilutions)	
Thyroid index See Free thyroxine index.			
Thyroid resin uptake (TRU, TU, T_3RU, T_4RU): A number (normal range 0.6–1.2) derived from the ability of serum to bind either T_3 or T_4. This provides an approximation of the serum's thyroid-binding ability (see Chapter 5). The number may be expressed as a decimal by which to divide the total serum thyroxine to obtain a "free thyroxine index."			
Thyroid-stimulating hormone (TSH)			
Polyclonal antibody	Serum	µU/mL	
		Cord: < 40	
		Neonate: < 20	
		Adult: < 10	
Monoclonal antibody	Serum		Adult: 0.4–4.8 µIU/mL

Thyroid-stimulating hormone response to TRH *See* TRH test protocol. *Condition:* not taking exogenous thyroid hormone. *Indications:* euthyroid Graves' ophthalmopathy; questionable thyrotoxicosis.

	µU/mL	mU/L
Women: increment	> 6	> 6
Men < 40: increment	> 6	> 6
Men > 40: increment	> 2	> 2

Note: The TRH test is of limited usefulness in patients with hypothalamic-pituitary disease. Although unreliable in detecting hypothyroidism, hypopituitary patients with pituitary destruction generally have no TSH response, whereas patients with hypothalamic destruction have an increased TSH response and a high level at 120 min as opposed to a return to baseline in normals.

Thyroid-stimulating immunoglobulin (TSI)

Negative (< 2 µUEq TSH/mL). Assay based on cAMP generation in tissue culture. Levels 2–3 equivocal.

Thyroid uptake of radioactive iodine (RAIU) *See also* Chapter 5 and Tables 5–4 and 5–10.

Activity over thyroid gland

Fractional uptake:

2 h: < 6%	2 h: < 0.06
6 h: 3–20%	6 h: 0.03–0.20
24 h: 8–30%	24 h: 0.08–0.30

Note: Thyroid uptake of RAI diminishes with increased iodine ingestion or administration.

Thyrotropin-releasing hormone (TRH)

Plasma

5–60 pg/mL   14–165 pmol/L

Thyrotropin-releasing hormone stimulation test
Adult dose: 500 µg TRH, IV
See TSH response to TRH, PRL response to TRH, GH response to TRH.

Serum, baseline, and at 30 and 60 min following TRH

Note: flushing, nausea, urgency are frequent.

Thyroxine (T₄, RIA) *See* Chapter 5

Serum. Fasting recommended.

µg/dL	nmol/L
Cord: 4.6–13.0	59–167
1–3 d: 11.8–23.2	152–299

(cont'd.)

Testing Protocols & Normal Laboratory Values (cont'd.)

Test	Collection Procedure	Common Units (Conversion Factor → SI)	Système International (SI) Units
		3–10 d: 9.9–21.9	127–282
		10–45 d: 8.2–16.2	106–209
		45–90 d: 6.4–14.0	82–180
		3–12 mo: 7.8–16.5	100–212
		1–5 yr: 7.3–15.0	94–193
		5–10 yr: 6.4–13.3	82–171
		10–15 yr: 5.6–11.7	72–150
		15–20 yr: 4.2–11.8	54–152
		> 20 yr: 5.0–11.0	64–142
		(CF - 12.8717)	
See Table 5-1 for factors affecting serum T$_4$ levels without affecting clinical status.			
Thyroxine-binding globulin (TBG)	Serum	16.0–34.0 µg/mL	
Thyroxine, free (FT$_4$)	Serum	0.9–1.7 ng/dL	11.6–21.9 pmol/L
Thyroxine, free, index *See Free thyroxine index.*			
Transcortin (Binds cortisol and progesterone)	Serum	mg/dL	mg/L
		Male: 1.5–2.0	15–20
		Female: Follicular: 1.7–2.0	17–20
		Luteal: 1.6–2.1	16–21
		Postmenopausal: 1.7–2.5	17–25
		Pregnancy: 21–28 wk: 4.7–5.4	47–54
		33–40 wk: 5.5–7.0	55–70
Transferrin	Serum	Adults: 216–399 mg/dL	2.1–4.0 g/L
Note: may be used to follow nutritional status and screen for hemochromatosis but is also an acute-phase reactant.			

Triglycerides (triacylglycerols, TG)

Serum, after ≥ 12-h fast; 18-h fast recommended.

Values decrease slightly above age 60.
Levels for blacks are 10–20 mg/dL (0.10–0.20 g/L) lower.

Recommended (desirable) levels for adults:

	mg/dL		g/L	
	Male	Female	Male	Female
Cord blood:	10–98	10–98	0.10–0.98	0.10–0.98
0–5 yr:	30–86	32–99	0.30–0.86	0.32–0.99
6–11 yr:	31–108	35–114	0.31–1.08	0.35–1.14
12–15 yr:	36–138	41–138	0.36–1.38	0.41–1.38
16–19 yr:	40–163	40–128	0.40–1.63	0.40–1.28
20–29 yr:	44–185	40–128	0.44–1.85	0.40–1.28
30–39 yr:	49–284	38–160	0.49–2.84	0.38–1.60
40–49 yr:	56–298	44–186	0.56–2.98	0.44–1.86
50–59 yr:	62–288	55–247	0.62–2.88	0.55–2.47
	25–150	25–150	0.25–1.50	0.25–1.50

Triiodothyronine (T₃, RIA)
See Chapter 5.

Serum

	ng/dL	pmol/L
Cord:	15–75	230–1150
1–3 d:	32–216	490–3320
3–30 d:	50–250	770–3840
1–12 mo:	105–280	1610–4300
1–5 yr:	105–269	1610–4130
5–10 yr:	94–241	1440–3700
10–15 yr:	83–213	1270–3270
15–20 yr:	80–210	1230–3230
> 20 yr:	95–190	1460–2920
	(CF – 15.3610)	

Triiodothyronine, free (free T₃)

Serum   0.2–0.52 ng/dL   3–8 pmol/L

Triiodothyronine, reverse See Reverse T₃.

T₃ resin uptake (T₃RU, RT₃U) See Thyroid resin uptake. Note: See Chapter 5 for factors affecting T₃RU.

T₄ resin uptake (T₄RU, RT₄U) See Thyroid resin uptake.

(cont'd.)

Testing Protocols & Normal Laboratory Values (cont'd.)

Test	Collection Procedure	Common Units (Conversion Factor → SI)	Système International (SI) Units
Tubular reabsorption of phosphate (TRP) *Protocol:* low-phosphate diet for 3 days before test	Urine, 4-h (8–12 AM) for phosphate and creatinine Serum (during above interval) for phosphorus and creatinine Formula:	80–90%; lower in hyperparathyroidism	Fraction reabsorbed: 0.80–0.90

$$TRP = 1 - (\text{Urine phosphate/Serum phosphate}) \times (\text{Serum creatinine/Urine creatinine})$$

Test	Collection Procedure	Common Units (Conversion Factor → SI)	Système International (SI) Units
Urea nitrogen	Serum or plasma	mg/dL Cord: 21–40 Adult: 10–24	mmol urea/L 7.5–14.3 3.6–8.5
	Urine	10–20 g/d Varies with diet	355–710 mmol/d
Urea nitrogen/creatinine ratio	Serum	12/1 to 20/1	
Uric acid	Serum Overnight fast recommended	mg/dL Adult male: 2.4–7.4 Adult female: 1.4–5.8 Child: slightly lower	μmol/L 140–440 83–340
	Urine (24-h)	mg/d Purine-free diet, male: < 420 Female: slightly lower Low-purine diet, male: < 480 Female: < 400 High-purine diet: < 1000	mmol/d < 2.5 < 2.86 < 2.38 < 5.9
Urine volume	Urine (24-h)	Male: 800–1800 mL/d Female: 600–1600 mL/d Varies with intake and other factors	Male: 0.800–1.800 L/d Female: 0.600–1.600 L/d

Vanillylmandelic acid (VMA)	Urine (24-h). No preservative required; compatible with 6 N HCl used for catecholamines.	mg/d	µmol/d
		Newborn: < 1.0	< 5.0
		Infant: < 2.0	< 10.1
		Child: 1–3	5–15
		Adolescent: 1–5	5–25
		Thereafter: 2–7	10–35
		(CF - 5.0454)	
	Urine (24-h) or "spot"	µg VMA/mg creatinine	mmol VMA/mol creatinine
		1–12 mo: ≤ 36	≤ 20.5
		1–2 yr: ≤ 31	≤ 17.7
		2–5 yr: ≤ 17	≤ 9.7
		5–10 yr: ≤ 15	≤ 8.6
		> 10 yr: ≤ 11	≤ 6.3
		(CF - 0.5706)	
Vasoactive intestinal peptides (VIP)	Plasma (heparin). Draw only with special refrigerated collection kit. Mix well. Process immediately.	< 70 pg/mL	< 21 pmol/L
Vasopressin See Antidiuretic hormone.			
Viscosity	Serum	1.4–1.8 relative to water at 37°C	
Vitamin A	Serum. Protect from light.	30–95 µg/dL	1.05–3.32 µmol/L
Vitamin B_{12} (cobalamin)	Serum	190–950 pg/mL	140–700 pmol/L
	Note: Some patients with documented megaloblastic anemia or neuropathy due to B_{12} deficiency have normal serum levels.		
		< 170 pg/mL (< 125 pmol/L) represents definite deficiency.	

(cont'd.)

Testing Protocols & Normal Laboratory Values (cont'd.)

Test	Collection Procedure	Common Units (Conversion Factor → SI)	Système International (SI) Units
Vitamin D, 25-hydroxy (both vitamins D_2 and D_3)	Serum Freeze in plastic tube at −20°C.	10–50 ng/mL (CF - 2.4963)	25–125 nmol/L
Note: Heavy milk drinkers may have slightly elevated levels. Some patients with vitamin D deficiency may have low-normal serum levels.			
Vitamin D, 1,25-hydroxy (both vitamins D_2 and D_3)	Serum Freeze in plastic tube at −60°C.	20–76 pg/mL (CF - 2.4004)	48–182 pmol/L
Water deprivation test See Antidiuretic hormone—water deprivation test.			
Xylose absorption test Adults must be fasting overnight Children < 2 yr old fast 4 h Dose: 1 g/kg (6.6 mmol/kg) Maximum 25 g (167 mmol)	Whole blood (Na fluoride) at 1 h. Do not centrifuge. Urine (5-h). Refrigerate.	mg/dL Adult: 29–72 Child: 16–40 Adults: 16–33% of dose or 4.8–8.2 g excreted in 5 h Children: 9–27% of dose excreted in 5 h	mmol/L 1.93–4.80 1.07–2.67

Index